300

W9-BSN-856

UPDATE

II

THE HEART

UPDATE II

THE HEART

Bypass Surgery for Obstructive Coronary Disease

Editor

J. Willis Hurst, M.D.

Professor of Medicine (Cardiology)
Chairman, Department of Medicine
Emory University School of Medicine
Atlanta, Georgia

McGraw-Hill Book Company

New York   St. Louis   San Francisco   Auckland   Bogotá   Düsseldorf
Johannesburg   London   Madrid   Mexico   Montreal   New Delhi
Panama   Paris   São Paulo   Singapore   Sydney   Tokyo   Toronto

UPDATE II: THE HEART

Copyright © 1980 by McGraw-Hill, Inc. All rights reserved. Printed in the United States of America. No part of this publication may be reproduced, stored in a retrieval system, or transmitted, in any form or by any means, electronic, mechanical, photocopying, recording, or otherwise, without the prior written permission of the publisher.

ISBN 0-07-031491-8

1 2 3 4 5 6 7 8 9 0   MUMU   7 8 3 2 1 0 9

This book was set in Times Roman by Waldman Graphics, Inc. The editors were Richard S. Laufer and Henry C. De Leo; the designer was Elliot Epstein; the production supervisor was Jeanne Selzam.
The Murray Printing Company was printer and binder.

NOTICE

Library of Congress Cataloging in Publication Data

Main entry under title:

Bypass surgery for obstructive coronary disease.

    Update 2 to the Heart, arteries, and veins,
edited by J. W. Hurst.
    Includes index.
    1. Aortocoronary bypass. 2. Myocardial revascularization. I. Hurst, John Willis, date II. Hurst, John Willis, date ed.
Heart, arteries, and veins. [DNLM:
1 Aortocoronary bypass. 2. Coronary disease—Surgery. W1 UP57 v. 2 (P) / WG168.3 B994]
RD598.B96   617'.412   79-9421
ISBN 0-07-031491-8

To F. Mason Sones, Jr., M.D.,
who developed coronary arteriography
and opened the door to the modern
recognition and management of
coronary atherosclerotic heart disease.

Contents

THE CONDUCT OF A PATIENT THROUGH CORONARY BYPASS SURGERY

THE COST OF CORONARY BYPASS SURGERY

List of Contributors

Ezra A. Amsterdam, M.D.
Associate Professor of Medicine, Chief, Coronary Care Unit, Section of Cardiovascular Medicine, University of California, School of Medicine and Sacramento Medical Center, Davis and Sacramento, California

Djavad T. Arani, M.D.
Clinical Assistant Professor of Medicine, State University of New York at Buffalo; Assistant Physician, Buffalo General Hospital, Buffalo, New York

Najam A. Awan, M.D.
Assistant Professor of Medicine, Director, Clinical Pharmacology, Section of Cardiovascular Medicine, University of California, School of Medicine and Sacramento Medical Center, Davis and Sacramento, California

John M. Bozer, M.D.
Clinical Associate Professor of Medicine, State University of New York at Buffalo; Attending Physician, Buffalo General Hospital, Buffalo, New York

Ivan L. Bunnell, M.D.
Clinical Professor of Medicine, State University of New York at Buffalo; Director, Angiology Laboratory, Attending Physician, Buffalo General Hospital, Buffalo, New York

Robert A. Chahine, M.D.
Associate Professor of Medicine, Chief of Cardiology, Baylor College of Medicine, Houston, Texas

Stephen D. Clements, Jr., M.D.
Associate Professor of Medicine (Cardiology), Department of Medicine, Emory University School of Medicine, Atlanta, Georgia

John J. Collins, Jr., M.D.
Professor of Surgery, Chief, Division of Thoracic and Cardiac Surgery, Peter Bent Brigham Hospital, Boston, Massachusetts

Carlos M. de Castro, M.D.
Director, Clayton Foundation, Noninvasive Cardiology Laboratory, St. Luke's Episcopal Hospital, Houston, Texas

Anthony N. DeMaria, M.D.
Associate Professor of Medicine, Director, Noninvasive Cardiology, Section of Cardiovascular Medicine, University of California, School of Medicine and Sacramento Medical Center, Davis and Sacramento, California

Timothy A. DeRouen, Ph.D.
Associate Professor of Biostatistics, University of Washington, Seattle, Washington

Harold T. Dodge, M.D.
Co-Chairman, Division of Cardiology, and Professor of Medicine, University of Washington, Seattle, Washington

Efrain Garcia, M.D.
Assistant Medical Director, Texas Heart Institute; Director, Clayton Foundation Cardiovascular Laboratories, St. Luke's Episcopal Hospital, Houston, Texas

David G. Greene, M.D.
Professor of Medicine and Associate Professor of Physiology, State University of New York at Buffalo; Attending Physician, Buffalo General Hospital, Buffalo, New York

Rolf M. Gunnar, M.D.
Professor of Medicine, Chief, Section of Cardiology, Loyola University Stritch School of Medicine, Maywood, Illinois; Consultant Program Director in Cardiology, Veterans Administration Edward J. Hines Medical Center, Hines, Illinois

Robert J. Hall, M.D.
Medical Director, Texas Heart Institute, Houston, Texas

K. E. Hammermeister, M.D.
Assistant Chief, Cardiology, Veterans Administration Hospital; Associate Professor of Medicine, University of Washington, Seattle, Washington

J. Willis Hurst, M.D.
Professor of Medicine (Cardiology), Chairman of the Department of Medicine, Emory University School of Medicine, Atlanta, Georgia

Ellis L. Jones, M.D.
Associate Professor of Surgery (Thoracic and Cardiovascular), Department of Surgery, Emory University School of Medicine, Atlanta, Georgia

James A. Joye, M.D.
Assistant Professor of Medicine, Director, Nuclear Cardiology, Section of Cardiovascular Medicine, University of California, School of Medicine and Sacramento Medical Center, Davis and Sacramento, California

Kenneth M. Kent, M.D.
Head, Section on Cardiovascular Diagnosis, Cardiology Branch, National Heart, Lung and Blood Institute, Bethesda, Maryland

Spencer B. King III, M.D.
Associate Professor of Medicine (Cardiology) and Department of Radiology (Cardiac Radiology), Emory University School of Medicine; Director, Cardiovascular Laboratory, Emory University Hospital, Atlanta, Georgia

Robert M. Kohn, M.D.
Clinical Professor of Medicine, State University of New York at Buffalo; Attending Physician, Buffalo General Hospital, Buffalo, New York

Thomas Z. Lajos, M.D.
Associate Professor of Surgery, State University of New York at Buffalo; Attending Surgeon, Buffalo General Hospital, Buffalo, New York

Gerald M. Lawrie, M.D.
Associate Professor of Surgery, Baylor College of Medicine, Houston, Texas

Arthur B. Lee, M.D.
Assistant Professor of Surgery, State University of New York at Buffalo; Assistant Attending Surgeon, Buffalo General Hospital, Buffalo, New York

Garrett Lee, M.D.
Assistant Professor of Medicine, Director, Cardiac Catheterization Laboratory, Section of Cardiovascular Medicine, University of California, School of Medicine and Sacramento Medical Center, Davis and Sacramento, California

Henry S. Loeb, M.D.
Professor of Medicine, Loyola University Stritch School of Medicine, Maywood, Illinois; Program Director in Cardiology, Veterans Administration Edward J. Hines Medical Center, Hines, Illinois

Reginald Low, M.D.
Fellow in Cardiovascular Medicine, Section of Cardiovascular Medicine, University of California, School of Medicine and Sacramento Medical Center, Davis and Sacramento, California

Joseph D. Marco, M.D.
Southwest Cardio-Thoracic Surgery, Ltd., 5200 East Grant Road, Suite 200-A, Tucson, Arizona

Dean T. Mason, M.D.
Professor of Medicine and Physiology, Chief, Section of Cardiovascular Medicine, University of California, School of Medicine and Sacramento Medical Center, Davis and Sacramento, California

Virendra S. Mathur, M.D.
Director, Clayton Foundation, Invasive Laboratories, St. Luke's Episcopal Hospital, Houston, Texas

George C. Morris, Jr., M.D.
Professor of Surgery, Baylor College of Medicine, Houston, Texas

Robert Palac, M.D.
Medical Resident, Rush-Presbyterian-St. Luke's Medical Center, Chicago, Illinois

Roque Pifarre, M.D.
Professor of Surgery, Chief, Section of Cardio-Thoracic Surgery, Loyola University Stritch School of Medicine, Maywood, Illinois; Chief, Thoracic Surgery Section, Veterans Administration Edward J. Hines Medical Center, Hines, Illinois

William L. Proudfit, M.D.
Senior Consultant, Department of Cardiology, Cleveland Clinic Foundation, Cleveland, Ohio

Albert E. Raizner, M.D.
Associate Professor of Medicine, Baylor College of Medicine, Houston, Texas

Charles E. Rackley, M.D.
Professor of Medicine, Department of Medicine, University of Alabama Medical Center, Birmingham, Alabama

George G. Rowe, M.D.
Professor of Medicine, Cardiology Section, The University of Wisconsin, Medical School, Madison, Wisconsin

George Schimert, M.D.
Professor of Surgery, State University of New York at Buffalo; Attending Surgeon, Buffalo General Hospital, Buffalo, New York

Gretchen L. Smith, R.N., M.S.
Research Nurse, Angiology Laboratory, Buffalo General Hospital, Buffalo, New York

Joan L. Smith, M.A.
Research Associate in Cardiac Rehabilitation, Section of Cardiovascular Medicine, University of California, School of Medicine and Sacramento Medical Center, Davis and Sacramento, California

Ravinder N. Tandon, M.D., M.R.C.P.
Professor of Medicine, University of Kanpur, Kanpur, India

Zakauddin Vera, M.D.
Assistant Professor of Medicine, Director, Clinical Electrophysiology, Section of Cardiovascular Medicine, University of California, School of Medicine and Sacramento Medical Center, Davis and Sacramento, California

John P. Visco, M.D.
Assistant Professor of Medicine, State University of New York at Buffalo; Assistant Physician, Buffalo General Hospital, Buffalo, New York

Walter T. Zimdahl, M.D.
Clinical Associate Professor of Medicine, State University of New York at Buffalo; Attending Physician, Buffalo General Hospital, Buffalo, New York

Preface to Update II

The preface to *Update I: The Heart* is reprinted here; in it are discussed the objectives of the Updates. Note that two different types of Updates are planned: One will be journallike, where a number of different topics will be discussed; the other will be thematic, where one subject is discussed in great depth. This second Update is thematic and is subtitled *Bypass Surgery for Obstructive Coronary Disease*.

The larger edition of *The Heart* has been published every 4 years since 1966. I recognized in the early sixties that one author could not write a complete textbook on the heart. This is as true today as it was then. Knowledge in every aspect of the field increases so rapidly that one person cannot master it all. Accordingly, I decided then to write what I could and I asked friends and colleagues *with whom I agree* to contribute to the book. In this way the book became personalized. In *Update II: Bypass Surgery for Obstructive Coronary Disease*, I authored or coauthored three chapters and friends and colleagues *with whom I agree* have written the remainder of the book. The book makes a case for the use of coronary bypass surgery for carefully selected patients. The book also supports the view that coronary bypass surgery relieves angina pectoris in 90 percent of patients and prolongs the life of certain subsets of patients when the operative risk is 0.5 to 2 percent. It should interest the reader to realize that the *majority of the authors are medical cardiologists and the miniority are surgeons.*

I wish to thank Carol Miller in my office for typing my own manuscripts, keeping order and meeting deadlines, recognizing the importance of accuracy, and enjoying her work. I wish to thank Rich Laufer, Hank De Leo, and Dereck Jeffers of the McGraw-Hill Book Company for their competence and kindness.

J. Willis Hurst, M.D.

Preface to Update I

I began the preparation for the first edition of THE HEART in 1962 and the first edition was published in 1966. The fourth edition was published in 1978. The objective of *The Heart* has always been to present in one or two volumes a complete treatise on the heart and blood vessels with the patient and the practicing physician as the focal point. Since the field is vast, it is necessary to use every method of editing in order to limit the size of the book(s). Accordingly, the allocation of space to a discussion of new advances that have not been tested by practicing physicians must be limited. For example, only a few pages were allocated to radionuclide imaging of the heart in the fourth edition. Similarly, the space allocated to a relatively small but important subject must be limited. For example, arrhythmias related to abnormal repolarization of the myocardium were not discussed in great detail in the fourth edition of the book, whereas a great deal is known about the subject. Finally, it has been necessary to limit the number of illustrations and references in *The Heart* in order to conserve space. This always concerns good teachers and good writers since such restraints may blunt their ability to express themselves as freely as they would like to do.

Toward the end of the preface of the fourth edition of *The Heart*, I wrote:

> Now that the fourth edition of *The Heart* is completed, the fifth edition is underway. The gestation period will be 3 or 4 years. The product of this gestation, the fifth edition, will be different from the first, second, third, and fourth editions. This is true because new information is being generated at such a rapid pace. I and the other authors who contribute to the book will evolve new ideas as new data dictate we should.

Since publication of the fourth edition the rapidly expanding body of knowledge has compelled me to search for an additional medium of communication. At times, just after a new edition of *The Heart* has been published, a new concept or a new procedure has come to my attention. Since the book is on a 4-year cycle, the new concept or procedure could not be presented for 4 years. Although this has never been a major problem, developments are coming at an ever-increasing pace, and it seems appropriate now to develop a method of assuring readers of *The Heart* that they will be apprised of every significant advance in the subject in the shortest possible period of time.

If one reflects carefully on this, one is led to the idea of periodic updates. I am eternally grateful for

the worldwide acceptance *The Heart* has enjoyed (it has been translated into Spanish, Portuguese, Italian, and Japanese), and its objective will not be changed. It will remain a complete treatise on the heart and blood vessels contained in one or two volumes and, as always, will be written with the patient and the practicing physician in mind. The Updates will be used to fulfill the needs stated above. Accordingly, four to six will be created to appear between editions of *The Heart*. Some of them will have no particular theme and will be journallike, containing a number of articles on a variety of subjects, while others will be thematic minibooks and will contain a number of articles on the same subject. The reader should see the continuity of the Updates and their umbilical attachment to the mother of them all, *The Heart*. The material presented in detail in the Updates will then be "summarized" in the subsequent edition of *The Heart*.

This, then, is the first of the Updates. It is of the journal nature. There is no particular theme expressed in it. Two articles deal with medical history. This fascinating aspect of our heritage not only brings enjoyment to us all but is essential to one who desires to be a logical thinker and needs to know if current thought is an appropriate extension of the beliefs of our predecessors. Regrettably, the limitation of space will not permit most textbooks to include such vital information. The discussion of radionuclide imaging of the heart presented in this Update is quite long compared to the few pages allocated to the subject in the fourth edition of *The Heart*. Although the field is still developing, it seems appropriate to give a progress report on this important subject since the procedure is being used by an ever increasing number of institutions. On the other hand, there are four articles that deal with old subjects such as the use of the patient's history, the electrocardiogram, the echocardiogram and blood level of digoxin. The thrust of these articles is different from the usual discussion, however, since the authors emphasize the *limitations* of the methods of examination as well as the value of the methods. Finally, a number of articles, including arrhythmias related to abnormal repolarization, are presented in greater detail than space permitted in *The Heart*. These subjects were chosen by me by simply asking—if I had unlimited space in *The Heart* what would I add?

The Heart and its daughters, the Updates, will, I hope, assure the reader that he or she has access to all of the important information regarding the cardiovascular system. *The Heart* was conceived in 1962 and delivered in 1966. It then developed and matured through four editions and now—not surprisingly—it plans to have daughters.

I wish to thank Carol Miller in my office. She keeps order, translates and types my own unique brand of shorthand, detects and corrects errors, and does so with a smile. I also wish to thank my publisher McGraw-Hill for its interest in these Updates. The very talented Dereck Jeffers and Rich Laufer deserve my special thanks.

J. Willis Hurst, M.D.

Chapter 1

A Note of Appreciation to F. Mason Sones*

J. WILLIS HURST, M.D.

In the early 1940s, Blumgart, Schlesinger, and Zoll developed a technique for visualizing the coronary arteries,[1] and many new concepts regarding coronary atherosclerotic heart disease emerged as a result of their work. However, since their work was done on hearts obtained at autopsy, it was not possible to visualize the effect of obstructive coronary disease on myocardial contractility. In addition, the useful information they obtained could not be translated to a treatment plan that might benefit the individuals they studied. The enormous benefit of their work was conceptual, and as such, they deserve much credit, because the new concepts they formulated paved the way for many investigators who followed them.

F. Mason Sones and his colleagues at the Cleveland Clinic deserve the credit for developing coronary arteriography. Julius Comroe discusses Sones' contribution in his delightful book, *Retrospectroscope*. The chapter entitled "Roast Pig and Scientific Discovery" is a literary gem.[2] The reader will recall Charles Lamb's classic essay entitled "Dissertation upon Roast Pig," in which Bo-Bo discovered roast pig after he accidentally burned down his father's house and barn and in the doing roasted nine pigs. Comroe then discusses a large number of discoveries that were the result of accidents. Obviously, the accidents could have gone unnoticed except for momentary irritation to those who observed them. Instead, however, new and useful scientific discoveries were born, because the men and women who observed the accidents were able to visualize some extremely useful consequences. It was, in reality, their insight that made the discovery. F. Mason Sones' "discovery" of coronary arteriography was such a serendipitous event. Comroe[2] introduces Litwak's[3] story of Sones' discovery in the following manner.

Physiologists had for many decades perfused the coronary arteries of animals with Ringer solution, modified Ringer solutions, or blood (even hypoxemic blood) but were apprehensive about sending a block of an unoxygenated foreign fluid through the coronary circulation for fear of inducing serious arrhythmias. Yet successful coronary arteriography

required flow of a highly concentrated, radiopaque solution through the coronary circulation. How did visualization of the coronary arteries become a diagnostic test? Litwak tells this story:

In 1958 an event transpired in Cleveland which was destined to have virtually unparalleled influence on medicine's understanding of coronary artery disease. F. Mason Sones, Jr. and his colleagues at the Cleveland Clinic were studying a young adult and had withdrawn their catheter from the left ventricle into the supravalvular area in preparation for an aortogram. Their equipment at this time did not allow them to precisely visualize the catheter tip immediately prior to injection of the contrast material. The usual dose of 35 ml. of a 90 percent diatrizoate compound was injected and, to Sones' horror, the right coronary artery and its distal branches were clearly visualized. Obviously, the catheter had accidentally entered the right coronary orifice and dye injected. The patient had remained stable through the entire procedure. That fortuitous event taught Sones that, contrary to views held at that time concerning electrical instability of the heart, non-oxygen carrying fluid could be injected into a major coronary artery without untoward event. Secondly, Sones realized that with proper equipment he could reduce the coronary artery injectate by ten-fold and he would then be able to sequentially study the entire coronary circulation of man and visualize vessels with a dimension of 100 microns or larger.**

The birth of coronary arteriography was accidental. Or was it? The minds of Sones and his colleagues were prepared, perhaps by the work of Blumgart, Schlesinger, Zoll, and others, and because of it they realized the great importance of the accident.[1] To continue the analogy with Lamb's essay, one should recall that following the fire that led to the discovery of roast pig, others tried to duplicate the event by burning down their houses to create their own roast pig. Over the years, however, it became obvious that other techniques could be used to roast a pig. Perhaps this sequence compares to the efforts that were spent to improve the technique of coronary arteriography. Sones led the way in this research. He and others refined the technique of coronary arteriography until it is currently a very safe and almost painless procedure. The risk of the procedure in most active laboratories is 0.1 percent. When the procedure is done in patients who are not seriously ill with shock, heart failure, arrhythmia, the risk is almost zero.

Coronary arteriography is a great teacher. It has,

*From the Department of Medicine, Emory University School of Medicine, Atlanta.

**Reproduced with the permission of Julius Comroe and the Von Gehr Press and R. Litwak and *Cardiovascular Clinics*.

to our consternation, taught us our error rate.[4] Our current understanding of coronary atherosclerotic heart disease would have been enhanced considerably if coronary arteriography had been available to Heberden.[5] Remember, we do not know what diseases Heberden's patients had, since there was only one autopsy performed, and the prosector did not report obstructive coronary disease. One could calculate that the clock of knowledge would have been turned forward by 200 years if coronary arteriography had been available to Heberden,[5] Hunter,[6] Parry,[7] Jenner,[7] and Burns.[7]

Coronary bypass surgery could not have been developed without coronary arteriography. Coronary arteriography provides all the information, and more, that Schlesinger, Blumgart, and Zoll obtained by their injection of the coronary arteries at autopsy. The difference between the techniques is profound, however.

Coronary arteriography reveals important information on an individual *living* patient, making it possible to design a *specific treatment plan for that individual.*

Coronary arteriography is one of the great medical advances of this century, and F. Mason Sones and his associates deserve the credit for its discovery and development. We all should remember the Chinese proverb—"Those who drink the water should not forget who dug the well." Sones and associates will remember the proverb, too, as they recall well-diggers such as Forssmann,[8] who dug the first well when he performed cardiac catheterization on himself, and Cournand and Richards,[9] Dexter, McMichael, Bing, Stead, Warren, Weens, Brannan, and others who further refined and developed cardiac catheterization.[10,11] They prepared the way so that Sones' "accident" could happen.

Mason, we are all indebted to you.

REFERENCES

1 Blumgart, H. L., Schlesinger, M. J., and Zoll, P. M.: Angina Pectoris, Coronary Failure and Acute Myocardial Infarction, *J.A.M.A.*, 116 (2):91, 1941.

2 Comroe, J. H., Jr.: "Retrospectroscope: Insights into Medical Discovery," Von Gehr Press, Menlo Park, Calif., 1977, p. 610.

3 Litwak, R.: The Growth of Cardiac Surgery: Historical Notes, *Cardiovasc. Clin.*, 3:5, 1951.

4 Douglas, J. S., and Hurst, J. W.: Limitations of Symptoms in the Recognition of Coronary Atherosclerotic Heart Disease, in J. W. Hurst (ed.) "Update I: The Heart," McGraw-Hill Book Company, New York, 1979.

5 Heberden, W.: Commentaries on the History and Cure of Diseases, in "Angina Pectoris," T. Tayne, Mews-Gate, London, 1802, chap. 7.

6 Home, E.: "A Treatise on the Blood, Inflammation, and Gun Shot Wounds by the Late John Hunter. To Which Is Prefixed an Account of the Author's Life by His Brother-in-Law, Everard Home," Thomas Bradford,

Philadelphia, 1796. (An earlier edition was published in England in 1794.)

7 Burns, A.: "Observations on Some of the Most Frequent and Important Diseases of the Heart," Hafner Publishing Company, New York, 1964, p.137.

8 Forssmann, W.: "Experiments on Myself. Memoirs of a Surgeon in Germany," Droste, Dusseldorf, 1972 (English ed., St. Martin's Press, New York, 1974).

9 Cournand, Baldwin, and Himmelstein: "Cardiac Catheterization in Congenital Heart Disease—Clinical and Physiological Study in Infants and Children," Common Wealth Fund, New York, 1949.

10 Cournand, A.: Cardiac Catheterization. Development of the Technique, Its Contributions to Clinical Medicine and Its Initial Applications in Man, *Acta Med. Scand.* [*Suppl.*], 579:1, 1975.

11 Franch, R. H.: Cardiac Catheterization, in J. W. Hurst (ed.). "The Heart," 4th ed., McGraw-Hill Book Company, New York, 1978, p. 479.

Chapter 2

Methods Used to Compare the Medical Management of Coronary Atherosclerotic Heart Disease with Coronary Bypass Surgery*

WILLIAM L. PROUDFIT, M.D.

Coronary atherosclerotic heart disease is manifested clinically by symptoms secondary to myocardial ischemia, and therefore the clinical diagnosis is not suspected until the disease is far advanced. The clinician ordinarily deals with obstructive symptomatic coronary disease, which is a subset of the primary condition. Most long-term studies of the natural history of coronary disease have been restricted to symptomatic patients. A proper study might involve evaluation of symptoms, signs, laboratory abnormalities, electrocardiographic manifestations, and the occurrence of myocardial infarction, cardiac arrhythmias, congestive failure, and embolism, as well as repeated demonstration of anatomic changes in the coronary circulation and variations in left ventricular function. Even if all these variables were described, there would still only be limited information about prognosis because of incomplete knowledge of the cause or causes of coronary disease. Furthermore, the patient has completed a successful experiment in survival before he or she arrives in the laboratory for study. So, in addition to the selection of primarily symptomatic patients, clinicians also necessarily select survivors, and therefore, their view is not that of the entire spectrum of coronary disease.

Obviously, a complete natural history of coronary disease cannot be written, even for the surviving symptomatic fraction. Ethical considerations dictate that some form of therapy must be utilized in the majority of patients, and treatment may modify the natural history. Indeed, it is the obligation of the physician to make the history as desirably unnatural as possible. Because of the complexity of analysis, most studies have focused on an easily definable end point—death. However, some information is available on the occurrence of myocardial infarction and persistence of angina pectoris.

The methods used to compare results of two or more therapeutic regimens depend on the objective.

Symptomatic relief would be the primary objective in studies of medical and surgical treatment of conditions such as cholelithiasis and tic douloureux, but in the case of many malignancies, improved longevity may be the primary objective. Confusion about the aim of treatment in obstructive disease of the coronary circulation has given rise to strong differences of opinion relating to the merits of medical and surgical treatment. Some who think that operative treatment should be reserved for those who fail to respond to medical measures evaluate the surgical results primarily in terms of longevity, whereas others who believe that improved survival is the surgical goal emphasize symptomatic results. Regardless of the attitude of the physician, the patient is interested in both symptomatic relief and increased longevity.

In some studies, one treatment might be a placebo, but in the case of arteriographically demonstrated coronary disease, this approach is seldom used. No detailed, long-term investigation comparing placebo therapy to any treatment of obstructive coronary disease has been reported. Studies that examined the effect of beta blockade therapy on survival following acute myocardial infarction have had somewhat divergent results.[1-3] The study of sulfinpyrazone in the same clinical condition has been reported, but the results are confusing.[4] In none of these studies has the coronary anatomy been demonstrated arteriographically. Many investigators think that vasodilator therapy has no effect on survival. There have been studies of arteriographically investigated patients who were selected during the years when this form of therapy was the only therapeutic approach commonly used.[5-14]

Comparison of two treatments might be expressed in terms of the simple formula shown below:

$$\frac{\text{Morbidity with treatment 1}}{\text{Morbidity with treatment 2}} \times \frac{\text{mortality with treatment 1}}{\text{mortality with treatment 2}} = K$$

where K represents the relative therapeutic efficacy. A valid comparison of two forms of therapy requires

*From Cleveland Clinic Foundation, Cleveland.

that each be carried out in an optimum manner. Otherwise, a study merely demonstrates the expertise of the physician or surgeon rather than the value of the treatment. Assuming optimum therapy, morbidity with two forms of treatment is an important component of the formula illustrated above. In the case of coronary disease, morbidity might be expressed in terms of pain of various clinical categories, myocardial infarction, embolism, cardiac arrhythmia, and congestive failure; criteria for clinical diagnosis of these conditions should be defined. The fact that most bypass surgery is carried out in referral centers in which it is not convenient to follow each patient at frequent intervals makes complete evaluation of morbidity difficult. The usual approach is to select angina pectoris for evaluation, although other kinds of morbidity might be analyzed. The other component of the formula is relatively simple to study, because deaths are easy to identify and count. However, incomplete follow-up information may cause serious distortions of survival figures.

It is apparent from the formula that there might be great differences between two forms of therapy based on morbidity or mortality or both. If the difference in morbidity is sufficient, a certain amount of operative mortality might be tolerated. If mortality is the focus of a study, surgical risk must be minimal, especially in short-term studies of groups of patients whose expected mortality with medical treatment is low. It is likely that improved survival would be associated with decreased morbidity, but symptomatic relief might not necessarily indicate the likelihood of increased longevity. It should be recalled that neither medical nor surgical treatment of coronary disease affects the basic cause, nor does either provide strong hope of prevention of progression. Since most patients die as a result of anatomic progression, which may occur at an unpredictable rate and episodically, long-term studies are required for rational evaluation of survival, although early results may justify operation in severely symptomatic or high-risk patients.

Because it is not known whether treatment of coronary disease increases longevity, the question of medical treatment in those who have had bypass operations cannot be settled. Certain measures such as control of weight and blood pressure and avoidance of tobacco seem reasonable, but the efficacy of dietary measures for modifications of serum lipids, programmed exercise, and medicinal therapy has not been defined.

Certain clinical tests may reflect changes in myocardial perfusion and may be necessary in forming a rational basis for treatment or for following progression of disease, but they are not required in a comparison of two forms of treatment. Stress tests before and after treatment are informative and interesting but are not essential in studies of morbidity or mortality. Determination of myocardial uptake of radioactive

material is not required for comparative therapeutic studies. Postoperative arteriography and visualization of grafts are useful in showing the progress of obstructive disease and in reflecting the quality of the surgery, but these procedures have no direct bearing on evaluation of morbidity and mortality. Naturally it would be disturbing if symptomatic relief and improved survival were found in patients whose grafts were nonfunctioning, but it would also be unlikely.

Partial relief of angina pectoris is common after medical treatment, but well controlled long-term studies are lacking. Most investigators will admit that it is unusual to eliminate angina with medical therapy, but the frequency of attacks is often reduced, at least temporarily. Spontaneous subsidence of anginal pain may occur over a long period of time with or without treatment. There is a wide divergence of opinion about the effect of medical therapy on survival, ranging from no effect to moderate improvement. This issue is not likely to be settled soon, but it is probable that the principal benefit of medical therapy results from decreased myocardial demand. Survival is related to progressive impairment of coronary blood supply, and bypass operation is designed to improve coronary blood supply to the myocardium. If it can be shown that graft patency is maintained and that distal progression in grafted arteries is uncommon, surgical treatment might be preferable to medical treatment. However, surgical technique must be excellent. This may be evaluated in terms of operative mortality, perioperative infarction rate, and graft patency. High operative mortality and perioperative infarction rate and low graft patency show lack of surgical skill and prevent adequate evaluation of results. It has been pointed out that the surgeon is a risk factor.[15,16] Some studies of survival have been done during a period in which the learning curve for surgery had not neared its zenith, and these have little bearing on current therapeutic decisions.

Mention should be made of evaluation of functional limitation prior to the institution of treatment. It is clear that few patients are totally disabled by coronary disease, although many are disabled by the idea that they have the condition. Few patients are unable to tolerate sedentary occupations, although many, even asymptomatic, patients decide to retire. The patient who has truly severe limitation of ability to exercise as well as nonexertional anginal pain is unusual, although many have nocturnal pain occasionally. However, the latter should not be considered class IV patients by the former New York Heart Association criteria.[17] Often these patients do not have severe limitation of ability to exercise during the day, and the occurrence of nocturnal pain has little bearing on prognosis.[18] On the other hand, severe limitation of ability to walk without angina does have prognostic significance.[18] The majority of patients have mild or moderate limitation of activity and would be content with medical treatment if one could assure them that death from coronary disease would not occur. If bypass surgery is to have an important place in the management of coronary disease, it must be shown that increased survival results. Only a small percentage of patients will require surgery as a result of the failure of severe symptoms to respond to medical therapy to an extent that life is tolerable.

Multicenter cooperative studies have a certain intellectual and emotional appeal. In cases of rare diseases, there is no alternative, but for common conditions, it would be preferable for institutions to report individual studies and analyze the comparative results independently. It is unusual for reports based on multicenter studies to show the variation among participating institutions, and when such variation is reported, striking discrepancies may be evident. Interinstitutional variations in several studies have been questioned, and incomplete responses to these questions have lessened confidence in the conclusions. Examples are the study of anticoagulant treatment of myocardial infarction, the University Group Diabetes Program, and the Veterans Administration (VA) study of chronic stable angina.[19-25] With the best of intentions, it is difficult for investigators in several institutions to adhere to a rigid protocol, which is a compromise not wholly acceptable and which must be applied over many years, often by successive investigators, each with his or her own ideas. Furthermore, even if rigid application of protocol is successful, one must assume skillful techniques in selection of patients and optimum medical and surgical therapy.

In comparing results from various studies, it is important to note the degree of narrowing of the arterial diameter that was considered "significant." A 50 percent decrease in diameter is a 75 percent decrease in cross-sectional area. If one study tabulates lesions narrowing the diameter by 50 percent and another by 80 percent, no direct comparison can be made. In the former case, obstructions of 50 to 70 percent in two arteries and 90 percent in the third would be considered three-artery disease, but if 80 percent is the standard, the same patient would be classified as having a single-artery obstruction. This confusion has affected experienced critics of reported studies.[26,27] In natural history studies, it is preferable to use 50 percent diameter reduction as the minimum standard because such lesions are significant prognostically. Until recently, however, few surgeons bypassed arteries with less than 70 percent narrowing of the diameter. Now lesions of lesser severity are bypassed with considerable success. Many previous surgical studies have used 70 or 80 percent narrowing of the diameter as a minimum standard, and one natural history study used 80 percent.[14] It is apparent that these studies cannot be compared with the VA study in which 50

percent diameter narrowing was the standard, although lesions of that magnitude were not bypassed at the time the study was done.

Knowledge of the cause or causes of coronary disease is incomplete. Most patients die as a result of progression of obstructive disease because ways of preventing progression are unknown, unproven, unused, or only partially effective. The patient has demonstrated that he or she can live with the disease as presented. If a guarantee could be given that progression would not occur, few would seek operative treatment, and many would endure the symptoms they experience. Unfortunately, it is difficult to predict when progression is likely to occur, although in time progression is the rule. Progression of coronary arterial obstruction complicates evaluation of therapeutic response. A treatment may be adequate for the anatomic and physiologic condition the patient has today but inappropriate a year later. A good symptomatic response may result from therapy, only to fail later as a result of progression of disease. One might consider this a failure of the disease rather than a failure of treatment, but the patient reacts in the same way. Late recurrence of symptoms in surgical patients is often the result of disease progression rather than graft failure. Fortunately, obstructive disease tends to affect the proximal portions of the coronary arteries, and surgeons graft as distally as convenient, but distal lesions may appear later and new lesions may develop or previously demonstrated minor abnormalities may progress. Furthermore, not all seriously narrowed arteries are amenable to bypass grafting. If progression of obstructive disease could be predicted in relation to time and site, more rational therapy might be planned.

MORBIDITY

If surgical candidates are selected on the basis of resistance to medical treatment, the primary objective of therapeutic assessment should be symptomatic relief. There have been no adequate large-scale, detailed studies of comparative symptomatic response to medical and surgical patients who have angina pectoris. Such a study would require a rigid protocol for medical therapy, operative treatment either alone or combined with a definite medical regimen in comparable groups of patients, and long-term follow-up. It is generally accepted that angina is relieved in most patients by an optimum bypass operation. Clinical experience indicates that less satisfactory results are obtained with medical therapy. Revascularization was followed by disappearance of angina in 65 percent of an early series of patients reported by Sheldon et al.[28] Many others have reported similar responses. Mathur and Guinn found that symptomatic relief was much better in 56 surgical than in 60 medical patients followed for 5 years in a randomized prospective study.[29] The published Veterans Administration reports do not include symptomatic response. A recent abstract indicates improvement in angina in 60 percent of patients after operation.[30] Studies must be carried out over many years, because the initial response to therapy may not persist, problems may arise with patient compliance in taking medication, medical patients may have bypass operation, obstructive coronary disease may progress, and angina may gradually disappear over a period of years with or without therapy. Even in the absence of satisfactory investigation, it seems quite clear that in short-term studies, angina pectoris is more regularly relieved by bypass grafting than by standard medical therapy. Myocardial infarction and other causes of morbidity requiring hospitalization have been reported to be less frequent in surgical patients after the initial postoperative period than in medically treated patients.[31] The total incidence of myocardial infarction obviously depends on the perioperative infarction rate. If the rate is high, such as the 18 percent figure in the VA study,[22] a long-term follow-up will be necessary to overcome the initial handicap imposed on the surgical group. However, a perioperative infarction rate of 1 or 2 percent is realistic now, and 4 to 6 percent was reasonable in 1972 to 1974; even lower rates might be anticipated in view of new techniques in myocardial preservation. With such rates, a better comparison might be made in the future. It is likely that the incidence of myocardial infarction may be reduced if graft patency is preserved and severe distal disease is uncommon.

In the cooperative study of unstable angina, patients were selected on the basis of a symptomatic clinical syndrome and were evaluated in terms of symptoms and early mortality.[32] Late mortality must be related to the anatomic features of the disease and would be expected to be similar to that of patients who did not have the same clinical picture initially. A high rate of crossover from medical to surgical treatment obscures long-term survival data. Symptomatic relief was better in the surgical group. Operative mortality and perioperative infarction rate were rather high.

The problem of working status in patients who have coronary disease is complex. Clinicians recognize that motivation is an important aspect. The suspicion or knowledge that coronary disease exists is enough for some individuals to seek retirement, especially if the economic returns are adequate, even though symptoms may be absent or minimal. Enforced prolonged absence from work as a result of acute myocardial infarction decreases motivation in some patients, and this may be true for prolonged absence following bypass operation. Adequate compensation and nearness to retirement age are complicating factors. Women are especially difficult to evaluate because often they have not been employed outside the home, and those who have been may be able to afford to quit work because of any health problem and be supported by their husbands. Other patients are instructed by their physicians not to work. Some patients return to work after surgery, even though their preoperative abstention from employment was not enforced by symptoms. If patients do not return to work after operation, it may be difficult to determine the exact reason, so that a statement about the percentage of patients returning to work after bypass operation is of limited value unless an extensive investigation has been carried out.

SURVIVAL

If determination of longevity is the object of investigation, the technique of construction of survival curves must be considered. Ideally it would be simple if, in a single institution, a large group of patients demonstrated to have coronary disease amenable to bypass surgery were entered into a study simultaneously and divided into two or more treatment groups, the surgical group being operated on after a brief interval, and all were followed for a fixed and uniform interval. Obviously, this is not possible. If almost all patients are followed for a fixed period, a direct calculation of survival may be made. If patient access to a study group extends over a considerable period of time, which is the usual situation, and if there is some urgency about acquisition of results, a life table technique (actuarial curve) is used. This type of analysis permits construction of curves when the minimum and maximum follow-up vary greatly. The assumption is made that those not followed will survive in the same manner as those who have been traced, which is not necessarily true. Incomplete attempts to follow patients may be buried in the investigation unless specifically described, which is an unusual occurrence. The smaller the number of patients lost or "withdrawn alive" (patient's last known living date), the more reliable the curve, but there is always an opportunity for error. If all patients are followed for the required minimum time period, the curve is the same as that constructed by the direct method, but this is seldom the case. If a small difference is expected in the results of two treatments, it is mandatory that all or almost all patients be followed adequately.

The size of the sample population must be considered. Because coronary disease is not a single problem and subsets must be studied, a rather large population is required, especially if differences in survival are expected to be small and the time period of study short.

Small study groups are appropriate only for conditions in which the anticipated mortality is high with one form of treatment. There are statistical methods for determining the size of the patient population. In the VA study of stable angina pectoris, it was estimated that 1,000 patients would be required and 1,015 were selected.[33] However, after the first 2 years of patient selection were excluded because of high surgical mortality and after certain patients were excluded for other reasons, only 686 patients remained before patient compliance was considered. The European cooperative study included 760 patients, and it excluded those who had obstruction of single arteries because of the expected low mortality.[34] If other considerations are equal, the larger number of patients in the European study is an advantage.

In some investigations, the total number of patients is so limited that only composite curves can be constructed. In larger series, subsets of patients may be so small that meaningful figures are not possible. This is true in the VA study, but perhaps not so much so in the European multicenter coronary artery bypass graft (CABG) trial, although the number of arteries obstructed was the principal variable in both cases. The condition of the left ventricle was given some consideration in both studies; patients who had severe ventricular impairment were excluded. The information available is limited to men who had stable angina pectoris and relatively good left ventricular function. The numbers of patients in various subsets are sufficient for analysis in only 4 of the 12 subsets of patients in the VA study, excluding those who had left main coronary artery lesions.[19]

Composite survival curves have limited utility and are of no value in clinical practice. There are no composite patients but only individuals who have certain clinical or laboratory characteristics that affect survival, not all of which are known at this time. These individuals may be grouped into subsets having various characteristics or combinations of characteristics. A few features known to affect survival are age, degree of functional limitation, duration of the history of cardiac symptoms, congestive heart failure, myocardial infarction, family history, hypertension, diabetes, obesity, certain arrhythmias, abnormalities of electrical depolarization, cardiac enlargement, the number and status of seriously obstructed coronary arteries, the functional condition of the left ventricular myocardium, valvular defects, ventricular aneurysm, and, at least in a few, medical treatment. It is apparent that all combinations of these factors will not be studied. Concentration on subsets of patients who have combinations of several of these features is required. Often the clinician is interested in the survival of nonsurgically treated patients who have been candidates for bypass surgery if it had been offered or accepted. Such a study might eliminate the very old, the very obese, patients who had anatomically unfavorable lesions, those who had severe impairment of left ventricular function, and individuals who had comorbidity factors that might result in severe limitation of life expectancy. One could not simply compare an unselected nonsurgical subset with patients who had operative treatment, for the survival in the former group certainly would be lower than that in the latter. The two factors of prognostic significance known to be most useful are the number of arteries obstructed and the status of the left ventricle. Because surgeons have tended to avoid operating on patients who had severe impairment of left ventricular function, surgical candidates may be divided conveniently into subsets characterized by the number of arteries seriously obstructed. This is an extremely simple classification, but even this requires large subsets of patients. It would be most useful to designate the number of arteries narrowed by 50 percent or more, because the prognosis for patients with 50 to 70 percent obstruction is about the same as those with 70 to 90 percent.[8] The completeness of surgical revascularization might be expressed in terms of the percentage of arteries obstructed by 50 percent or more that have been bypassed, the number of arteries supplying nonviable myocardium being subtracted from the total number. The adequacy of revascularization of viable myocardium could be measured in this way. The ideal is a bypass for every major artery seriously obstructed if the myocardium supplied by the artery is viable. This ideal cannot always be achieved for anatomic reasons. The long-term prognosis of surgical patients must depend on the adequacy of the attempt at revascularization and the continued patency of grafts.

Ultimately the place of bypass surgery for coronary disease will be determined by its effect on longevity. If operative mortality is high, it is evident that a group subjected to surgery suffers a disadvantage, especially in the early stage of an investigation. In the current VA study, the first 2 years of patient acquisition were excluded because of high operative mortality (16 percent), but even in the last 3 years the mortality was 6 percent, if an additional "late" operative death is included.[15] This mortality excludes those who had left main coronary artery disease. Some believe that average operative mortality should be a standard for comparison.[26,27] Operative mortality is a measure of surgical competence and not an index related to the clinical value of surgery. Poor survival stimulates surgeons to improve techniques if other surgeons report superior results. A low mortality can be achieved even in multicenter studies. A report of all pure bypass surgery in Australia recently showed an operative mortality of 2.5 percent (710 patients) and 2.1 percent for those who had chronic angina.[35] Our operative mortality for 1973, which is the middle year of the VA study, was 0.6 percent for elective operations, excluding left main coronary artery lesions as in the VA study. Others are also reporting low operative mortality.[36-38] If surgical treatment is to achieve its objective, the perioperative infarction rate must be low, for prognosis is related to ventricular impairment. Low infarction rates are possible, as noted above. Finally, a high percentage of graft patency is necessary. Patency rates of 85 to 95 percent are being reported for various types of grafts. A complicating factor in coronary disease is the possibility of progression of disease distal to the point of insertion of the graft or obstruction of the graft itself. Fortunately, obstructive lesions usually involve the proximal portion of coronary arteries predominantly, and late graft failure is uncommon for at least 5 or 6 years.[28,39] The existence of these complicating factors does not pevent evaluation of surgical results.

There are six principal methods for studying survival in coronary disease. The first is to investigate patients after the clinical diagnosis of angina pectoris or myocardial infarction has been made. It is apparent that this is an unsatisfactory method because of the possibility of error in diagnosis and the lack of information of prognostic significance, such as the number of arteries obstructed and the status of the left ventricle. The second technique involves the selection of a group of patients who had adequate cardiac catheterization during a period in which only a minority of patients had surgical treatment, such as internal mammary artery implantation. The latter operation was applicable to patients who had severe obstruction of the anterior descending artery, so removal of this group would somewhat bias the survival curve of the remaining patients and would have a specific effect in the study of single-artery disease. Other subsets would be little influenced. Selection of such a group means that the initial therapy would have been limited to vasodilators, but later some would receive beta blockade. If a fixed date, such as the date of catheterization, is selected and patients are followed from that date onward, the study is not retrospective but a retrospective-prospective or retrolective cohort study. Feinstein has pointed out that such studies may be valid for prognosis.[40] Retrolective cohort studies of the prognosis of coronary disease have been reported.[5-14] It must be assumed that there have been no striking changes in the natural history of the disease or in the response to medical therapy in terms of survival if studies of this type are to be used for comparison with subsequent surgical experience.

An important limitation of the use of these reports for comparison with surgical experience is the fact that only one of these studies was intended to be a surgical control, despite the fact that others have been used for that purpose. In only one study was an effort made to select patients who would have been candidates for bypass surgery on the basis of criteria developed subsequently.[14] In this study, 80 percent obstruction was the minimum considered, so the number of arteries significantly narrowed was underestimated, resulting in a relatively poor prognosis. A recent report analyzes the prognosis of various subsets of 388 patients who would have been candidates for bypass surgery but whose catheterizations were done in the 1963–1965 period.[18] An estimated 50 percent obstruction was considered significant, but 60 percent narrowing of at least one artery was required for surgical candidacy. All patients were followed until death, subsequent operation,[30] or for a minimum of 10 years. Although this was not an ideal study, it may serve as a control for survival after bypass operation. With the passage of time, it is difficult to repeat this type of retrolective cohort study because of selection bias.

The case control technique has not been applied extensively to the study of prognosis of coronary disease. This method entails the description of clinical characteristics thought to be of prognostic significance in a surgical group and a selection of a nonsurgical patient matching the important characteristics of each individual surgical patient. It is difficult to match individual patients precisely for factors such as age, sex, family history, hypertension, diabetes, smoking habits, serum lipid levels, symptoms, electrocardiographic findings, number of arteries obstructed, ventriculographic abnormalities, and anatomic candidacy for bypass operation, as well as many other variables. Hammermeister et al. used the case control technique in a study of late morbidity.[31]

The use of a data bank in prognostic studies has been advocated.[10] Multiple variables were compared in surgical and nonsurgical groups to show similarity. However, only a few of these characteristics were actually used in comparative prognostic studies of the two groups. The nonsurgical cases were not classified on the basis of surgical candidacy. Obviously, surgical candidates were not picked at random from the pool of catheterized patients. It would be necessary to select only patients who would have been candidates for bypass operation and study subsets of these patients. This could be done, but it would require considerable effort if meaningful results are to be expected. High operative mortality was another problem in this study.

A similar method of study that avoids some of these pitfalls involved selection of a group of patients who, anatomically, were surgical candidates but who did not have operation because of misgivings of the patient or the attending physicians. This group was compared with a similar group in which operation was done during the same time frame. The groups were compared for baseline characteristics and survival in a study by

Vismara et al.[41] With this method, the possible effect of changing medical therapy with time is avoided, and the study can be carried out in a single large institution in a reasonable period of time, thereby affording the advantage of uniformity. If operative mortality and morbidity are low, reasonable conclusions might be drawn. The crossover rate (noncompliance) might be low in such a study because the attitudes of the physicians concerned are not likely to change much in a reasonably short period. In this particular investigation, there was no noncompliance. Like other studies, it can be done only once, because future therapeutic attitudes are strongly influenced by the result of the investigation.

The randomized prospective study has been utilized for a long time and has been promoted as the only valid method of therapeutic research.[26] In theory, it appears to be the ideal approach. Patients are selected randomly from a large group eligible for study and are divided randomly into two or more treatment groups. The nature of the study is explained to the patient and informed consent given. Full information is rarely supplied to the patient, and sometimes it may be difficult for the patient to comprehend. Patient groups are subjected to various forms of treatment and the therapeutic effect is observed, with or without the knowledge of the patient or the investigator of the treatment assigned. Of course, the use of surgical treatment is obvious. If all bypasses became occluded in a reasonably large group, this subset of patients might be used as a "control" group for further study, but a large group would indicate poor operative technique. After a predetermined interval, the therapeutic result is observed in reference to either morbidity or mortality or both. In clinical application, problems arise. First, patients are not randomly selected, although assignment of treatment might be random. After receiving therapeutic assignment, the patient may refuse to accept it; that is, he or she becomes noncompliant. In some cases, compliance may occur initially and the patients may later change their minds unless they have accepted surgical treatment and operation has been performed. A late change from medical to surgical treatment is particularly frequent if the surgical approach is thought to be more effective in the relief of symptoms. Physicians participating in studies may even encourage noncompliance. If a poor therapeutic response in the medical subset occurs, noncompliance is an increasing problem. In the VA study of stable angina pectoris, 17 percent of the nonsurgical patients had operations within 3 years, and most had severe symptoms.[19]

One of the major problems associated with randomized prospective studies is that these investigations are usually multicenter in nature. Problems with multicenter studies have been mentioned. The two large American multicenter randomized prospective studies of coronary disease suffer from problems in execution.[19,32] Nonuniformity of results is a serious problem in the VA trial.[15,42] Other prospective studies in single institutions have involved such small groups of patients that conclusions cannot be drawn, and other problems have blurred the focus of these studies. If small series are followed for many years, differences in survival may emerge. The European cooperative study may have advantages over most of the randomized prospective studies reported, although the published details of its organization are incomplete.[34] There is no evidence in any major study that medical treatment has been optimum, so all reports should be considered comparisons between nonsurgical and surgical therapy. In the VA study, propranolol therapy was known to have been used in only 19 percent of nonsurgical patients, and even in these, there are no data relative to the regularity of treatment or the dosage employed. Other defects in the VA study have been mentioned and reviewed.[15] The problems of the VA study have been recognized by the participants, and they have suggested that it might be necessary to initiate a new and better investigation,[19,22] but this is not likely.

Recently, Greene et al.[43] and Lawrie et al.[44] compared survival data for surgical patients with survival of age-comparable individuals based on U.S. Vital Statistics or insurance actuarial curves. Berkson and Gage used a similar technique many years ago for a somewhat different reason.[45] The great advantage of such a comparison is that it eliminates the necessity of starting a new randomized prospective study with the introduction of each new form of therapy or modification of an old treatment. Most would admit that if survival approaches predicted survival for the whole United States population, it could be assumed that treatment is effective. However, as with all techniques of study, there are complicating factors. About half the deaths in the United States may be ascribed to coronary disease in the 50- to 60-year age group. Some, perhaps many, of the other half died of a disease the existence of which may have been detected a year or more prior to death, and if such detection were made in patients who had serious coronary disease, these patients might have been excluded from study. Therefore, noncoronary deaths might be less frequent in the year or two following selection for operation, creating a climate favorable for survival of the surgical group early in an investigation. On the other hand, all surgical patients have severe coronary disease, whereas only a minority of the age-comparable general population has seriously obstructive coronary disease. Not only is coronary disease likely to progress over a period of years, but also the patient who is known to have serious obstructive disease is more likely to have vascular disease elsewhere than is the "average" person of the same age. Therefore, in long-term studies the gross mortality may be higher in surgical cases than in the general population even if the initial surgical result is ideal. For a limited period of time, perhaps for 5 years or more, this method of comparison might be useful. It is not likely that subsets of patients known to be at highest risk with medical or surgical treatment will have survival curves that closely duplicate the U.S. Vital Statistics curves. It is possible that with improving surgical techniques, some subsets may exceed expected survival for some period of time.

SUMMARY

There are problems with all methods of comparison of medical and surgical treatment of patients who have symptomatic obstructive coronary artery disease, and there is no practical, ethical, ideal method of study. All the methods described for arteriographically documented patients may prove useful, and reports should be critically reviewed. It is likely that all major methods will yield somewhat similar results if the investigations are on a large scale and are well performed.

REFERENCES

1 Green, K. G. (coordinating secretary): Improvement in Prognosis of Myocardial Infarction by Long-term β-Adrenoreceptor Blockage Using Practolol: A Multicenter International Study, *Br. Med. J.*, 3:735, 1975.

2 Vedin, A., Wilhelmsson, C., and Wenko, L.: Chronic Alprenolol Treatment of Patients with Acute Myocardial Infarction After Discharge from the Hospital, *Acta Med. Scand.* [Suppl.] 575:19, 1975.

3 Barber, J. M., Boyle, D. M., Chaturved, N. C., Singh, N., and Walsh, M. J.: Practolol in Acute Myocardial Infarction, *Acta Med. Scand.* [Suppl.], 587:213, 1976.

4 The Anturane Reinfarction Trial Research Group, Sherry, S. (chairman): Sulfinpyrazone in the Prevention of Cardiac Death After Myocardial Infarction, *N. Engl. J. Med.*, 298:289, 1978.

5 Friesinger, G. C., Page, E. E., and Ross, R. S.: Prognostic Significance of Coronary Arteriography, *Trans. Assoc. Am. Physicians.*, 83:78, 1970.

6 Oberman, A., Jones, W. B., Riley, C. D., et al.: Natural History of Coronary Artery Disease, *Bull. N.Y. Acad. Med.*, 48:1109, 1972.

7 Lichtlen, P. R., and Moccetti, T.: Prognostic Aspects of Coronary Arteriography, *Circulation*, 46 (suppl. 2): II-7, 1972. (Abstract.)

8 Bruschke, A. V. G., Proudfit, W. L., and Sones, F. M., Jr.: Progress Study of 590 Consecutive Nonsurgical Cases of Coronary Disease Followed 5–9 Years. I. Arteriographic Correlations, *Circulation*, 47:1147, 1973.

9 Bruschke, A. V. G., Proudfit, W. L., and Sones, F. M., Jr.: Progress Study of 590 Consecutive Nonsurgical Cases of Coronary Disease Followed 5–9 years. II. Ventriculographic and Other Correlations, *Circulation*, 47: 1154, 1973.

10 McNeer, J. F., Starmer, C. F., Bartel, A. G., et al.: The Nature of Treatment Selection in Coronary Artery Disease. Experience with Medical and Surgical Treatment of a Chronic Disease, *Circulation*, 49:606, 1974.

11 Brymer, J. F., Buter, T. H., Walton, J. A., Jr., et al.: A Natural History Study of the Prognostic Role of Coronary Arteriography, *Am. Heart J.*, 88:139, 1974.

12 Humphries, J. O., Kuller, L., Ross, R. S., et al.: Natural History of Ischemic Heart Disease in Relation to Arteriographic Findings: A Twelve-Year Study of 224 Patients, *Circulation*, 49:489, 1974.

13 Burggraf, G. W., and Parker, J. O.: Prognosis in Coronary Artery Disease: Angiographic, Hemodynamic and Clinical Factors, *Circulation*, 51:146, 1975.

14 Webster, J. S., Moberg, C., and Rincon, G.: Natural History of Severe Proximal Coronary Artery Disease as Documented by Coronary Cineangiography, *Am. J. Cardiol.*, 33:195, 1974.

15 Proudfit, W. L.: Criticisms of the VA Randomized Study of Coronary Bypass Surgery, *Clin. Res.*, 26:236, 1978.

16 Fielding, L. P., Stewart-Brown, S., and Dudley, H. A. D.: Surgeon-related Variables and the Clinical Trial, *Lancet*, 1:778, 1978.

17 The Criteria Committee of the New York Heart Association, Kossman, C. E. (chairman): "Diseases of the Heart and Blood Vessels: Nomenclature and Criteria for Diagnosis," 6th ed., Little, Brown and Company, Boston, 1964.

18 Proudfit, W. L., Bruschke, A. V. G., and Sones, F. M., Jr.: Natural History of Obstructive Coronary Artery Disease. Ten-Year Study of 601 Nonsurgical Cases, *Prog. Cardiovasc. Dis.*, 21:53, 1978.

19 Murphy, M. L., Hultgren, H. N., and Detre, K., et al.: Treatment of Chronic Stable Angina. A Preliminary Report of Survival Data of the Randomized Veterans Administration Cooperative Study, *N. Engl. J. Med.*, 297:621, 1977.

20 Hultgren, H. N., Takaro, T., and Detre, K.: Medical Versus Surgical Treatment of Stable Angina Pectoris: Progress Report of a Large-scale Study, *Postgrad. Med. J.*, 52:757, 1976.

21 Detre, K., Hultgren, H, and Takaro, T.: Veterans Administration Cooperative Study of Surgery for Coronary Arterial Occlusive Disease. III. Methods and Baseline Characteristics, Including Experience with Medical Treatment, *Am. J. Cardiol.*, 40:212, 1977.

22 Read, R. C., Murphy, M. L., Hultgren, H. N., et al.: Survival of Men Treated for Chronic Stable Angina Pectoris: A Cooperative Randomized Study, *J. Thorac. Cardiovasc. Surg.*, 75:1, 1978.

23 Hultgren, H. N., Takaro, T., and Detre, K.: Veterans Administration Cooperative Study of Surgical Treatment of Stable Angina. Preliminary Results, *Cardiovasc. Clin.*, 8:119, 1977.

24 Hultgren, H. N., Detre, K. M., and Takaro, T., et al.: The VA Cooperative Study of Coronary Arterial Surgery. Baseline Characteristics of Study Population and Survival in Subgroups with Medical Versus Surgical Treatment, *Prog. Cardiol.*, 6:67, 1977.

25 Detre, K., Murphy, M. L., and Hultgren, H. N.: Effect of Coronary Bypass Surgery on Longevity in High and Low Risk Patients. Report from the VA Cooperative Coronary Surgery Study, *Lancet*, 2:1243, 1977.

26 Chalmers, T. C., Smith, H., Ambroz, A., Reitman, D, and Schroeder, B.: In Defense of the VA Randomized Control Trial of Coronary Artery Surgery, *Clin. Res.*, 26:230, 1978.

27 Braunwald, E.: Coronary Artery Surgery at the Crossroads, *N. Engl. J. Med.*, 297:661, 1977.

28 Sheldon, W. C., Rincon, G., Pichard, A. D., et al.: Surgical Treatment for Coronary Artery Disease. Pure Graft Operations, with a Study of 741 Patients Followed 3 to 7 Years, *Prog. Cardiovasc. Dis.*, 18:237, 1975.

29 Mather, V. S., and Guinn, G. A.: Sustained Benefit from Aorto-coronary Bypass Surgery Demonstrated for 5 Years. A Prospective Randomized Study, *Circulation*, 56 (suppl. 3):III-190, 1977. (Abstract.)

30 Hultgren, H. N., Peduzzi, D., and Pfeifer, J.: VA Cooperative Study of Stable Angina. Comparison of Medical Versus Surgical Treatment upon Symptoms, *Circulation*, 58 (suppl. 2):II-151, 1978. (Abstract.)

31 Hammermeister, K. E., DeRouen, T. A., Cure, H., et al.: Evidence for Reduction in Rate of Hospitalization for Cardiac Causes as a Result of Coronary Bypass Surgery, *Circulation*, 58 (suppl. 2):II-18, 1978. (Abstract.)

32 Unstable Angina Pectoris: National Cooperative Study Group to Compare Surgical and Medical Therapy: II. Inhospital Experience and Initial Follow-up Results in Patients with One, Two and Three Vessel Disease, *Am. J. Cardiol.*, 42:839, 1978.

33 Detre, K.: The VA Cooperative Study of Surgical Treatment for Coronary Arterial Occlusive Disease: III. Characterization of the Study Population, *1975 Computers in Cardiology,* IEEE, pp. 59–63, 1975.

34 Varnauskas, E., and Olsson, S. B.: The European Multicenter CABG Trial, *Prog. Cardiol.*, 6:83, 1977.

35 Coronary Artery Surgery in Australia — 1974–1976, *Med. J. Aust.*, 1:241, 1978.

36 Tector, A. J., Davis, L., Gabriel, R., et al.: Experience with Internal Mammary Artery Grafts in 298 Patients, *Ann. Thorac. Surg.*, 22:515, 1976.

37 Wisoff, B. G., Fogel, R., Voleti, C., et al. Survival After Cardiac Surgery, *J. Thorac. Cardiovasc. Surg.*, 76:108, 1978.

38 Hurst, J. W., King, S. B., Logue, R. B., et al.: Value of Bypass Surgery: Controversies in Cardiology: Part I, *Am. J. Cardiol.*, 42:308, 1978.

39 Compeau, L., Lesperance, J., Corbara, F., et al.: Patency of Aortocoronary Saphenous Vein Bypass Grafts 5 to 7 Years After Surgery, *Can. J. Surg.*, 21:118, 1978.

40 Feinstein, A. R.: XXXII. Biological Dependency, "Hypothesis Testing," Unilateral Probabilities, and Other Issues in Scientific Direction vs. Statistical Duplexity, *Clin. Pharmacol. Ther.*, 17:499, 1975.

41 Vismara, L. A., Miller, R. R., Price, J. E., et al.: Improved Longevity Due to Reduction of Sudden Death by Aortocoronary Bypass in Coronary Atherosclerosis. Prospective Evaluation of Medical Versus Surgical Therapy in Matched Patients with Multivessel Disease, *Am. J. Cardiol.*, 39:914, 1977.

42 Piffare, R., Loeb, H., Sullivan, H., et al.: Improved Survival After Surgical Therapy for Chronic Angina Pectoris. One Hospital's Experience in a Randomized Trial, *Circulation*, 51–58 (suppl. 2):II-96, 1978. (Abstract.)

43 Green, D. G., Bunnell, L. L., Arani, D. T., et al.: Long-term Survival After Coronary Bypass Surgery. Buffalo General Hospital State University of New York (brochure for exhibit at American Heart Association Meeting, Miami, 1977).

44 Lawrie, G. M., Morris, G. C., Howell, J. F., et al.: Improved Survival After 5 Years in 1,144 Patients After Coronary Bypass Surgery, *Am. J. Cardiol.*, 42:709, 1978.

45 Berkson, J., and Gage, R. P.: Calculation of Survival Rates for Cancer, *Proc. Staff Mtg., Mayo Clin.*, 25:270, 1950.

Chapter 3

Myocardial Perfusion by Coronary Artery Bypass*

JOSEPH D. MARCO, M.D.

The objective of myocardial revascularization over the past decades has been to reestablish blood flow that is adequate to sustain the metabolism of viable muscle compromised by obstructive coronary atherosclerosis. Forty years of ingenious work included multiple techniques for the creation of epicardial adhesions to indirectly increase myocardial perfusion. The coronary sinus has been partially ligated, and an aortocoronary sinus-vein graft was used in an attempt to reverse flow through a valve-free sinusoidal bed. A breakthrough appeared when intramyocardial implantation of the internal thoracic artery stemmed from laboratory work in 1946 and culminated in clinical use in 1951. A great impetus occurred in 1959 when cineangiography demonstrated patency of the internal thoracic myocardial implant. Although this gave rise to the largest surge of clinical use up to that time, experimental data continued to be gathered. Closed, open, and gas endarterectomy followed with vein patch grafts. The next extension was the use of vein interposition grafts, followed by aortocoronary saphenous vein bypass grafting in 1964. In 1967, coronary artery bypass grafting with the internal thoracic artery was done by direct anastomosis.

The importance of the foregoing history and development of coronary bypass to the evaluation of myocardial perfusion is the distinct lack of experimental and clinical data to substantiate the efficacy of these procedures.

The initial goal of coronary surgery was to relieve angina pectoris. Using this as an end point for proof of myocardial perfusion is fraught with hazard, however, since early procedures that are now considered to be without merit have been associated with symptomatic relief in 60 to 80 percent of patients.[1] Coronary artery bypass grafting has achieved even better results, with 75 percent of patients totally free of pain and 90 percent gaining benefit.[2] Benefit is further clinically demonstrated by the fact that 22 percent of postoperative patients require nitrates, while 97 percent without operation require this medication, and that 9 percent of postoperative patients are on propranolol, while 77 percent of random patients without operation

require beta blockade.[3] In spite of this enthusiastic result, laboratory and clinical data proving myocardial perfusion must be shown.

The most readily accessible data come from the laboratory abnormalities associated with coronary atherosclerosis and ischemic myocardium. The most obvious is the occlusive lesion in the coronary artery, as demonstrated by cineangiography. Coronary artery bypass must negate this lesion and is only possible by a procedure that provides prolonged patency. The result of an occluded graft can only be evaluated in the negative, and vein grafts that later occlude have been shown to occasionally induce rapid progression of previously tight coronary lesions to total occlusions. Thus, one must document a satisfactory patency as the first stage in the evaluation of coronary vein grafting, followed by proof of improved myocardial perfusion attributable to the procedure.

A delivery of metabolically useful blood flow through a patent channel is necessary for beneficial myocardial perfusion. Vein graft flow is well documented and has been shown to be significant when compared to the myocardial muscle volume supplied by normal coronaries. Flow would be the second stage of evaluating vein grafts.

The destination of patent vessel flow is the third step. Coronary arteriovenous shunting is of no benefit, and if such shunting steals flow from other capillary beds, it would be harmful. Radioactive tracers can determine the fate of blood traveling these routes in regard to its flow through shunts, smaller arteries, and into the myocardial capillaries and sinusoids. However, it is only the appropriate functional utilization of myocardial flow that sets an operation apart from its predecessors, and for this final aspect, metabolic effects must be examined.

Other parameters, such as the cineventriculogram, left ventricular end-diastolic pressure, systolic time intervals, ejection fraction, segmental wall motion, maximal rate of ventricular contraction, and left atrial and pulmonary arterial pressures, have been evaluated, but these, along with symptoms, longevity, and infarction rate, are far from providing definitive answers. For this reason, the three aforementioned factors will provide the basis for this discussion—patency, flow, and metabolism.

*From 7200 East Grant Road, Tucson, Arizona 85712.

13

PATENCY

Patency has already been mentioned as the first mandatory result of bypass surgery. Internal thoracic artery implantation was shown to remain patent in 85 to 95 percent of cases.[4] The myocardial sinusoids prevent hematoma formation but also contain a low volume capacity. Systolic contraction provides a to-and-fro movement of blood, preventing clotting of the graft, but this type of patency can no longer be accepted as proof of the worth of a procedure. The present author has shown the internal thoracic artery to remain patent in the dog heart while supplying only a miniscule branch to its own pedicle. The internal thoracic artery implanted into normal myocardial muscle will also remain patent and can hardly be assumed to be supplying needed myocardial perfusion. Bjork[5] and Gott[6] found no correlation between clinical internal thoracic artery implants that were patent and the patient's symptoms, but these findings are not universal.[7] Internal thoracic artery implants had an acceptable patency, but this in itself is of no inherent value. Significant disadvantages included the unpredictable flow and the fact that several weeks were required for channels to develop while the heart had no support in the postoperative period.

Initial work for the saphenous vein bypass graft has shown early patency ranging from 79 to 95 percent.[8,9] Most studies involving patency are inadequate, since patients are frequently selected for catheterization on the basis of return of symptoms; since they are catheterized at variable intervals, with early, one-year, and up to six-year data being grouped together to accumulate adequate numbers; and since only a small percentage of the entire bypassed patients are catheterized. There is also very little control as a study group. Another source of differing statistics is the experience of the group involved; subsequent studies by identical groups will usually show an improved patency that can only be attributed to improved technique and experience.

Grondin has reported an excellent series of patients followed for 5 to 7 years.[10] These results reflect the improvements in surgery in that two groups are available for examination: one that had surgery early and one that benefited from more recent and modified techniques. The results are impressive when one realizes that the cumulative patency of early patients is 57.7 percent at a mean of 6.7 years, while that of the later patients is 83.2 percent at a mean of 5 years. The yearly attrition rate of early grafts was shown to be 2.7 percent per year, while that of the later techniques is 0.7 percent. Others have found that 10 to 20 percent of veins occlude after the first year in addition to the early occlusion rate. Rimm found that 23 percent of vein grafts occluded after 2 years and believed that

they close independently of each other.[11] The chance of all three grafts of a triple bypass procedure occluding was determined to be 1 percent, while the chance of both grafts of a double bypass procedure occluding was 5 percent.

Two definite periods are evident in patency follow-up: early closure within 2 to 4 weeks and late closure. The immediate postoperative closure of a graft is related to selectivity of the recipient artery, size of the artery grafted, flows, type of conduit used, and technical expertise. Late occlusion is secondary to fibrous proliferation and atheromatous disease.[11,12] Microscopic examination of autopsy-harvested grafts show degenerative changes with the presence of extracellular lipid particles, accumulation of extracellular material and cellular debris, and loss of normal morphology as demonstrated in grafts 37 to 59 months old.[12]

The internal thoracic–coronary artery bypass is an attempt to increase conduit patency. The use of a conduit with structural identity, one already supplying arterial pressure and of a size approximating the coronary artery, and with a natural origin having decreased turbulence as opposed to a proximal anastomosis, a higher velocity of flow, a lack of subintimal hyperplasia, and the occurrence of fewer atheromatous changes all seem beneficial to thoracic patency. The disadvantages of a somewhat more difficult and tedious technique, the occasional smaller size, a lower potential flow, and sometimes a diseased subclavian system must be balanced against improving the patency of the standard saphenous vein graft. Patency has ranged to 99 percent.[13,14] Barner, in examining 180 internal thoracic artery grafts, found 96 percent early and 93 percent late patency as opposed to 86 percent and 82 percent patency for veins. Most authors' data suggest 5 percent early occlusion and 3 percent late occlusion.[16] Although Jahnke found a great increase in patency for internal thoracic arteries to the circumflex and right coronary arteries,[13] most surgeons use the internal thoracic artery only for the left anterior descending coronary system. Initially, some authors recommended using internal thoracic arteries for all grafts, but a national study has shown that 50 percent of surgeons use it selectively and 3 percent use it routinely for left anterior descending coronary bypass.[17]

Other arterial conduits have been used as well. A reverse internal thoracic artery with the distal end in continuity with the epigastric artery has been proposed for reaching areas beyond the length of the fifth intercostal space, where the artery generally becomes quite small and unsuitable for coronary grafts.[18] Other arteries have been suggested, and the radial artery found some popularity because it was easily accessible. Patency was a problem, and although the difficult aortic anastomosis was feasible, it appears that translocated arteries need their vasa vasorum intact at one end to preserve their superiority over vein grafts.[19] Thus, both translocated internal thoracic arteries and radial arteries have fallen into disuse.

Other attempts have been made to improve single saphenous vein bypass graft patency. One aortic anastomosis for multiple coronary anastomoses has been called a jump graft, a serpigenous graft, and bridge, sequential, and circular grafts. All employ a single proximal anastomosis with one or more side-to-side anastomoses before an end-to-side anastomosis. Grondin reported sequential grafts of which 24 percent were placed to 1-mm arteries, having an attrition rate of 2.3 percent for side-to-side anastomoses and 13 percent for all grafts.[20] The early occlusion rates were 6 percent and 20 percent, respectively. In a later series, Grondin reported 96 percent patency in circular grafts, which he attributed to the higher total flow of multiple anastomoses and to the avoidance of angulation and right-angle anastomosis as seen with some double anastomotic sequential grafts.[21] Cheanvechai et al. showed an 86 percent 1-year patency of sequential grafts, which was the same as that for single coronary artery bypass grafts.[22] They did, however, reserve the sequential graft for smaller arteries, but if the 3-year patency approaches 70 percent, as found by others, the overall result will be similar for all types of saphenous bypass grafts, differing only according to technical abilities. Their biggest advantage is the requirement of less total vein.[23] The disadvantages include venous dilatation and hyperplasia from high flow, risk of atheromatous deposition aggravated by high flow, and the possibility of proximal lesions in a multipurpose conduit.

Another area of controversy has been Y-grafts and their patency.[24,25] The author performed experimental and clinical research to evaluate the use of such grafts.[26] Although the flow dynamics of a Newtonian fluid in a rigid perfect cylinder are well established by Poiseuille's equation, the consideration of blood through an arterial or venous conduit affects many other variables. However, these multiple forces are of little consequence when compared to the relative quantity of change seen between the theoretical and the actual values. With this in mind, the calculations presented in Fig. 3-1 demonstrate that flow potential through the parent vessel is greater than the combined flows possible through either of the two Y grafts when the square of the length of the parent branch is less than the product of the length of the arm grafts. If one makes the anastomosis of a Y graft so that the common channel is as short as possible, then there is no theoretical reason for a significant change in flow as opposed to using a single graft.

This theory was examined in a laboratory procedure. Dogs underwent induction of anesthesia and

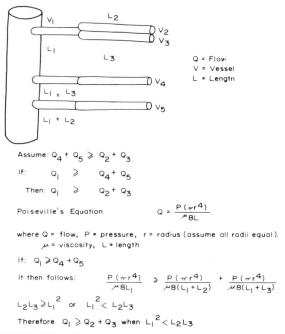

Assume: $Q_4 + Q_5 \geqslant Q_2 + Q_3$

If: $Q_1 \geqslant Q_4 + Q_5$

Then: $Q_1 \geqslant Q_2 + Q_3$

Poiseuille's Equation

$$Q = \frac{P(\pi r^4)}{\mu 8L}$$

where Q = flow, P = pressure, r = radius (assume all radii equal).
μ = viscosity, L = length

If: $Q_1 \geqslant Q_4 + Q_5$

It then follows: $\dfrac{P(\pi r^4)}{\mu 8L_1} \geqslant \dfrac{P(\pi r^4)}{\mu 8(L_1+L_2)} + \dfrac{P(\pi r^4)}{\mu 8(L_1+L_3)}$

$L_2 L_3 \geqslant L_1{}^2$ or $L_1{}^2 < L_2 L_3$

Therefore $Q_1 \geqslant Q_2 + Q_3$ when $L_1{}^2 < L_2 L_3$

FIGURE 3-1 These calculations demonstrate the circumstances under which the flow potential through the parent vessel is greater than the combined flows possible through either of the two Y grafts.

after heparinization, a 6-cm section of human saphenous vein was sewn onto the abdominal aorta with standard technique. A 42-cm section of 2.5-mm internal diameter tubing was then added to each vein for the purpose of collection and was considered as a constant peripheral resistance. This had no effect on the actual numerical values obtained, as the flow in the experimental situation was within or above the ranges utilized by coronary bypass grafts. The free volumetric flow was then measured for 5-s intervals and repeated to increase accuracy. A standard bifid anastomosis with a Y graft was also constructed (Fig. 3-2). The aorta-to-vein graft length remained 6 cm, and the 42-cm tubing was added to each as a collection technique. A partially occluding vascular clamp was then used to ensure that the starting and stopping of flows would simultaneously affect all grafts concerned. Flow measurements were then serially taken for grafts singularly and in combination by clamping and unclamping the desired collection tubing and releasing the aortic hood flow. Continuous intraarterial blood pressure monitoring was performed, and blood reinfusion was maintained to keep the preparation stable. Resistance of a single vein preparation was calculated by dividing electronically determined mean arterial pressure by graft flow. These resistances were then used to calculate the expected flow of the bifid Y graft for each

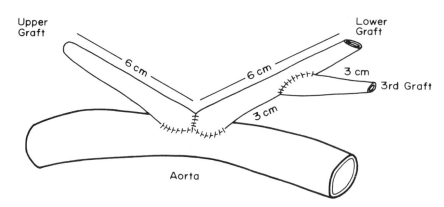

FIGURE 3-2 Schematic drawing of the saphenous vein bypass technique utilizing a bifid hood with bidirectional flow and a Y graft.

branch individually and in combination. This was utilized to allow for the varying blood pressures that existed during the experiments. The measured Y graft flow was compared with calculated graft flow for each graft (Table 3-1). Flows from bifid grafts and Y grafts were not significantly different from those of single grafts. When mean graft flow was calculated, there was minimal difference between the theoretical and actual flow obtained. To evaluate clinical results, the 1-year postoperative catheterization in 171 patients having coronary reverse saphenous bypass was analyzed. The patency rate for single vein grafts to the right and left anterior descending coronary arteries was not significantly different. These patency rates were compared to those for the bifid hood and the Y graft as well as for a combination of these techniques. Patency rates were not statistically different for any of these methods (Table 3-2).

TABLE 3-1
Actual and anticipated flow through Y grafts

Type of Graft	Average expected flow range (ml/5 s)	Average measured flow (ml± 0.5/5 s)		
		Upper graft	Lower graft	Third graft
Bifid hood, simultaneous flows	28–29	28	30	
Y graft, simultaneous lower limb and third graft flows	25–27		26	27
Bifid hood with Y graft, Simultaneous flows				
All three grafts	23–25	25	24	25
Upper graft alone	31–35	33		
Lower graft alone	32–34		32	
Third graft alone	32–34			32

Although many authors have expressed preference for single grafts and some work has been done showing unfavorable data for the Y grafts, there appears to be no theoretical disadvantage to their use. A simplified application of fluid dynamics shows that within certain requirements the flow of a common graft is greater than that needed to supply its own branches in parallel. The laboratory preparation to duplicate the clinical situation substantiated this and showed that flows measured in both branches of a bifid hood, as well as Y grafts, were comparable. These observations showed no difference in flow between the primary, secondary, and tertiary branches. Since this does not evaluate the different flow requirements and peripheral resistance as found within a diseased coronary bed, the clinical aspect was examined as well, and the results at 1-year catheterization show no statistical difference between the different methods of grafting. This analysis does not include the extent of disease of each vessel, the dominance of the particular anatomy, or the progression of disease during the postoperative year. The variance in patency between the three most commonly grafted coronary arteries can probably be explained by these factors. The theoretical objection to the use of a Y graft because of segmental intimal proliferation in the common channel, as well as atherosclerotic development in the proximal channel, is indeed real. However, there is no clinical evidence to show that this occurs in the very short (1 cm) common channel or that it would not occur if grafts had been placed individually. Griffith[27] and Hutchins[28] examined grafts at autopsy and found no narrowing at the Y anastomosis. The major advantage for the use of Y grafts occurs when inadequate vein is available for reaching the aorta or in the presence of a short aortic arch that cannot support sites for multiple anastomoses; under these conditions, the use of a Y graft is justified.

The option of endarterectomizing grafted vessels is available, and many have found this satisfactory when restricted to the right coronary artery. Most experience shows that grafting to a lower area free of disease is preferable. Griffith found on autopsy examination a 50 percent recurrence rate of new significant disease.[27] Walters reported endarterectomized patency of 59 percent in the right coronary artery, 58 percent in the left anterior descending coronary artery, and 74 percent in the circumflex coronary artery.[29]

Several factors contribute to patency. Most important is technical ability. Campeau found a high follow-up occlusion rate of patients whose grafts at 6 to 18 months had localized stenosis in the anastomosis or trunk, and he believed that these were related to unsatisfactory surgical technique.[10] Graft pressure and tension may cause changes in the walls of the veins, possibly stretching smooth muscle and initiating the development of degenerative changes as found in some vein grafts. Other factors are present as well. The problem of choosing a recipient artery with a bed of sufficient quality to support flow and maintain patency is currently an area with no prospective evaluation, although some radioactive scanning techniques offer promise. A great advantage will be the ability to determine scar versus graft-sustaining functional myocardium. The lack of wall motion on ventriculogram in conjunction with coincidental old infarction on electrocardiogram is currently used as suggestive of scar. The site of angina in conjunction with the area of scar and the ischemic muscle–normal myocardium interface is unknown. Blumlein, in evaluating preoperative factors, found a high diastolic blood pressure and a high-grade coronary occlusion to result in increased patency,[30] but this has not been a consistent finding.

Several studies have examined causes of graft occlusion. Zajtchuk examined 59 occluded grafts with flows ranging from 35 to 90 ml/min and found patients to have a high degree of blood hypercoagulability with low levels of antithrombin III and a high level of factor VIII, a high thrombin generation index, and increased platelet adhesiveness.[31] It would appear that some patients have such predisposing factors to account for graft occlusion. The postcardiotomy syndrome has been suggested as causing graft failure, and Urschel found a better patency if these patients were vigorously treated with steroids.[32] Griffith examined 95 grafts post mortem and found that most changes occurred adjacent to the anastomosis.[27] These were compression, thrombosis, and mural dissection. Patency was more favorable if the recipient vessel was greater than 1.2 mm in diameter. An anastomosis at a branch frequently compromised the lumen. Hutchins also examined postmortem grafts of an end-to-side and side-to-side technique and found changes in the recipient artery lumen, especially when an atheroma was present in the anastomosis.[28] There was also frequent dissection of the coronary artery wall. Y grafts and aortic anastomoses were no problem.

Pathophysiologic factors influencing patency are

TABLE 3-2
Coronary vein graft patency in 171 patients undergoing catheterization 1 year postoperatively

Type of graft	RCA*	LAD	CCA
Single	7 (9)†	8 (12)	0
Bifid hood	61 (78)	62 (79)	0
Y graft	0	11 (18)	11 (16)
Bifid hood with Y graft	38 (52)	40 (53)	34 (52)

*RCA, right coronary artery; LAD, left anterior descending coronary artery; CCA, circumflex coronary artery.

†Total number of patients is given in parentheses. Of populations large enough for analysis, there is no statistical difference at the chi-square level ($p < 0.050$).

competitive flow between artery and graft and between different grafts, the extent of outflow disease, and collateral circulation. There is no doubt that saphenous vein grafts are subject to atherosclerosis (Fig. 3-3). The rate of development seems quite variable, as does the progression of distal disease. However, intimal proliferation does not appear to progress after the first year.[10] Coronary recipients of less than 1.5 mm seem less likely to stay patent,[33] and whether this is a limitation of our surgical technique, a product of stasis and low flow, or a reflection of the distal runoff is not known. Certainly distal runoff capacity is of significant importance, and some feel this can be evaluated by angiography.[34] Infection has also been implicated in graft occlusion. However, most authors find little difference in the patency of patients having proven graft status.[35] Walters has evaluated patency in relation to the technique of grafting vessels while not on cardiopulmonary bypass.[29] If one uses cardiopulmonary bypass, patency increases from 52 percent to 78 percent for saphenous vein bypass and from 78 percent to 86 percent for internal thoracic artery anastomosis. Patients under 40 years of age have been found to have 85 percent for vein grafts and 96 percent for internal thoracic arteries, suggesting that the age of the patient does not affect graft patency.[36] Aintablain examined 28 patients with subendocardial infarctions and studied the influence of operating in the face of acute infarction as compared to surgery while the patient was unstable or stable.[37] None of these factors affected graft patency.

FLOWS

The measurement of flow through arterial bypasses had its development in the evolution of peripheral vascular surgery. Much work has been done in this regard for coronary surgery. Flow is dependent on the lumenal size of the conduit relative to the recipient ar-

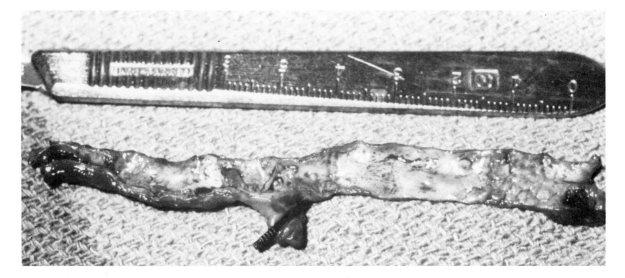

FIGURE 3-3 An occluded saphenous vein graft showing severe atheromatous disease.

tery, the degree of stenosis, the size of the recipient artery, and the status of the perfused bed.[38,39] Flow can be manipulated and markedly increases with hypoxic hyperemia, papaverine injection, Isuprel infusion, and administration of nitroglycerin.[40,41] Flows have been most commonly measured at surgery, but they have also been measured postoperatively by videodensitometry, K_{45}, and xenon flow. Pressure traces and flows have been shown to duplicate those of normal arteries.[38] To evaluate the operative flow and its relation to coronary graft patency, the author performed a study in which patients were selected on the basis of having a postoperative and 1-year postoperative catheterization performed.[42] In all instances, surgery was performed for relief of angina pectoris. In the study, 142 patients had 310 coronary bypasses with reversed saphenous vein. There were 134 grafts to the left anterior descending coronary artery (LAD), 59 to the circumflex coronary artery (CCA), and 117 to the right coronary artery (RCA). At the time of surgery, graft flows were measured with a Carolina Medical Electronics electromagnetic flow-

meter and recorded on a direct writing recorder. Flows were measured after baselines had been established, and reactive hyperemia was recorded after a 30-s graft occlusion. After the resumption of baseline flow, 15 mg of papaverine was injected into the graft over 5 s, and the pulsatile and mean graft flows were again measured.

Early catheterization revealed a patency of 85.5 percent (265 of 310 grafts). Patency rates for individual arteries were RCA, 86 percent; LAD, 85 percent; and CCA, 81 percent. Catheterization after 1 year revealed 193 of the original 310 grafts to be patent (76.8 percent). For individual arteries, these were RCA, 75 percent; LAD, 78 percent; and CCA, 76 percent patency.

Examination of basal flows (Table 3-3) showed that 42 percent of grafts with basal flows of less than 20 ml/min were occluded at 1 week of catheterization, whereas 63 percent were occluded at 1 year. Similarly, grafts with basal flows between 20 and 40 ml/min had a 25 percent occlusion rate at 1 week and 28 percent cumulative occlusion rate.

Reactive hyperemia was examined as percentage of flow over the basal values (Table 3-4). Absence of reactive hyperemia was associated with a 19 percent early occlusion rate and a 12 percent late occlusion rate. The presence of reactive hyperemia was associated with a 16 percent early and a 5 percent late occlusion rate, which was not influenced by the magnitude of change.

The flow response to papaverine was evaluated in increments of a onefold to over fourfold increase in flow above basal values (Table 3-5). When the flow increase was less than 100 percent, there was a 20 percent early and a 30 percent cumulative failure rate.

TABLE 3-3
Vein graft basal flows

Basal flow (ml/min)	Total	Occluded 1 week	Occluded 1 year	Cumulative occlusion
0–19	19	8	4	12
20–39	61	12	5	17
40–59	87	9	7	16
60–99	102	13	8	21
100–149	35	3	2	5
≥ 150	5	0	0	0

Greater flow responses to papaverine were associated with early and cumulative failure rates of 7 to 22 percent without correlation between the magnitude of change and patency.

These data were collected from a consecutive series of surgical patients, 90 percent of whom had early postoperative catheterization, with 50 percent returning for a 1-year coronary angiogram. The patients were catheterized on a routine follow-up basis and do not reflect any selectivity for symptomatic patients. The obvious association of increased occlusion in the early postoperative period with low flows is recognized by other authors as well and is related to the various causes for early graft occlusion.[33,42-46] The relationship between flow of less than 40 ml/min and late occlusion is not statistically significant but is also consistent with current thinking. The factors involved in the determination of coronary bed flow and its acceptance of graft flow are such that the effect is seen initially and would affect the early postoperative patency. The accepted reasons for late postoperative graft occlusion are generally graft intimal proliferation and graft atherosclerosis, neither of which are particularly affected by the coronary bed flow capacity. These data indicate that the absence of reactive hyperemia is associated with higher early and late occlusion rates; however, neither is related to the magnitude of reactive hyperemia. The various components of a myocardial perfusion bed that are affected by the change in the available flow of an immediate nature, such as seen by placement of a coronary graft, and the affect of temporary occlusion of this graft in relation to the changes seen in the capillary bed are unknown. It is also unknown whether this is a fixed and permanent reflection of the bed status or whether this is just an extension of the flow capabilities. Since the obtaining of reactive hyperemia is part of the mandatory occlusion for the measurement of basal mean flow, it is obtained without additional procedure or potential harm to the patient. It is, however, of minimal usefulness.

Initially, papaverine-induced vasodilatation was used in peripheral vascular reconstruction, and it was found that this procedure was not of value in predicting graft patency.[47] Whether it produced increased perfusion capabilities or increased shunting is unknown. Again, in the present study, the flow response to papaverine was not helpful in determining either early or late graft patency. On the basis of these observations we continue to measure basal graft flow in all coronary bypass grafts for proof of graft function and prognosis. If the flow is less than 40 ml/min, there is a 36 percent chance that the graft will fail within 1 year. As mentioned, although reactive hyperemia is not separately sought, it is created by the procedure of obtaining zero flow for the measurement of basal

TABLE 3-4

Vein graft reactive hyperemia to 30-s occlusion

Reactive hyperemia (% of basal flow)	Total	Occluded 1 week	Occluded 1 year	Cumulative occlusion
0	134	26	16	42
1–10	17	2	0	2
11–20	25	3	1	4
21–50	49	4	6	10
51–100	48	7	1	8
> 100	28	2	1	3

flow itself. Despite complete occlusion of the proximal coronary artery and graft, the collateral flow is frequently so abundant that with the resumption of graft flow, reactive hyperemia does not occur. Papaverine-induced vasodilatation is no longer utilized.

These data were similarly evaluated for the different components of the cardiac and flow cycles in the hope of finding hemodynamic parameters measurable at operation which would indicate more precisely the severity of diffuse distal coronary artery disease and graft prognosis. Physiologically, the cardiac cycle in conjunction with Poiseuille's law relating pressure and resistance also affects graft flow. Examination of different coronary arteries during the cardiac cycle shows different intramural pressure developed by the ventricles, with a high wall tension in the left ventricle preventing much systolic flow compared to the diastolic component, while the right ventricle produces much less effect. Predominant flow occurs during diastole and differs for right and left coronary arteries (Fig. 3-4). Increased tissue pressure decreases flow, and low blood pressure may aggravate this situation. Moran found left grafts to carry 73 ml/min mean flow, while right grafts supplied 53 ml/min mean flow.[44] These were consistent with resistances of 1.2 for the left and 2.6 peripheral resistance units for the right coronary artery. Endocardial pressure has been shown by flow cessation techniques to be less than epicardial pressure, which explains the greater endocardial flow as

TABLE 3-5

Vein graft flows after papaverine (0.15 mg)

Papaverine-induced flow (% of basal flow)	Total	Occluded 1 week	Occluded 1 year	Cumulative occlusion
0–100	76	15	8	23
101–200	114	17	8	25
201–300	69	8	7	15
301–400	29	2	3	5
> 400	20	3	1	4

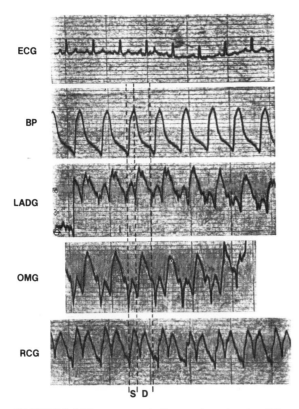

ECG

BP

LADG

OMG

RCG

S D

FIGURE 3-4 Electromagnetic flow tracings showing different flow ratios during a cardiac cycle for the right anterior descending and circumflex coronary artery grafts. BP, systemic blood pressure; LADG, left anterior descending coronary bypass graft; OMG, obtuse marginal coronary bypass graft; RCG, right coronary bypass graft; D, diastolic; S, systolic.

shown by radioactive microsphere, rubidium, and potassium techniques.[48] Similarly, it has been shown that a fixed partial obstruction in the distal coronary artery or graft would change the phasic flow and might be of predictive value in graft prognosis.[45,50] Lack of reactive hyperemia may be secondary to myocardial scar, sufficient collateral, sufficient flow through the obstruction, or maximally dilated vessels. Grafts without predominant diastolic flow may have a partial obstructing anastomosis, obstructed distal coronary artery, or poor runoff and have an increased chance of occlusion. For these reasons, the author examined mean flow, reactive hyperemia, peak-to-peak amplitude, diastolic flow, systolic flow, and diastolic/systolic flow ratio and difference but could find no correlation with early or late patency for anything but mean coronary flow (Table 3-6). This was not in support of early findings and initial thinking but has held up with further investigation.[49-51] The only significant findings were related to different flow patterns for the right and left coronary systems. The right coronary

artery had a systolic flow volume 29 percent greater than the left coronary artery and the diastolic/systolic flow ratio was 2.9 for the right and 3.9 and 4.0 for the circumflex and anterior descending coronary arteries, respectively, which supports the physiology of flow as it is now understood.

The flow of the internal thoracic artery bypass graft has been an area of great discussion. Pulsatile flows experimentally have been shown to be very different from the ascending aorta grafts, not because of time lag of pulse propagation, but because of differing pressure contours.[52] Clinically, this may translate into some of the different and conflicting data on internal thoracic artery grafts. Flows through the open end of an internal thoracic artery range from 60 to 270 ml/min and average 138 ml/min, showing a capacity greater than the average flow through either the internal thoracic artery or the saphenous vein coronary graft.[53] The internal thoracic artery is generally used only if free flow is greater than 60 ml/min. This level has been chosen by several authors versed in the use of the internal thoracic graft. When anastomosed to a coronary artery the flow will be less than free flow, as determined by coronary resistance and internal thoracic artery size and length. Shorter grafts may increase flow by 20 ml/min.[14] Velocities range from 20 to 37 cm/s, as compared to 4 to 14 cm/s for vein grafts.[38] An internal thoracic artery of 2 mm diameter, with a flow of 50 ml/min, has a velocity of 25 cm/s, while a 5-mm vein with the same flow would have a velocity of 7 cm/s.[54] This is one reason given for the improved patency of internal thoracic artery grafts; however, smaller veins also give higher velocity, but not all investigators believe that this affects patency.[55] It has also been pointed out that an anastomosis affording bidirectional flow will have increased flow and patency.

The internal thoracic artery may increase in size by as much as twofold.[14] Coronary flow remains within a relatively constant range, so increasing the size of a conduit can increase pressure through less graft resistance and can maximize flow up to a point, beyond which decreased velocity and stasis result. This may explain some variation in reports regarding different-sized veins. The most frequently recognized reason for failure of the internal thoracic artery anastomosis is fracture of the intima at the time of surgery.[14,16] Mean basal flows of the right, left anterior descending, and the circumflex coronary arteries are not significantly different whether one uses an internal thoracic artery or reverse saphenous vein graft.[16,56] Patency, however, differs by 10 to 15 percent. If known low-flow situations, such as an area of likely scar, are encountered, an internal thoracic artery graft will give superior results.[57]

The use of the internal thoracic artery as a graft

TABLE 3-6
Phasic flow measurements in which only basal mean flow is of value

	Vessel:	LAD*				CCA				RCA			
	Conduit:	Vein		ITA		Vein		ITA		Vein		ITA	
	Patency:	P	O	P	O	P	O	P	O	P	O	P	O
Flows	Basal mean	73.1	47.8	52.5	36.7	83.0	59.9	42.5	—	83.9	49.3	57.2	20.0
mm²/cycle	Systolic	55.4	55.4	55.8	47.6	53.4	81.6	20.0	—	76.9	77.3	65.5	12.0
of tracing	Diastolic (+) systolic	251.6	160.5	201.7	146.3	142.8	258.0	120.5	—	281.2	196.3	231.9	59.0
	Diastolic (−) systolic	152.6	68.3	86.1	53.9	112.8	98.0	78.5	—	132.3	83.9	107.2	35.0
	Diastolic/ systolic	4.9	3.0	3.3	2.5	4.3	2.5	4.7	—	3.1	2.7	2.8	3.9

*LAD, left anterior descending coronary artery; CCA, circumflex coronary artery; RCA, right coronary artery; ITA, internal thoracic artery; P, patent; O, occluded.

rather than an implant has been proven superior. Barner reported a marked difference in total coronary flow and other physiological parameters.[58] Thoracic artery implantation showed a change of only 1.2 to 5.8 percent of total coronary flow, and at 4 to 9 months postoperatively, one could occlude the implant in a laboratory preparation and show no change in ventricular function, ventricular function curve, and *dp/dt* and no consistent change in the total coronary flow.

Functionally the internal thoracic artery appears to be adequate, since symptoms are relieved and patency approaches 99 percent.[59] Physiologically, exercise testing has shown that results are similar between internal thoracic artery and saphenous vein grafts, implying adequate flow.[60]

Flow has been evaluated for other coronary bypass grafts. Szilagyi has shown that an end-to-side anastomosis is less efficient hemodynamically than an end-to-end anastomosis or normal vessel but that a small angle between the graft and recipient and a bell-mouthed anastomosis decreases this difference.[61] Also, the optimal ratio between recipient and graft vessels is 1:1.4 to 1:1.6, which makes smaller veins and internal thoracic arteries seem ideal conduits. Grondin showed mean flows in side-to-side grafts to be 70 ml/min, which is quite similar to that of end-to-side grafts. Although never demonstrated, there is a possibility of sequential grafts demonstrating a "steal" syndrome, especially if obstructive lesions were to develop in the graft.

Coronary collateralization is an important determinant of graft flow, fate, and patency. Many investigators believe that coronary collaterals are genetically determined. A significant stenosis makes collaterals increase and become visible on routine coronary angiography at a diameter of 100 μm.[62] Valle found the degree of collateralization proportional to the degree of obstruction, requiring at least 50 percent,

and after successful coronary bypass, these may disappear with return after graft occlusion.[63] It has also been shown that sufficient collateralization can make a total occlusion hemodynamically similar to that of a 90 percent occlusion and thus affect pressure and graft flow.[64]

The possibilities of varied flows with different subsets of clinical groups have been examined. It has been shown that the phasic flow of coronary artery bypass grafts in patients with diabetes mellitus is 12 percent in systole, and the mean arterial pressures, flows, and coronary resistances have been shown to equal those of nondiabetic patients.[65] These data do not support the theory that microangiopathy affects the flow in the myocardium of a diabetic patient.

Females, as a group, also frequently seem to have small coronary arteries and hearts. A series of 241 women were evaluated and found to have a similar mortality for surgery but better ventricular preservation requiring fewer coronary artery bypass grafts.[66] The important finding was a significantly lower patency rate of postoperative, 1-year, and 3-year catheterization, and the recipient arteries were statistically smaller in diameter than in men.

We began by first discussing the patency of the conduit and then the volumes of conduit blood delivery and have shown that hemodynamics of coronary artery bypass grafts are capable of mimicking normal coronary arteries.[67] We will, however, continue beyond the anastomosis. Myocardial scanning has been helpful in following the flow of blood through the anastomosis into the myocardium. In a recent study, macroaggregates of human serum albumin labeled with [131]I- and ^{99m}Tc-labeled microspheres were injected preoperatively into the right and left coronary arteries, respectively, of 82 patients.[68] Two weeks postoperatively, similar injections were carried out into the coronary arteries and bypass grafts. Compar-

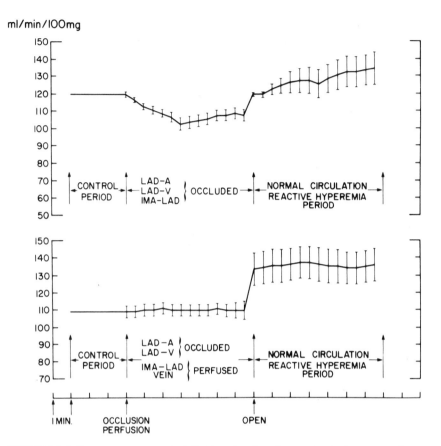

FIGURE 3-5 Coronary venous arterialization showing changes in total coronary flow. *(From J. D. Marco et al., Coronary Venous Arterialization: Acute Hemodynamic, Metabolic, and Chronic Anatomical Observations, Ann. Thorac. Surg., 23:449, 1977.)*

ison of data showed 67 normal perfusion scans with 34 abnormal wall motions in which left ventricular function significantly improved postoperatively. Fifteen patients had abnormal perfusion scans. Left ventricular function improved postoperatively only if a coronary bypass graft was placed to an area that preoperatively had normal regional perfusion. The conclusion drawn was that a normal regional perfusion scan meant an adequate capillary bed for grafting regardless of the degree of coronary stenosis by angiography and was thus predictive that abnormal wall motion with a normal capillary bed would improve after coronary artery bypass. The distribution of biodegradable particles reflects the blood flow to each region containing these particles as detected by external radionuclide imaging and thus substantiates coronary grafts perfusing myocardium. Although not all perfusion defects can be reversed by coronary grafting, there has not been sufficient evaluation to answer questions of graph patency, graft flow, adequacy of graft flow, and presence of scar with need of regional

perfusion. These must be evaluated as to the presence of grafts to adjacent and differing regional areas as well as symptomatic relief. Since regional obstruction of blood flow is associated with a corresponding area of diminished concentration of radioactivity in the perfusion image, and since a relief of this obstruction does not always correct the perfusion defect, there is more to the aspect of coronary artery disease than we can evaluate on the coronary angiogram alone.

^{43}KCl myocardial imaging has myocardial uptake which is a function of regional distribution of blood flow, and 79 percent clearing is accomplished at each passage of blood. This has been used to show abnormal preoperative scans reverting to normal scans postoperatively.[69] Patients with exercise-induced angina were evaluated by ^{81}Rb myocardial imaging and had exercise-induced scan defects indicative of decreased myocardial perfusion, since ^{81}Rb, a radioactive isotopic analogue of potassium, is also cleared by the myocardium in proportion to relative coronary blood flow. All symptomatically improved patients had improved treadmill exercise tests and heart rate–blood pressure products. Most importantly, after coronary bypass grafting the scans were improved in all patients and were normal in 6 patients.[70]

Thallium 201 myocardial imaging has improved the quality of scans over previous agents and studies support the thesis that exertional deficits represent regional ischemia and that the disappearance postoperatively represents improved regional blood flow.[77] Improved scans have been associated with angiographically patent grafts. Patients who developed a new defect postoperatively had only 54 percent patency of coronary artery bypass grafts, and each was associated with regional graft closure or ungrafted residual disease.

The predictive value of ^{201}Tl has been compared to stress scintigraphy, cardiac catheterization, chest pain, and exercise electrocardiography.[72] Chest pain was neither sensitive nor specific. The stress electrocardiogram was not sensitive but was specific. The scan has good sensitivity and is highly specific. Evidence of perfusion was seen in patients with successful revascularization and can reliably predict graft patency, as shown by other authors.[71,73,74]

Another study of coronary bypass patients with ^{201}Tl myocardial perfusion imaging showed that 70 percent of preoperative underperfused myocardial segments improved after coronary bypass grafting and that 85 percent of the patients had demonstrable improvement in myocardial perfusion.[75] Sixty percent of patients had some residual perfusion abnormalities. Most notably the improved scans correlated with clinical improvement, and patients with a history of myocardial infarction had more residual perfusion defects postoperatively. Cox showed experimentally that collateral was sufficient during rest to prevent changes in subendocardial flow supplied by obstructed coronary arteries as shown by radioactive microsphere techniques.[76] However, pharmacologic stress caused differences, suggesting underperfusion in the distribution

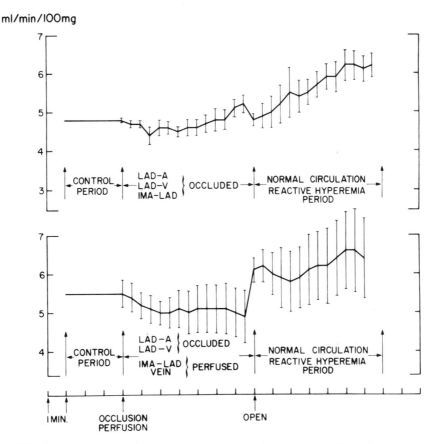

FIGURE 3-6 Coronary venous arterialization showing lactate consumption. *(From J. D. Marco et al., Coronary Venous Arterialization: Acute Hemodynamic, Metabolic, and Chronic Anatomical Observations, Ann. Thorac. Surg., 23:449, 1977.)*

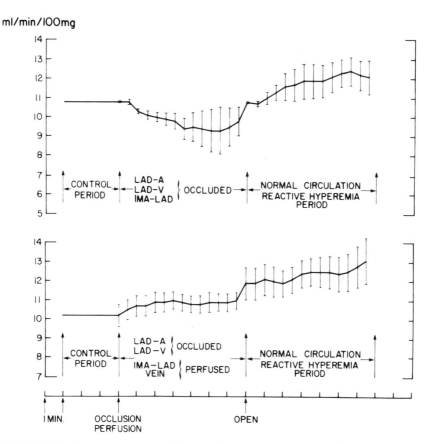

FIGURE 3-7 Coronary venous arterialization showing oxygen consumption. *(From J. D. Marco et al., Coronary Venous Arterialization: Acute Hemodynamic, Metabolic, and Chronic Anatomical Observations, Ann. Thorac. Surg., 23:449, 1977.)*

of blocked coronary arteries. A functioning coronary artery bypass graft returned the model to that of normal coronary perfusion.

An indirect method of evaluating myocardial perfusion by coronary artery bypass grafting is the result of myocardial function and activity. Some investigators conclude that resting left ventricular hemodynamics are unchanged.[74] Starr studied internal thoracic artery ligation, internal thoracic artery implantation and coronary artery bypass grafting with force ballistocardiograms and carotid pulse derivative.[77] He concluded that internal thoracic artery ligation had no effect, that internal thoracic artery implantation had little to no effect, but that most coronary artery bypass patients showed significant improvement. Although Nordstrom reported relief of refractory ventricular fibrillation and ventricular tachycardia in 2 patients by coronary artery bypass grafting,[78] the relation in general remains unclear.

Anderson evaluated the first derivative of the ventricular pressure (*dp/dt*) as compared to a common peak developed isovolumetric pressure (CPIP).[80] This ratio was used to cancel effects on contractility of preload and afterload. Nine of 14 patients demonstrated a decrease in this ratio with temporary acute occlusion of the bypass graft. Five patients were unaffected. Pacing-induced tachycardia was used to increase oxygen requirements, and most patients again showed benefit by coronary artery bypass graft perfusion.

Santos compared patients with patent and occluded grafts.[81] Pressures and indexes were essentially the same between the groups. There was a trend toward improved functional values of values abnormal preoperatively, but normal values were maintained even in the face of total graft occlusion.

MYOCARDIAL PERFUSION—
METABOLISM

The ability of the heart to move its preload against an afterload and the governing contractile state is dependent upon the availability of oxygen.[79] Oxygen requirements are assessed by measuring left ventricular oxygen consumption. Oxygen delivery is considered adequate if no signs of metabolic, histochemical, or functional damage are present. The evaluation of metabolic parameters has been carried out for various methods of coronary revascularization. Right-sided heart bypass in laboratory preparations has been useful for these studies. Studies of the internal thoracic–coronary artery bypass and saphenous vein–coronary artery bypass show no difference between the two groups. The hemodynamics and metabolic response to graft occlusions were similar to but less dramatic than those obtained in normal dogs after coronary artery occlusion.[82] Twelve to 22 months after surgery, the veins showed irregularities and narrowing, while the internal thoracic arteries were smooth and clear.[82]

Some patients are not suitable candidates for coronary bypass because of diffuse or distal coronary disease. Because of the discouraging results obtained with endarterectomy and combined bypass, the consideration of coronary vein arterialization has not only been suggested but has received surprisingly frequent clinical use. Although this concept underwent a significant amount of research in various aspects applied to the coronary sinus, its clinical use was begun prior to established laboratory justification.[83-86]

To this end, acute and chronic studies were performed by the author.[87] The technique used was one well established for right-sided heart bypass and the utilization of hemodynamic and metabolic data.[88] After the establishment of this technique, the animal was placed on total cardiopulmonary bypass. The proximal left anterior descending coronary artery and vein were then surrounded with a snare. Under aortic cross-clamping and topical hypothermia a coronary vein–internal thoracic artery anastomosis was made with standard surgical technique. At its completion, obvious apical venovenous shunts were ligated. Bypass was then discontinued, and the preparation was allowed to return to a stable state. Right-sided heart bypass was then instituted, and again a stable state

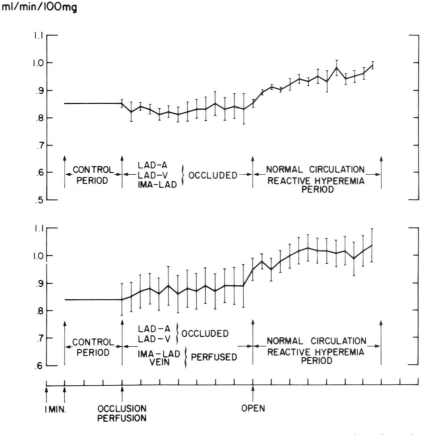

FIGURE 3-8 Coronary venous arterialization showing pyruvate consumption. *(From J. D. Marco et al., Coronary Venous Arterialization: Acute Hemodynamic, Metabolic, and Chronic Anatomical Observations, Ann. Thorac. Surg., 23:449, 1977.)*

was established. After a 10-min control with the internal thoracic artery graft occluded, the snare around the anterior descending vein and artery was occluded for 7 min of controlled ischemia. The snare was then released, restoring coronary circulation and evaluating reactive hyperemia. Once again, the snare was occluded, and the internal thoracic artery–coronary vein graft was simultaneously released. Again, there was a 7-min test period, after which the snare on the anterior descending artery and vein was released, the graft occluded, and reactive hyperemia evaluated. At the completion of each procedure, the internal thoracic artery was injected with methylene blue to identify the adequacy of perfusion. The left ventricle was weighed for calculations of myocardial oxygen consumption.

The hemodynamic and metabolic data are shown in Figs. 3-5 to 3-8 and summarized in Table 3-7. Without venous arterialization, occlusion of the anterior descending artery resulted in a significant decrease of stroke work, total coronary flow, and myocardial oxygen consumption, while left ventricular end-diastolic pressures and lactate and pyruvate uptake did not change. Reactive hyperemia produced by arterial occlusion was associated with no change in total coronary flow or myocardial oxygen consumption, but there was a significant increase in pyruvate and lactate uptake with venous arterialization. Occlusion of the anterior descending artery did not change hemodynamic or metabolic measurements. The only change during reactive hyperemia was an increase in total coronary flow secondary to arteriovenous shunting.

A chronic experiment was also undertaken in which dogs underwent thoracotomy and mobilization of the right internal thoracic artery with a pedicle of soft tissue. Under heparinization the anterior descending vein was anastomosed to the end of the internal thoracic artery using standard surgical technique without the aid of cardiopulmonary bypass. The anterior descending artery was then ligated distal to the first diagonal branch, and anterior descending vein perfusion begun after the proximal vein had similarly been ligated. Heparin was reversed, and the chest was closed in the standard manner. Control dogs underwent thoracotomy and anterior descending artery and vein ligation. This produced a 40 percent mortality, while the dogs with venous arterialization had a 14 percent mortality, substantiating the acute benefit shown by the metabolic study. Angiography was performed in nine dogs prior to their death and revealed patency of the internal thoracic artery to the heart, with no significant filling of the coronary veins. Postmortem examination of both control and treated animals revealed transmural infarcts in both groups involving the anterior wall of the left ventricle, the apex, and the adjacent septum (Fig. 3-9). These infarcts were significantly more extensive in control animals. The infarcts had a definite apical localization in treated animals. The internal thoracic artery was patent to the heart in all instances, but the anastomosis appeared occluded by tissue grossly indistinguishable from artery and vein. There was no gross evidence of acute or chronic thrombosis in the internal thoracic artery or anastomosis. Microscopy revealed occlusion of all anastomoses at 6 weeks by obliteration of the lumen with mature fibrous tissue with minimal inflammatory reaction, good preservation of the internal thoracic artery at the anastomosis, and frequent loss of definition of the vein (Fig. 3-10). Smooth muscle was absent and pigment containing macrophages and fibrin were generally not found. Remote from the anastomosis, two types of changes were noted in the coronary veins. In a few instances, there was uniform thickening of the media as a result of increased smooth muscle. Most commonly, there was encroachment on the lumen by focal intimal proliferation or subintimal foci of mature

TABLE 3-7

Hemodynamic and metabolic data from acute coronary venous arterialization experiments

Measurement	No venous arterialization			With arterialization		
	Control	Occlusion of LAD*	Reactive hyperemia	Control	Occlusion of LAD	Reactive hyperemia
LVEDP (mm Hg)	10.1	11.9 ± 4.7	. . .	10.0	11.2 ± 3.2	. . .
Stroke work (g-m)	6.0	4.9 ± 1.6†	. . .	6.0	5.9 ± 1.4	. . .
TCF (ml · 100 g · min)	120 ± 1.5	108 ± 3.0+	133 ± 8.7	109 ± 3.5	111 ± 3.2	135 ± 9.3‡
O₂ uptake (ml · 100 g · min)	10.8 ± 0.1	9.4 ± 0.6	12.3 ± 0.7	10.2 ± 6.9	10.9 ± 0.5	12.4 ± 0.9
Lactate uptake (mg · 100 g min)	4.8 ± 0.1	4.8 ± 0.3	6.2 ± 0.4‡	5.5 ± 0.4	5.1 ± 0.6	6.6 ± 1.0
Pyruvate uptake (mg · 100 g · min)	0.85 ± 0.01	0.85 ± 0.05	0.94 ± 0.02†	0.84 ± 0.06	0.87 ± 0.06	1.60 ± 0.05

*LAD, left anterior descending artery; LVEDP, left ventricular end-diastolic pressure; TCF, total coronary flow.

†$p < .005$.

‡$p < 0.05$.

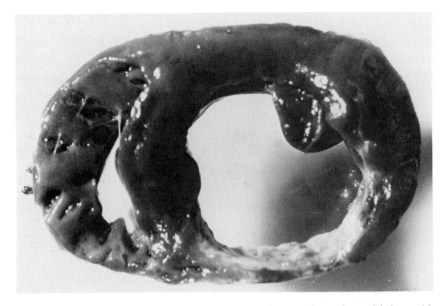

FIGURE 3-9 Cross-sectional view of the heart showing anterior and septal infarct with scarring and loss of muscle.

collagen. Study of the infarcts in both groups revealed no significant microscopic differences other than the observations seen grossly of smaller infarct size and less thinning of the myocardium in the animals receiving venous arterialization.

This study found that acute arterialization of the anterior descending vein prevents the same degree of hemodynamic and metabolic changes associated with ligation of the left anterior descending coronary artery, but long-term patency is in jeopardy of fibrosis and intimal proliferation and requires further clarification before clinical use.

The foregoing demonstration and other similar experiments for coronary artery bypass have provided the capacity to evaluate the metabolic benefit derived from various procedures. We have seen the multitude of data supporting the patency and flow of coronary artery bypass grafts. Scanning techniques follow this flow into the nutrient area of the myocardium, and metabolic evaluation provides further support for the acceptance of symptomatic and physiologic improvement as secondary to coronary artery bypass surgery. Knowing that coronary disease progresses, grafts occlude, and new disease occurs in the natural circulation makes the potential deterioration of patient status and ventricular function more easily understood. However, this cannot detract from the proof shown for justifying the use of coronary bypass to improve myocardial perfusion. As techniques improve, so will conduit patency, whether it be vein, internal thoracic

artery, or prosthesis. Until scanning techniques can differentiate perfusable muscle from scar, arteries over 1 mm in diameter will remain the minimal recipient, since unselected use of smaller arteries is associated with unacceptable occlusion rates. Given the relationship of resistance to diameters and lengths, a vein of reasonable size should be selected. The use of the internal thoracic artery appears appropriate for the left anterior descending coronary and its diagonal branches if certain criteria are met. The vessel should be 2 mm or greater in diameter, at least as large as the recipient, have free flow of 60 ml/min or more, and be free of occlusive disease in its origin. Immediate and urgent bypass may also preclude its use. The graft should be as short as feasible to provide greater diameter and decreased resistance. The most important aspect of its use and the largest factor in its occlusion is the absolute avoidance of any intimal injury at the time of surgery. The use of sequential grafts remains unclear, but the angle, direction, and size of anastomosis remain critical technical concerns. Y grafts continue to be acceptable when appropriate for vein length or available anastomotic sites. The graft length, avoiding pressure, kinking, or tension, continues to be of importance. Anastomoses at branches or at the site of an atherosclerotic plaque should be avoided, as lumen compromise or intimal damage and dissection will result.

The area of greatest potential is that of identifying arteries appropriate for grafting for both symptomatic

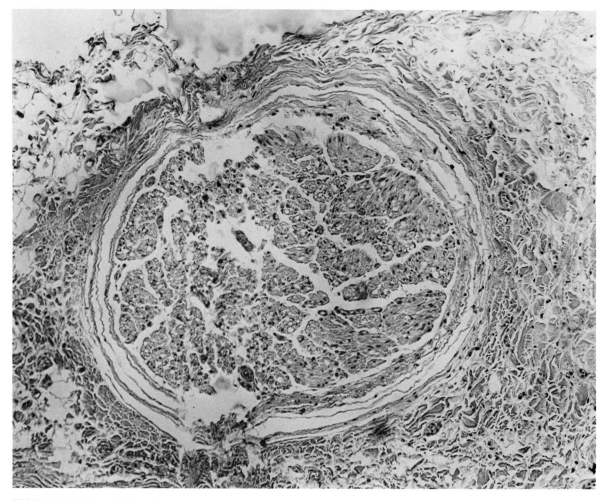

FIGURE 3-10 Internal thoracic artery–coronary artery anastomosis showing tissue occlusion.

relief and ventricular functional improvement, as well as selecting myocardial beds capable of handling sufficient flow and sustaining patency. Strides are being made in multiple scanning techniques coupled with cardiac stressing. When these areas are elucidated and when technical factors realized from the multitude of research and evaluation are put to maximal use, graft function and attrition rate will be limited only by the development of intimal proliferation and new atherosclerotic disease. Whether this will be affected by aspirin and other drugs currently under investigation is only conjecture. It is apparent, however, that all of these steps, used to their maximum, will have an effect on coronary artery disease that can only be exceeded by its prevention.

REFERENCES

1 McIntosh, H. D., Wright, K. E., and Wray, N. P.: Indications for Saphenous Vein Aortocoronary Bypass Surgery, in R. Paoletti and A. M. Giotto (eds.), "Atherosclerosis Reviews," Vol. 1, Raven Press, New York, 1976, p. 183.

2 McIntosh, H. D.: Benefit from Aortocoronary Bypass Graft. *J.A.M.A.,* 239:1197, 1978.

3. Guinn, G. A., and Matthews, V. S.: Surgical Versus Medical Treatment for Stable Angina Pectoris: Prospective Randomized Study with One to Four Year Follow-up, *Ann. Thorac. Surg.,* 22:524, 1976.

4 Spencer, F. C.: A Critique of Implantation of a Systemic Artery for Myocardial Revascularization, *Prog. Cardiovasc. Dis.,* 11:351, 1969.

5 Bjork, L., Cullhed, I., Hallen, A., and Strom, G.: Results of Internal Mammary Artery Implantation in Patients with Angina Pectoris, *Scand. J. Thorac. Cardiovasc. Surg.*, 2:1, 1968.

6 Gott, V. L., Brawley, R. K., Donahoo, J. S., and Griffith, L. S. C.: Current Surgical Approach to Ischemic Heart Disease, *Curr. Probl. Surg.*, May 1973.

7 Fergusson, D. J., Shirey, E. K., Sheldon, E. B., Effler, D. B., and Sones, F. M.: Left Internal Mammary Artery Implant—Postoperative Assessment, *Circulation*, 37:24, 1968.

8 Boloki, H., Thurer, R. J., Ghahramani, A., Vargas, A., Williams, W., and Kaiser, G.: Objective Assessment of Late Results of Aortocoronary Bypass Operation, *Surgery*, 76:925, 1974.

9 Wisoff, B. G., Aintablian, A., Hartstein, M. L., and Hamby, R. I.: Unified Diagnostic and Surgical Approach for Unstable Angina, *Ann. Thorac. Surg.*, 18:5, 1974.

10 Campeau, L., Lesperance, J., Corbara, F., Hermann, J., Grondin, C., and Bourassa, M. G.: Patency of Aortocoronary Saphenous Vein Bypass Grafts 5 to 7 Years After Surgery, *Can. J. Surg.*, 21:118, 1978.

11 Rimm, A. A., Blumlein, S., Barboriak, J. J., Anderson, A. J., Walker, J. A., and Johnson, W. D.: The Probability of Closure in Aortocoronary Vein Bypass Grafts, *J.A.M.A.*, 236:2637, 1976.

12 Barboriak, J. J., Batayias, G. E., Pintar, K., Tieu, T. M., VanHorn, D. L., and Korns, M. E.: Late Lesions in Aortocoronary Artery Vein Grafts, *J. Thorac. Cardiovasc. Surg.*, 73:596, 1977.

13 Jahnke, E. J., and Love, J. W.: Bypass of the Right and Circumflex Coronary Arteries with the Internal Mammary Artery, *J. Thorac. Cardiovasc. Surg.*, 71:58, 1976.

14 Kay, E. B., Naraghipour, H., Beg, R. A., DeManey, M., Tambe, A., and Zimmerman, H. A.: Internal Mammary Artery Bypass Graft—Long-term Patency Rate and Follow-up, *Ann. Thorac. Surg.*, 18:269, 1974.

15 Mark, A. L., Ahmad, N., Mudd, J. G., Dickens, J. F., and Barner, H. B.: Patency of Internal Mammary–Coronary Grafts, *Circulation*, 51,52 (suppl. 2):142, 1975.

16 Barner, H. B.: Value of Internal Mammary Artery Bypass, *Adv. Cardiol.*, 15:170, 1975.

17 Miller, D. W., Hessel, E. A., Winterscheid, L. C., Merendino, K. A., and Dillard, D. H.: Current Practice of Coronary Artery Bypass Surgery—Results of a National Survey, *J. Thorac. Cardiovasc. Surg.*, 73:75, 1977.

18 Florian, A., Lamberti, J. J., Cohn, L. H., and Collins, J. J.: Revascularization of the Right Coronary Artery by Retrograde Perfusion of the Mammary Artery, *J. Thorac. Cardiovasc. Surg.*, 70:19, 1975.

19 Chiu, C. J.: Why Do Radial Artery Grafts for Aortocoronary Bypass Fail? A Reappraisal, *Ann. Thorac. Surg.*, 22:520, 1976.

20 Grondin, C. M., and Limet, R.: Sequential Anastomoses

in Coronary Artery Grafting: Technical Aspects and Early and Late Angiographic Results, *Ann. Thorac. Surg.*, 23:1, 1977.

21 Grondin, C. M., Vouhe, P., Bourassa, M. G., Lesperance, J., Bouvier, M., and Campeau, L.: Optimal Patency Rates Obtained in Coronary Artery Grafting with Circular Vein Grafts, *J. Thorac. Cardiovasc. Surg.*, 75:161, 1978.

22 Cheanvechai, C., Groves, L. K., Surakiatchanukul, S., Tanaka, N., Effler, D. B., Shirey, E. K., and Sones, F. M.: Bridge Saphenous Vein Graft, *J. Thorac. Cardiovasc. Surg.*, 70:63, 1975.

23 Bigelow, J. C., Bartley, T. D., Page, U. S., and Krause, A. H.: Long-term Follow-up of Sequential Aortocoronary Venous Grafts, *Ann. Thorac. Surg.*, 22:507, 1976.

24 Loop, F. D.: Sequential Coronary Artery Anastomoses, *Ann. Thorac. Surg.*, 17:637, 1974. (Editorial.)

25 Hammond, G. L., and Poirier, R. A.: Early and Late Results in Direct Coronary Reconstruction Surgery for Angina, *J. Thorac. Cardiovasc. Surg.*, 65:1973.

26 Marco, J. D., Orszulak, T. L., Barner, H. B., and Kaiser, G. C.: In Favor of the Y-Graft for Aortocoronary Bypass, *Ann. Thorac. Surg.*, 21:519, 1976.

27 Griffith, L. S. C., Bulkley, B. H., Hutchins, G. M., and Brawley, R. K.: Occlusive Changes at the Coronary Artery-Bypass Graft Anastomosis, *J. Thorac. Cardiovasc. Surg.*, 73:668, 1977.

28 Hutchins, G. M., and Bulkley, B. H.: Mechanisms of Occlusion of Saphenous Vein–Coronary Artery "Jump" Grafts, *J. Thorac. Cardiovasc. Surg.*, 73:660, 1977.

29 Walters, M. B., and Aneke, C.: Graft Patency in Coronary Bypass Surgery, *Ann. Thorac. Surg.*, 26:228, 1978.

30 Blumlein, S. L., Anderson, A. J., Barboriak, J. J., Rimm, A. A., Walker, J., and Flemma, R.: Preoperative Risk Factors and Aortocoronary Bypass Graft Patency, *J. Thorac. Cardiovasc. Surg.*, 72:778, 1976.

31 Zajtchuk, R., Collins, G. J., Holley, P. W., Heydorn, W. H., Schuchmann, G. F., and Hamraker, W. R.: Coagulation Factors Influencing Thrombosis of Aorto-coronary Bypass Grafts, *J. Thorac. Cardiovasc. Surg.*, 73:309, 1977.

32 Urschel, H. C., Razzuk, M. A., and Gardner, M.: Coronary Artery Bypass Occlusion Secondary to Postcardiotomy Syndrome, *Ann. Thorac. Surg.*, 22:528, 1976.

33 Walker, J. A., Friedberg, H. D., Flemma, R. J., and Johnson, W. D.: Determinants of Angiographic Patency of Aorto-coronary Vein Bypass Grafts, *Circulation* 45,46(suppl. 1):86, 1972.

34 Lesperance, J., Bourassa, M. G., and Biron, P.: Aortocoronary Artery Saphenous Vein Grafts. Preoperative Angiographic Criteria for Successful Surgery, *Am. J. Cardiol.*, 30:459, 1972.

35 Macmanus, Q., and Okies, J. E.: Mediastinal Wound Infection and Aortocoronary Graft Patency, *Am. J. Surg.*, 132:558, 1976.

36 Laks, H., Kaiser, G. C., Barner, H. B., Codd, J. E., and Willman, V. L.: Coronary Revascularization Under Age 40 Years, *Am. J. Cardiol.*, 41:584, 1978.

37 Aintablian, A., Hamby, R. I., Weisz, D., Hoffman, I., Voleti, C., and Wisoff, B. G.: Results of Aortocoronary Bypass Grafting in Patients with Subendocardial Infarction: Late Follow-up, *Am. J. Cardiol.*, 42:183, 1978.

38 Furuse, A., Klopp, E. H., Brawley, R. K., and Gott, V. L.: Hemodynamics of Aortocoronary Artery Bypass, *Ann. Thorac. Surg.*, 14:282, 1972.

39 Kakos, G. S., Oldham, H. N., and Dixon, S. H.: Coronary Artery Hemodynamics After Aortocoronary Artery Vein Bypass, *J. Thorac. Cardiovasc. Surg.*, 63:849, 1972.

40 Greenfield, J. C., Rembert, J. C., and Young, W. G.: Studies of Blood Flow in Aortocoronary Venous Bypass Grafts in Man, *J. Clin. Invest.*, 51:2724, 1972.

41 VanderMark, F., Frank, H. L. L., and Buis, B.: Significance of Blood Flow Measurements in Implanted Aortocoronary Bypass Grafts, *Circulation,* 46 (suppl. 2):232, 1972.

42 Marco, J. D., Barner, H. B., Kaiser, G. C., Codd, J. E., Mudd, J. G., and Willman, V. L.: Operative Flow Measurements and Coronary Bypass Graft Patency, *J. Thorac. Cardiovasc. Surg.*, 71:545, 1976.

43 Urschel, H. C., Razzuk, M. A., Wood, R. E., and Paulson, D. L.: Factors Influencing Patency of Aortocoronary Saphenous Vein Grafts, *Surgery,* 72:1048, 1972.

44 Moran, J. M., Chen, Y., and Rheinlander, D. F.: Coronary Hemodynamics Following Aorto-coronary Bypass Graft, *Surgery,* 103:539, 1971.

45 Grondin, C. M., Lepage, G., Castonguay, Y. R., Meere, C., and Grondin, P.: Aortocoronary Bypass Graft: Initial Blood Flow Through the Graft and Early Postoperative Patency, *Circulation,* 44:817, 1971.

46 Danielson, G. K., Gau, G. T., and Davis, G. D.: Early Results of Vein Bypass for Coronary Artery Disease, *Mayo Clin. Proc.*, 48:487, 1973.

47 Barner, H. B., Kaminski, D. L., Codd, J. E., Kaiser, G. C., and Willman, V. L.: Hemodynamics of Autogenous Femoropopliteal Bypass Grafts, *Arch. Surg.*, 109:219, 1974.

48 Baird, R. J., Adiseshiah, M., and Okumori, M.: The Gradient in Regional Myocardial Tissue Pressure in the Left Ventricle During Diastole: Its Relationship to Regional Flow Distribution, *J. Surg. Res.*, 20:11, 1976.

49 Furuse, A., Klopp, E. H., Braiwoley, R. K., and Gott, V. L.: Hemodynamic Determinations in the Assessment of Distal Coronary Artery Disease, *J. Surg. Res.*, 19:25, 1975.

50 Folts, J. D., Kahn, D. R., Bittar, N., and Rowe, G. G.: Effects of Partial Obstruction on Phasic Flow in Aortocoronary Grafts, *Circulation,* 51,52(suppl. 1):148, 1975.

51 Bittar, N., Kroncke, G. M., Dacumos, G. C., Rowe, G. G., Young, W. P., Chopra, P. S., Folts, J. D., and Kahn, D. R.: Vein Graft Flow and Reactive Hyperemia in the Human Heart, *J. Thorac. Cardiovasc. Surg.*, 64:855, 1972.

52 Wakabayashi, A., Beron, E., Lou, M. A., Mino, J. Y., daCosta, I. A., and Connolly, J. E.: Physiological Basis for the Systemic-to-Coronary Artery Bypass Graft, *Arch. Surg.*, 100:17, 1970.

53 Green, G. E.: Rate of Blood Flow from the Internal Mammary Artery, *Surgery,* 70:809, 1971.

54 Klopp, E. H., Furuse, A., and Gott, V. L.: Normogram for the Determination of Blood Velocity in Aortocoronary Bypass Grafts, *Surg. Gynecol. Obstet.*, 135:795, 1972.

55 Grondin, C. M., Castonguay, Y. R., Lesperance, J., Bourasa, M. G., Campeau, L., and Grondin, P.: Attrition Rate of Aorta-to-Coronary Artery Saphenous Vein Grafts After One Year, *Ann. Thorac. Surg.*, 14:3, 1972.

56 Geha, A. S., Krone, R. J., McCormick, J. R., and Baue, A. E.: Selection of Coronary Bypass. Anatomic, Physiological and Angiographic Considerations of Vein and Mammary Artery Grafts, *J. Thorac. Cardiovasc. Surg.*, 70:414, 1975.

57 Geha, A. S., Baue, A. E., Krone, R. J., Kleiger, R. E., Oliver, G. C., McCormick, J. R., and Salimi, A.: Surgical Treatment of Unstable Angina by Saphenous Vein and Internal Mammary Artery Bypass Grafting, *J. Thorac. Cardiovasc. Surg.*, 71:348, 1976.

58 Barner, H. B., Barnhorst, D. A., Jellinek, M., Tara, A., and Mudd, J. G.: Ventricular Function Coronary Flow and Oxygen Consumption After Telescopic Internal Mammary–Coronary Anastomosis, *Surgery,* 65:127, 1969.

59 Vogel, J. H. K., McFadden, R. B., Spence, R., Jahnke, E. J., and Love, J. W.: Quantitative Assessment of Myocardial Performance and Graft Patency Following Coronary Bypass with the Internal Mammary Artery, *J. Thorac. Cardiovasc. Surg.*, 75:487, 1978.

60 Siegel, W., Loop, F. D., Proudfit, W. L., and Sheldon, W. C.: Comparison of Internal Mammary Artery and Saphenous Vein Grafts for Myocardial Revascularization by Exercise Testing, *Circulation,* 51,52 (suppl. 2):142, 1975.

61 Szilagyi, E., Whitcomb, J. G., Schenker, W., and Waibel, P.: The Laws of Fluid Flow and Arterial Grafting, *Surgery,* 47:55, 1960.

62 Jochem, W., Soto, B., Karp, R. B., Russell, R. O., Holt, J. H., and Barcia, A.: Radiographic Anatomy of the Coronary Collateral Circulation, *Am. J. Roentgenol.*, 116:50, 1972.

63 Valle, M., Wiljasalo, M., Frick, M. H., Korhola, O., Suoranta, A., and Tallroth, K.: Collateral Circulation Before and After Coronary Artery Reconstruction, *Ann. Clin. Res.*, 7:251, 1975.

64 Flaming, W., Schwarz, R., and Hehrlein, F. W.: Intraoperative Evaluation of the Functional Significance of Coronary Collateral Vessels in Patients with Coronary Artery Disease, *Am. J. Cardiol.*, 42:187, 1978.

65 Barner, H. B., Kaiser, G. C., Codd, J. E., and Willman, V. L.: Coronary Graft Flow and Glucose Tolerance: Evi-

dence Against the Existence of Myocardial Microvascular Disease, *Vasc. Surg.*, 9:220, 1975.

66 Tyras, D. H., Barner, H. B., Kaiser, G. C., Codd, J. E., Laks, H., and Willman, V. L.: Myocardial Revascularization in Women, *Ann. Thorac. Surg.*, 25:449, 1978.

67 Kakos, G. S., Oldham, H. N., Dixon, S. H., Davis, R. W., Hagen, P. O., and Sabiston, D. C.: Coronary Artery Hemodynamics After Aortocoronary Artery Vein Bypass, *J. Thorac. Cardiovasc. Surg.*, 63:849, 1972.

68 Kostuk, W. J., and Chamberlain, M. J.: Predictive Value of Myocardial Perfusion Imaging for Aortocoronary Bypass Surgery, *Can. J. Surg.*, 20:112, 1977.

69 Termini, B. A., Scherlis, L., Singleton, R. T., McLaughlin, J. J., and Cooper, M.: Myocardial Scanning in Patients Undergoing Coronary Bypass Surgery, *Arch. Surg.*, 109:648, 1974.

70 Lurie, A. J., Salel, A. F., Berman, D. S., DeNardo, G. L., Hurley, E. J., and Mason, D. T.: Determination of Improved Myocardial Perfusion After Aortocoronary Bypass Surgery by Exercise Rubidium-81 Scintigraphy, *Circulation*, 54(suppl. 3):20, 1976.

71 Ritchie, J. L., Narahara, K. A., Trobaugh, G. B., Williams, D. L., and Hamilton, G. W.: Thallium-201 Myocardial Imaging Before and After Coronary Revascularization, *Circulation*, 56:830, 1977.

72 Greenberg, B. W., Hart, R., Botvinick, E. H., Werner, J. A., Bundage, B. H., Shames, D. M., Chatterjee, K., and Parmley, W. W.: Thallium-201 Myocardial Perfusion Scintigraphy to Evaluate Patients After Coronary Bypass Surgery, *Am. J. Cardiol.*, 42:167, 1978.

73 Sbarbaro, J. A., Harischandra, K., and Cantez, S.: Thallium-201 Imaging in the Assessment of Coronary Artery Bypass Graft Patency, *Circulation*, 55,56 (suppl. 3):231, 1977.

74 Chatterjee, K., Swan, H. J. C., Parmley, W. W., Sustaita, H., Marcus, H. S., and Matloff, J.: Influence of Direct Myocardial Revascularization on Left Ventricular Asynergy and Function in Patients with Coronary Heart Disease With and Without Previous Myocardial Infarction, *Circulation*, 47:276, 1973.

75 Verani, M. S., Marcus, M. L., Spoto, G., Rossi, N. P., Ehrhardt, J. C., and Razzak, M. A.: Thallium-201 Myocardial Perfusion Scintigrams in the Evaluation of Aortocoronary Saphenous Bypass Surgery, *J. Nucl. Med.*, 19:765, 1978.

76 Cox, J. L, Pass, H. I., Oldham, H. N., Wechsler, A. S., and Sabiston, D. C.: Coronary Collateral Circulation During Stress and the Effects of Aortocoronary Bypass Grafts, *J. Thorac. Cardiovasc. Surg.*, 71:540, 1976.

77 Starr, I., and MacVaugh, H.: Early and Late Effects of the Coronary Bypass Operation on Cardiac Contractility and Coordination, *Am. Heart J.*, 90:179, 1975.

78 Nordstrom, L. A., Lillehei, J. P., Adicoff, A., Sako, Y., and Gobel, F. L.: Coronary Artery Surgery for Recurrent Ventricular Arrhythmias in Patients with Variant Angina, *Am. Heart J.*, 89:236, 1975.

79 Sonnenblick, E. H., Ross, J., and Braunwald, E.: Oxygen Consumption of the Heart: Newer Concepts of Its Multifactoral Determination, *Am. J. Cardiol.*, 22:328, 1968.

80 Anderson, R. P., and Bonchek, L. I.: Enhancement of Ventricular Performance by Pacing Induced Tachycardia: A Means of Assessing the Immediate Effect of Coronary Bypass Grafts, *J. Surg. Res.*, 14:490, 1973.

81 Santos, A. D., Benchimol, A., Desser, K. B., and Graves, C.: Effects of Coronary Artery Bypass Surgery on Hemodynamic Parameters and Derived Indices of Myocardial Function, *J. Thorac. Cardiovasc. Surg.*, 73:231, 1977.

82 Barner, H. B., Kaiser, G. C., Jellinek, M., Hahn, J. W., Amako, H., Ohtsubo, M., and Willman, V. L.: Aortocoronary Vein Graft and Internal Mammary–Coronary Anastomosis, *Arch. Surg.*, 105:908, 1972.

83 Park, S. B., Magovern, G. J., and Lieber, G. A.: Direct Selective Myocardial Revascularization by Internal Mammary Artery–Coronary Vein Anastomosis, *J. Thorac. Cardiovasc. Surg.*, 69:63, 1975.

84 Benedict, J. S., Buhl, T. L., and Henhey, R. P.: Cardiac Vein Myocardial Revascularization: An Experimental Study and Report of Three Clinical Cases, *Ann. Thorac. Surg.*, 20:550, 1975.

85 Benedict, J. S., Buhl, T. L., and Henhey, R. P.: Cardiac Vein Myocardial Revascularization of the Coronary Veins in Diffuse Coronary Arteriosclerosis, *J. Cardiovasc. Surg. (Torino)*, 16:520, 1975.

86 Moll, J. W., Dziatkowiak, A. J., and Edelman, M.: Arterialization of the Coronary Veins in Diffuse Coronary Arteriosclerosis, *J. Cardiovasc. Surg. (Torino)*, 16:520, 1975.

87 Marco, J. D., Hahn, J. W., Barner, H. B., Jellinek, M., Blair, O. M., Standeven, J. W., and Kaiser, G. C.: Coronary Venous Arterialization: Acute Hemodynamic Metabolic and Chronic Anatomical Observations, *Ann. Thorac. Surg.*, 23:449, 1977.

88 Jellinek, M., Barner, H. B., and Kaiser, G. C.: Continuous in Vivo Analysis Using a Mobile Autoanalyzer, in "Advances in Automated Analysis," Mediad, White Plains, N.Y., 1970, p. 171.

Chapter 4

The Improvement of Cardiac Performance by Coronary Bypass Surgery*

KENNETH M. KENT, M.D.

Myocardial contraction is exquisitely sensitive to ischemia. Detectable changes in the pattern of myocardial contraction occur within 10 s after coronary occlusion and precede changes in the endocardial or epicardial electrograms[1] (Fig. 4-1). This ischemia-induced reduction of myocardial contraction appears to be caused by an inhibition of the contractile process by ischemia rather than being the consequence of exhausted energy stores. A model of this inhibition has been proposed by Katz[2] in which hydrogen ions compete with calcium in the acidotic intracellular milieu resulting from ischemia. When perfusion is interrupted, myocardial anoxia leads to accelerated glycolysis, and intracellular pH falls because of the accumulation of lactic acid. The increase in hydrogen ion concentration results in the displacement by hydrogen ions of the calcium bound to troponin. Since the tropomyosin-troponin complex regulates tension development by actin-myosin interaction, this acidosis-induced decrease in the calcium tropomyosin-troponin interaction may be responsible for the abrupt cessation of contraction that occurs well before high-energy phosphate stores are depleted. The inhibition of contraction prior to the exhaustion of energy stores may serve as a protective mechanism by which the high energy requirements of the myocardial cell, the contraction process, are eliminated and energy consumption is reduced rather than exhausting the energy supply. Thus, although myocardial contraction decreases in the first few seconds after coronary occlusion, cell function and structural integrity are preserved for up to 20 to 30 min after temporary interruption of flow.[3] From a teleologic viewpoint, the inhibition of contraction soon after coronary occlusion may preserve the more fundamental aspects of myocardial cell integrity and prevent irreversible cell damage from occurring during transient ischemic episodes. A schematic presentation of the temporal events that follow experimental coronary occlusion are depicted in Fig. 4-2.

Since myocardial contraction abnormalities are common in patients with ischemic heart disease who are undergoing aortocoronary bypass operations, a number of studies have been performed in patients prior to and after coronary revascularization to determine if the restoration of blood flow to diseased myocardium improves the function of the heart. The purpose of this chapter is to review the findings of such studies and to describe the more recent studies of myocardial function in patients with coronary artery disease during periods of stress rather than only under basal conditions.

GLOBAL FUNCTION

Ejection fraction, the ratio of stroke volume to end-diastolic volume, is a commonly used index of global systolic function of the left ventricle. The ejection fraction can be calculated from the left ventricular cineangiogram in which left ventricular end-diastolic (EDV) and end-systolic volumes (ESV) are determined. The ratio EDV−ESV/EDV is the ejection fraction. Ejection fraction has been calculated for most of the groups of patients reviewed, and this index of systolic function will be used to characterize the effect of aortocoronary bypass on global ventricular function.

Initial expectations that coronary revascularization would improve myocardial function in patients with ischemic heart disease were supported by the early report of Saltiel et al., in which 23 patients with patent aortocoronary bypass grafts who were studied 2 to 3 weeks after operation demonstrated improved patterns of left ventricular contraction.[4] Ejection fractions were not measured; however, abnormalities of left ventricular motion were improved in two-thirds of the patients who had patent grafts. Another report on patients studied within the first few weeks after operation was that of Rees et al., in which 8 patients with patent grafts manifested an increased ejection fraction.[5] The ejection fraction of this group of patients was 61 percent preoperatively and increased to 72 percent postoperatively. Of course, the average preoperative ejection fraction was normal and the postoperative ejection fraction of 72 per cent was rather high. That this apparent enhancement of ventricular function could have been caused by an increase in the sympathetic tone in the early postoper-

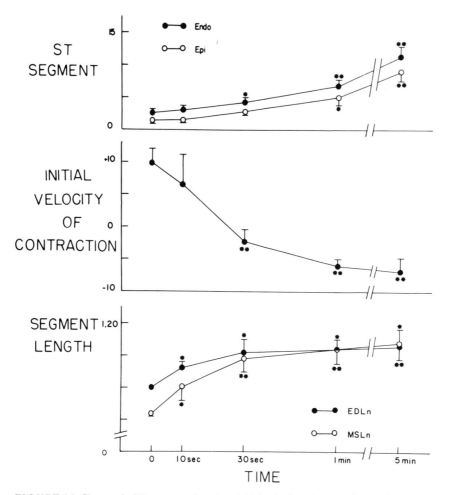

FIGURE 4-1 Changes in ST-segment elevation, initial velocity of contraction, and segment length. ST segments were recorded from endocardial (Endo) and epicardial (Epi) electrodes. Contractile function was measured with a pair of ultrasonic crystals sutured to the myocardium in the distribution of the left anterior descending coronary artery which provided segment length from which end-diastolic (EDLn) and mean systolic length (MSLn) were calculated. Velocity of shortening over the first one-third of systole (initial) was determined. Occlusion of the left anterior descending coronary artery at time 0 was accompanied by a significant lengthening of the segment at 10 s and a significant decrease in initial velocity of shortening at 30 s. At 30 s, only endocardial ST segments had significantly increased. *(Adapted from H. J. Smith, et al. Relationship Between Regional Contractile Function and ST-Segment Elevation After Experimental Coronary Artery Occlusion in the Dog, Cardiovasc. Res., 12:444, 1978, and reproduced by permission of Cardiovascular Research.)* (* p < .005, ** p < .01)

ative period was supported by the trend toward faster heart rates and larger cardiac outputs during the postoperative study. Chatterjee et al. reported two groups of patients that demonstrated enhanced postoperative left ventricular function within 2 weeks after operation.[6,7] The first group of six patients had preinfarction angina, and in all patients, ejection fraction increased following aortocoronary bypass.[6] In the second report by these authors, 19 of the patients who had abnormal ejection fraction preoperatively manifested a signifi-

cant improvement after operation from an initial value of approximately 45 percent to a normal postoperative value: 74 percent in those patients without previous myocardial infarction and 59 percent in those with previous myocardial infarction.[7] Many of the patients in whom ejection fraction increased were those with preinfarction angina. However, improvement of left ventricular function in the early postoperative period was found in the other patients with chronic stable angina. Thus the subgroup of patients with transient myocardial dysfunction resulting from ischemia were invariably improved after successful coronary revascularization, but improvement also occurred in patients with chronic ischemic heart disease. The extent to which the results of these three studies were affected by factors in the early postoperative period is unclear,[8,9] but subsequent studies in which global function was examined several months after aortocoronary bypass demonstrated no systematic improvement of global myocardial function after coronary revascularization. Young et al. reported 7 patients who were restudied several months following coronary revascularization.[10] Although there was no significant improvement of the ejection fraction in the group as a whole, 2 patients with subnormal preoperative ejection fractions did have an increased ejection fraction after operation. However, 4 patients with preoperatively normal ejection fractions manifested a decrease after operation. Arbogast et al. reported the results in 51 patients undergoing aortocoronary bypass procedures who were studied 1 year after operation.[11] The ejection fraction in the group as a whole was not changed after operation, nor was there any improvement in any of the subgroups, for example, those patients with patent vein grafts. Those patients who had occluded vein grafts, particularly in the distribution of the left anterior descending coronary artery, manifested a deterioration of systolic function. Hammermeister et al. examined 40 patients before and after aortocoronary bypass and found the ejection fraction was 53 ± 11 percent preoperatively and 50 ± 13 percent postoperatively.[12] No change in the ejection fraction was found in any of the subgroups, such as those patients with all grafts patent or those patients with subnormal preoperative systolic function. Similarly, She-

pard et al. studied 22 consecutive patients undergoing aortocoronary bypass 3 to 9 months previously and found no change in ejection fraction in those patients with all grafts patent, but there was a significant reduction of ejection fraction—59 percent to 49 percent—in the patients with one or more of the grafts occluded.[13] Chesebro et al. reported similar results in 52 patients in whom ejection fraction was unchanged by operation.[14] In contrast, there was no deterioration of function in the 22 of their patients who had one or more occluded grafts. Righetti et al., using a first pass radionuclide technique to measure ejection fraction, demonstrated no change in the ejection fraction in the early postoperative period (10 days or later) even in those patients who sustained a perioperative myocardial infarction.[15] Hemodynamic indexes of left ventricular function were unchanged after aortocoronary bypass even in the group of patients with all grafts patent.[16] Partridge et al. have more recently demonstrated a small but statistically significant increase in the ejection fraction from 44 percent to 53 percent in patients with patent grafts who had a subnormal ejection fraction preoperatively.[17] Similarly, Wolf et al. have demonstrated an increase in ejection fraction from 53 percent to 65 percent after aortocoronary bypass in patients who had preoperative myocardial dysfunction and who subsequently had all grafts patent.[18] These last two reports were published in 1978 and represent patients operated on more recently. The extent to which these two studies represent a trend that will develop over the next few years as the operative techniques improve is uncertain. Alternatively, selection factors may account for these differences, since all of these reports are based on a relatively few patients. In a group of 23 patients that we have recently studied

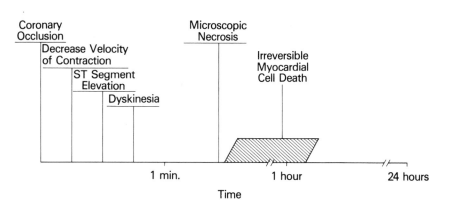

FIGURE 4-2 A schematic representation of the temporal events that follow coronary occlusion. The pattern of myocardial contraction changes within 10 s after coronary occlusion. Microscopic necrosis is noted if reperfusion occurs 20 to 30 min after coronary occlusion.[3] Irreversible myocardial damage occurs if occlusion is extended for longer periods of time, the exact duration being dependent on myocardial metabolic demands (i.e., temperature, workload, etc.) and collateral flow.

preoperatively and postoperatively,[19] there was no significant change in ejection fraction at rest in the group as a whole or in the subgroup of patients with subnormal preoperative ejection fraction.

The lack of a major effect of aortocoronary bypass on global left ventricular function was supported by the findings that coronary revascularization failed to improve chronic left ventricular decompensation in the initial studies by Spencer et al.[20] and Kouchoukos et al.[21] In the former study, 40 patients had signs and symptoms of congestive heart failure, mild to severe. Thirty-seven percent of the patients died either at operation or soon after discharge from the hospital. A good result was present in 8 of the 40 patients, and 13 other patients had some improvement. Kouchoukos et al. reported 9 patients with severe congestive heart failure; 3 patients died at operation and 4 died within 4 months after operation.[21] Neither of the 2 survivors were improved postoperatively. This excessively high operative mortality has been reduced by intraaortic balloon counterpulsation.[22] Thus, greater attention to myocardial preservation during operation and in the postoperative period may lead to more encouraging results of aortocoronary bypass procedures in patients with severely depressed myocardial function.

In summary, little or no improvement of global left ventricular function measured at rest has been observed after successful aortocoronary bypass grafting procedures. Occasionally, patients with preoperatively depressed left ventricular function who subsequently have patent grafts demonstrate some improvement of systolic function. However, the responses of such patients are not the general rule, and from the previously published results, one should not expect marked improvement of global left ventricular function after successful coronary revascularization. Since most patients undergoing aortocoronary bypass have normal global function at rest, improved global function postoperatively in such patients would be unlikely. Whether or not newer techniques of myocardial preservation during operation or in the postoperative period will result in more favorable results in patients with abnormal preoperative left ventricular function is unknown.

REGIONAL FUNCTION

Since occlusive coronary disease is segmental in nature, regional abnormalities of left ventricular contraction, *asynergy*, distal to obstruction of the coronary arteries are frequently seen in patients with coronary disease.[23] These regional wall motion abnormalities are characterized by reduced motion of the segment, *hypokinesis*; no motion, *akinesis*; or systolic expansion of the segment, *dyskinesis*. It is important to note that while regional abnormalities of left ventricular contraction are common in patients with coronary artery disease, the overall left ventricular function may remain normal despite the regional abnormalities. In a recent review of the contrast left ventricular cineangiograms in 100 patients with coronary artery disease at the National Institutes of Health, 67 percent manifested regional wall motion abnormalities, but the ejection fraction was normal in 64 percent of the patients. Since all patients with normal regional function had normal global function, 31 patients had some regional abnormality but manifested a normal ejection fraction (≥55 percent). The maintenance of global left ventricular function despite regional dysfunction probably is the result of enhanced contraction of the remaining undepressed segments. Furthermore, it is important to note that regional function measured at rest may be entirely normal, even in the distribution of coronary vessels with high-grade obstructions. Thus, in the group cited above, 33 patients had normal regional function despite the fact that all patients had significant occlusions of one or more coronary vessels.

Since it is unlikely that segments with normal function at rest would be improved by coronary revascularization, most of the reports demonstrating improved left ventricular function after aortocoronary bypass have focused on segments that were abnormal in the preoperative study. Bourassa et al. initially reported on 87 patients studied 1 year after aortocoronary bypass.[24] Of the preoperative abnormal segments that subsequently received a patent graft, 51 percent were improved postoperatively. However, if one excluded the more severe forms of asynergy and examined only hypokinetic segments, 70 percent were improved postoperatively and half of those segments were normal. Not unexpectedly, segments that were normal preoperatively were unchanged even when they received a patent graft, but 42 percent had abnormal function if the grafts were occluded. Griffith et al. found that one-third of the myocardial segments supplied by patent grafts were improved, one-third were unchanged, and one-third had diminished function postoperatively.[25] When supplied by occluded grafts, the function of myocardial segments was unchanged in half the patients and worse in the other half. Of note, these authors found that 38 percent of the segments supplied by a vessel that was not grafted had diminished function postoperatively. Jacob et al. demonstrated that the electrocardiogram could be used to further characterize those myocardial segments that were improved by coronary revascularization.[26] Seventy-seven percent of the hypokinetic segments in which there was no preoperative electrocardiographic evidence of infarction manifested improvement after aortocoronary bypass, with normal function being restored in most. In contrast, half of the preoperative hypokinetic segments with electrocardiographic evidence of infarction improved but only rarely normalized. No improvement was noted in those segments that were akinetic preoperatively almost all of which had electrocardiographic abnormalities.

Hammermeister et al. reported their experience in patients undergoing aortocoronary bypass[12] and found no change in wall motion in 63 percent of the patients, improvement in 15 percent, and deterioration in 22 percent. Shepard et al. examined the segments supplied by patent grafts and found that approximately half were unchanged, 21 percent had improved, and the remainder had deteriorated.[13] However, of the preoperative hypokinetic segments, 39 percent improved. Chesebro et al. utilized a quantitative videometric analysis of wall motion and demonstrated that 71 percent of preoperative hypokinetic segments that received patent grafts were improved postoperatively, and in about half of the improved segments, function normalized.[14] Of the myocardial segments that received a patent graft but did not normalize, half were associated with myocardial infarction during or after the surgery. The remainder of the segments that received a patent graft but did not normalize had a graft flow estimated at less than 60 ml/min. Furthermore, these investigators demonstrated a relation between the graft flow and the effect of coronary revascularization on myocardial function. The function of hypokinetic segments receiving grafts with a flow of less than 40 ml/min was unchanged postoperatively. When the graft flow was estimated at between 40 and 60 ml/min, half of the hypokinetic segments improved, and if the graft flow was greater than 60 ml/min, function of the previously hypokinetic segments invariably improved. The function of almost all the myocardial segments receiving occluded grafts deteriorated after the operation. No increase in segmental shortening occurred in preoperatively normal segments that received patent grafts, but two normal segments receiving grafts with flows <40 ml/min became hypokinetic.

Brower et al. have reported a technique for noninvasively assessing regional myocardial function in patients after aortocoronary bypass operations.[27] Radiopaque markers were sutured in the areas of the myocardium perfused by coronary arteries receiving grafts as well as control areas. In 56 patients, there was a progressive improvement in fractional shortening that occurred from 1 week to 6 months postoperatively in the segments receiving aortocoronary grafts.

DYNAMIC ASYNERGY

Wechsler et al. demonstrated that the beneficial effect of coronary revascularization on myocardial function may be evident only during conditions of metabolic stress induced by catecholamine stimulation.[28] In the basal state, myocardial function of experimental animal and human hearts receiving bypass grafts was independent of the patency of the grafts. However, during catecholamine administration, myocardial function deteriorated when the grafts were occluded and returned to augmented levels when the grafts were open. From these studies, it was evident that myocardial function distal to critical stenoses in human beings or to occluded arteries in experimental animals may remain normal under basal conditions when perfused through the limited antegrade and collateral flow channels. However, during increased oxygen and blood flow requirements of metabolic stress, myocardial function deteriorated when it exceeded the adequacy of perfusion. Restoring blood flow through aortocoronary bypass grafts ameliorated the stress-induced myocardial dysfunction.

A similar concept of stress-induced myocardial dysfunction has proved useful in evaluating patients with coronary artery disease by radionuclide cineangiography during supine bicycle exercise.[23-32] To study patients with this technique, human serum albumin labeled with 10 mCi of technetium (^{99m}Tc) is administered intravenously. After equilibration of the tracer in the blood pool, with the patient in the supine position, an Anger camera is positioned over the patient's chest in a modified left anterior oblique position to isolate the left ventricle from other cardiac structures. Electrocardiographic gating is used in the organization of acquired data by a computer into a series of images that span an average cardiac cycle. The data are then displayed in two formats. In the first, the images are displayed in rapid sequence as an endless-loop flicker-free movie, so that wall motion can be evaluated qualitatively. Function of the inferior and anterobasal walls, which are not border forming in this projection, is evaluated by examining a "difference image,"[31-33] which is created by subtraction of the end-systolic from the end-diastolic image. Global ventricular function is then assessed by determining the ejection fraction, which is calculated from the ratio of radioactive emissions (counts), after background correction, collected from the left ventricle in end-diastole (ED) minus end-systolic (ES) counts to end-diastolic (ED) counts, (ED−ES)/ED. Global and regional function are evaluated at rest, and then the patient begins to pedal a supine bicycle ergometer at increasing loads until the patient reaches the desired heart rate or until symptoms limit the exercise. Patients with coronary artery disease evaluated by this technique often have normal global function at rest. During exercise, however, global function almost invariably deteriorates.[19,31,32] The exercise-induced global dysfunction occurs even in those patients with coronary artery disease who remain asymptomatic during the test.[32] Furthermore, regional wall motion abnormalities develop during exercise in over 90 percent of the patients with coronary artery disease previously studied.[19,31,32] This technique documents the fact that the function of myocardium distal to coronary arterial obstructions may be normal when the patient is at rest but will become abnormal when myocardial oxygen and perfusion requirements are increased during exercise.

Radionuclide cineangiograms obtained during exercise have proved useful in evaluating patients after aortocoronary bypass,[19] and those results will be discussed in a subsequent section.

REVERSIBLE ASYNERGY

In contrast to normal function at rest that becomes abnormal during stress is *reversible asynergy* in which abnormal function of myocardial segments under basal conditions may improve after certain interventions.[34] Nitroglycerin, which reduces impedance to left ventricular outflow and augments collateral blood flow, enhances the contraction of some myocardial segments that, under basal conditions, are abnormal. Helfant et al. demonstrated that approximately three-fourths of hypokinetic areas improved following nitroglycerin administration, whereas only 57 percent of akinetic areas improved.[35] No dyskinetic areas improved. Similarly, nitroglycerin improved exercise-induced myocardial dysfunction.[32]

The increase in the contractile force of the heart that follows a premature ventricular contraction, *postextrasystolic potentiation,* also improves the systolic function not only of normal hearts but also of areas of the heart that manifest abnormal function in the basal state. Dyke et al. divided the heart into four axes in normal patients as well as in those with coronary artery disease.[36] Postextrasystolic potentiation enhanced segmental function in 51 of 55 axes with normal function and in 15 of 17 axes with abnormal function. In experimental myocardial infarction, postextrasystolic potentiation consistently augments myocardial contraction, whereas inotropic stimulation with calcium or isoproterenol fails to improve segmental function.[37] The ability of myocardial segments with abnormal function under basal conditions to improve with nitroglycerin and premature ventricular contractions denotes that such segments contain viable myocardium rather than scar tissue. Those segments containing potentially viable myocardium that manifest reversible asynergy would be likely to improve after successful aortocoronary bypass. Conversely, those segments in which function was unchanged by nitroglycerin or postextrasystolic potentiation probably consist mainly of scar tissue and would be unexpected to improve after coronary revascularization.

EFFECTS OF AORTOCORONARY BYPASS ON DYNAMIC ASYNERGY

Helfant et al. demonstrated that evaluation of reversible asynergy provides important prognostic information as to the fate of the regional function after aortocoronary bypass.[35] Ninety-three percent of the regions demonstrating reversible asynergy with nitroglycerin that subsequently received a patent graft had improved function under basal conditions postoperatively. Conversely, none of the segments that were unresponsive to nitroglycerin improved. Similarly, Popio et al. found that 69 percent of the regions in which reversible asynergy was demonstrated and that subsequently received a patent graft had improved postoperative function.[38]

More recently, we have studied the effect of aortocoronary bypass on exercise-induced left ventricular dysfunction in patients undergoing coronary revascularization at our institution.[19] Since the exercise-induced abnormalities of left ventricular function would be expected to respond to an augmentation in coronary blood flow after coronary artery revascularization, these abnormalities were examined to determine if the increased blood flow occurring in regions of myocardial revascularization[39] would be sufficient to maintain function during exercise. Using the technique of electrocardiographic-gated ^{99m}Tc blood pool scans, global and regional left ventricular function were evaluated in 23 consecutive patients undergoing coronary revascularization at rest and during exercise, both preoperatively and 2 to 6 months postoperatively, at the same level of exercise. Ejection fraction was calculated as described above. Regional function was semiquantitatively assessed by developing an index of regional wall dysfunction and assigning a score of 0 for normal function, 1 for hypokinesia, 2 for akinesia, and 3 for dyskinesia. Using this function score, the anteroseptal and anterobasal borders of the cardiac silhouette in the left anterior oblique projection were assessed. The inferior and anterobasal regions were evaluated by the difference image and assigned the score of 0 if normal or 1 if abnormal. Preoperatively the ejection fraction of the group was 51 at rest, which was in the range previously established for normal subjects. During exercise, however, ejection fraction was abnormal for all subjects in that it was lower than the previously established normal range and averaged 39 percent (Fig. 4-3). Analysis of the movie display of the radionuclide cineangiogram demonstrated that 13 of the 23 patients had normal regional function at rest, 5 patients had one region of hypokinesia, and the remainder had more severe regional dysfunction. However, during exercise, 21 of 23 patients had at least one new area of regional dysfunction that had appeared during exercise. The regional function index

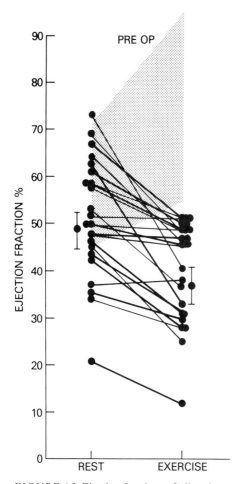

FIGURE 4-3 Ejection fractions of all patients at rest and during exercise prior to operation. The shaded area is the limit of ejection fraction measurements of a group of 25 normal subjects (⊢—•—⊣ denotes the mean and standard error of the mean).[32] The ejection fractions of the patients with coronary artery disease overlap the measurements of ejection fraction of normal subjects at rest, but there is a clear separation of the two groups during exercise. *(Reprinted by permission. From New England Journal of Medicine, 298:1434, 1978.)*

postoperatively. All 17 of these patients were symptomatically improved during exercise, with 12 being asymptomatic. Although 2 of the remaining 6 patients were asymptomatic after the operation, the ejection fraction was not increased during exercise in any of the 6. Five of these 6 patients in whom there was no increase in ejection fraction during exercise manifested new regional wall abnormalities at rest. Only one of these new regional rest wall abnormalities was in the distribution of an occluded graft, two were in the distribution of patent graft, and three were in the distribution of ungrafted vessels.

The salutary effect of aortocoronary bypass grafting on symptoms could be related to perioperative infarction of previously ischemic segments or neural deafferentation of the ischemic segments secondary to the operative procedure. However, the present study demonstrates that improved symptoms in most cases is related to a functionally important augmentation of coronary perfusion which is sufficient to sustain the increased metabolic demands of the myocardium during exercise. Most patients that we studied demonstrated improved myocardial function in segments that, prior to operation, had subnormal function during exercise. No significant effect on resting global or segmental function was observed after aortocoronary bypass grafting. This was anticipated, since preoper-

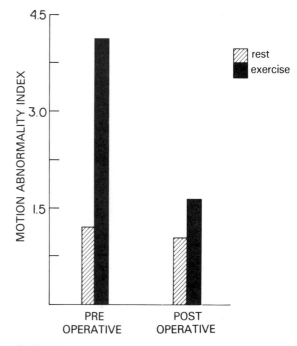

FIGURE 4-4 Wall motion abnormality index derived from the movie display of the radionuclide cineangiogram obtained at rest and during exercise, before and after operation for three regions of the left ventricle. The index increases with increasing degrees of asynergy. (0 = normal, 1 = hypokinesis, 2 = akinesis, 3 = dyskinesis.)

was 1.1 at rest and increased to 3.9 during exercise (Fig. 4-4). At the postoperative study 2 to 6 months after the operation, there was no significant change in the ejection fraction measured at rest (Fig. 4-5). The ejection fraction during exercise of the entire group of 23 patients increased from 38 to 53 percent postoperatively (Fig. 4-5). In addition, the regional function index during exercise decreased in all patients from 3.9 preoperatively to 1.6 postoperatively (Fig. 4-4). Seventeen of 23 patients demonstrated a marked improvement of the ejection fraction during exercise from 39 ± 3 percent preoperatively to 59 ± 4 percent

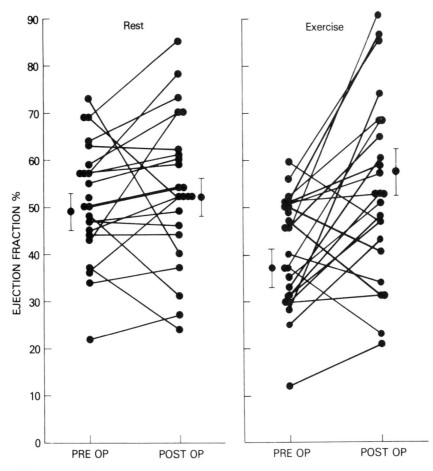

FIGURE 4-5 Ejection fraction prior to and after operation in 23 patients at rest and during exercise. Although no consistent improvement occurred in the ejection fraction measured at rest, the ejection fraction of 17 of the 23 patients was greater during exercise postoperatively. All 17 patients were improved symptomatically, with 12 being asymptomatic.

atively, 17 of the 23 patients had normal ejection fraction at rest and 56 of the 69 segments examined in the 23 patients (3 segments: anteroapical, lateral, and inferior) were normal at rest.

The previously cited studies using contrast ventriculography at rest demonstrated that normal segments cannot improve but can only get worse. The improvement of regional function in those studies occurred exclusively in segments with mild abnormalities. In the present study, since exercise-induced global dysfunction occurred in all patients, and since almost all patients had new regional wall motion abnormalities that developed during exercise, a salutary effect of revascularization on global and regional function was demonstrated in most of the patients. Those patients in whom myocardial function did not improve during exercise were usually those who had evidence of new myocardial damage present at rest. Presumably, these

abnormalities in rest function were the result of perioperative myocardial infarction or "silent" infarction occurring prior to the return of the patient for the postoperative studies. It is possible that newer techniques of cardiac preservation during revascularization and prior to unloading the heart on cardiopulmonary bypass will reduce the incidence of operative myocardial damage.

The sensitivity of myocardial function to ischemia should provide an index to evaluate the effectiveness of aortocoronary bypass in restoring physiologically important myocardial blood flow in patients with coronary artery disease. Uniform improvement of functional abnormalities occurring at rest does not occur after successful myocardial revascularization. In some subgroups of patients with mild resting abnormalities, improvement of function may occur. In addition, more sophisticated assessments of regional function may unmask improvement in rest abnormalities not noted by less sensitive techniques. However, the concept of *dynamic asynergy* has provided a new framework with which to examine this important aspect of aortocoronary bypass. Myocardial segments that are abnormal at rest but that contain potentially viable myocardium demonstrate improved function after nitroglycerin administration or postextrasystolic potentiation. The function of those segments that manifest reversible asynergy is usually improved after aortocoronary bypass. Similarly, myocardial segments having normal function at rest that develop stress-induced dysfunction are generally improved after aortocoronary bypass. Further advances in myocardial protection in the perioperative and operative periods will undoubtedly enhance the salutary effect of aortocoronary bypass on myocardial function.

REFERENCES

1 Smith, H. J., Kent, K. M., and Epstein, S. E.: Relationship Between Regional Contractile Function and S-T Segment Elevation After Experimental Coronary Artery Occlusion in the Dog, *Cardiovasc. Res.,* 12:444, 1978.

2 Katz, A. M., and Hecht, H. H.: The Early "Pump" Failure of the Ischemic Heart, *Am. J. Med.,* 47:497, 1969.

3 Jennings, R. B., Sommers, H. M., Smyth, G. A., Flack, H.A., and Linn, H.: Myocardial Necrosis Induced by Temporary Occlusion of a Coronary Artery in the Dog, *Arch. Pathol.,* 70:82, 1960.

4 Saltiel, J., Lesperance, J., Bourassa, M. G., Castonguay, Y., Campeau, I. and Grondin, P.: Reversibility of Left Ventricular Dysfunction Following Aortocoronary Bypass Grafts, *Am J. Roentgenol.,* 110:739, 1970.

5 Rees, G., Bristow, J. D., Kremkau, E. L., Green, G. S., Herr, R. H., Griswold, H. E., and Starr, A.: Influence of Aortocoronary Bypass Surgery on Left Ventricular Performance, *N. Engl. J. Med.,* 284:1116, 1971.

6 Chatterjee, K., Swan, H. J. C., Parmley, W. W., Sustaita, H., Marcus, H., and Matloff, J.: Depression of Left Ventricular Function Due to Acute Myocardial Ischemia and Its Reversal After Aortocoronary Saphenous-Vein Bypass, *N. Engl. J. Med.,* 286:1117, 1972.

7 Chatterjee, K., Swan, H. J. C., Parmley, W. W., Sustaita, H., Marcus, H. S., and Matloff, J.: Influence of Direct Myocardial Revascularization on Left Ventricular Asynergy and Function in Patients with Coronary Heart Disease, *Circulation,* 47:276, 1973.

8 Bourassa, M. G.: Left Ventricular Performance Following Direct Myocardial Revascularization, *Circulation,* 48:915, 1973. (Editorial.)

9 Apstein, C. S., Kline, S. A., Levin, D. C., Baltaxe, H. A., and Killip, T.: Left Ventricular Performance and Graft Patency After Coronary Artery–Saphenous Vein Bypass Surgery: Early and Late Follow-up, *Am. Heart J.,* 93:547, 1977.

10 Young, W. G., Sabiston, D. C., Jr., Ebert, P. A., Oldham, H. N., Behar, V. S., Kong, Y., Peter, R. H., and Morris, J. J., Jr.: Preoperative Assessment of Left Ventricular Function in Patients Selected for Direct Myocardial Revascularization, *Ann. Thorac. Surg.,* 11:395, 1971.

11 Arbogast, R., Solignac, A., and Bourassa, M. G.: Influence of Aortocoronary Saphenous Vein Bypass Surgery on Left Ventricular Volumes and Ejection Fraction, *Am. J. Med.,* 54:290, 1973.

12 Hammermeister, K. E., Kennedy, J. W., Hamilton, G. W., Stewart, D. K., Gould, K. L., Lipscomb, K., and Murray, J. A.: Aortocoronary Saphenous-Vein Bypass. *N. Engl. J. Med.,* 290:186, 1974.

13 Shepherd, R. L., Itscoitz, S. B., Glancy, D. L., Stinson, E. B., Reis, R. L., Olinger, G. N., Clark, C. C., and Epstein, S. E.: Deterioration of Myocardial Function Following Aorto-coronary Bypass Operation, *Circulation,* 49:467, 1974.

14 Chesebro, J. H., Ritman, E. L., Frye, R. L., Smith, H. C., Connolly, D. C., Rutherford, B. D., Davis, G. D., Danielson, G. K., Pluth, J. R., Barnhorst, D. A., and Wallace, R. B.: Videometric Analysis of Regional Left Ventricular Function Before and After Aortocoronary Artery Bypass Surgery, *J. Clin. Invest.,* 58:1339, 1976.

15 Righetti, A., Crawford, M. H., O'Rourke, R. A., Schlebert, H., Daily, P. O., and Ross, J., Jr.: Interventricular Septal Motion and Left Ventricular Function After Coronary Bypass Surgery, *Am. J. Cardiol.,* 39:372, 1977.

16 Santos, A. D., Benchimol, A., Desser, K. B., and Graves, C.: Effects of Coronary Artery Bypass Surgery on Hemodynamic Parameters and Derived Indices of Myocardial Function. *J. Thorac. Cardiovasc. Surg.,* 73:231, 1977.

17 Partridge, J. B., Brandt, P. W., and Whitlock, R. M. L.: The Underfilled Coronary Artery: Some Pre- and Postoperative Observations on Recipient Arterial Quality and Left Ventricular Function After Coronary Artery Surgery, *Clin. Radiol.,* 29:5, 1978.

18 Wolf, N. M., Kruelen, T. H., Bove, A. A., McDonough, M. T., Kessler, K. M., Strong, M., LeMole, G., and Spann J. F.: Left Ventricular Function Following Coronary Bypass Surgery, *Circulation,* 58:63, 1978.

19 Kent, K. M., Borer, J. S., Green, M. V., Bacharach, S. L., McIntosh, C. L., Conkle, D. M., and Epstein, S. E.:

Effects of Coronary-Artery Bypass on Global and Regional Left Ventricular Function During Exercise, *N. Engl. J. Med.*, 298:1434, 1978.

20 Spencer, F. C., Green, G. E., Tice, D. A., Wallsh, E., Mills, N. L., and Glassman, E.: Coronary Artery Bypass Grafts for Congestive Heart Failure, *J. Thorac. Cardiovasc. Surg.*, 62:529, 1971.

21 Kouchoukos, N. T., Doty, D. B., Buettner, L. E., and Kirklin, J. W.: Treatment of Postinfarction Cardiac Failure by Myocardial Excision and Revascularization, *Circulation* 45 (suppl. 1):I-72, 1972.

22 Feola, M., Wiener, L., Walinksy, P., Kasparian, H., Duca, P., Gottlieb, R., Brest, A., and Templeton, J.: Improved Survival After Coronary Bypass Surgery in Patients with Poor Left Ventricular Function: Role of Intraaortic Balloon Counterpulsation, *Am. J. Cardiol.*, 39:1021, 1977.

23 Herman, M. V., Heinle, R. A., Klein, M. D., and Gorlin, R.: Localized Disorders in Myocardial Contraction, *N. Engl. J. Med.*, 23:222, 1967.

24 Bourassa, M. G., Lesperance, J., Campeau, L., and Saltiel, J.: Fate of Left Ventricular Contraction Following Aortocoronary Venous Grafts, *Circulation,* 46:724, 1972.

25 Griffith, L. S. C., Achuff, S. C., Conti, C. R., Humphries, J. O., Brawley, R. K., Gott, V. L., and Ross, R. S.: Changes in Intrinsic Coronary Circulation and Segmental Ventricular Motion After Saphenous-vein Coronary Bypass Graft Surgery; *N. Engl. J. Med.*, 288:589, 1973.

26 Jacob, K., Chabot, M., Saltiel, J., and Campeau, L.: Improvement of Left Ventricular Asynergy Following Aortocoronary Bypass Surgery Related to Preoperative Electrocardiogram and Vectorcardiogram, *Am. Heart J.*, 86:438, 1973.

27 Brower, R. W., Katen, H. J., and Meester, G. T.: Direct Method for Determining Regional Myocardial Shortening After Bypass Surgery from Radiopaque Markers in Man, *Am. J. Cardiol.*, 41:1222, 1978.

28 Wechsler, A. S., Gill, C., Rosenfeldt, F., Oldham, H. N., and Sabiston, D. C., Jr.: Augmentation of Myocardial Contractility by Aorto-coronary Bypass Grafts in Patients and Experimental Animals, *J. Thorac. Cardiovasc. Surg.*, 64:861, 1972.

29 Green, M. V., Ostrow, H. G., Douglas, M. A., Myers, R. W., Scott, R. N., Bailey, J. J., and Johnston, G. S.: High Temporal Resolution ECG-gaged Scintigraphic Angiocardiography, *J. Nucl. Med.*, 16:95, 1975.

30 Bacharach, S. L., Green, M. V., Borer, J. S., Douglas, M. A., Ostrow, H. G., and Johnston, G. S.: A Real-time System for Multi-image Gated Cardiac Studies., *J. Nucl. Med.*, 18:79, 1977.

31 Borer, J. S., Bacharach, S. L., Green, M. V., Kent, K. M., Epstein, S. E., and Johnston, G. S.: Real-time Radionuclide Cineangiography in the Noninvasive Evaluation of Global and Regional Left Ventricular Function at Rest and During Exercise in Patients with Coronary-Artery Disease, *N. Engl. J. Med.*, 296:839, 1977.

32 Borer, J. S., Bacharach, S. L., Green, M. V., Kent, K. M., Johnston, G. S., and Epstein, S. E.: Effect of Nitroglycerin on Exercise-induced Abnormalities of Left Ventricular Regional Function and Ejection Fraction in Coronary Artery Disease, *Circulation,* 57:314, 1978.

33 Green, M. V., Bacharach, S. L., Douglas, M. A., Line, B. R., Ostrow, H. G., Redwood, D. R., Bailey, J. J., and Johnston, G. S.: The Measurement of Left Ventricular Function and the Detection of Wall Motion Abnormalities with High Temporal Resolution ECG-Gated Scintigraphic Angiocardiography, *IEEE Trans. Nucl. Sci.*, 23:1257, 1976.

34 Helfant, R. H., Bodenheimer, M. M., and Banka, V. S.: Asynergy in Coronary Heart Disease, *Ann. Intern. Med.*, 87:475, 1977.

35 Helfant, R. H., Pine, R., Meister, S. G., Feldman, M. S., Trout, R. G., and Banka, V. S.: Nitroglycerin to Unmask Reversible Asynergy: Correlation with Postcoronary Bypass Ventriculography, *Circulation,* 50:108, 1974.

36 Dyke, S. H., Cohn, P. F., Gorlin, R., and Sonnenblick, E. H.: Detection of Residual Myocardial Function in Coronary Artery Disease Using Post-extrasystolic Potentiation, *Circulation* 50:694, 1974.

37 Dyke, S. H., Urschel, C. W., Sonnenblick, E. H., Gorlin, R., and Cohn P. F.: Detection of Latent Function in Acutely Ischemic Myocardium in the Dog, *Circ. Res.*, 36:490, 1975.

38 Popio, K. A., Gorlin, R., Bechtel, D., and Levine, J. A.: Postextrasystolic Potentiation as a Predictor of Potential Myocardial Viability: Preoperative Analyses Compared with Studies After Coronary Bypass Surgery,. *Am. J. Cardiol.*, 39:944, 1977.

39 Lurie, A. J., Salel, A. F., Berman, D. S., DeNardo, G. L., Hurley, E. J., and Mason, D. T.: Determination of Improved Myocardial Perfusion After Aortocoronary Bypass Surgery by Exercise Rubidium-81 Scintigraphy, *Circulation,* 54(suppl. 3):20, 1976.

Chapter 5

The Improvement of Hemodynamic Abnormalities by Coronary Bypass Surgery*

GEORGE G. ROWE, M.D.

Much of the current popularity of aortocoronary by-pass surgery is based upon angiographic evidence that symptomatic coronary disease is primarily a mechanical problem of vascular obstruction that can be bypassed successfully. This concept and the procedure have grown progressively as an extension of a long history of surgical successes in relieving the occlusion of various biologic conduits, including blood vessels, to many other areas of the body. We have divided the subject into four parts. First, we consider the anatomic and hemodynamic abnormalities that are created by coronary disease. Second, we discuss which of these functional abnormalities should be treatable by surgery. Third, we examine the evidence that the theoretical objectives of treatment can be achieved. Finally, it is important to point out what cannot be done by reconstructive surgery.

ABNORMALITIES PRODUCED BY CORONARY DISEASE

Pathologic Anatomy

Careful pathologic studies of the hearts of many who have died from symptomatic coronary disease reveal a truly surprising degree of coronary obstruction,[1-4] and similar changes may be found in those who have died suddenly without cardiovascular symptoms.[5] Indeed, it is reported that postmortem examination of the coronary arteries cannot differentiate those who have had myocardial infarction from those who have had angina or from those who have died suddenly apparently without symptoms.[3] Nor can the vascular lesions found at autopsy be used successfully to separate the hearts of those who have had unstable, moderate, or severe angina.[6,7] The degree of coronary destruction seen in some pathologic specimens is difficult to believe, and yet the myocardium may be very well preserved.

Arteriographic Anatomy

The advent of coronary arteriography[8] and its progressive improvement has now made it possible to study the coronary anatomy of the living. It comes as no surprise that the extent and the severity of coronary artery disease found in the living is comparable to that which has been documented in the dead. And, again, in looking at the coronary arteriogram, it is not possible to guess the clinical picture. Indeed, in many individuals who have just recognized the onset of angina pectoris, very severe and extensive three-vessel obstructive coronary disease is found. Furthermore, among those who are considered to have a preinfarction state with such severe chest pain that they are confined to intensive care units and receiving continual treatment for myocardial ischemia, a significant number are found to have normal coronary arteries, normal left ventricular contraction, and no hemodynamic evidence of ischemia.[9,10] Similarly, among asymptomatic individuals with positive exercise test results, either normal coronary arteries or very extensive and severe coronary disease may be found.[11] Yet the extent and severity of coronary disease found by arteriography and the status of the myocardium revealed by left ventriculography are directly related to prognosis, and life expectancy is directly dependent upon the severity of the abnormalities found.[12-15] These data are admirably reviewed by Wilson.[16] It is therefore apparent that serious studies of coronary artery disease need an anatomic base of reference.

Coronary Collaterals

Over the years, observations by many methods have shown that reduction in flow through obstructed arteries is related directly, but not linearly, to the severity of obstruction.[17] However, the blood supply to the myocardium is not as simple as the usual situations that have been studied by objective methods because of intercoronary arterial connections or collaterals. Although there has been considerable debate, as summarized recently,[18-20] it seems clear that the reason for survival of the left ventricle in the presence of severe coronary arterial obstruction in animals[20-24]

*From Department of Medicine, University of Wisconsin Medical School, Madison.

and in human beings[19] is the presence of extensive interarterial collateral networks through the myocardium. These collateral pathways are present in the normal heart[25] but rapidly undergo additional development when coronary occlusion occurs as evidenced by postmortem examination,[1,5,26] by detailed anatomic study showing the proliferation of cells in the collateral vessel walls as they undergo hypertrophy,[24] by radiographic demonstration of their steadily increasing visibility,[19,27] by physiologic data revealing improved distal arterial pressure in occluded arteries as collateral develops,[28,29] and by hemodynamic observations confirming improved peripheral distribution of radionuclides in the myocardium distal to complete arterial obstructions.[30,31]

Coronary Blood Flow

Despite the extensive collateral network and the data indicating that total coronary flow tends to be within the normal range when measured directly in the coronary sinus[32] in patients subject to angina or indirectly by the inert gas method,[33-45] some have found resting coronary blood flow to be somewhat reduced in patients who develop angina on exertion.[46] Most investigators believe that the capacity to increase coronary flow is limited and fails to increase further in response to pacing when angina occurs[47,48] or when angina occurs with the hand grip test.[49] It has now been established directly at operation by clearance of locally injected radioactive materials[50] and by many other methods that there are localized areas in the myocardium of patients with coronary disease that have clearly reduced coronary flow[51-62] and that during angina the measured deficit in flow is greater.[60] Reduced perfusion has been demonstrated by direct injection of radioactive xenon through the coronary bypass grafts and thence into the myocardium at operation, utilizing the washout curve as an index of coronary flow.[51] It has also been done by following the washout of radioactive materials injected through the coronary artery and followed by multiple scintillation crystals which form a grid over the heart and describe multiple simultaneous washout curves.[52,54,55,59] These data can then be ingeniously superimposed on a coronary arteriographic image so that areas of reduced flow can be correlated with areas of vascular obstruction.[52,54,55,59] Similarly, the distribution of ^{201}Tl can be used as an index of myocardial perfusion and the heterogeneity of myocardial flow revealed.[58] All of these results can be supported by the inequality of the rate of flow of contrast material down adjacent branches of the same coronary artery when some are severely obstructed and others are not. When all of these lines of evidence are considered, irregular myocardial perfusion no longer seems to be contestable. It is not clear, however, that the areas of reduced flow supply normal, viable cardiac muscle rather than areas of mixed myocardium and fibrous scar. Indeed, it seems unlikely that normal myocardial cells will long endure flow inadequate to sustain them in their resting state.[45] Some have concluded after extensive study of the problem that coronary flow per unit of normally functioning myocardium is actually increased as coronary disease advances because the remaining normal muscle cells are required to do not only their own share of the cardiac work but also that which cannot be done by ineffective or dead muscle cells in the more ischemic areas.[63] Furthermore, cardiac dilatation occurs in the presence of severe ischemia,[64] increasing the volume of the left ventricle and stretching the myocardial fibers, thereby increasing their oxygen requirement and reducing their mechanical advantage during contraction. This thesis is supported by data which demonstrate that in the early phase after myocardial revascularization (2 weeks to 6 months) and while the hemoglobin is still reduced (14.5 to 11.7), coronary sinus blood flow tends to be slower at rest and is significantly reduced at the patient's maximum pacing rate,[65] even though postoperatively the pacing rate was more rapid and did not produce angina. Left ventricular function improved postoperatively as judged by better wall motion and a higher ejection fraction and the ventricles extracted rather than produced lactate as they had preoperatively. In spite of the lower hemoglobin, the coronary sinus blood oxygen content increased.[65] The simplest explanation seems to be that better distribution of flow in the myocardium improved the performance of ischemic segments, thus improving overall cardiac efficiency so that less total blood flow and oxygen consumption was required. It may well be that the "intermediate coronary syndrome" occurs when a significant number of myocardial fibers are in the process of being converted individually from myocardium into fibrous tissue because blood flow is inadequate to support the myocardium at rest in a localized area; at least presently available data support such a concept without actually proving it.

Distal Coronary Blood Pressure and Flow Distribution

It has been demonstrated that the pressure in the coronary arterial bed distal to the proximal obstruction can be very seriously reduced.[51,66-72] This distal coronary pressure is somewhat improved by collaterals.[67,71] These data must mean that significant portions of the myocardium in individuals with coronary artery disease are perfused by reduced arterial pressure even at rest. Furthermore, when collateral vessels arise from the distal end of a partially obstructed coronary artery and supply the terminal end of a completely obstructed artery, the hemodynamic basis exists for coronary steal to occur.[73-75] Under these circumstances, flow through the collateral to the distal end of the completely obstructed artery depends very heavily, if not totally, on the perfusion pressure at the origin of the collateral. If the proximal partial stenosis is severe enough to limit flow, vasodilatation will decrease the distal coronary arterial pressure and flow through collaterals will decrease.[76-78] Thus, administration of therapeutic vasodilators[79] or even coronary autoregulation itself occurring during exercise or increased cardiac rate may be detrimental to the bed perfused through the collateral, and anything that lowers distal coronary arterial blood pressure may precipitate ischemia.

The same problem must be recognized to exist between the epicardium and the endocardium. Normally during the systolic compression of the perforating branches of the coronary arteries, blood flow to the subendocardial tissue is interrupted temporarily, but during diastole, flow increases and the transient deficit is made up. When there is critical epicardial arterial constriction, however, the vasodilatory capacity of the subendocardial tissue may be exhausted first while the epicardial vessels continue to have some vasomotor tone.[80] Under these circumstances, vasodilators increase epicardial flow and decrease endocardial flow, producing in effect localized and layered ''coronary steal,''[76-78,80] which could critically reduce subendocardial flow and precipitate subendocardial infarction while the relatively less jeopardized epicardium remains viable. Although the preceding data have been accumulated in dogs, there is a very strong possibility that they apply to human beings as well, and this could explain the high incidence of subendocardial myocardial infarction in those with coronary artery disease. It could also explain why subendocardial infarction may be regarded as an incomplete lesion that is at high risk of extending and becoming a transmural infarct.[81]

Evidence of Myocardial Ischemia

It is widely accepted that the most important phenomenon produced by coronary artery obstruction is myocardial ischemia. This has been demonstrated directly at operation by using a mass spectrometer that revealed a decrease in the P_{O_2} and an increase in P_{CO_2} in the myocardium distal to the coronary arterial obstruction.[82] Metabolic study of arterial and coronary sinus blood specimens has confirmed that anaerobic myocardial metabolism takes place with localized production of lactate[83-87] and acute reduction in P_{O_2} of blood draining from the ischemic section of the heart.[87] It has been known since the classic experiments by Tennant and Wiggers[64] that myocardial ischemia leads

very quickly to reduced contractility in the ischemic segment, and this has readily been confirmed in human beings on a daily basis in clinical cardiovascular catheterization laboratories. As a result of myocardial ischemia the systolic early relaxation phenomenon is identified in which a portion of the ventricle appears to be unable to sustain systolic contraction for as long as the surrounding tissue. This results in early relaxation with sudden interruption of the uniform pattern of contraction along the wall of the ventricle.[88,89] Sometimes, ischemic segments delay in contraction and do not reach their full systolic shortening until after their radius of curvature has been reduced by contraction of the rest of the ventricle. More severe ischemia can result in complete failure to contract or actual localized bulging of the myocardium.[90-113] Left ventricular ischemia, either acute or chronic, is frequently associated with increased left ventricular end-diastolic pressure.[86,90,93,96,97,99,103,109,114-119] This hallmark of inadequacy of left ventricular function can frequently be precipitated by increasing left ventricular work through exercise,[99,105,111] increased blood pressure,[120] or cardiac pacing.[105,115] Left ventricular end-diastolic pressure is also elevated in left ventricular failure for any other reason, as well as in patients with left ventricular aneurysm. The capacity to increase cardiac output in response to exercise is also limited in patients with coronary artery disease.[121]

End Results of Ischemia

As ischemia becomes more severe, cardiac muscle fibers are replaced by connective tissue, with ensuing myocardial fibrosis.[113] It is presumed that if the process occurs more acutely and widely, large sections of muscle are destroyed at once, and the clinical state known as myocardial infarction occurs. With myocardial infarction, there follows a series of events that may lead to mitral valvular insufficiency. Several important factors are believed to be involved in this process, including valve ring dilatation, malposition, malfunction, stretching, and/or rupture of the papillochordal structures.[122] Animal studies have shown that destruction of the left ventricular wall at the site of papillary muscle insertion is important in producing mitral insufficiency through papillochordal dysfunction.[123] This pattern of wall and papillary muscle change occurs frequently in human beings. Since the valve ring contracts vigorously in systole,[124,125] dilatation or failure of adequate contraction of the mitral valve ring may also contribute to mitral insufficiency.[122] In addition, since the left atrial endocardium is continuous with the mitral valve, with progressive left atrial enlargement, sliding of the endocardium over the valve ring may produce tension on the posterior cusp of the mitral valve and progressively greater insufficiency, and thus "mitral insufficiency begets mitral insufficiency."[126] If the process of myocardial destruction is hyperacute and exceeds the rate of repair, dissolution in the continuity of the myocardial fibers may occur, with rupture of the heart into the pericardium or with internal rupture of the ventricular septum or of the papillary muscles.

THEORETICAL, SURGICAL, THERAPEUTIC POSSIBILITIES

Having described briefly the events which follow progressive occlusion of the coronary arteries, it is reasonable to consider which of the abnormalities should be treatable by surgery. Obstructions in the coronary arteries are frequently located proximally.[127] Since the major coronary arteries are usually of sufficient size, a skilled surgeon can produce an anastomosis from the aorta or internal thoracic artery to the distal part of the coronary vessel and bypass coronary arterial obstruction. Even secondary branches are frequently large enough to permit bypass of more distal disease. It has now been confirmed many times that this can usually be done, and although uniform patency of such bypasses has not as yet been achieved, and no doubt never will be, as the technical problems are solved, the frequency of graft patency continues to rise. Since the coronary obstructions can be bypassed, it seems reasonable to believe that the areas of myocardial ischemia can be relieved.[128] Clearly, for the best results, this should be done before the myocardial ischemia has been so severe and prolonged that permanent damage is done to the myocardium or the papillochordal structures.[128] When actual myocardial destruction has taken place, surgical resection of aneurysms and scars must usually sacrifice further cardiac tissue, since infarction is seldom complete and since some viable cells are present in most areas of the heart that are resected.[26,30] Those muscle cells trapped in the center of a scar or aneurysm may be removed, and those at the periphery of a scarred area that is resected are almost invariably damaged where normal tissue must be rejoined by sutures.

EVIDENCE THAT THEORETICAL, SURGICAL POSSIBILITIES CAN BE ACHIEVED

Increased Coronary Blood Flow

Many of the hemodynamic studies that yielded discouraging results as to what could be achieved hemodynamically by revascularization were done early, when surgical technique was less adequate than today, in patients with chronic stable angina who presumably had minimal or no resting ischemia, and in those who had residuals of myocardial infarction that could not reasonably be expected to change. Many of these studies were also done before it was widely accepted that nitrates,[129-135] postextrasystolic potentiation,[108,136] and epinephrine[137] could at least partially differentiate ischemic dysfunction from permanent destruction. It seems likely that much of the discouragement that resulted from these early studies was based on the unrealistic expectation that improvement could take place in tissue that was no longer ischemic at rest and that was not known then to be irreversibly damaged and fibrotic. Consequently, the literature on the hemodynamic results of coronary bypass is widely scattered and reports of good and bad results abound. Postoperative evidence of decreased functional capacity, reduced contraction, or impaired blood flow at rest is clearly a bad result, and there are many such failures. A "bad result" may occur in only one area of the heart, while other areas have a good result, in which case the situation must be regarded as mixed. No change in function at rest is still compatible with a good result, since what happens under duress is crucial. Finally, clear improvement at rest is a good result and is usually achieved only in the face of ischemia so severe that abnormality of function was demonstrated at rest. A good result has far more theoretical significance than a bad result, because it provides proof that improvement is achievable and hope that the frequency of good results can be increased when the proper solution is found. Examined in this light, there is a great deal of evidence that many of the theoretical objectives of coronary revascularization can be achieved.

It is routine during myocardial revascularization surgery, after cardiopulmonary bypass is terminated and when the circulation is stable, to measure the flow through coronary bypass grafts. The total flow measured through these grafts is very impressive when large arteries with severe proximal obstruction are bypassed and progressively less impressive if smaller, more distal vessels are bypassed.[16,51,66,67,69,70,128] But there can be no doubt that if the anastomoses are well constructed, blood may flow rapidly through a reversed saphenous vein graft into the distal coronary artery to which it is attached. The flow through grafts is related directly to the size of the lumen of the graft and inversely to the size of the artery.[138] Graft flow increases directly with increasing severity of the proximal coronary arterial stenosis.[138,139] Furthermore, if two grafts go to adjacent coronary arteries, flow has been shown to increase somewhat through one graft when the other is temporarily obstructed, and to decrease when both grafts are open.[66,140] This could mean that flow can go either way through intercoronary collaterals, but pressure measurement in the distal end of an occluded vessel has shown that when an adjacent graft is opened, the rise in pressure transmitted through collateral from the opened graft is inadequate, and thus all major obstructed vessels need to be grafted.[69]

Increased Distal Coronary Blood Pressure

It is known in experimental animals that pressure in the superficial coronary arteries is almost the same as it is in the aorta. Catheterization of human coronary arteries has confirmed repeatedly that this is also true in human beings. In the presence of obstructed proximal coronary arteries, the distal vessels are less accessible, and the reduced pressure recorded beyond a coronary obstruction when a retrograde aortic catheter measures distal intracoronary pressure directly is vitiated by the obstruction that the catheter produces as it passes through the partially obstructing lesion. But at operation, accurate pressures may be obtained directly through inserting a cannula into the distal obstructed artery at the site where a bypass graft is to be attached. It has been shown by this technique that the pressure gradient at the coronary lesion is related directly to the degree of stenosis.[67,68] Furthermore, when collected directly at operation, the flow of blood from the proximal end of the artery through the stenosis is inversely related to the severity of the obstruction.[67,68] Conversely, flow from the distal end of an obstructed artery (retrograde flow) tends to be greater as the severity of the proximal stenosis increases, suggesting that more severe proximal stenosis is associated with more distal collateral development.[67] As might be expected in subjects with preinfarction angina, the distal coronary pressure and the antegrade and retrograde flow are less than in others with angina.[68] This suggests that in the "preinfarction state" the proximal stenosis is more severe, the distal collaterals are less adequate, and the degree of ischemia is more pronounced.

Many have taken a more circuitous approach to the problem that has provided similar but more plentiful results. Thus, pressure is found to be essentially the same as that in the aorta when it is measured in a graft after it is attached from the aorta to the coronary artery and while blood is flowing into the distal artery. However, when the proximal end of the graft is clamped and flow is stopped, pressure in the distal end of the graft reflects that in the coronary artery to which it is attached. This distal coronary pressure is frequently low and is inversely related to the severity of coronary stenosis.[66-72,139] Opening of an aortocoronary artery graft, then, can return the distal coronary artery pressure and flow to the level that was present before coronary artery obstruction developed.

Intraoperative Coronary Flow Distribution and Response to Vasoactive Drugs

The restitution of normal distal coronary pressure and flow would be of limited interest if there were no evidence that additional nutrient blood flow is provided. So let us examine the evidence that this does occur. It has been concluded that blood flow through the bypass grafts supplies actively contracting myocardium, because the same pattern of phasic flow is recorded in the graft as is recorded in a normal coronary artery supplying the actively contracting left ventricle.[69,140-145] This pattern consists of a sudden reduction in flow during systole and a marked increase in flow during diastole and is attributed to the compression of the coronary arterial perforating branches as they pass from the surface of the myocardium through the wall to the endocardium. This pattern of flow does not occur in arteries that supply other tissues in the body, although similar interruption of flow may occur during forceable contraction of skeletal muscle. Furthermore, it is confirmed that the blood nourishes actively contracting myocardium, because when the graft is clamped for 10 to 30 s and then released, a prolonged and pronounced increase in coronary flow frequently occurs as the blood passes through the graft to repay the oxygen and nutrient debt acquired and to wash away the metabolites that accumulated in the contracting myocardium while the graft was clamped.[70,144-151] This reproduces the classical hyperemic response recorded after clamping the coronary arteries of normal animals.[152] It is no surprise that the hyperemic response does not occur on all occasions and in all grafts, since the blood flow available through the proximal stenosis and the distal collateral bed may be adequate for the resting myocardium, and it may not become sufficiently ischemic when the graft is clamped at rest to produce a typical response.[144-147,151] Nevertheless, the response is seen often and can be sufficiently dramatic as to leave little doubt that actively metabolizing myocardium is supplied through the vein graft. If reactive hyperemia does not occur, it is still possible, indeed likely, that it will occur if the graft is clamped while compressing and obstructing the proximal end of the coronary artery to which it is attached.[147] Not only do these data confirm that active myocardium is supplied by the graft, but they also show that when added flow is required, it is available. The reactive hyperemic response predicts long-range patency of aortocoronary bypass grafts, with good hyperemic response increasing the chances the graft will remain open.[150,151,153] This constitutes a clear extension of the widely accepted observation that long-range graft patency is related to total graft flow.[66,128,144,150,154-156] Furthermore, a good phasic pattern of graft flow predicts long-term graft patency,[153] since phasic flow can demonstrate the presence of a partial obstruction which limits the normal high diastolic flow rate.[141] In addition, the graft flow response at operation was measured in the fibrillating, the nonfibrillating, the resting, and the working heart.[142] As compared to the stable working heart, graft flow to the nonworking heart in sinus rhythm was reduced to 50 percent. Fibrillation in the nonworking heart increased flow by 33 percent above that during sinus rhythm, but there was still significantly less flow than in the working heart.[142] These results are just as would be expected to occur, supporting the idea that normal hemodynamics is restored.

It is also reassuring to observe that vasoactive drugs produce the expected response when injected through vein grafts into the coronary circulation, implying that the supplied vascular bed responds normally to pharmacologic agents. Thus, it has been demonstrated that when nitroglycerin is injected into a bypass graft at operation, coronary flow increases,[70,145,149] as would be expected. Similarly, increases occur with papaverine,[66,144,149,150,156] Isuprel,[145,157,158] epinephrine,[157] and phenylephrine.[157] Inhalation of amyl nitrate produced increased velocity of flow, as measured by a Doppler flowmeter,[143,160] and norepinephrine given into a graft reduced coronary flow,[145] as does administration of propranolol.[142]

When radioactive materials are injected into a vein graft intraoperatively, it can be demonstrated that they are distributed into the peripheral portion of the myocardium to which the grafted artery goes[51] and may extend into adjacent areas of myocardium as well, apparently through collaterals.[161] The estimated mass of myocardium supplied by the graft is variable but may be very large.[161,162] Furthermore, if an injection of radioactive tracer is made into an area of myocardium supplied by an aortocoronary graft and the rate of its clearance determined while the graft is clamped, graft release is followed by a sudden and clear increase in the rate of clearance of tracer.[51] This may be equated with an increase in nutrient blood flow provided by the graft.

Postoperative Coronary Flow

It could be argued that the bulk of the hemodynamic data presented so far has been collected in the operating room from the open chest human subject and bears little relation to the real world. This cannot be denied; however, additional data have been collected postoperatively that support the idea that the bulk of hemodynamic conclusions is correct. Thus, it has been demonstrated by direct recording for 6 days postoperatively with an electromagnetic flowmeter that graft flow remains considerable and that it responds to pharmacologic intervention as the normal coronary circulation does.[158] Postoperative isotopic studies in some patients show that blood continues to flow to sections of the myocardium that have been revascularized, suggesting that considerble portions of myocardium are well supplied which on preoperative studies were demonstrated to be ischemic.[161-168] One study showed not only wide postoperative distribution of flow but also increased flow and a direct relation between increased flow and increased exercise tolerance.[169] In addition, it has been shown that myocardial flow increased with exercise after myocardial revascularization to an extent comparable to that seen in normal subjects.[170,171] Roentgen videodensitometry has confirmed, by measuring the lumen diameter of the bypassed graft and the rate of transit of contrast material down the graft, that considerable flow continues in the postoperative period.[172-174] In addition, catheter-tip flow-measuring devices have been inserted into vein bypass grafts postoperatively and have demonstrated persistence of the velocity profile of phasic flow seen in normal human coronary arteries.[160]

Finally, many patients have now had a second operation for coronary artery disease to repair new coronary obstruction, to bypass vessels not previously bypassed, or to repair grafts that have failed. When there are grafts that are thought angiographically to be functioning normally, direct flow measurements have been made in these normal grafts utilizing the electromagnetic flowmeter. These studies have confirmed that grafts may continue to carry a vigorous flow of blood to the myocardium long after they were placed.[175] Similarly prolonged angiographic follow-up has shown that grafts can remain open for many years.[176] Contrast material which flows down the graft lumen passes into the coronary arteries, travels through their peripheral distribution into the myocardial capillary bed, and drains through the myocardial venous channels. Frequently, the myocardium is densely opacified while the contrast material is in its capillary bed and can be seen to contract vigorously, so there can be no reasonable doubt that actively contracting myocardium continues to receive nutrients through the surgically created accessory pathway.

Myocardial Metabolism

Many metabolic studies conducted both at and after operation have shown considerable evidence for relief of myocardial ischemia. Thus, it has been shown directly that the P_{CO_2} falls and the P_{O_2} in the myocardium increases when a graft is opened into an ischemic area.[82] In addition, the P_{O_2} of venous blood from bypassed regions is higher postoperatively than it was preoperatively both at rest and during stress.[65,87,177]

The increased O_2 delivery reaches the nutrient circulation and improves myocardial metabolism, as confirmed by the data, which show that after effective coronary bypass, lactate is consumed normally rather than produced, and aerobic metabolism is improved.[87,177-183]

Myocardial Contractility

There is also much evidence that shows improved mechanical function of the left ventricle produced by aortocoronary bypass grafts. Thus, it has been shown that if a strain gauge arch is sewed to the myocardium in the area supplied by a stenotic coronary artery and if a vein graft is then attached into the artery distal to the stenosis, myocardial contractility increases when the graft is open and decreases when the graft is closed.[98,184] Similarly, left ventricular function is impaired at operation when a graft is clamped and improved again when the graft is reopened.[114,149,185-187] It is reported that contractility is adversely affected by clamping the bypass graft in those who have normal function but not in those with depressed function,[187] and further data indicate that during the stress of norepinephrine infusion, the adverse effect of bypass clamping is accentuated.[186] This is compatible with the data already presented that reactive hyperemia occurs sometimes but not always when a temporarily obstructed graft is reopened,[144-151,156] and therefore not all subjects who have revascularization have myocardial ischemia at rest. It also suggests that heavily damaged tissue that is replaced by fibrous scar[113] will not be improved in function by providing an improved blood supply. In addition, there will always be imperfections and failures in such a complex technical procedure, and although many studies have reported improved contractility of ischemic segments of myocardium during operation and at postoperative study, the data are always mixed, with both good and bad results reported.

Additional mechanical studies have shown an increase in the velocity of ventricular pressure rise (dp/dt), long considered a rough index of contractility.[69,114,187,188] A decrease in left ventricular end-diastolic pressure is reported at rest,[101,114,159,188-191,193] but this is not seen in all cases,[97] especially not in those who were normal before bypass[99,192] or severely dyskinetic.[99] Segmental contraction is commonly reported to increase in postoperative angiographic studies repeated after successful revascularization,[88,101,107,112,129,188,192,200] but it does not if the local graft is occluded.[91,92,94,100,107,197,199-201] Asynergy and hypokinesis can improve also, as shown by many investigators,[91,92,94,101,189,202,203] and even akinesis can improve,[91,94,189,198] especially if found in

subjects with the severe ischemia of the preinfarction state.[189,192,197,198] But akinesis does not improve if it was caused by infarction rather than being secondary to ischemia.[194] The left ventricular systolic ejection fraction may improve subsequent to revascularization if it is well done,[87,101,112,189,190,192,198,200-212] but no improvement occurs in some, and some are worse.[190,192,197,199-201,208]

Postoperative Cardiac Function

Probably the most significant hemodynamic change as far as the patient is concerned is improved exercise tolerance. This has been measured objectively, and improvement has been demonstrated and reviewed by many investigators.[16,214-222] Also, it has been shown that the rate pressure product, which is a reasonable measure of myocardial oxygen consumption,[223,224] is improved.[87,177,200,221,222,225,226] More importantly to the investigator is the cardiac output response to exercise. Early data concerning cardiac output showed that there was no change in postoperative patients.[208] However, these studies were done in subjects with chronic stable angina or old healed myocardial infarctions, and when those with acute ischemia of the intermediate syndrome were recatheterized postoperatively, considerable increase in cardiac output was demonstrated.[226,227] Furthermore, when cardiovascular response to exercise was tested before and after operation, it was clear that individuals who had received adequate revascularization could achieve a considerable increase in cardiac work and output postoperatively. This was achieved by an increase in rate, but stroke volume does not rise[226,227] and in most subjects is reduced.[211]

Prediction of Improved Ventricular Function

Since the data on ventricular function are so widely scattered, attempts have been made preoperatively to predict improvement, assuming revascularization will be done well and without infarction. The fundamental thesis states that if a portion of depressed myocardium can be made to increase its vigor of contraction during preoperative study, it is depressed because of ischemia rather than because of myocardial fibrosis and/or infarction, and that there is a reasonable chance that normal function can be restored by revascularization. Improved contraction frequently does occur postoperatively in those segments that preoperatively improve their contractility following nitroglycerin administration.[100,129,132,195] Postextrasystolic potentiation of contraction also indicates viable myocardium,[108,136] as does improved contractility during the administration of epinephrine.[137] This subject of predicting myocardial viability has been reviewed recently, and the utility of such tests seems clearly established.[202,203] As might be expected, the degree of hemodynamic improvement that has been obtained in patients with rapidly advancing chest pain syndromes or so-called preinfarction angina is much greater than that obtained in patients with chronic angina and with healed infarcts.[189,208,210,211] Postoperative hemodynamic studies also indicate very clearly that improvement in the left ventricular function curve is directly related to the amount of scar in the ventricle.[213] Thus, 77 percent of those having only grade I scarring showed improvement, and 77 percent of those having grade IV scarring remained unchanged.[228] Medically treated patients are reported not to improve their ventricular contraction and frequently to become worse, whereas improvement occurs frequently in surgical[229] patients. Similarly, it is shown that contractile abnormalities that are not present at rest but that are produced by pacing the heart can be relieved by bypass grafting that provides an adequate blood supply.[214] Thus the data support the idea that abnormalities of ventricular contraction that are caused by reversible ischemia can be treated successfully but those caused by myocardial destruction cannot.

Intercoronary Collaterals

Additional data indicate that a functionally normal circulatory state is restored in the myocardium by successful revascularization, since postoperatively intracoronary collaterals disappear as long as the patent graft nourishes a circulatory bed originally supplied by collateral.[230,231] If the graft becomes occluded, the collaterals appear again, indicating that they were present all along but were rendered nonfunctional when an adequate blood supply was brought to the area.[230,232] These studies confirm the functional significance of collateral and demonstrate that bypass grafting can supply an area previously dependent on collateral.

Symptomatic Relief

In addition to direct hemodynamic observations, it has been shown that there is marked relief of angina pectoris postoperatively. Relief of anginal pain is notably difficult to evaluate;[220,233-235] however, the degree of relief of anginal pain and the degree of postoperative increase in exercise capacity correlate well with the presence of patent vein grafts and especially with total revascularization.[206,212] It is admitted that the correlation is not perfect and that there are exceptions in which the patients appear to be improved sympto-

matically when there are no patent vein grafts.[233] Usually the degree of improvement in patients without patent grafts is not as great as it is in those with all areas adequately revascularized.[225]

Improvement when no grafts are patent has been well discussed, and many possible mechanisms for its occurrence have been considered, including the denervation, infarction, and placebo effect of surgery.[234,235] We may also consider that it may result from scarring of the cardiac surface, which may tend to increase collaterals between obstructed vessels, but this seems unlikely. There are clinical reports of decreased angina from numerous surgical procedures in which the heart was exposed, powdered, abraded, and grafted with arteries that subsequently clotted, and reasonable explanations have also been suggested to explain these observations, including a placebo effect.[234,235] During all of these cardiac operations and coronary bypass, the pericardium is opened wide but remains in place, quickly healing closed, and there is very extensive postoperative fibrosis of the pericardium and epicardium. This reaction is severe enough to complicate second operations by constricting the heart and obscuring surface landmarks. Indeed, pericardial constriction with purulent tamponade has been reported as a fatal complication of myocardial revascularization.[236] Furthermore, postoperative hemodynamic studies of the response to exercise have shown a decrease in stroke work[211] and stroke volume.[193,194,211,226,227] A reasonable additional explanation for symptomatic postoperative improvement could be built upon the dense pericarditis which arises postoperatively in all patients who have cardiac surgery. It could limit the oxygen consumption of the heart in general and the ischemic sections in particular by reducing their capacity to dilate. Since the contractile force required of the heart is related to its diastolic size, relative or actual constriction could have an important overall effect on ischemia and myocardial oxygen requirement and could considerably improve the mechanical advantage of the remaining myocardium, thus reducing angina. This thesis is supported by long-accepted data which showed that pericardiectomy of the heart-lung preparation was followed by larger heart volume and increased left ventricular oxygen consumption.[237]

RECONSTRUCTIVE PROCEDURES

Surgical procedures can be done for patients with coronary artery disease and left ventricular destruction even though complete myocardial revascularization is not always possible, and clearly measurable hemodynamic benefits can be shown that are entirely independent of improved myocardial blood flow. For example, aneurysmectomy[238-240] can reduce the amount of work required of the left ventricle by eliminating paradoxical expansion of the devitalized segment. Also, the mechanical advantage of the ventricle can be increased, as just discussed, when the size of its cavity is reduced by removing a noncontractile scar or segment of myocardium produced by an infarct.[241] Similarly, when papillochordal dysfunction has created severe valvular insufficiency or when the papillary muscles actually rupture, leaving a flail valve leaflet, the mitral valve can be replaced or sometimes repaired so that it becomes competent and thereby directly reduces the left ventricular load.[242] Also, septal defects can sometimes be repaired, thus eliminating a left-to-right shunt and the useless work done by the left ventricle in continually recirculating blood through the lungs to the detriment of the systemic arterial flow.[241] When the heart ruptures externally and the pericardial cavity is obliterated, a localized intrapericardial blood pool results, and after healing of the edges of the defect, direct myocardial suture is not a major surgical problem. If the visceral and parietal pericardial layers are nonadherent, however, an acute emergency of greater magnitude is produced. If the myocardial leak were chronic and slow and only terminally became catastrophic, further exploration could indicate hope for such individuals when clinicians are sufficiently alert to define the premonitory signs of impending cardiac rupture.[243]

LIMITATIONS OF SURGERY

In the vast number of patients who have myocardial revascularization, it has become progressively clearer that there are many things that cannot be done by surgery. Clearly, dead muscle cannot be revived, and fibrous tissue cannot be made to contract. Although these principles are obvious and simple, as is invariably true, the practical problems are not obvious and simple. Most hearts, even with extensive ischemic damage, have a mixture of myocardial cells and fibrous tissue without clear gross separation of normal and pathological areas.[26] Direct biopsies at the time of surgery have invariably revealed the same mixture of muscle and fibrous tissue that has been found at postmortem.[113] Consequently, the practical problem becomes that of determining how much tissue is viable and how much is scar. As indicated before, the administration of nitroglycerin[100,129,132,195] and epinephrine[137] and the induction of premature contractions[136] have helped to elucidate this problem,[202,203] but obviously, there is no present solution that is foolproof. There is no problem in selecting patients who are excellent candidates for myocardial revascularization in that the procedure should usually be straightforward,

easily done, and produce a good postoperative result. Nor is there any problem in determining which candidates are very poor surgical risks; such candidates will usually be difficult to operate on, have a high incidence of complications, a stormy postoperative course, and a high probability of death or a poor result.[244,245] It is in these latter situations, with essentially infinite but largely uncontrollable variables, that clinical judgment becomes very important, and its importance to the outcome of the patient is strongly shared by all who are involved in the care of the patient, as well as in the technique and completeness with which bypass is accomplished. It is also clear that the metabolic and structural factors that cause coronary disease and its progression cannot be changed by surgery directed at the heart or the coronary arteries. Myocardial revascularization remains basically a plumbing procedure which cannot be expected to alter a metabolic disease. The surgical intervention, even though it is major and disabling, cannot permanently alter the destructive life-style so prevalent in those who develop coronary disease, and all too frequently those who are given a reprieve by successful myocardial revascularization return as soon as they feel well to the same destructive pattern of living, resuming eating, drinking, and smoking habits that many believe was etiologic in their atheromatous problem. Finally, destroyed distal vessels cannot be remade and turned into normal coronary arteries. In those individuals with a good ventricle in whom the coronary disease is predominantly localized in the proximal ends of the coronary arteries[127] and in whom the distal vessels remain normal or essentially clear of atherosclerosis, truly excellent results may be expected and obtained by coronary bypass. However, there are many individuals with badly impaired ventricles and extensive peripheral coronary disease who can have very significant relief of symptoms, improvement in myocardial blood flow, and partial restoration of normal hemodynamics. It should not surprise anyone that such patients have more occluded grafts, and the short- and long-range results obtained in these individuals are not as good.

THE THERAPEUTIC DILEMMA OF MEDICAL VERSUS SURGICAL THERAPY

It is hoped that by now the reader is convinced that myocardial revascularization is based on sound principles, both anatomically and physiologically. Nevertheless, in myocardial revascularization, as in every surgical procedure, both patient and physician face a familiar therapeutic dilemma. Gamblers have long lived with the fact that the more they choose to risk, the more they may gain and the more they may lose; conversely, the less they choose to risk, the less they may gain and the less they may lose. It is the same with cardiovascular surgery. If patients with heart disease follow a careful medical regimen until they can no longer be maintained by digitalis, diuretics, restriction of salt and fluid, and marked reduction in activity, they may have a reasonably long life. By foregoing their desire ever to be well, they may lead a limited existence for many years. However, it is unreasonable when close to death to expect that replacement of a defective valve, repair of a congenital cardiac defect, or myocardial revascularization will restore normal health. The residual abnormalities of damaged pulmonary vessels, dilated and hypertrophied ventricular chambers, hepatic dysfunction, and chronic tissue wasting result in a high-risk surgical procedure with limited gain expected. By choosing surgery at this terminal state, a patient has little to lose and little to gain. Thus, if a patient with angina is treated medically with nitrites and beta blockers until he or she has had one or more myocardial infarctions and has developed extensive myocardial fibrosis and valvular insufficiency,

it is not very likely that a miraculous result will be achieved from cardiovascular surgery, regardless of how skillfully and completely it is done. It is true that the patient has less to lose at this stage, but there is also less to gain, and no matter how well the surgical procedure is done, the patient will never have a normal heart. On the other hand, individuals who have just developed angina pectoris, who have not had any myocardial infarction, and who show no evidence of resting myocardial dysfunction or fibrosis may have coronary bypass surgery with very little risk and with considerable expectancy that they will be returned to essentially normal cardiovascular function by the operation. Prudent individuals can then expect a period of several years in which they may alter their life-style, change their diet, stop smoking, exercise regularly, lose weight, and do all of those things that they should have done before but that they did not consider to be necessary. It is not reasonable to expect any uniform agreement as to which of these courses should be followed, but it does seem reasonable for this therapeutic dilemma to be explained to patients so that they may choose wisely which course they wish to take when they make an informed decision.

REFERENCES

1 Schlesinger, M. J., and Zoll, P. M.: Incidence and Localization of Coronary Artery Occlusions, *Arch. Pathol.*, 32:176, 1941.

2 Baroldi, G., and Scomazzoni, G.: "Coronary Circulation in the Normal and Pathologic Heart," U.S. Government Printing Office, Washington, D. C., 1966.

3 Baroldi, G.: Acute Coronary Occlusion as a Cause of Myocardial Infarct and Sudden Coronary Heart Death, *Am. J. Cardiol.*, 16:859, 1965.

4 Baroldi, G.: Myocardial Infarct and Sudden Coronary Heart Death in Relation to Coronary Occlusion and Collateral Circulation, *Am. Heart J.*, 71:826, 1966.

5 Viel, B., Donoso, S., and Salcedo, D.: Coronary Atherosclerosis in Persons Dying Violently, *Arch. Intern. Med.*, 122:97, 1968.

6 Vlodaver, Z., Neufeld, H. N., and Edwards, J. E.: Pathology of Angina Pectoris, *Circulation*, 46:1048, 1972.

7 Guthrie, R. B., Vlodaver, Z., Nicoloff, D. M., and Edwards, J. E.: Pathology of Stable and Unstable Angina Pectoris, *Circulation*, 51:1059, 1975.

8 Sones, F. M., Jr., and Shirey, E. K.: Cinecoronary Arteriography, *Mod. Concepts Cardiovasc. Dis.*, 31:735, 1962.

9 Cairns, J. A., Fantus, I. G., and Klassen, G. A.: Unstable Angina Pectoris, *Am. Heart J.*, 92:(3):373, 1976.

10 Scanlon, P. J., Nemickas, R., Moran, J. F., Talano, J. V., Amirparviz, F., and Pifarre, R.: Accelerated Angina

Pectoris: Clinical, Hemodynamic, Arteriographic and Therapeutic Experience in 85 Patients, *Circulation*, 47:19, 1973.

11 Redwood, D. R., and Epstein, S. E.: Uses and Limitations of Stress Testing in the Evaluation of Ischemic Heart Disease, *Circulation*, 46:1115, 1972.

12 Bruschke, A. V. G., Proudfit, W. L., and Sones, F. M., Jr.: Progress Study of 590 Consecutive Nonsurgical Cases of Coronary Disease Followed 5 to 9 Years. I. Arteriographic Correlations, *Circulation*, 47:1147, 1973.

13 Bruschke, A. V. G., Proudfit, W. L., and Sones, F. M., Jr.: Progress Study of 590 Consecutive Nonsurgical Cases of Coronary Disease Followed 5 to 9 Years. II. Ventriculographic and Other Correlations. *Circulation*, 47:1154, 1973.

14 Burgraff, G. W., and Parker, J. D. Prognosis in Coronary Artery Disease. Angiographic, Hemodynamic, and Clinical Factors, *Circulation*, 51:146, 1975.

15 Lichtlen, P., and Steinbrunn, W.: Natural History of Coronary Artery Disease Based on Coronary Angiography. Complete 5-Year Survival Rates in 244 Unselected Unoperated Coronary Patients Undergoing Angiography, *Cleve. Clin. O.*, 45:153, 1977.

16 Wilson, W. S.: Aortocoronary Bypass—State of the Art 1974. Cardiovascular Diseases, *Bull. Texas Heart Inst.*, 1:271, 1974.

17 Mann, F. C., Herrick, J. F., Essex, H. E., and Baldes, E. J.: The Effect on the Blood Flow of Decreasing the Lumen of a Blood Vessel, *Surgery*, 4:249, 1938.

18 McGregor, M.: The Coronary Collateral Circulation, a Significant Compensatory Mechanism or a Functionless Quirk of Nature, *Circulation*, 52:529, 1975.

19 Rowe, G. G.: An Angiographic and Clinical Study of Coronary Collateral Circulation, *Basic Res. Cardiol.*, in press.

20 Khouri, E. M., Gregg, D. E., and Lowensohn, H. S.: Flow in the Major Branches of the Left Coronary Artery During Experimental Coronary Insufficiency in the Unanesthetized Dog, *Circ. Res.*, 23:99, 1968.

21 Khouri, E. M., Gregg, D. E., and McGranakan, G. M., Jr.: Regression and Reappearance of Coronary Collaterals, *Am. J. Physiol.*, 220:655, 1971.

22 Menick, F. J., White, F. C., and Bloor, C. M.: Coronary Collateral Circulation: Determination of an Anatomical Index of Functional Collateral Flow Capacity, *Am. Heart J.*, 82:503, 1971.

23 Becker, L. C., and Pitt, B.: Collateral Blood Flow in Conscious Dogs with Chronic Coronary Artery Occlusion, *Am. J. Physiol.*, 221:1507, 1971.

24 Schaper, W., and Pasyk, S.: Influence of Collateral Flow on the Ischemic Tolerance of the Heart Following Acute and Subacute Coronary Occlusion, *Circulation*, 53 (suppl. 1):57, 1976.

25 Robbins, S. L., Solomon, M., and Bennett, A.: Demonstration of Intercoronary Anastomoses in Human Hearts with a Low Viscosity Perfusion Mass, *Circulation*, 33:733, 1966.

26 Morgan Jones, A.: The Functional Role of Intercoronary Anastomoses, *Acta Cardiol. (Brux.)*, (suppl. 2):130, 1965.

27 Marlon, A. M., Adams, M. H., Wexler, L., and Harrison, D. C.: Angiographic Demonstration of Collateral Development in Experimental Coronary Artery Occlusion with Ameroid Constrictors, *Invest. Radiol.*, 8:131, 1973.

28 Elliot, E. C., Jones, E. L., Bloor, C. M., Leon, A. S., and Gregg, D. E.: Day-to-Day Changes in Coronary Hemodynamics Secondary to Constriction of Circumflex Branch of Left Coronary Artery in Conscious Dogs, *Circ. Res.*, 22:237, 1968.

29 Scheel, K. W., Banet, M., Ott, C., and Lehan, P. H.: A Quantitative Approach to Collateral and Antegrade Flows After Coronary Occlusion, *Am. J. Physiol.*, 222(3):687, 1972.

30 Prinzmetal, M., Bergman, H. C., Kruger, H. E., Schwartz, L. L., Simkin, B., and Sobin, S. S.: Studies on the Coronary Circulation. III. Collateral Circulation of Beating Human and Dog Hearts with Coronary Occlusion, *Am. Heart J.*, 35(5):689, 1948.

31 Becker, L. C., and Pitt, B.: Collateral Blood Flow in Conscious Dogs with Chronic Coronary Artery Occlusion, *Am. J. Physiol.*, 221(5):1507, 1971.

32 Ganz, W., Tamura, K., Marcus, H. S., Donoso, R., Yoshida, S., and Swan, H. J. C.: Measurement of Coronary Sinus Blood Flow by Continuous Thermodilution in Man, *Circulation*, 44:181, 1971.

33 Ito, I., et al.: Studies on Coronary Circulation in Man by Method of Coronary Sinus Catheterization, *Jpn. Circ. J.*, 20:299, 1956.

34 Rowe, G. G., Maxwell, G. M., Castillo, C. A., Crumpton, C. W., Botham, R. J., and Young, W. P.: Evaluation of Effect of Bilateral Internal Mammary Artery Ligation on Cardiac Output and Coronary Blood Flow, *N. Engl. J. Med.*, 261:653, 1959.

35 Gorlin, R., Brachfeld, N., Messer, J. V., and Turner, J. D.: Physiologic and Biochemical Aspects of the Disordered Coronary Circulation, *Ann. Intern. Med.*, 51:698, 1959.

36 Gorlin, R., Brachfeld, N., MacLeod, C., and Bopp, P.: Effect of Nitroglycerin on Coronary Circulation in Patients with Coronary Artery Disease or Increased Left Ventricular Work, *Circulation*, 19:705, 1959.

37 Brachfeld, N., and Gorlin, R.: Physiologic Evaluation of Angina Pectoris, *Dis. Chest*, 38:658, 1960.

38 Gorlin, R.: Measurement of Coronary Flow in Health and Disease, in A. M. Jones (ed.), "Modern Trends in Cardiology," Butterworth & Co. (Publishers), Ltd., London, 1961.

39 Bing, R. J.: "The Anoxic Heart." (Lecture at the Henry Ford Symposium on Coronary Artery Disease, Henry Ford Hospital, Detroit, Michigan, November, 1961.)

40 Rowe, G. G., Chelius, C. J., Afonso, S., Gurtner, H. P., and Crumpton, C. W.: Systemic and Coronary Hemodynamic Effects of Erythrol Tetranitrate, *J. Clin. Invest.*, 40:1217, 1961.

41 Cohen, L. S., Elliott, W. C., Klein, M. D., and Gorlin, R.: Coronary Heart Disease: Clinical Cinearteriographic and Metabolic Correlations, *Am. J. Cardiol.*, 17:153, 1966.

42 Holmberg, S., Paulin, S., Prerovsky, I., and Varnauskas, E.: Coronary Blood Flow in Man and Its Relation to the Coronary Arteriogram, *Am. J. Cardiol.*, 19:486, 1967.

43 Rowe, G. G.: Nitrous Oxide Method for Determining Coronary Blood Flow in Man, *Am. Heart J.*, 58:268, 1959.

44 Ross, R. S., Ueda, K., Lichtlen, P. R., and Rees, J. R.: Measurement of Myocardial Blood Flow in Animals and Man by Selective Injection of Radioactive Inert Gas into Coronary Arteries, *Cir. Res.*, 15:28, 1964.

45 Rowe, G. G., Thomsen, J. H., Stenlund, R. R., McKenna, D. H., Sialer, S., and Corliss, R. J.: A Study of Hemodynamics and Coronary Blood Flow in Man with Coronary Artery Disease, *Circulation*, 39:139, 1969.

46 Klocke, F. J., Bunnell, I. L., Wittenberg, S. M., Greene, D. G., and Falsetti, H. L.: Validation of Inert Gas Measurements of Coronary Blood Flow and Contrasting Findings in Patients With and Without Coronary Artery Disease, in A. Maseri (ed.), "Myocardial Blood Flow in Man, Methods and Significance in Coronary Disease," Minerva Medica, Torino, 1972.

47 Yoshida, S., Ganz, W., Donoso, R., Marcus, H. S., and

Swan, H. J. C.: Coronary Hemodynamics During Successive Elevation of Heart Rate by Pacing in Subjects with Angina Pectoris, *Circulation,* 44:1062, 1971.

48 Macleod, C. A., Bahler, R. C., and Davies, B.: Pacing-induced Changes in Cardiac Venous Blood Flow in Normal Subjects and Patients with Coronary Artery Disease, *Am. J. Cardiol.,* 32:686, 1973.

49 Lowe, D. K., Rothbaum, D. A., McHenry, P. L., Corya, B. C., and Knoebel, S. B.: Myocardial Blood Flow Response to Isometric (Handgrip) and Treadmill Exercise in Coronary Artery Disease, *Circulation,* 51:126, 1975.

50 Sullivan, J. M., Taylor, W. J., Elliott, W. C., and Gorlin, R.: Regional Myocardial Blood Flow, *J. Clin. Invest.,* 46:1402, 1967.

51 Smith, S. C., Jr., Gorlin, R., Herman, M. V., Taylor, W. J., and Collins, J. J.: Myocardial Blood Flow in Man: Effects of Coronary Collateral Circulation and Coronary Artery Bypass Surgery, *J. Clin. Invest.,* 51:2556, 1972.

52 Cannon, P. J., Dell, R. B., and Dwyer, E. M.: Regional Myocardial Perfusion Rates in Patients with Coronary Artery Disease, *J. Clin. Invest.,* 51(4):978, 1972.

53 Ritchie, J. L., Hamilton, G. W., Gould, K. L., Allen, D., Kennedy, J. W., and Hammermeister, K. E.: Myocardial Imaging with Indium-113m- and Technetium-99m-Macro-Aggregated Albumin, *Am. J. Cardiol.,* 35:380, 1975.

54 Cannon, P. J.: Radioisotopic Studies of the Regional Myocardial Circulation, *Circulation,* 51:955, 1975.

55 Cannon, P. J., Sciacca, R. R., Fowler, D. L., Weiss, M. B., Schmidt, D. H., and Casarella, W. J.: Measurement of Regional Myocardial Blood Flow in Man: Description and Critique of the Method Using Xenon-133 and a Scintillation Camera, *Am. J. Cardiol.,* 36:783, 1975.

56 Maseri, A.: Pathophysiologic Studies of the Pulmonary and Coronary Circulations in Man, *Am. J. Cardiol.,* 38:751, 1976.

57 Holman, B. L., Cohn, P. F., Adams, D. F., See, J. R., Roberts, B. H., Idoine, J., and Gorlin, R.: Regional Myocardial Blood Flow During Hyperemia Induced by Contrast Agent in Patients with Coronary Artery Disease, *Am. J. Cardiol.,* 38:416, 1976.

58 Pitt, B., and Strauss, H. W.: Myocardial Perfusion Imaging and Gated Cardiac Blood Pool Scanning: Clinical Application, *Am. J. Cardiol.,* 38:739, 1976.

59 Schmidt, D. H., Weiss, M. B., Casarella, W. J., Fowler, D. L., Sciacca, R., and Cannon, P. J.: Regional Myocardial Perfusion During Atrial Pacing in Patients with Coronary Artery Disease, *Circulation,* 53(5):807, 1976.

60 Maseri, A., L'Abbate, A., Pesola, A., Michelassi, C., Marzilli, M., and De Nes, M.: Regional Myocardial Perfusion in Patients with Atherosclerotic Coronary Artery Disease, at Rest and During Angina Pectoris Induced by Tachycardia, *Circulation,* 55(3):423, 1977.

61 Maseri, A., and Mancini, P.: The Evaluation of Regional Myocardial Perfusion in Man by a Scintillation Camera Computer System, in A. Maseri (ed.)., "Myocardial Blood Flow in Man, Methods and Significance in Coronary Disease," Minerva Medica, Torino, 1972.

62 Dwyer, E. M., Jr., Dell, R. B., and Cannon, P. J.: Regional Myocardial Blood Flow in Patients with Residual Anterior and Inferior Transmural Infarction, *Circulation,* 48:924, 1973.

63 Rowe, G. G.: Observations in Coronary Blood Flow with N_2O Method in Man with Coronary Artery Disease, in A. Maseri (ed.), "Myocardial Blood Flow in Man, Methods and Significance in Coronary Disease." Minerva Medica, Torino, 1972, p. 297.

64 Tennant, R., and Wiggers, C. J.: The Effect of Coronary Occlusion on Myocardial Contraction, *Am. J. Physiol.,* 112:351, 1935.

65 Chatterjee, K.: Global and Regional Myocardial Metabolism Before and After Successful Aortocoronary Artery Bypass Surgery, *Cleve. Clin. Q.,* 45:112, 1977.

66 Urschel, H. C., Razzuk, M. A., Wood, R. E., and Paulson, D. L.: Factors Influencing Patency of Aortocoronary Artery Saphenous Vein Grafts, *Surgery,* 72(6):1048, 1972.

67 Webb, W. R., Parker, F. B., Jr., and Neville, J. F., Jr.: Retrograde Pressures and Flows in Coronary Arterial Disease, *Ann. Thorac. Surg.,* 15(3):256, 1973.

68 Parker, F. B., Jr., Neville, J. F., Jr., Hanson, E. L., and Webb, W. R.: Collateral Pressures and Flows in the Preinfarction Syndrome, *Circulation,* 48(suppl. 4):92, 1973.

69 Johnson, W. D., Flemma, R. J., Manley, J. C., and Lepley, D., Jr.: The Physiologic Parameters of Ventricular Function as Affected by Direct Coronary Surgery, *J. Thorac. Cardiovasc. Surg.,* 60(4):483, 1970.

70 Borkenhagen, D. M., Kirk, E. S., Lamberti, J. J., Cohn, L. H., Collins, J. J., and Gorlin, R.: Low Saphenous Vein Graft Blood Flow and Absence of Reactive Hyperemia in Non-occlusive Coronary Artery Disease, *Circulation,* 48(suppl. 4):59, 1973.

71 Scherer, J. L., Goldstein, R. E., Stinson, E. B., Seningen, R. P., Grehl, T. M., and Epstein, S. E.: Correlation of Angiographic and Physiologic Assessment of Coronary Collaterals in Patients Receiving Bypass Grafts, *Circulation,* 8(suppl. 4):88, 1973.

72 Bodenheimer, M. M., Banka, V. S., Trout, R. G., and Helfant, R. H.: Relationship Between Angiographically Determined Coronary Artery Lesions and Their Distal Pressure and Flow in Man, *Clin. Res.,* 26:598A, 1978.

73 Rowe, G. G.: Coronary Vasodilator Therapy for Angina Pectoris, *Am. Heart J.,* 68(5):691, 1964.

74 Fam, W. M., and McGregor, M.: Effect of Coronary Vasodilator Drugs on Retrograde Flow in Areas of Chronic Myocardial Ischemia, *Cir. Res.,* 15:355, 1964.

75 Rowe, G. G.: Inequalities of Myocardial Perfusion in Coronary Artery Disease ("Coronary Steal"), *Circulation,* 42:193, 1970.

76 Flameng, W., Wusten, B., and Schaper, W.: On the Distribution of Myocardial Flow. Part II: Effects of Arterial Stenosis and Vasodilation, *Basic Res. Cardiol.,* 69:435, 1974.

77 Flameng, W., Schaper, W., and Lewi, P.: Multiple Experimental Coronary Occlusion Without Infarction, *Am. Heart J.,* 85(6):767, 1973.

78 Schaper, W., Lewi, P., Flameng, W., and Gijpen, L.: Myocardial Steal Produced by Coronary Vasodilation in Chronic Coronary Artery Occlusion, *Basic Res. Cardiol.,* 68:3, 1973.

79 Cohen, M. V., Sonnenblick, E. H., and Kirk, E. S.: Coronary Steal: Its Role in Detrimental Effect of Isoproterenol After Acute Coronary Occlusion in Dogs, *Am. J. Cardiol.,* 38:880, 1976.

80 Gallagher, K. P., Folts, J. D., Shebuski, R. J., Rankin, J. H., and Rowe, G. G.: Epicardial Vasodilator Reserve in the Presence of Critical Stenosis in Dogs, submitted for publication.

81 Hutter, A. M., Yeatman, L. A., Flynn, T., and DeSanctis, R. W.: Long-term Course of Subendocardial Myocardial Infarction Compared to That of Anterior and Inferior Transmural Infarction. A Controlled Study, *Am. J. Cardiol.,* 41:398, 1978.

82 Gardner, T. J., Brantigan, J. W., Perna, A. M., Bender, H. W., Brawley, R. K., and Gott, V. L.: Intramyocardial Gas Tensions in the Human Heart During Coronary Artery–Saphenous Vein Bypass, *J. Thorac. Cardiovasc. Surg.,* 62:844, 1971.

83 Krasnow, N., Neill, W. A., Messer, J. V., and Gorlin, R.: Myocardial Lactate and Pyruvate Metabolism, *J. Clin. Invest.,* 41(11):2075, 1962.

84 Neill, W. A.: Myocardial Hypoxia and Anaerobic Metabolism in Coronary Heart Disease, *Am. J. Cardiol.,* 22:507, 1968.

85 Parker, J. O., West, R. O., Case, R. B., and Chiong, M. A.: Temporal Relationships of Myocardial Lactate Metabolism, Left Ventricular Function, and S-T Segment Depression During Angina Precipitated by Exercise, *Circulation,* 40:97, 1969.

86 Bourassa, M. G., Campeau, L., Bois, M. A., and Rico, O.: Myocardial Lactate Metabolism at Rest and During Exercise in Ischemic Heart Disease, *Am. J. Cardiol.,* 23:771, 1969.

87 Chatterjee, K., Matloff, J. M., Swan, H. J. C., Ganz, W., Kaushik, V. S., Magnusson, P., Henis, M. M., and Forrester, J. S.: Abnormal Regional Metabolism and Mechanical Function in Patients with Ischemic Heart Disease. Improvement After Successful Regional Revascularization by Aortocoronary Bypass, *Circulation,* 52:390, 1975.

88 Wilson, C. S., Krueger, S., Forker, A. D., and Weaver, W. F.: Correlation Between Segmental Early Relaxation of the Left Ventricular Wall and Coronary Occlusive Disease, *Am. Heart J.,* 89(4):474, 1975.

89 Hamby, R. I., Aintablian, A., Tabrah, F., et al.: Late Systolic Bulging of Left Ventricle in Patients with Angina Pectoris, *Chest,* 65:169, 1974.

90 Dwyer, E. M., Jr.: Left Ventricular Pressure-Volume Alterations and Regional Disorders of Contraction During Myocardial Ischemia Induced by Atrial Pacing, *Circulation,* 42:1111, 1970.

91 Saltiel, J., Lesperance, J., Bourassa, M. G., Castonguay, Y., Campeau, L., and Grondin, P.: Reversibility of Left Ventricular Dysfunction Following Aorto-coronary By-pass Grafts, *Am. J. Roentgenol. Radium Ther. Nucl. Med.,* 110:739, 1970.

92 Chatterjee, K., Parmley, W. W., Sustaita, H., Matloff, J. M., and Swan, H. J. C.: Influence of Aortocoronary Artery Bypass on Left Ventricular Asynergy, *Am. J. Cardiol.,* 29:256, 1972.

93 Feild, B. J., Russell, R. O., Dowling, J. T., and Rackley, C. E.: Regional Left Ventricular Performance in the Year Following Myocardial Infarction, *Circulation,* 46:679, 1972.

94 Bourassa, M. G., Lesperance, J., Campeau, L., and Saltiel, J.: Fate of Left Ventricular Contraction Following Aortocoronary Venous Grafts, *Circulation,* 46:724, 1972.

95 Levin, D. C., and Baltaxe, H. A.: Role of Coronary Collateral Circulation and Distal Runoff in Preserving Myocardial Contractility, *Circulation,* 8(suppl. 4):88, 1973.

96 Linhart, J. W.: Atrial Pacing in Coronary Artery Disease, Including Preinfarction Angina and Postoperative Studies, *Am. J. Cardiol.,* 30:603, 1972.

97 Linhart, J. W., Hildner, F. J., Barold, S. S., Lister, J. W., and Samet, P.: Left Heart Hemodynamics During Angina Pectoris Induced by Atrial Pacing, *Circulation,* 40:483, 1969.

98 Hairston, P., Newman, W. H., and Daniell, H. B.: Myocardial Contractile Force as Influenced by Direct Coronary Surgery, *Ann. Thorac. Surg.,* 15:364, 1973.

99 Campeau, L., Elias, G., Esplugas, E., Lesperance, J., and Bourassa, M. G.: Left Ventricular Performance During Exercise Before and One Year After Saphenous Vein Graft Surgery for Angina Pectoris, *Circulation,* 48 (suppl.4):53, 1973.

100 Pine, R., Meister, S. G., Banka, V. S., Feldman, M. S., Trout, R., and Helfant, R. H.: Detection of Reversible Ventricular Contraction Abnormalities with Nitroglycerin: Correlation with Post Coronary Bypass Ventriculography, *Circulation,* 48 (suppl. 4):104, 1973.

101 Hamby, R. I., Aintablian, A., Tabrah, F., Hartstein, M. L., and Wisoff, B.G.: Determinants of Reversibility of

Left Ventricular Function After Aortocoronary Bypass Surgery, *Am. J. Cardiol.,* 33:142, 1974.

102 Tyberg, J. V., Forrester, J. S., Wyatt, H. L., Goldner, S. J., Parmley, W. W., and Swan, J. H. C.: An Analysis of Segmental Ischemic Dysfunction Utilizing the Pressure-Length Loop, *Circulation,* 49:748, 1974.

103 Brundage, B. H., and Cheitlin, M. D.: Ventricular Function Curves from the Cardiac Response to Angiographic Contrast: A Sensitive Detector of Ventricular Dysfunction in Coronary Artery Disease, *Am. Heart J.,* 88 (3):281, 1974.

104 Burggraf, G. W., and Parker, J. O.: Prognosis in Coronary Artery Disease, Angiographic, Hemodynamic, and Clinical Factors, *Circulation,* 51:146, 1975.

105 Krayenbuehl, H. P., Schoenbeck, M., Rutishauser, W., and Wirz, P.: Abnormal Segmental Contraction Velocity in Coronary Artery Disease Produced by Isometric Exercise and Atrial Pacing, *Am. J. Cardiol.,* 35:785, 1975.

106 Wyatt, H. L., Forrester, J. S., Tyberg, J. V., Goldner, S. J., Logan, S. E., Parmley, W. W., and Swan, J. H. C.: Effect of Graded Reductions in Regional Coronary Perfusion on Regional and Total Cardiac Function, *Am. J. Cardiol.,* 36:185, 1975.

107 Leighton, R. F., Pollack, M. E. M., and Welch, T. G.: Abnormal Left Ventricular Wall Motion at Mid-ejection in Patients with Coronary Heart Disease, *Circulation,* 52:238, 1975.

108 Zir, L. M., Pohost, G. M., Gold, H. K., Leinbach, R. C., and Dinsmore, R. E.: The Significance of Reversal of Left Ventricular Asynergy by Postextrasystolic Potentiation: A Comparison of Left Ventriculography and Thallium-201 Myocardial Scans, *Circulation,* 54(suppl. 2):5, 1976.

109 Flessas, A. P., Connelly, G. P., Handa, S., Tilney, C. R., Kloster, C. K., Rimmer, R. H., Keefe, J. F., Klein, M. D., and Ryan, T. J.: Effects of Isometric Exercise on the End-Diastolic Pressure, Volumes, and Function of the Left Ventricle in Man, *Circulation,* 53(5):839, 1976.

110 Borer, J. S., Bacharach, S. L., Green, M. V., Kent, K. M., Epstein, S. E., and Johnston, G. S.: Real-time Radionuclide Cineangiography in the Noninvasive Evaluation of Global and Regional Left Ventricular Function at Rest and During Exercise in Patients with Coronary-Artery Disease, *N. Engl. J. Med.,* 296:839, 1977.

111 Tomoike, H., Franklin, D., McKown, D., Kemper, W. S., Guberek, M., and Ross, J., Jr.: Regional Myocardial Dysfunction and Hemodynamic Abnormalities During Strenuous Exercise in Dogs with Limited Coronary Flow; *Circ. Res.,* 42(4):487, 1978.

112 Wolf, N. M., Kreulen, T. H., Bove, A. A., McDonough, M. T., Kessler, K. M., Strong, M., LeMole, G., and Spann, J. F.: Left Ventricular Function Following Coronary Bypass Surgery, *Circulation,* 58(1):63, 1978.

113 Ideker, R. E., Behar, V. S., Wagner, G. S., Starr, J. W., Starmer, C. F., Lee, K. L., and Hackel, D. B.: Evaluation of Asynergy as an Indicator of Myocardial Fibrosis, *Circulation,* 57(4):715, 1978.

114 Enright, L. P., Marlon, A. M., Daily, P. O., Adams, M., and Shumway, N. E.: Human Coronary Artery Bypass Grafts and Left Ventricular Function, *Surgery,* 72(3):404, 1972.

115 Mann, T., Brodie, B. R., Grossman, W., and McLaurin, L. P.: Effect of Angina on the Left Ventricular Diastolic Pressure-Volume Relationship, *Circulation,* 55(5):761, 1977.

116 McCallister, B. D., Yipintsoi, T., Hallermann, F. J., Wallace, R. B., and Frye, R. L.: Left Ventricular Performance During Mild Supine Leg Exercise in Coronary Artery Disease, *Circulation,* 37:922, 1968.

117 Bristow, J. D., Van Zee, B. E., and Judkins, M. P.: Systolic and Diastolic Abnormalities of the Left Ventricle in Coronary Artery Disease: Studies in Patients with Little or No Enlargement of Ventricular Volume, *Circulation,* 42:219, 1970.

118 Parker, J. O., Ledwich, J. R., West, R. O., and Case, R. B.: Reversible Cardiac Failure During Angina Pectoris: Hemodynamic Effects of Atrial Pacing in Coronary Artery Disease, *Circulation,* 39:745, 1969.

119 Parker, J. O., Di Giorgi, S., and West, R. O.: A Hemodynamic Study of Acute Coronary Insufficiency Precipitated by Exercise: With Observations on the Effects of Nitroglycerin, *Am. J. Cardiol.,* 17:470, 1966.

120 Cohen, L. S., Elliott, W. C., Rolett, E. L., and Gorlin, R.: Hemodynamic Studies During Angina Pectoris, *Circulation,* 31:409, 1965.

121 McDonough, J. R., Danielson, R. A., Wills, R. E., and Vine, D. L.: Maximal Cardiac Output During Exercise in Patients with Coronary Artery Disease, *Am. J. Cardiol.,* 33:23, 1974.

122 Roberts, W. C., and Perloff, J. K.: Mitral Valvular Disease, *Ann. Intern. Med.,* 77:939, 1972.

123 Tsakiris, A. G., Rastelli, G. C., Amorin, D., Titus, J. L., and Wood, E. M: Effect of Papillary Muscle Damage on Mitral Valve Closure in Intact Anesthetized Dogs, *Mayo Clin. Proc.,* 45:275, 1970.

124 Smith, H. L., Essex, H. E., and Baldes, E. J.: A Study of Movements of the Heart Valves and of Heart Sounds, *Ann. Intern. Med.,* 33:1357, 1950.

125 Tsakiris, A. G., Sturm, R. E., and Wood, E. H.: Experimental Studies on the Mechanism of Closure of Cardiac Valves with Use of Roentgen Videodensitometry, *Am. J. Cardiol.,* 32:136, 1973.

126 Edwards, J. E., and Burchell, H. B.: Pathologic Anatomy of Mitral Insufficiency, *Proc. Staff Mtg. Mayo Clin.,* 33(21):497, 1958.

127 Blumgart, H. L., Zoll, P. M., and Kurland, G. S.: Discussion of the Direct Relief of Coronary Occlusion: The Anatomic Pathologic Problems, *Arch. Intern. Med.,* 104:862, 1959.

128 Johnson, W. D.: Surgical Techniques of Myocardial Revascularization: An Overview, *Bull. N. Y. Acad. Med.*, 48(9):1146, 1972.

129 Dumesnil, J. G., Ritman, E. L., Frye, R. L., Davis, G. D., Gau, G. T., Sturm, R. E., and Wood, E. H.: Regional Left Ventricular Wall Dynamics Before and After the Administration of Oral Nitroglycerin, *Circulation*, 48(suppl. 4):104, 1973.

130 Helfant, R. H., Pine, R., Meister, S. G., Feldman, M. S., Trout, R. G., and Banka, V. S.: Nitroglycerin to Unmask Reversible Asynergy. Correlation with Post Coronary Bypass Ventriculography, *Circulation*, 50:108, 1974.

131 Matthews, R. G., Reddy, S. P., O'Toole, J. D., Salerni, R., and Shaver, J. A.: Reversibility of Left Ventricular Asynergy Assessed by Post-Nitroglycerin Left Ventriculography, *Am. J. Cardiol.* 33:156, 1974.

132 Bryson, A. L., Aycock, A. C., Flamm, M. D., Zaret, B. L., Ratshin, R. A., and McGowan, R. L.: Changes in Regional Ventricular Contraction of the Arteriosclerotic Heart Following Nitroglycerin Administration — Surgical Correlation, *Circulation*, 50 (suppl. 3):44, 1974.

133 Banka, V. S., Bodenheimer, M., and Helfant, R. H.: Effects of Nitroglycerin on Regional Left Ventricular Length-Tension Relations After Coronary Occlusion, *Am. J. Cardiol.*, 33:124, 1974.

134 McAnulty, J. H., Hattenhauer, M. T., Rosch, J., Kloster, F. E., and Rahimtoola, S. H.: Improvement in Left Ventricular Wall Motion Abnormalities After Nitroglycerin, *Am. J. Cardiol.*, 33:153, 1974.

135 Bodenheimer, M. M., Banka, V. S., Hermann, G. A., Trout, R. G., Parker, H., and Helfant, R. H.: Reversible Asynergy, Histopathologic and Electrographic Correlations in Patients with Coronary Artery Disease, *Circulation*, 53:792, 1976.

136 Dyke, S. H., Cohn, P. F., Gorlin, R., and Sonnenblick, E. H.: Detection of Residual Myocardial Function in Coronary Artery Disease Using Postextrasystolic Potentiation, *Circulation* 50:694, 1974.

137 Horn, H. R., Teichholz, L. E., Cohn, P. F., Herman, M. V., and Gorlin, R.: Augmentation of Left Ventricular Contraction Pattern in Coronary Artery Disease by an Inotropic Catecholamine. The Epinephrine Ventriculogram, *Circulation*, 49:1063, 1974.

138 Furuse, A., Klopp, E. H., Brawley, R. K., and Gott, V. L.: Hemodynamics of Aorta-to-Coronary Artery Bypass, *Ann. Thorac. Surg.*, 14:282, 1972.

139 Kakos, G. S., Oldham, H. N., Dixon, S. H., Davis, R. W., Hagen, P., and Sabiston, D. C., Jr.: Coronary Artery Hemodynamics After Aorto-Coronary Artery Vein Bypass, *J. Thorac. Cardiovasc. Surg.*, 63(6):849, 1972.

140 Mitchel, B. F., Adam, M., Lambert, C. J., Sungu, U., and Shiekh, S.: Ascending Aorta-to-Coronary Artery Saphenous Vein Bypass Grafts, *J. Thorac. Cardiovasc. Surg.*, 60(4):457, 1970.

141 Folts, J. D., Kahn, D. R., Bittar, N., and Rowe, G. G.: Effects of Partial Obstruction on Phasic Flow in Aortocoronary Grafts, *Circulation*, 51,52 (suppl. 1):148, 1975.

142 Tyers, G. F. O., O'Neill, M. J., Messner, J. T., and Waldhausen, J. A.: Nonmechanical Factors Affecting Aortocoronary Vein Graft Flow, *Circulation*, 51,52 (suppl. 1):178, 1975.

143 Benchimol, A., Desser, K. B., and Schumacher, J. A.: New Method to Measure Aortocoronary Bypass Graft Blood Flow Velocity, *Am. J. Cardiol.*, 31:120, 1973.

144 Moran, J. M., Chen, P. Y., and Rheinlander, H. F.: Coronary Hemodynamics Following Aorta-Coronary Bypass Graft, *Arch. Surg.*, 103(5):539, 1971.

145 Greenfield, J. C., Rembert, J. C., Young, W. G., Jr., Oldham, H. N., Jr., Alexander, J. A., and Sabiston, D. C., Jr.: Studies of Blood Flow in Aorta-to-Coronary Venous Bypass Grafts in Man, *J. Clin. Invest.*, 51: 2724, 1972.

146 Bittar, N., Kroncke, G. M., Dacumos, G. C., Rowe, G. G., Young, W. P., Chopra, P. S., Folts, J. D., and Kahn, D. R.: Vein Graft Flow and Reactive Hyperemia in the Human Heart, *J. Thorac. Cardiovasc. Surg.*, 64(6):885, 1972.

147 Webb, W. R., Jr.: Discussion following article by N. Bittar, et al., *J. Thorac. Cardiovasc. Surg.*, 64:855, 1972.

148 Sabiston, D. C., Jr.: Direct Revascularization Procedures in the Management of Myocardial Ischemia, *Circulation*, 43:175, 1971.

149 Rickards, A., Wright, J., and Balcon, R.: Observations on the Effect of Occlusion, Nitroglycerin and Papaverine on Coronary Artery Bypass Grafts, *Am. J. Cardiol.*, 33:164, 1974.

150 Kaiser, G. C., Barner, H. B., Willman, V. L., Mudd, J. G., Westura, E. W., and Alves, L. E.: Aortocoronary Bypass Grafting, *Arch. Surg.*, 105(2):319, 1972.

151 van der Mark, F., Frank, H. L. L., Buis, B., Brom, A. G., Bos, E., and Nauta, J.: Significance of Blood Flow Measurements in Implanted Aorta-Coronary Bypass Grafts, *Circulation*, 46(suppl. 2):232, 1972.

152 Gregg, D. E., and Fisher, L. C.: Blood Supply to the Heart, in "Handbook of Physiology," Sect. II. "Circulation," American Physiology Society, Washington, D. C., 1963, p. 1539.

153 Folts, J. D., Kahn, D. R., Bittar, N., and Rowe, G. G.: Effects of Partial Obstruction on Phasic Flow in Aortocoronary Grafts, *Circulation*, 51,52(suppl. 1):148, 1975.

154 Grondin, C. M., Castonguay, Y. R., Lesperance, J., Bourassa, M. G., Campeau, L., and Grondin, P.: Attrition Rate of Aorta-to-Coronary Artery Saphenous Vein Grafts After One Year, *Ann. Thorac. Surg.*, 14(3):223, 1972.

155 Walker, J. A., Friedberg, H. D., Flemma, R. J., and Johnson, W. D.: Determinants of Angiographic Patency

of Aortocoronary Vein Bypass Grafts, *Circulation*, 44(suppl. 2):108, 1971.

156 Grondin, C. M., Lepage, G., Castonguay, Y. R., Meere, C., and Grondin, P.: Aortocoronary Bypass Graft. Initial Blood Flow Through the Graft, and Early Postoperative Patency, *Circulation*, 44:815, 1971.

157 McCormick, J. R., Kaneko, M., Baue, A. E., and Geha, A. S.: Blood Flow and Vasoactive Drug Effects in Internal Mammary and Venous Bypass Grafts, *Circulation*, 51, 52(suppl. 1):72, 1975.

158 Bertranou, E., Ekestrom, S., Giraudo, N., Perez-Day, C., Ramponi, R., and Silva Iribarren, C.: Effect de l'Isoproterenol sur le Debit des Pontages Aorto-coronaires chez l'Humain, *Union Med. Can.*, 101:871, 1972.

159 Knoebel, S. B., McHenry, P. L., Phillips, J. F., and Lowe, D. K.: The Effect of Aortocoronary Bypass Grafts on Myocardial Blood Flow Reserve and Treadmill Exercise Tolerance, *Circulation*, 50:685, 1974.

160 Benchimol, A., and Desser, K. B.: Measurement of Phasic Aortocoronary Bypass Graft Blood Flow Velocity in Conscious Man, *Am. J. Cardiol.*, 32:895, 1973.

161 Kreulen, T. H., Kirk, E. S., Gorlin, R., Cohn, L. H., and Collins, J. J., Jr.: Coronary Artery Bypass Surgery: Assessment of Revascularization by Determination of Blood Flow and Myocardial Mass, *Am. J.Cardiol.*, 34(2):129, 1974.

162 Greene, D. G., Klocke, F. J., Schimert, G. L., Bunnell, I. L., Wittenberg, S. M., and Lajos, T.: Evaluation of Venous Bypass Grafts from Aorta to Coronary Artery by Inert Gas Desaturation and Direct Flowmeter Techniques, *J. Clin. Invest.*, 51(1):191, 1972.

163 Botti, R. E., and MacIntyre, W. J.: Evaluation of Surgical Revascularization of the Myocardium by Peripheral [43]K Injection, *Circulation*, 48(suppl. 4):118, 1973.

164 Zaret, B. L., Martin, N. D., McGowan, R. L., Wells, H. P., and Flamm, M. D.: Potassium-43 Myocardial Imaging for Noninvasive Assessment of Regional Perfusion Following Aortocoronary Bypass Surgery, *Circulation*, 48(suppl. 4):118, 1973.

165 Hamilton, G. W., Lapin, E. S., Murray, J. A., and Allen, D.: Evaluation of Coronary Artery Surgery by ^{99m}Tc MAA Myocardial Perfusing Imaging, *Circulation*, 48(suppl. 4):118, 1973.

166 Goldberg, A. D., Crawley, J. C. W., Raferty, E. B., and Yacoub, M. H.: Myocardial Blood Flow Following Saphenous Vein Bypass Surgery, *Circulation*, 52(suppl. 1):215, 1975.

167 Lurie, A. J., Salel, A. F., Berman, D. S., DeNardo, G. L., Hurley, E. J., and Mason, D. T.: Determination of Improved Myocardial Perfusion After Aortocoronary Bypass Surgery by Exercise Rubidium-81 Scintigraphy, *Circulation*, 54(6):III-20, 1976.

168 Ritchie, J. L., Narahara, K. A., Trobaugh, G. B., Williams, D. L., and Hamilton, G. W.: Thallium-201 Myocardial Imaging Before and After Coronary Revascu-

larization. Assessment of Regional Myocardial Blood Flow and Graft Patency, *Circulation*, 56(5):830, 1977.

169 Korbuly, D. E., Formanek, A., Gypser, G., Moore, R., Ovitt, T. W., Tuna, N., and Amplatz, K.: Regional Myocardial Blood Flow Measurements Before and After Coronary Bypass Surgery. A Preliminary Report, *Circulation*, 52:38, 1975.

170 Lichtlen, P., Moccetti, T., Halter, J., Schonbeck, M., and Senning, A.: Postoperative Evaluation of Myocardial Blood Flow in Aorta-to-Coronary Artery Vein Bypass Grafts Using the Xenon-Residue Detection Technic, *Circulation*, 46:445, 1972.

171 Lichtlen, P., Moccetti, T., Halter, J., and Galliker, K.: Coronary Heart Disease, in Kaltenback, P. Lichtlen, and G. C. Fresinger (eds.), "Second International Symposium at Frankfurt," George Thieme Publishers, Stuttgart, 1972, p. 286.

172 Rutishauser, W., Noseda, G., Bussmann W-D, and Preter, B.: Blood Flow Measurement Through Single Coronary Arteries by Roentgen Densitometry, *Am. J. Roentgenol. Radium Ther. Nucl. Med.*, 109(1):21, 1970.

173 Smith, H. C., Frye, R. L., Wood, E. H., Davis, G. D., Danielson, G. K., Pluth, J. R., and Wallace, R. B.: Sequential Measurement of Saphenous Vein Graft Flows and Dimensions, *Circulation*, 46(suppl. 2):68, 1972.

174 Smith, H. C., Frye, R. L., Donald, D. E., Davis, G. D., Pluth, J. R., Sturm, R. E., and Wood, E. H.: Roentgen Videodensitometric Measure of Coronary Blood Flow. Determination from Simultaneous Indicator-Dilution Curves at Selected Sites in the Coronary Circulation and in Coronary Artery–Saphenous Vein Grafts, *Mayo Clin. Proc.*, 46:800, 1971.

175 Diettrich, F. B.: Discussion of Grondin et al., *Ann. Thorac. Surg.*, 14:223, 1972.

176 Sheldon, W. C.: Factors Influencing Patency of Coronary Bypass Grafts, *Cleve. Clin. Q.*, 45:109, 1978.

177 Chatterjee, K., Matloff, J. M., Swan, J. H. C., Ganz, W., Sustaita, H., Magnusson, P., Buchbinder, N., Henis, M., and Forrester, J. S.: Improved Angina Threshold and Coronary Reserve Following Direct Myocardial Revascularization, *Circulation*, 51,52 (suppl. 1):81, 1975.

178 Hammond, G. L.: Metabolic Response of the Myocardium to Aorta-Coronary Artery Vein Grafting, *Circulation*, 41, 42(suppl. 3):163, 1970.

179 Kremkau, E. L., Kloster, F. E., and Neill, W. A.: Influence of Aortocoronary Bypass on Myocardial Hypoxia, *Circulation*, 44(suppl. 2):103, 1971.

180 Beer, N., Keller, N., Apstein, C., Kline, S., Tarjan, E., Carlson, R. G., and Brachfeld, N.: The Cardiac Hemodynamic and Metabolic Responses to Coronary Arteriovenous Bypass Surgery, *Am. J. Cardiol.*, 29:252, 1972.

181 Smullens, S. N., Wiener, L., Kasparian, H., Brest, A. N., Bacharach, B., Noble, P. H., and Templeton, J. Y.: Evaluation and Surgical Management of Acute Evolving

Myocardial Infarction, *J. Thorac. Cardiovasc. Surg.,* 64(4):495, 1972.

182 Carlson, R. G., Kline, S., Apstein, C., Scheidt, S., Brachfeld, N., Killip, T., and Lillehei, C. W.: Lactate Metabolism After Aorto-Coronary Artery Vein Bypass Grafts, *Ann. Surg.,* 176:680, 1972.

183 Piccone, V., Sawyer, P., LeVeen, H., Manoli, A., Thompson, E., Oran, E., Sass, M., Lauterstein, J., and Summers, D.: The Mechanism of Anginal Relief Following Direct Cardiac Revascularization, *Chest,* 64(3):405, 1973.

184 Moran, S. V., Tarazi, R. C., Urzua, J. U., Favaloro, R. G., and Effler, D. B.: Effects of Aorto-coronary Bypass on Myocardial Contractility, *J. Thorac. Cardiovasc. Surg.,* 65(3):335, 1973.

185 Anderson, R. P.: Effects of Coronary Bypass Graft Occlusion on Left Ventricular Performance, *Circulation,* 46:507, 1972.

186 Wechsler, A. S., Gill, C., Rosenfeldt, F., Oldham, H. N., and Sabiston, D. C., Jr.: Augmentation of Myocardial Contractility by Aorto-coronary Bypass Grafts in Patients and Experimental Animals, *J. Thorac. Cardiovasc. Surg.,* 64(6):861, 1972.

187 Bolooki, H., Rubinson, R. M., Michie, D. D., and Jude, J. R.: Assessment of Myocardial Contractility After Coronary Bypass Grafts, *J. Thorac. Cardiovasc. Surg.,* 62:543, 1971.

188 Boudoulas, H., Lewis, R. P., Karayannacos, P. E., and Vasko, J. S.: Effect of Saphenous Vein Graft Surgery Upon Left Ventricular Function, *Am. J. Cardiol.,* 31:122, 1973.

189 Chatterjee, K., Swan, H. J. C., Parmley, W. W., Sustaita, H., Marcus, H. S., and Matloff, J.: Influence of Direct Myocardial Revascularization on Left Ventricular Asynergy and Function in Patients with Coronary Heart Disease, With and Without Previous Myocardial Infarction, *Circulation,* 47:276, 1973.

190 Young, W. G., Jr., Sabiston, D. C., Jr., Ebert, P. A., Oldham, H. N., Behar, V. S., Kong, Y., Peter, R. H., and Morris, J. J., Jr.: Preoperative Assessment of Left Ventricular Function in Patients Selected for Direct Myocardial Revascularization, *Ann. Thorac. Surg.,* 11(5):395, 1971.

191 Rutherford, B. D., Gau, G. T., Danielson, G. K., Pluth, J. R., Davis, George D., Wallace, R. B., and Frye, R. L.: Left Ventricular Haemodynamics Before and Soon After Saphenous Vein Bypass Graft Operation for Angina Pectoris, *Br. Heart J.,* 34:1156, 1972.

192 Bolooki, H., Mallon, S., Ghahramani, A., Sommer, L., Vargas, A., Slavin, D., and Kaiser, G. A.: Objective Assessment of the Effects of Aorto-coronary Bypass Operation on Cardiac Function, *J. Thorac. Cardiovasc. Surg.,* 66:916, 1973.

193 Roskamm, H., Rentrop, P., Schnellbacher, K., Lonne, E., Hahn, C., Schmuziger, M., and Faidutti, B.: Factors

Influencing Hemodynamic Improvement After Aortocoronary Bypass Surgery, in P. R. Lichtlen (ed.) "Coronary Angiography and Angina Pectoris," Thieme Edition/Publishing Sciences Group, Inc., Stuttgart, 1976.

194 Bourassa, M. G.: Left Ventricular Performance Following Direct Myocardial Revascularization, *Circulation,* 48(5):915, 1973.

195 Hellman, C., and Schmidt, D.: First Pass RAO Radionuclide Angiography After Nitroglycerin to Assess Myocardial Viability, *Clin. Res.,* 26:239A, 1978.

196 Jacob, K., Chabot, M., Saltiel, J., and Campeau, L.: Improvement of Left Ventricular Asynergy Following Aortocoronary Bypass Surgery Related to Preoperative Electrocardiogram and Vectorcardiogram, *Am. Heart J.,* 86(4):438, 1973.

197 Arbogast, R., Solignac, A., and Bourassa, M. G.: Influence of Aortocoronary Saphenous Vein Bypass Surgery on Left Ventricular Volumes and Ejection Fraction, *Am. J. Med.,* 54:290, 1973.

198 Neuhaus, K. L., Bornikoel, K., Kreuzer, H., and Niessen, H. W.: Left Ventricular Myocardial Function Before and After Coronary Surgery, in P. R. Lichtlen (ed.), "Coronary Angiography and Angina Pectoris," Thieme Edition/Publishing Sciences Group, Inc., Stuttgart, 1976, p. 249.

199 Suzuki, A., Kaye, E. B., and Hardy, J. D.: Direct Anastomosis of the Bilateral Internal Mammary Artery to the Distal Coronary Artery, Without a Magnifier, for Severe Diffuse Coronary Atherosclerosis, *Circulation,* 48 (suppl. 3):190, 1973.

200 Merrill, A. J., Jr., Thomas, C., Schechter, E., Cline, R., Armstrong, R., and Stanford, W.: Coronary Bypass Surgery. Value of Maximal Exercise Testing in Assessment of Results, *Circulation,* 51,52 (suppl. 1):173,1975.

201 Rees, G., Bristow, J. D., Kremkau, E. L., Green, G. S., Herr, R. H., Griswold, H. E., and Starr, A.: Influence of Aortocoronary Bypass Surgery on Left Ventricular Performance, *N. Engl. J. Med.,* 284(20):1116, 1971.

202 Bodenheimer, M. M., Banka, V. S., Fooshee, C., Hermann, G. A., and Helfant, R. H.: Relationship Between Regional Myocardial Perfusion and the Presence, Severity and Reversibility of Asynergy in Patients with Coronary Heart Disease, *Circulation,* 58(5):789, 1978.

203 Bodenheimer, M. M., Banka, V. S., and Helfant, R. H.: Reversible Asynergy and Its Determinants, *Chest,* 69(1):87, 1976.

204 Lea, R. E., Tector, A. J., Flemma, R. J., Johnson, W. D., Beddingfield, G. W., and Lepley, D., Jr.: Prognostic Significance of a Reduced Left Ventricular Ejection Fraction in Coronary Artery Surgery, *Circulation,* 46(suppl. 2):49, 1972.

205 Solignac, A., Gueret, P., and Bourassa, M. G.: Influence of Left Ventricular Function on Survival 3 to 4 Years After Aortocoronary Bypass, *Eur. J. Cardiol.,* 2(4):421, 1975.

206 Siegel, W., Lim, J. S., Proudfit, W. L., Sheldon, W. C., and Loop, F. D.: The Spectrum of Exercise Test and Angiographic Correlations in Myocardial Revascularization Surgery, *Circulation,* 51,52 (suppl. 1):156, 1975.

207 Fischl, S. J., Herman, M. V., and Gorlin, R.: The Intermediate Coronary Syndrome, *N. Engl. J. Med.,* 288(23):1193, 1973.

208 Hammermeister, K. E., Kennedy, J. W., Hamilton, G. W., Stewart, D. K., Gould, K. L., Lipscomb, K., and Murray, J. A.: Aortocoronary–Saphenous Vein Bypass. Failure of Successful Grafting to Improve Resting Left Ventricular Function in Chronic Angina, *N. Eng. J. Med.,* 290(4):186, 1974.

209 Meester, G. T., Van den Brand, M., Hugenholtz, P. G., Tiggelaar-de Widt, I., Bos, E., and Nauta, J.: Angiocardiographic and Functional Aspects of the Left Ventricle After Coronary Bypass Surgery, in P. R. Lichtlen (ed.), "Coronary Angiography and Angina Pectoris," Thieme Edition/Publishing Sciences Group, Inc., Stuttgart, 1976, p.228.

210 Sustaita, H., Chatterjee, K., Matloff, J. M., Marty, A. T., Swan, H. J. C., and Fields, J.: Emergency Bypass Surgery in Impending and Complicated Acute Myocardial Infarction, *Arch. Surg.,* 105(1):30, 1972.

211 Brundage, B. H., Anderson, W. T., Davia, J. E., Cheitlin, M. D., and deCastro, C. M.: Determinants of Left Ventricular Function Following Aorto-coronary Bypass Surgery, *Am. Heart J.,* 93(6):687, 1977.

212 Najmi, M., Ushiyama, K., Blanco, G., Adam, A., and Segal, B. L.: Results of Aortocoronary Artery Saphenous Vein Bypass Surgery for Ischemic Heart Disease, *Am. J. Cardiol.,* 33:42, 1974.

213 Bourassa, M. G., Campeau, L., Lesperance, J., Saltiel, J., Castonguay, Y., Grondin, P., and David, P.: Etude des Modifications de la Dynamique et de la Fonction Ventriculaire Gauche Après Pontage Aorto-coronarien, *Arch Mal. Coeur,* 65(4):417, 1972.

214 Lapin, E. S., Murray, J. A., and Bruce, R. A.: A New Hypothesis to Improve Selection of Patients for Saphenous Vein Graft Surgery, *Am. J. Cardiol.,* 31:144, 1973.

215 Matlof, H. J., Alderman, E. L., Wexler, L., Shumway, N. E., and Harrison, D. C.: What Is the Relationship Between the Response of Angina to Coronary Surgery and Anatomical Success?, *Circulation,* 47,48(suppl. 3):168, 1973.

216 Vlietstra, R. E., Chesebro, J. H., Frye, R. L., and Wallace, R. B.: Exercise Hemodynamic Improvement After Aorto-coronary Artery Bypass Surgery, *Am. J. Cardiol.,* 41:410, 1978.

217 Miller, D. W., Jr., and Dodge, H. T.: Benefits of Coronary Artery Bypass Surgery, *Arch. Intern. Med.,* 137:1439, 1977.

218 Bartel, A. G., Behar, V. S., Peter, R. H., Orgain, E. S., and Kong, Y.: Exercise Stress Testing in Evaluation of Aortocoronary Bypass Surgery. Report of 123 Patients, *Circulation,* 48:141, 1973.

219 Barry, W. H., Pfiefer, J. F., Lipton, M. J., Tilkian, A. G., and Hultgren, H. N.: Effects of Coronary Artery Bypass Grafting on Resting and Exercise Hemodynamics in Patients with Stable Angina Pectoris: A Prospective Randomized Study, *Am. J. Cardiol.,* 37:823, 1976.

220 Miller, S. E. P., Johnson, W. D., Tector, A. J., Manley, J. C., and Gale, H. H.: The Effect of Myocardial Revascularization on Anginal Symptoms, Ventricular Function and Exercise Performance, *Circulation,* 46(suppl. 2): 24, 1972.

221 Amsterdam, E. Z., Hughes, J. L., Demaria, A. N., Zelis, R., and Mason, D. T.: Indirect Assessment of Myocardial Oxygen Consumption in the Evaluation of Mechanisms and Therapy of Angina Pectoris, *Am. J. Cardiol.,* 33:737, 1974.

222 Amsterdam, E. A., and Mason, D. T.: Preop and Postop Stress Evaluation in the Assessment of Coronary Artery Bypass Grafts, *Cleve. Clin. Q.,* 45:121, 1977.

223 Kitamura, K., Jorgensen, C. R., Gobel, F. L., Taylor, H. L., and Wang, Y.: Hemodynamic Correlates of Myocardial Oxygen Consumption During Upright Exercise, *J. Appl. Physiol.,* 32(4):516, 1972.

224 Gobel, F. L., Nordstrom, L. A., Nelson, R. R., Jorgensen, C. R., and Wang, Y.: The Rate-Pressure Product as an Index of Myocardial O_2 Consumption During Exercise in Patients with Angina Pectoris, *Circulation,* 57:549, 1978.

225 Mnayer, M., Chahine, R. A., and Raizner, A. E.: Mechanisms of Angina Relief in Patients After Coronary Artery Bypass Surgery, *Br. Heart J.,* 39:605, 1977.

226 McDonough, J. R., Danielson, R. A., and Foster, R. K.: Maximal Cardiac Output Before and After Coronary Artery Surgery in Patients with Angina, *Am. J. Cardiol.,* 33:154, 1974.

227 McDonough, J. R., Foster, R. K., Danielson, R. A., and Wills, R. E.: Maximal Cardiac Output in Angina Patients Before and After Coronary Artery Surgery, *Jpn. Circ. J.,* 40:343, 1976.

228 Manley, J. C.: Postoperative Assessment of Left Ventricular Function, *Cleve. Clin. Q.,* 45:116, 1978.

229 Thompson, R., Ahmed, R., Sabra-Gomez, R., Richards, A., Towers, M., and Yacoub, M.: The Effect of Surgical vs. Medical Treatment on L. V. Function in Patients with Stable Angina. A Prospective Randomized Study, *Circulation,* 50:729, October 1977. (Abstract.)

230 McLaughlin, P. R., Berman, N. D., Morton, B. C., McLoughlin, M. J., Aldridge, H. E., Adelman, A. G., Goldman, B. S., Trimble, A. S., and Morch, J. E.: Saphenous Vein Bypass Grafting. Changes in Native Circulation and Collaterals, *Circulation,* 51,52(suppl. 1):66, 1975.

231 Glassman, E., Krauss, K. R., Wissinger, B., and Spencer, F. C.: The Effect of Bypass Grafting on the Coronary Circulation, *Circulation*, 48(suppl. 4):53, 1973.

232 Solignac, A., Campeau, L., and Bourassa, M.: Regression and Appearance of Coronary Collaterals in Humans During Life, *Circulation*, 48(suppl. 4):92,1973.

233 Block, T., English, M., and Murray, J. A.: Changes in Exercise Performance Following Unsuccessful Coronary Artery Bypass Grafting, *Am. J. Cardiol.*, 37:122, 1976.

234 Ross, R. S.: Ischemic Heart Disease: An Overview, *Am. J. Cardiol.*, 36:496, 1975.

235 Bulkley, B. H., and Ross, R. S.: Coronary-Artery Bypass Surgery: It Works, But Why?, *Ann. Intern. Med.*, 88:835, 1978.

236 Bulkley, B. H., Humphries, J.O., and Hutchins, G. M.: Purulent Pericarditis with Asymmetric Cardiac Tamponade: A Cause of Death Months After Coronary Artery Bypass Surgery, *Am. Heart J.*, 93(6):776, 1977.

237 Evans, C. L., and Matsoutka, Y.: The Effects of Various Mechanical Conditions on the Gaseous Exchange Metabolism and Efficiency of the Mammalian Heart, *J. Physiol.*, 49:378, 1915.

238 Bedard, P., Taylor, G., Kem, W. J., and Akyurekla, Y.: Surgery for Coronary Disease and Congestive Heart Failure, *Circulation*, 48(suppl. 4):143, 1973.

239 Cooley, D. A.: Ventricular Aneurysms and Akinesis, *Cleve. Clin. Q.*, 45:130, 1978.

240 Rivera, R., and Delcan, J. L.: Ventricular Aneurysms and Akinesis, *Cleve. Clin. Q.*, 45:133, 1978.

241 DeWeese, J. A., Moss, A. J., and Yu, P. N.: Infarctectomy and Closure Ventricular Septal Defect Following Myocardial Infarction, *Circulation*, 43, 44(suppl. 2):108, 1971.

242 Grondin, P., Donzeau-Gouge, P., Bical, O., and Kretz, J. G.: Combined Valve Replacement or Valvulotomy and Bypass Graft Surgery, *Cleve. Clin. Q.*, 45:123, 1978.

243 Bates, R. J., Beutler, S., Resnekov, L., and Anagnospopoulos, C. E.: Cardiac Rupture—a Challenge in Diagnosis and Management, *Am. J. Cardiol.*, 40:429, 1977.

244 Kay, J. H., Redington, J. V., Mendez, A. M., Zubiate, P., and Dunne, E. F.: Coronary Artery Surgery for the Patient with Impaired Left Ventricular Function, *Circulation*, 46(suppl. 2):49, 1972.

245 Ghahramani, A., Bolooki, H., Sommer, L., Vargas, A., and Mallon, S.: Following Hemodynamic Studies and Survival in Patients Operated on for Intractable Congestive Failure After Acute Myocardial Infarction, *Circulation*, 48(suppl.):168, 1973.

Chapter 6

Effect of Coronary Artery Bypass Graft Surgery on the Exercise Electrocardiogram*

EZRA A. AMSTERDAM, M.D., GARRETT LEE, M.D., NAJAM AWAN, M.D., REGINALD LOW, M.D., ANTHONY N. De MARIA, M.D., and DEAN T. MASON, M.D.

Exercise testing is the most widely utilized noninvasive diagnostic procedure for the detection of coronary artery disease. Although this method encompasses the electrocardiographic, hemodynamic, functional, and symptomatic responses to stress, the exercise electrocardiogram is its principal component for the diagnosis of coronary disease. Based on characteristic electrocardiographic ST-segment displacement as objective evidence of myocardial ischemia and thereby clinically significant obstructive coronary lesions, this method provides objective data that can be applied to both the diagnosis of the disease and the assessment of therapeutic interventions. Because of the well-known placebo response to medical and surgical interventions for angina,[1,2] and because there are data that indicate beneficial effects of myocardial revascularization on anginal symptoms by mechanisms unrelated to enhanced myocardial perfusion,[3-5] exercise testing has been utilized as an objective, indirect means for determining the efficacy of surgery in augmenting coronary blood flow and diminishing myocardial ischemia. This chapter reviews the basis for application of this method in assessing the results of myocardial revascularization and analyzes current data on this subject.

BASIS OF EXERCISE ELECTROCARDIOGRAPHY IN CORONARY ARTERY DISEASE

Methodology

The principle underlying exercise testing is the provocation, in the presence of coronary artery disease, of electrocardiographic evidence of myocardial ischemia not present at rest by imposing on the patient a stress sufficient to elevate myocardial oxygen requirements beyond the delivery capacity of a restricted coronary circulation. The consequent imbalance between myocardial oxygen supply and demand results in ischemia, which is reflected in the exercise electrocardiogram by ST-segment depression that reverts to control shortly after the stress is terminated. A controlled stress, such as graded treadmill or bicycle exercise, is employed to augment myocardial oxygen requirements. The latter are principally determined by heart rate, myocardial contractility, blood pressure, and ventricular volume,[6] the first three of which are consistently increased by exercise. The criterion for a positive response in the exercise electrocardiogram is horizontal or downsloping ST-segment depression of at least 0.1 mV for 80 ms or more in an ST segment that is normal at rest (Fig. 6-1).

Diagnostic Accuracy

Considerable experience with exercise electrocardiography in the assessment of coronary artery disease has confirmed its usefulness as a noninvasive method that has wide applicability, acceptable diagnostic accuracy, and minimal risk when properly applied. In correlative studies utilizing coronary angiography as the standard of reference and defining a significant coronary artery stenosis as a 70 percent or more decrease in luminal diameter of at least one major coronary vessel, exercise electrocardiography has a diagnostic sensitivity (proportion of patients with coronary artery disease who have positive test results) of approximately 60 to 70 percent and a specificity (proportion of individuals without coronary artery disease who have negative test results) of 85 to 90 percent.[6,7] A number of important clinical factors can be correlated with the occurrence of positive test results. The sensitivity of the method increases with increasing extent of coronary disease and may be 80 percent or more in patients with disease of all three coronary arteries and

*From the Section of Cardiovascular Medicine, Departments of Medicine and Physiology, University of California at Davis School of Medicine and Sacramento Medical Center, Davis and Sacramento.

Supported in part by Research Program Project Grant HL 15780 from the National Heart, Lung and Blood Institute, Bethesda, Maryland and research grants from the Golden Empire Chapter of the American Heart Association.

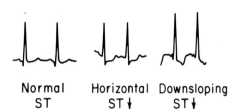

Normal   Horizontal Downsloping
ST   ST↓   ST↓

FIGURE 6-1 ST-segment responses to exercise. Horizontal and downsloping ST↓ are positive responses.

less than 50 percent in those with involvement of only one artery.[7] The predictive accuracy of a positive test result rises with increasing degree of ST-segment depression. Thus, it is highly unusual for a test with more than 2 mm ST-segment depression to give a false positive result.[7] Further, there is a positive correlation between the degree of ST-segment depression and the number of diseased arteries.[7,8] Ischemic ST-segment depression during exercise has also been correlated with increased prognostic risk compared to absence of ischemic response,[9-11] a finding that follows from the relationship of exercise-induced ischemia to the presence and extent of coronary disease[7,8] and the relationship of the latter factors to prognosis.[12]

Assessment of Therapy

Exercise electrocardiography has a number of characteristics of particular importance for serial application in the assessment of a therapeutic intervention. It is a convenient, standardized, relatively inexpensive method, and it provides objective, quantifiable data that are highly reproducible if the disease state is unaltered. Further, the test can be readily repeated to afford long-term evaluation. Consistency in the results of any method employed to assess efficacy of a therapeutic modality is a prerequisite to its application for this purpose. In this regard, several studies have demonstrated excellent reproducibility of the ischemic electrocardiographic response to exercise 1 year after an initial test.[13,14] These findings are in accord with the high degree of consistency of our own results of serial exercise electrocardiography.

Application in Assessment of Coronary Bypass Surgery

On the basis of the foregoing features, exercise electrocardiography has been utilized as an objective means of assessing the efficacy of coronary artery bypass graft surgery in reducing myocardial ischemia. Thus, conversion of an exercise-induced ischemic ST-segment response to normal is consistent with enhanced myocardial perfusion and oxygen delivery and alleviation of ischemia. Although not yet documented, such an effect may also have beneficial implications for prognosis because of the relation of the latter to the ST-segment response to exercise, as previously noted.[9-11]

It must be emphasized that exercise electrocardiography is an indirect method for assessing the presence or absence of myocardial ischemia. This approach, therefore, provides no direct evidence regarding coronary blood flow or myocardial oxygen supply. Furthermore, the ST-segment response to exercise can be affected by a number of nonspecific factors.[7,8] Thus, alterations in the exercise electrocardiogram by nontherapeutic variables must be considered in the application of this method to assessment of therapeutic modalities for coronary artery disease. The results of exercise electrocardiography should therefore be interpreted with caution and awareness of its limitations. Nevertheless, when the test is applied in the absence of nonspecific factors that can influence the ST-segment response to exercise,[7,8] this method provides meaningful data for objective assessment of the physiological efficacy of coronary bypass graft surgery. As with all diagnostic methods, optimal application of exercise electrocardiography is predicated on an appreciation of its values and limitations, an understanding of its indications and contraindications, and an interpretation of results in the context of the total clinical evaluation.

EXERCISE ELECTROCARDIOGRAPHY IN THE ASSESSMENT OF CORONARY ARTERY BYPASS GRAFT SURGERY

Criteria of Improvement

Conclusions regarding electrocardiographic evidence of decrease or absence of exercise-induced myocardial ischemia following coronary bypass graft surgery require fulfillment of the following criteria: diminution in the degree of ST-segment depression as compared to the preoperative result at a level of myocardial stress equivalent to or greater than that at which evidence of ischemia developed preoperatively. Myocardial stress is reflected by the heart rate or, preferably, the heart rate–blood pressure product, both of which are indirect indexes of myocardial oxygen demand.[15] In this regard, the external work presented to the skeletal muscles, in terms of treadmill speed and grade, does not reflect the stress on the heart, since the circulatory response to an external workload may differ from that of the body's, depending on factors such as conditioning.[15] Therefore, although it is important to perform preoperative and postoperative exercise testing according to the same protocol, the duration of exercise and the work achieved cannot be utilized as indications of comparative cardiac stress in assessing the exercise electrocardiogram. Ideally, the latter should be compared before and after surgery at the same heart rate–blood pressure product or, at least, at the same heart rate.

Clinical Studies

Investigations of the comparative results of exercise electrocardiography before and after coronary artery bypass surgery have demonstrated a favorable effect of this therapy in a large majority of patients, many of whom have had striking, objective evidence of improvement. Exercise-induced myocardial ischemia is commonly abolished or diminished at a higher level of cardiac performance, as indicated by the heart rate or product of heart rate and systolic blood pressure (double product),[15] in comparison to the preoperative threshold for ischemic ST-segment depression, as indicated by these variables. The data in Fig. 6-2 demonstrate a successful result of coronary bypass graft surgery on symptoms, functional capacity, exercise electrocardiogram, and hemodynamic determinants of myocardial oxygen consumption (double product of heart rate and systolic blood pressure). The favorable alteration of each of these parameters is consistent with enhanced myocardial oxygen delivery and decreased ischemia. Similarly, most reports of improvement in the exercise electrocardiogram also demonstrate beneficial effects on other preoperative clinical limitations resulting from coronary heart disease. However, the importance of the exercise electrocardiogram derives from the objective data it provides that is so closely related to myocardial ischemia.

Studies of the effect of coronary artery bypass graft surgery on the exercise electrocardiogram have been presented in the literature in several ways. Most have reported the results of preoperative and postoperative exercise electrocardiography in terms of the proportion of patients whose test results have changed from positive to negative following surgery.[5,16-21] A number of investigations have further analyzed these results in relation to graft patency, providing essential data from which to infer the potential of the surgical procedure, when anatomically successful, to augment myocardial nutritional blood flow and reduce ischemia.[5,18-22] Quantitation of group mean ST-segment depression before and after surgery has also been reported.[14,21] These studies have usually included exercise heart rate, blood pressure, or double product, as well as functional capacity, as indicated by intensity and duration of exercise. The results herein reviewed are obtained primarily from studies that present preoperative and postoperative exercise electrocardiographic data in relation to a hemodynamic measurement of myocardial oxygen demand, thereby affording a means of relating the relative level of myocardial stress to the electrocardiographic result before and after surgery.

EFFECT ON QUANTITATIVE ST-SEGMENT DEPRESSION

In a study comparing medical and surgical treatment of angina, the quantitative effects of therapy on the exercise electrocardiogram were analyzed.[14] As indicated in Table 6-1, exercise-induced ST-segment depression was equivalent in 42 medical and 42 surgical patients at entry into the study. After 1 year, repeat exercise testing demonstrated that ST-segment depression in the coronary bypass graft group was significantly less than at entry and also significantly less than that demonstrated in the medical group after 1 year of therapy. Furthermore, the diminution of evidence of exercise-induced myocardial ischemia in the surgical patients was associated with a significantly

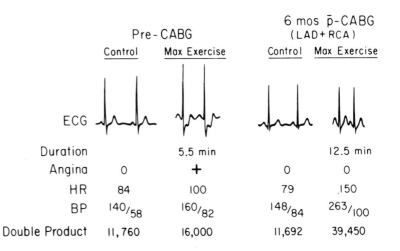

FIGURE 6-2 Preoperative and postoperative treadmill exercise tests in a patient with coronary heart disease who received coronary bypass grafts to the left anterior descending and right coronary arteries. Blood pressure was measured by brachial artery catheter. *(From E. A. Amsterdam et al., Exercise Testing in the Indirect Assessment of Myocardial Oxygen Consumption: Application for Evaluation of Mechanisms and Therapy of Angina Pectoris, in E. A. Amsterdam, J. H. Wilmore, and A. N. DeMaria (eds.), "Exercise in Cardiovascular Health and Disease," Yorke Medical Books, New York, 1977, Chap. 15, pp. 218-233.)*

	Pre-CABG		6 mos p̄-CABG (LAD+RCA)	
	Control	Max Exercise	Control	Max Exercise
ECG				
Duration		5.5 min		12.5 min
Angina	O	+	O	O
HR	84	100	79	150
BP	140/58	160/82	148/84	263/100
Double Product	11,760	16,000	11,692	39,450

TABLE 6-1

Exercise Electrocardiography in Medically and Surgically Treated Patients Initially and After 1 Year

	Medical (n=42)	Surgical (n=42)	p
ST-segment depression (mm)			
Initial	1.5	1.7	n.s.
1 year	1.6	0.9	<0.005
p	n.s.	<0.0001	
Peak HR × SBP × 10^{-2}			
Initial	199	212	n.s.
1 year	195	253	<0.0001
p	n.s.	<0.0001	

Source: Tilkian et al.[14]

greater exercise heart rate–systolic blood pressure product, whereas the double product was unchanged in the medical group. Thus, coronary bypass graft surgery resulted in less evidence of myocardial ischemia at a greater level of cardiac oxygen demand, consistent with enhanced oxygen delivery to previously ischemic myocardium.[15] This study also demonstrates the reproducibility of exercise-related ST-segment depression if the physiologic defect in the myocardium is not alleviated, as in the medical patients.

Our results at the University of California, Davis, Medical Center are consistent with these findings (Table 6-2). Of 27 patients with preoperative positive exercise electrocardiograms, ST-segment depression was absent in 17 and decreased in 8 following coronary bypass graft surgery.[21] Heart rate–blood pressure product was significantly elevated after surgery as compared to that achieved preoperatively (24,221 vs. 21,132 p.<0.05). Furthermore, in 3 patients with significantly positive ST-segment responses (2.5 to 4.0 mm depression) before surgery, the abnormality was reduced to 1.0 mm after revascularization. However, on the basis of this ST-segment depression, the test results in these patients are still defined as positive. Thus, evaluation limited only to qualitative analysis of the test may fail to detect quantitative evidence of improvement in some patients. Although most data in the literature are reported only in terms of the sign (positive or negative) of the exercise electrocardiogram, it is apparent that quantitative determination of the ST-segment response is important in assessing the results of surgery on this diagnostic index.

NORMALIZATION OF POSITIVE TEST RESULTS

Abolition of an abnormal exercise test result was reported in 30 of 35 patients evaluated 3 to 8 months after surgery.[23] However, in this investigation an ab-

normality was defined as either exercise-induced ST-segment displacement or angina, and the number of patients with each finding was not indicated. Improvement was documented in 20 patients by absence of the preoperative exercised-induced abnormality at a higher heart rate–blood pressure product than that prior to surgery and in 10 patients by occurrence of angina or ST-segment depression only at a higher double product. Although indicative of beneficial effects of surgery on the exercise electrocardiogram, this report did not specify the actual number of patients demonstrating improvement in this parameter.

The results of seven series dealing specifically with the effect of surgery on the exercise electrocardiogram are summarized in Table 6-2.[5,16-21] These series include 297 patients evaluated 2 to 29 months (average 3 to 9 months) after surgery. It is apparent that coronary artery bypass graft surgery is followed in a relatively high proportion of patients (approximately two-thirds) by conversion to normal of preoperative ischemic ST-segment response to exercise. In addition, this elimination of electrocardiographic evidence of ischemia is consistently manifested at an elevated heart rate or heart rate–blood pressure product after surgery, reflecting abolition of ischemia at a greater level of myocardial oxygen demand.

In assessing this evidence of benefit from coronary bypass graft surgery, influences other than additional blood flow to ischemic myocardium must be considered. Improvement in the stress electrocardiogram cannot be attributed to inadequate intensity of exercise in the foregoing studies, since the heart rate–blood pressure data reflect a higher level of myocardial oxygen demand postoperatively. Although the placebo effect[1,2] and cardiac denervation[24] may influence symptoms, there is no physiological basis for reduction of exercise-induced electrocardiographic evidence of ischemia by these factors. On the other hand, perioperative myocardial infarction is commonly considered a factor that can, by "silencing" segmental areas of myocardial ischemia, contribute to postoperative improvement of clinical status and exercise electrocardiography in some patients.[3-5] However, infarction can also produce additional areas of myocardial ischemia that augment signs and symptoms of the disease and can contribute to deterioration of the exercise electrocardiogram. Thus, it has been shown that loss of preexisting angina following myocardial infarction is actually quite uncommon.[25,26]

A positive exercise electrocardiogram persisted in one-third of patients following surgery (Table 6-2). Although this finding raises the question of graft occlusion or failure of the procedure, other possibilities merit consideration. These alternative explanations include ST-segment depression elicited because a higher heart rate–blood pressure product was reached after

TABLE 6-2
Effect of Coronary Artery Bypass Graft Surgery on Exercise Electrocardiogram

	ST↓			ST↓		
	+ Pre-S	− Post-S	HR or DP Post-S	− Pre-S	+ Post-S	HR or DP Post-S
Lapin et al.[16]	32	20 (63%)	↑	0	1 (100%)	↑
Bartel et al.[17]	68	38 (56%)	↑	11	0 (0%)	
Dodek et al.[18]	32	14 (44%)	↑	13	3 (3%)	↑
Knoebel et al.[19]	13	10 (77%)	↑			
Siegel et al.[20]	114	84 (74%)	↑			
Block et al.[5]	11	6 (55%)		8	1 (13%)	
U. California, Davis[21]	27	21 (78%)	↑	1	1 (100%)	
Total	297	193 (65%)		33	6 (18%)	

HR, heart rate; DP, double product (heart rate × systolic blood pressure); S, coronary bypass graft surgery; +, ST↓ present; −, ST↓ absent; ↑, HR or DP greater post-S than pre-S; (no arrow indicates data not available).

surgery; reduced but residual ST-segment depression of 1.0 mm; ischemia resulting from disease in coronary arteries not technically suitable for grafting; and progression of native coronary disease in grafted or ungrafted coronary vessels. The elevated double product achieved in the studies reviewed suggests the possibility that improvement might have been detected in some of these patients if the ST segment were measured at comparable levels before and after surgery rather than at maximum performance in each of the tests.

The exercise test results changed from negative to positive following surgery in less than 20% of patients (Table 6-2). Possible causes of this finding, in addition to increased myocardial ischemia related to graft occlusion (which may also involve the grafted coronary vessels), are progression of disease in the native coronary circulation, perioperative myocardial infarction, and exercise to a higher heart rate–blood pressure product than preoperatively, with resultant provocation of myocardial ischemia at a level of myocardial oxygen demand not attained prior to surgery. In this regard, in the two studies in which data were available, heart rate or double product increased in association with conversion of the exercise test results from negative to positive.[16,18] Data regarding perioperative infarction were not available in these studies.

RELATIONSHIP OF GRAFT PATENCY TO THE EXERCISE ELECTROCARDIOGRAM

Data on the relationship of graft patency to alterations in the exercise electrocardiogram provide essential information on the potential of the surgical procedure to alleviate myocardial ischemia as reflected by this diagnostic method. Our findings, indicated in Fig. 6-3, demonstrate a close correlation between graft patency

and decreased electrocardiographic evidence of myocardial ischemia. As in our previously cited results, the postoperative normalization of preoperative, exercise-provoked ST-segment depression is associated with a higher heart rate than that achieved before surgery. In addition, the quantitative data in Fig. 6-3 reveal, in 2 patients with patent grafts and persistently positive test results, considerable reduction of ST-segment depression from 4.0 to 1.0 mm. Thus, all patients with one or more patent grafts in this series had objective findings consistent with decreased myocardial ischemia. In the group with occluded grafts, 2 patients demonstrated conversion of the exercise electrocardiogram from positive to negative, 2 had persistently positive results, and in 1 patient the test results changed from negative to positive. It is noteworthy

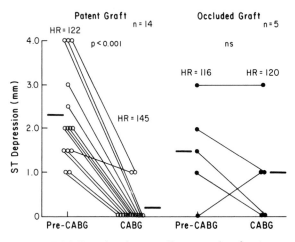

FIGURE 6-3 Exercise electrocardiogram and graft patency. Normalization or improvement in ST-segment response at elevated heart rate was associated with graft patency; with occluded grafts, results were inconsistent, and there was no increase in heart rate.

TABLE 6-3
Relation of Exercise Electrocardiogram to Status of Coronary Bypass Grafts

	Number of patients	Graft patency		+Pre, −post CABGs	−Pre, −post CABGs	+Pre, +post CABGs	−Pre, +post CABGs
Dodek et al.[18]	41	≥1 patent	34	12	9	10	3
		0 patent	7			7	
Knoebel et al.[19]	13	≥1 patent	11	10		1	
		0 patent	2			2	
Siegel et al.[20]	114	≥1 patent	112	84		28*	
		0 patent	2			2	
Hartman et al.[22]	22	≥1 patent	14	10		4	
		0 patent	8	3		5	
Block et al.[5]	19	≥1 patent	0	6	7	5	1
		0 patent	19				
U. California, Davis[21]	19	≥1 patent	14	12		2	
		0 patent	5	2		2	1
Total	228	≥ patent	185	128 (69%)	9 (5%)	45 (24%)	3 (2%)
		0 patent	43	11 (25%)	7 (16%)	23 (54%)	2 (5%)

*Postoperative exercise ST↓ associated with significantly higher heart rate x systolic blood pressure.

that in the group with occluded grafts, electrocardiographic improvement was not associated with elevation of the postoperative exercise heart rate. None of these patients had perioperative infarctions, and the explanation for the improvement in two is thus not apparent.

In six reports of 228 patients with correlative exercise and angiographic data (Table 6-3), more than two-thirds of patients with one or more patent grafts demonstrated postoperative abolition of preoperative, exercise-induced ST-segment depression.[15,18-22] Furthermore, in Siegel's study, in which 29 patients had positive preoperative and postoperative tests, the latter were recorded at higher heart rate–blood pressure products,[20] suggesting the possibility of a negative test result at exercise to the preoperative double product. Of considerable interest and practical importance are the data in Table 6-3 indicating that conversion of a positive preoperative exercise electrocardiogram to negative postoperatively in the total group of 139 patients with this result was associated with patency of one or more coronary bypass grafts in 128 patients (92 percent). Thus, normalization of an ischemic ST-segment response to exercise is a strong indicator of graft patency. However, the converse is not true to a similar degree; that is, 69 percent of patients with patent grafts demonstrated conversion of a positive exercise electrocardiogram to negative.

The study of Block et al. deals with a group of patients in whom all coronary artery bypass grafts were occluded (Table 6-3).[5] In six of 11 patients, a positive preoperative exercise electrocardiogram converted to a negative result. The authors conclude that interim myocardial infarction, by eliminating zones of myocardial ischemia, may have been an important factor in favorably altering exercise performance in pa-

tients postoperatively. However, only 2 of the 6 patients with improved exercise electrocardiograms had had infarction. It is also possible that these patients exercised to a lower heart rate–blood pressure product after surgery than before, and thus the threshold for myocardial ischemia may not have been reached. However, this cannot be determined, since individual double product data during exercise are not presented.

Nuclear Cardiologic Stress Studies

It is of interest that the findings of exercise electrocardiography consistent with physiologic efficacy of coronary bypass surgery have been confirmed and extended by nuclear cardiologic techniques that reflect segmental myocardial perfusion and function. Thus, evidence of augmented myocardial perfusion to previously ischemic areas of the left ventricle has been demonstrated by exercise myocardial scintigraphy,[27] radionuclide cineangiography in patients following bypass surgery has documented improvement in exercise-induced left ventricular regional wall motion abnormalities, presumably as a result of increased myocardial blood flow to ischemic segments.[28] These findings are in accord with those of exercise electrocardiography in providing objective evidence consistent with increased myocardial perfusion following coronary artery bypass graft surgery.

SUMMARY

Exercise electrocardiography is an objective method of determining the efficacy of coronary artery bypass graft surgery in alleviating myocardial ischemia, as reflected by the response of the S-T segment to exercise. This indirect index must be interpreted with an appreciation of its limitations and the nonspecific factors that can influence it. In more than two-thirds of patients, coronary bypass graft surgery is associated with conversion to normal of a preoperative ischemic exercise electrocardiogram. Furthermore, normaliza-tion of the exercise electrocardiogram reliably predicts graft patency, as indicated by the more than 90 percent correlation in the series reviewed. Exercise electro-cardiographic data support the efficacy of coronary bypass graft surgery in reducing myocardial ischemia, and this diagnostic method is valuable in assessing surgical therapy for coronary artery disease.

REFERENCES

1 Dimond, E. G., Kittle, C. G., and Crockett, J. E.: Comparison of Internal Mammary Artery Ligation and Sham Operation for Angina Pectoris, *Am. J. Cardiol.*, 5:483, 1960.

2 Amsterdam, E. A., Wolfson, S., and Gorlin, R.: New Aspects of the Placebo Response in Angina Pectoris. (Editorial), *Am. J. Cardiol.*, 24:305, 1969.

3 Achuff S. C., Griffith L. S. C., Conti, C. R., et al.: The ''Angina Producing'' Myocardial Segment: An Approach to the Interpretation of Results of Coronary Bypass Surgery, *Am. J. Cardiol.*, 36:723, 1975.

4 DiLuzio, V., Roy, P. R., and Sowton, E.: Angina in Patients with Occluded Aortocoronary Vein Grafts, *Br. Heart J.*, 36:139, 1974.

5 Block, T. A., Murray, J. A., and English, M. T.: Improvement in Exercise Performance After Unsuccessful Myocardial Revascularization, *Am. J. Cardiol.*, 40:673, 1977.

6 Sonnenblick, E. H., and Skelton, C. L.: Oxygen Consumption of the Heart: Physiological Principles and Clinical Implications, *Mod. Concepts Cardiovasc. Dis.*, 40:9, 1971.

7 McHenry, P., and Morris, S. N.: Exercise Electrocardiography—Current State of the Art, in R. Schlant and J. W. Hurst (eds.), ''Advances in Electrocardiography,'' Vol. 2, Grune & Stratton, New York, 1976, p. 265.

8 Fortuin, N. J., and Weiss, J. L.: Exercise Stress Testing, *Circulation*, 56:699, 1977.

9 Robb, G. P., and Seltzer, F.: Appraisal of the Double Two-Step Exercise Test: A Long-term Follow-up of 3,325 Men, *JAMA*, 234:722, 1975.

10 Amsterdam, E. A., and Mason, D. T.: Prognostic Importance of Exercise Tests, in W. E. James and E. A. Amsterdam, (eds.), ''Coronary Heart Disease, Exercise Testing and Cardiac Rehabilitation,'' Symposia Specialists, Miami, 1977, pp. 183–193.

11 McNeer, J. F., Margolis, J. R., Lee, K. L., Kisslo, J. A., Peter, R. H., Kong, Y., Behar, V. S., Wallace, A. G., McCants, C. B., and Rosati, R. A.: The Role of the Exercise Test in the Evaluation of Patients for Ischemic Heart Disease, *Circulation*, 57:64, 1978.

12 Bruschke, A. V. G., Proudfit, W. G., and Sones, F. M.: Progress Study of 590 Consecutive Nonsurgical Cases of Coronary Disease Followed 5-9 Years. 1. Arteriographic Correlations, *Circulation*, 47:1147, 1973.

13 Doan, A. E., Peterson, D. R., Blackmon, J. R., and Bruce, R. A.: Myocardial Ischemia After Maximal Exercise in Healthy Men. One Year Follow-up of Physically Active and Inactive Men, *Am. J. Cardiol.*, 17:9, 1966.

14 Tilkian, A. G., Pfeifer, J. F., Barry, W. H., Lipton, M. J., and Hultgren, H. N.: The Effect of Coronary Bypass Surgery on Exercise-induced Ventricular Arrhythmias, *Am. Heart J.*, 92:707, 1976.

15 Amsterdam, E. A., Price, J. E., Berman, D., Hughes, J. L., Riggs, K., DeMaria, A. N., Miller, R. R., and Mason, D. T.: Exercise Testing in the Indirect Assessment of Myocardial Oxygen Consumption: Application for Evaluation of Mechanisms and Therapy of Angina Pectoris, in ''Exercise in Cardiovascular Health and Disease,'' E. A. Amsterdam, J. H. Wilmore, and A. N. DeMaria (eds.), Yorke Medical Books, New York, 1977.

16 Lapin, E. S., Murray, J. A., Bruce, R. A., and Winterscheid, L.: Changes in Maximal Exercise Performance in the Evaluation of Saphenous Vein Bypass Surgery, *Circulation*, 47:1164, 1973.

17 Bartel, A. G., Behar, V. S., Peter, R. H., Orgain, E. S., and Kong, Y.: Exercise Stress Testing in Evaluation of Aortocoronary Bypass Surgery. Report of 123 Patients, *Circulation*, 48:141, 1973.

18 Dodek, A., Kassebaum, D. G., and Griswold, H. E.: Stress Electrocardiography in the Evaluation of Aortocoronary Bypass Surgery, *Am. Heart J.*, 86:292, 1973.

19 Knoebel, S. B., McHenry, P., Phillips, J. E., and Lowe, D. K.: The Effect of Aortocoronary Bypass Grafts on Myocardial Blood Flow Reserve and Treadmill Exercise Tolerance, *Circulation*, 50:685, 1974.

20 Siegel, W., Lim, J. S., Proudfit, W. L., Sheldon, W. C., and Loop, F. L.: The Spectrum of Exercise Test and Angiographic Correlations in Myocardial Revascularization Surgery, *Circulation*, 51,52 (suppl. 1):156, 1973.

21 Grehl, T., Amsterdam, E. A., Matthews, E., DeMaria, A. N., Miller, R. R., Price, J. E., Lee, G., Lurie, A. J., Hurley, E. J., and Mason, D.T.: Evaluation of Coronary Bypass Graft Surgery by Exercise Testing: Objective Assessment by Effect on Ischemic ST Depression, Heart Rate–Blood Pressure Product and Correlation with Postoperative Angiography, *Am. J. Cardiol.*, 39:268, 1977.

22 Hartman, C. W., Kong, Y., Margolis, J. R., Warren, S. G., Peter, R. H., Behar, V. S., and Oldham, H. N.: Aortocoronary Bypass Surgery: Correlation of Angiographic, Symptomatic, and Functional Improvement at 1 Year, *Am. J. Cardiol.*, 37:352, 1977.

23 Guiney, T. E., Rubenstein, J. J., Sanders, C. A., and Mundth, E. D.: Functional Evaluation of Coronary Bypass Surgery by Exercise Testing and Oxygen Consumption, *Circulation*, 47, 48 (suppl. 3):141, 1973.

24 Soloff, L. A.: Effects of Coronary Bypass Procedure, *N. Engl. J. Med.*, 288:1302, 1973.

25 Amsterdam, E. A., Lee, G., Mathews, E. A., and Mason, D. T.: Relationship of Myocardial Infarction to Presence of Angina Pectoris in Patients with Coronary Heart Disease: Lack of Abolition of Angina by Infarction, *Clin. Cardiol.*, 1:31, 1978.

26 Kannel, W. B., and Feinlieb, M.: National History of Angina Pectoris in the Framingham Study: Prognosis and Survival, *Am. J. Cardiol.*, 29:154, 1972.

27 Lurie, A. J., Salel, A. F., Berman, D. S., Denardo, G. L., Hurley, E. J., and Mason, Dean T.: Determination of Improved Myocardial Perfusion After Aortocoronary Bypass Surgery by Exercise Rubidium-81 Scintigraphy, *Circulation,* 54:6, 1976.

28 Kent, K. M., Borer, J. S. Green, M. V., Bacharach, S. L., McIntosh, C. L., Conkle, D. M., and Epstein, S. E.: Effects of Coronary Artery Bypass on Global and Regional Left Ventricular Function During Exercise, *N. Engl. J. Med.*, 298:1434, 1978.

The technical assistance of Elizabeth Matthews and the secretarial assistance of Nancy Yudin are gratefully acknowledged by the author.

Chapter 7

The Relief of Angina Pectoris by Coronary Bypass Surgery*

SPENCER B. KING III, M.D., and
J. WILLIS HURST, M.D.

Sir William Osler said in 1910 that angina pectoris is a subject "full of knotty problems which lend themselves to speculation."[1] This best expresses the difficulty in assessing the effects of any therapy for the many symptom complexes that we call angina pectoris.

The first description of chest discomfort likely to have been angina pectoris was given by Lucius Annaeus Seneca (4 B.C.–65 A.D.), the Roman philosopher in describing his own symptoms.[2] It was, however, William Heberden's (1710–1801) description that has become "classic angina."[3]

But there is a disorder of the breast marked with strong and peculiar symptoms, considerable for the kind of danger belonging to it, and not extremely rare, which deserves to be mentioned more at length. The seat of it, and sense of strangling, and anxiety with which it is attended, may make it not improperly be called angina pectoris.

They who are afflicted with it, are seized while they are walking (more especially if it be up hill, and soon after eating), with a painful and most disagreeable sensation in the breast, which seems as if it would extinguish life, if it were to increase or to continue; but the moment they stand still, all this uneasiness vanishes.

In all other respects, the patients are, at the beginning of the disorder, perfectly well, and in particular have no shortness of breath, from which it is totally different. The pain is sometimes situated in the upper part, sometimes in the middle, sometimes at the bottom of the os sterni, and often more inclined to the left than to the right side. It likewise very frequently extends from the breast to the middle of the left arm. The pulse is, at least sometimes, not disturbed by this pain, as I have had opportunities of observing by feeling the pulse during the paroxysm. Males are most liable to this disease, especially such as have past [sic] their fiftieth year.

After it has continued a year or more, it will not cease so instantaneously upon standing still; and it will come on not only when the persons are walking, but when they are lying down, especially if they lie on the left side, and oblige them to rise up out of their beds. In some inveterate cases it has been brought on by the motion of a horse, or a carriage, and even by swallowing, coughing, going to stool, or speaking, or any disturbance of mind.

It was not Heberden but Edward Jenner who linked angina pectoris to coronary sclerosis in 1799.[4] The relationship of angina pectoris to myocardial ischemia

was brilliantly described by the anatomist, Allan Burns, in 1809.[5]

In health, when we excite the muscular system to more energetic action than usual, we increase the circulation in every part, so that to support this increased action, the heart and every other part has its power augmented. If, however, we call into vigorous action, a limb, round which we have with a moderate degree of tightness applied a ligature, we find that then the member can only support its action for a very short time; for now its supply of energy and its expenditure do not balance each other; consequently, it soon, from a deficiency of nervous influence and arterial blood, fails and sinks into a state of quiescence. A heart, the coronary vessels of which are cartilagenous or ossified, is in nearly a similar condition; it can, like the limb, be girt with a moderately light ligature, discharge its functions so long as its action is moderate and equal. Increase, however, the action of the whole body, and along with the rest, that of the heart, and you will soon see exemplified, the truth of what has been said; with this difference, that as there is no interruption to the action of the cardial nerves, the heart will be able to hold out a little longer than the limb.

Although any schoolchild given Burns' experiment could devise a surgical procedure to relieve the ischemia, that was not possible in the early nineteenth century, and in fact the theories of Burns were not widely accepted until well into the twentieth century. Sir James Mackenzie (1853–1925) accepted the ischemic origin of angina pectoris and its relationship to coronary artery obliterative disease.[6]

That a muscle should evoke disagreeable symptoms when overfatigued is a principle applicable to all muscular structures of the body. In looking at the coronary arteries in certain typical cases of angina pectoris, one can reasonably infer one way in which the attacks are brought about. In some cases the coronary arteries are so narrowed as scarce to permit the entrance of a pin. During life the stream of blood must have been greatly reduced, and if it were sufficient to supply the muscle during rest, it was demonstrably insufficient while the heart was in a state of activity. In this respect there seems to be a distinct affinity between the origin of the pain in these cases, and in those cases of what is called intermittent claudication.

Even though few would argue that the relief of leg claudication by removal or bypass of vascular obstructions results from improved perfusion of the limb, there continues today to be some doubt that coronary bypass surgery relieves angina pectoris by the same

*From Departments of Medicine and Radiology, Emory University School of Medicine, Atlanta, Georgia.

mechanism. After 12 years of direct coronary bypass surgery, we have now had the opportunity to test Allan Burns' theory that angina pectoris is caused by myocardial ischemia. Since we believe Osler's admonition that the evaluation of angina pectoris (a most subjective symptom complex) is "full of knotty problems," we will call on objective evidence for improved myocardial perfusion with direct coronary surgery as well as pure subjective results.

Most of our knowledge of the relationship between angina pectoris and coronary artery obstructive disease has been learned in the past 20 years. This was made possible by coronary arteriography. The angina syndrome has, however, become less and less "classic." Many expressions of myocardial ischemia that do not fit Heberden's description have been found, and there are many other patients with "classic angina" in whom no myocardial ischemia can be demonstrated. Accordingly, without coronary arteriography, we would not be much further along in our understanding of angina pectoris than Heberden, Burns, and Mackenzie had taken us.

HISTORY OF SURGERY FOR ANGINA PECTORIS

Surgical attempts to relieve angina pectoris began in 1916 with the first cervical sympathectomy by Thomas Jonnesto of France.[7] After the left sympathectomy was completed, the patient stopped the procedure and would not allow the right side to be done, announcing that the pain was completely relieved. Perhaps relief from the surgical procedure was more compelling than relief from his angina. This procedure was later discredited because it was hazardous and ineffective.

Since this first attempt, many surgical procedures intended to relieve angina pectoris have been devised. All have been enthusiastically put forward. In the mid-1930s, Claude Beck began performing various operations designed to bring increased blood flow to the heart by producing inflammation of the surface of the heart and attaching various vascular pedicles of omentum, pectoralis muscle, spleen, stomach, or jejunum.[8] The operative mortality was very high, as reported later by Feil.[9] There was a 37 percent surgical mortality and 24 percent mortality at the 6-year follow-up period. Symptomatic improvement was reported as excellent in 60 percent, and there was some improvement in 82 percent of the operative survivors, although complete relief of angina was unusual. Later, Beck reported improved operative survival and symptomatic improvement. Long-term symptomatic improvement was not reported, however, and of course, coronary arteriography was not performed in any of these patients.

Internal mammary artery ligation, introduced in 1955, was quickly discredited following excellent double-blind randomized studies by Cobb et al.[10] and by Diamond et al.[11] comparing the ligation procedure to a sham operation. They were unable to show any difference in symptomatic results even with a short follow-up, and Diamond found no improvement in the exercise ECG with the procedure. Symptomatic improvement was reported in about 60 percent of the patients in each group.

The technique of implanting the internal mammary artery with free bleeding by branches into the myocardium was introduced by Vineberg.[12] Early enthusiasm was great, with Vineberg reporting 79 percent improvement with surgery and very excellent survival. Sewell later reported surgical survival curves indicating a 6 to 7 percent annual mortality for operated patients.[13] Two studies showed that the grafts in most patients had little effect on increasing myocardial blood flow or improving symptoms on a long-term basis.[14,15] Dart et al. showed that 13 grafts studied 2 to 5 years after implantation had a mean flow of only 8 ml/min and occlusion of the grafts produced no ECG changes.

Why were these early attempts to relieve angina pectoris discredited? All of them relieved angina to varying degrees. By in large, they were discredited, not because carefully controlled randomized studies were performed, but primarily because physicians following patients could not document long-lasting improvement and the procedures did little to alleviate the basic defect Burns described; decreased myocardial perfusion. The one exception was the double-blind mammary artery ligation and sham operation studies, each involving less than 20 patients. Most physicians concluded that the improvement from the early operations was caused by a placebo effect.

How does coronary bypass surgery differ from the previous techniques? Before we explore the possible mechanisms of pain relief, we should examine the evidence that angina is improved by coronary bypass surgery. Mundt and Austin, in an extensive review in 1975, concluded that 95 percent of patients are improved symptomatically and 60 to 70 percent are relieved of their pain.[16]

EVIDENCE FOR RELIEF OF ANGINA

The Cleveland Clinic has had the largest experience with coronary artery bypass graft surgery. Sheldon et al. reported 741 patients with isolated vein bypass surgery.[17] When these patients were recatheterized 16 months following surgery, they were evaluated for complete relief from symptoms of angina pectoris. Relief of pain correlated closely with vein graft patency. Those patients who underwent bypass of all coronary arteries with greater than 75 percent narrowing and who had no lesions greater than 75 percent in the vein grafts and no new significant coronary lesions had an 87 percent incidence of freedom from angina. Patients with incomplete revascularization (i.e., at least one graft patent but some grafts closed or new coronary artery lesions that produced greater than 75 percent obstruction) had 56 percent freedom from angina, while only 42 percent of the patients with all grafts closed were relieved of angina.

The patients who were operated on at Emory University Hospital have been surveyed by mail and asked to answer a questionnaire. In so doing, 92 percent reported improved symptoms and 62 percent said they are free of angina an average of 18 months after surgery.[18] Laurie et al. found 93 percent of their patients improved and 51 percent completely free of angina more than 5 years following surgery.[19] A subgroup of patients operated at Emory University between 1973 and 1974 who had unstable angina and complete revascularization were evaluated. Of these, 63 percent were free of pain and only 1 individual reported no improvement 16 months following surgery.[18] Several review articles by Gott in 1974,[20] Ross in 1975,[21] and Macintosh in 1976[7] have concluded, based on reviews of the literature, that relief of angina occurs in 75 to 95 percent of patients.

Laks studied patients under 40 who had many risk factors for coronary atherosclerotic heart disease, including a strong family history, smoking, hyperlipi-

demia, and diabetes.[22] Despite these risks of disease progression, 67 percent remain pain free and 84 percent improved 26 months following surgery. Sustained symptomatic improvement is also documented by Anderson et al.[23] In approximately 500 patients operated on for stable disabling angina (class III and IV), 93 percent became functionally class I or II during the first year and 75 percent were similarly improved 4 years postoperatively. The authors point out that more recent results are better because many of the patients in the longest follow-up also had incomplete revascularization. When patients have recurrent symptoms, reoperation may not produce the same good results. Wukarch et al. reported a series of reoperations in which 67 percent were improved if revascularization was complete and 37 percent were improved if revascularization was incomplete.[24] The operative mortality was low, but the authors pointed out that there was less relief from angina in the patients undergoing reoperation than with initial surgery.

At Emory University Hospital, we have evaluated symptomatic improvement by questionnaire using a computerized data bank. A series of patients operated between 1973 and 1977 were evaluated based on certain baseline characteristics.[25] There was 92 percent overall improvement in angina, and 62 percent of patients were free of pain an average of 20 months after surgery. There was no difference in baseline characteristics except that those patients with single-vessel disease had less complete pain relief than the other subgroups. (See Fig.7-1.)

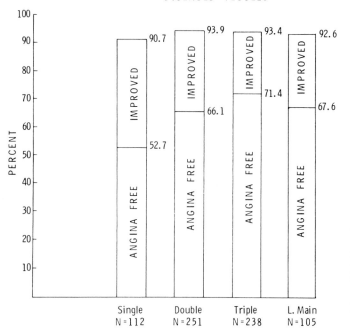

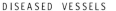

DISEASED VESSELS

FIGURE 7-1 Percentage of patients free of angina and those who are improved related to preoperative characteristics: *a.* number of vessels diseased; *b.* contractility of the left ventricle; *c.* ejection fraction; *d.* left ventricular end-diastolic pressure; *e.* the preoperative angina status of stable angina or the many subsets of unstable angina pectoris at a mean follow-up of 20 months.

How can we be sure that the pain relief obtained in these uncontrolled clinical situations could not just as well have occurred spontaneously or with medical therapy. Patients in the Framingham study [26,27] have been followed over the past 20 years. Among the patients who were followed clinically without coronary arteriography, there were 74 men and 84 women who developed new angina not complicated by other manifestations of coronary atherosclerotic heart disease. Remission occurred in 32 percent of the men and in 44 percent of the women. That is, pain that was present on one exam disappeared completely for a period of at least 2 years. If these patients were suffering from angina pectoris resulting from decreased myocardial perfusion, then the high remission rates are truly startling. Several points seem appropriate. First, it is odd that more women than men developed new angina in the Framingham study. It is also interesting that in 44 percent of the women, the pain disappeared. In our hospital, 37 percent of the women referred for coronary arteriography and thought to have angina pectoris in fact have normal coronary arteries on arteriography.[28] The Cleveland Clinic group found similar results. We believe that women whose angina completely disappears for a period of 2 years might also have a high incidence of normal coronary arteries.

The mortality in the Framingham patients with transient angina was 0 percent in men and 3 percent in women over 4 years, while it was 20 percent in men and 11 percent in women for those patients whose symptoms persisted. This also casts considerable doubt as to whether the patients who had a remission truly had coronary atherosclerotic heart disease.

The sensitivity of angina pectoris as an indicator of coronary artery disease is likewise imperfect. Two autopsy studies of patients with significant coronary artery disease showed that only 19 to 32 percent reported angina pectoris.[29,30] Of course, this kind of retrospective study would be expected to produce many false negative histories for angina pectoris. Angiographic studies at Emory University Hospital also showed that 32 percent of men and 18 percent of women with chest discomfort thought not to be angina pectoris had coronary atherosclerotic heart disease.[28]

RESULTS OF RANDOMIZED STUDIES OF MEDICAL VERSUS SURGICAL THERAPY FOR ANGINA PECTORIS

The symptomatic results of previous surgical attempts to relieve angina pectoris amply demonstrated the unreliability of the early assessment of relief of angina. As we can see from the preceding discussion, the initial relief of angina by coronary artery bypass graft surgery is not markedly different from that of previously discredited operations. The difference between the results of coronary artery bypass surgery and the previous techniques is in the duration of relief and the number of patients with complete relief of angina. Additional data are now available from randomized studies of medically and surgically treated patients.

Prospective randomized studies have been initiated at several centers. The Houston Veterans Administration group studied patients with chronic stable angina.[31] After a mean follow-up of 34 months, although 91 percent of surgical patients were improved as compared to 66 percent of the medical patients, 68 percent of the surgical patients were free of angina pectoris compared with only 8 percent of the medical patients. The Portland Veterans Administration Hospital initiated a similar study.[32] All patients were class III prior to entering the study. At 6 months, 34 percent of the medical patients were improved and 77 percent of the surgical patients were improved. No medical patients and 30 percent of the surgical patients were totally asymptomatic. At last follow-up, the number of improved surgical patients decreased to 64 percent.

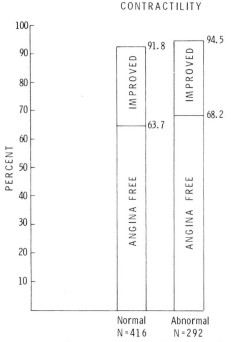

FIGURE 7-2 Percentage of patients free of angina and those who are improved related to the contractility of the left ventricle.

Patients with unstable angina have been similarly assessed. In a small series from Parkland Hospital in Dallas,[33] 58 percent of the operated patients were relieved as compared to 1 of 13 medical patients. Chronic stable angina persisted in 7 of these, and 5 had such severe unstable angina that they required surgery and were removed from the medical group.

The Duke University group, utilizing their data bank, matched and compared a medical group with a surgical group. Pain relief for the medical and surgical cohorts was 23 percent and 69 percent at 6 months, 21 percent and 62 percent at 12 months, and 26 percent and 53 percent at 24 months, respectively ($p >$ 0.001).[34]

The randomized studies that have received most interest deserve closer scrutiny. They are the Veterans Administration cooperative study of chronic stable angina[35,36] and the National Heart, Lung and Blood Institute study of unstable angina.[37]

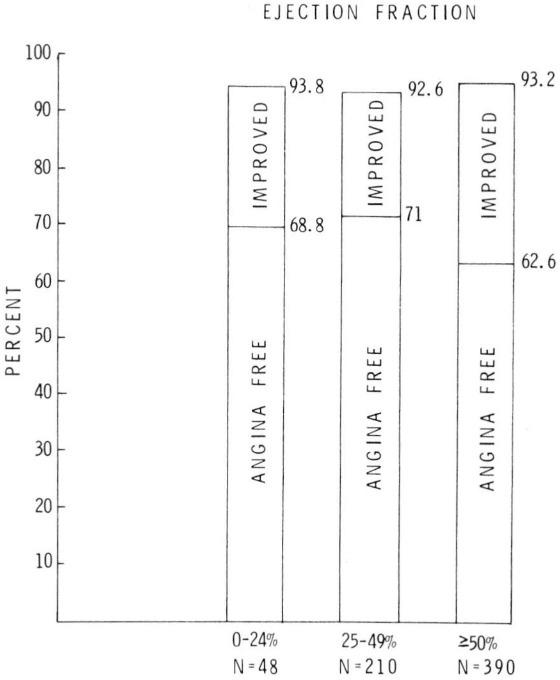

The Veterans Administration Study

Reports of the Veterans Administration study in the lay press and in medical editorials have concentrated on the survival data. Even though there are many valid criticisms of the study weighted toward the medical group, the symptomatic results clearly favor surgery. Our major criticisms of the study are included in the special section on coronary artery surgery in the *New England Journal of Medicine*.[38]

Four points make this study less than helpful in dealing with our patients today. The first is that the authors studied patients who were highly selected. They excluded patients with unstable angina, left-main-coronary-artery disease, ventricular aneurysm, generalized poor contraction, markedly increased end-diastolic pressure, large left ventricular size and poor ejection fraction. By systematically excluding "bad ventricles," one of the prime determinants of survival, have not the authors selected a group at lower risk than those forming the basis of the survival curves from earlier studies that do not exclude such patients?

Secondly, the surgical mortality of 5.6 percent has placed their surgical group at an initial disadvantage. Despite this drawback, the surgical curve catches and crosses the medical curve at 36 months. Could the factors of older and less effective operative technic, high perioperative infarction rate (18 percent), incomplete revascularization (many obstructed vessels were not bypassed), and poor graft patency (69 percent) have resulted in more late deaths in the surgical group than can be achieved with improved current methods?

Thirdly, of 310 patients assigned to the medical group, 54 had operations during the follow-up period. Could this fact have altered the medical survival curve in a favorable fashion?

Finally, despite the points listed, the group with three-vessel disease and some left ventricular abnormality (the

EJECTION FRACTION

FIGURE 7-3 Percentage of patients free of angina and those who are improved related to ejection fraction.

largest subgroup), when analyzed at 54 months in a further follow-up report on the same patients presented to the American Association of Thoracic Surgery, shows an 85 percent survival of the surgical group as compared to 76 percent survival of the medical group. Therefore, the Veterans Administration study itself is beginning to show improved surgical survival in certain subgroups of these already highly selected patients reported by Murphy and his colleagues.

Many medical centers can now cite much lower operative mortality rates (1.1 percent for the last 1000 patients at Emory University Hospital) with a perioperative infarction rate near 5 percent and 90 percent average graft patency. Several studies have shown a late mortality rate after bypass surgery in the range of 2 percent per year even for patients with triple-vessel disease. Although medical treatment may have improved survival, it is clear that surgical results are dramatically improved as well.

Even with these problems, substantial improvement or no angina occurred in 60 percent of the surgical group as compared to 16 percent of the medical group. Conversely, angina was unchanged or worse in 56 percent of the medical group and 14 percent of the surgical group.[36] These data were obtained by physician-administered questionnaires before therapy and 1 year following therapy. There were significant differences in frequency of pain, rest pain, dyspnea, and use of nitroglycerin, long-acting nitrites, and propranolol. The differences favored the surgical group.

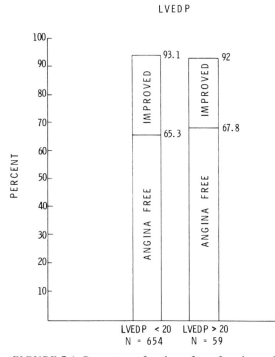

LVEDP

FIGURE 7-4 Percentage of patients free of angina and those who are improved related to the left ventricular end-diastolic pressure.

The National Heart, Lung and Blood Institute Study

The National Heart, Lung and Blood Institute trial of unstable angina was designed to test the concept that patients with unstable angina pectoris could be stabilized safely over the short term prior to any surgical intervention. A number of medical centers entered into the evaluation. The study was never designed to evaluate long-term survival. Nonetheless, this study has now been quoted as showing no significant difference in survival. The study has been invalidated for this purpose because many of the same problems that were encountered in the VA study also occurred in this study. The operative mortality was high, and one-third of the medical patients were operated on during the follow-up period because of refractory symptoms. In fact, of the patients with three-vessel disease, one-half of the medical group had to be removed from that group and operated on for this reason. There was no difference in the symptomatic status of either the medically treated patients with or without myocardial infarction or the surgical patients with myocardial infarction perioperatively; however, the surgical patients without myocardial infarction were much less symptomatic than the other three groups. (p <0.01). During the 2-year follow-up period, 45 percent of the medically treated group but only 15 percent of the surgi-

cally treated group developed class III or class IV symptoms. The authors concluded that ''during the first year of follow-up the data suggests that a major mechanism of symptomatic improvement in the group of patients with unstable angina pectoris is related to successful myocardial revascularization of previously ischemic myocardium.''[37]

The subgroup of patients in the Veterans Administration study with left main artery disease showed a dramatic improvement in survival in the surgical group. Relief of angina was also much better in the surgical group as compared to the medical survivors.[39]

These controlled studies all show that relief of angina is significantly more prevalent in the operated patients than in those treated with medications alone in contradistinction to all previous surgical efforts to control angina pectoris. Even though the operation is based on Allen Burns' physiologic principle of relieving the ischemic insult and even though controlled trials have shown surgery to be superior to medical therapy in achieving these ends, there remains skepticism regarding the mechanism by which surgery relieves angina pectoris.

MECHANISM OF ANGINA RELIEF

The mechanism of relieving angina for which the operation was designed is obvious. There is restoration of normal perfusion of previously ischemic myocardium. The evidence of this mechanism of relief will be presented later. However, let us first consider other explanations for angina relief that have been proposed. Buckley and Ross suggest three possible explanations for relief of angina in addition to relief of ischemia.[40] They are (1) denervation of the epicardial coronary vessels secondary to mobilization of the arteries, (2) perioperative infarction, and (3) placebo effect.

Perivascular Denervation

Perivascular denervation has been postulated by some as an explanation for relief of angina. However, those who have spent time in the operating room observing coronary bypass surgery are aware that very little mobilization of the epicardial coronary vessels is accomplished during coronary bypass surgery. Most surgeons who operate today do not pass ligatures around the artery nor remove it from its bed on the epicardial surface of the heart. They open the artery with very little dissection over a short segment immediately above the vessel. If denervation of the heart could prevent this sensation of angina pectoris, this explanation still would not be tenable, since no manipulation of the coronary vessels occurs during bypass surgery.

Following coronary bypass surgery, a varying percentage of patients will have positive exercise test results. It has been suggested that this is evidence that there is continuing myocardial ischemia and that it simply is no longer felt because of denervation. Our experience is that pericarditis is universal following coronary bypass surgery and the ST and T wave changes produced by this make subtle shifts of the ST segments and postoperative exercise tests hard to interpret. Recent studies of exercise test results and the addition of thallium scanning will be discussed later.

Perioperative Infarction

Perioperative infarction of ischemic myocardium is a possible mechanism of relief of angina. Most patients with angina pectoris have multiple-vessel disease and a potential for multiple areas of ischemia. However, when a single angina-producing segment of myocardium, as described by Achuff et al.,[41] becomes totally infarcted and organizes into scar tissue, previously existing angina may disappear. This does not mean, however, that every infarction results in relief of angina. In fact, in the Framingham study of 4,200 persons followed for 14 years, previously existing angina disappeared in only 11 percent of the male patients who had infarction, while angina appeared following new infarction in 50 percent.[42] In that series, angina was present prior to infarction in only 25 percent of the patients.

In a recent study of 146 patients with myocardial infarction, relief of angina as a result of infarction was not demonstrated.[43,44] Those patients who had angina prior to infarction continued to have angina after infarction. This was true in 86 percent of the group. New angina not present prior to infarction appeared for the first time following infarction in one-half of the patients, as it did in the Framingham study. Only 7 percent of the patients with infarction noted disappearance of previously existing angina pectoris. These findings are in agreement with previous studies. One of these assessed 212 survivors of their first myocardial infarction.[45] The incidence of angina went from 39 percent prior to myocardial infarction to 58 percent following the infarction. In patients with angina prior to the myocardial infarction, 77 percent had angina persisting following the infarction.

An additional argument against angina relief occurring as a result of perioperative infarction is that while relief of angina in most series is between 80 and 90 percent, perioperative infarction rates have dropped to 5 percent and below in many major centers. Some would argue that with newer techniques such as pyro-

phosphate scanning, smaller infarctions can be detected that would not be picked up on the electrocardiogram. While this is true, it does not seem reasonable that these small, localized areas of damage would be responsible for relief of angina pectoris considering the preceding data.

The Placebo Effect

The one explanation for angina relief, in addition to perfusion of previously ischemic myocardium, that cannot be discounted is the placebo effect. Indeed, this effect must be considered additive in all therapy of all diseases. Wolff defined placebo effect as "any effect attributable to a pill, potion, or procedure but not to its pharmaco-dynamic or specific properties."[46] Beecher studied the placebo effect in many clinical situations, such as postoperative wound pain, pain of angina pectoris, headache, seasickness, cough, mood changes, and anxiety.[47] He stated that in 15 studies involving 1,082 patients, satisfactory relief from placebos was produced in 35 percent of the cases. He contacted various groups performing internal mammary artery ligation. We have already seen that there was no difference regarding angina relief obtained by

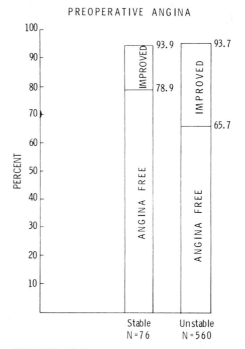

FIGURE 7-5 Percentage of patients free of angina and those who are improved related to the preoperative angina status of stable angina or the many subsets of unstable angina pectoris at a mean follow-up of 20 months.

this procedure compared to a sham operation. He stated that complete pain relief was reported to occur in 6 percent,[10] 36 percent,[48] 61 percent,[49] 39 percent,[50] and 28 percent of the patients.[11] Beecher also points out that the procedure was abandoned because the results were fleeting, lasting only for a number of weeks. Based on these early studies, the incidence of angina relief as a result of the placebo effect may be about one-third. It must be remembered, however, that none of these patients had selective coronary arteriography, and therefore it is likely that some of the patients were not suffering from coronary atherosclerotic heart disease. Also, there may be some spontaneous resolution of angina as a result of the previously discussed mechanisms.

Relief of angina has been noted in a certain percentage of patients whose grafts are all occluded. This occurred in 39 percent of patients in a series reported from Alabama.[51] This percentage is similar to the incidence of relief of angina that was found following the Vineberg procedure. Our experience is that patients reporting no angina following surgery who have no patent grafts are usually those who have severely limited their activity, or are those with single-vessel disease originally who, although having an occluded graft, still have good perfusion through the native circulation. It is unusual to see a patient with multivessel disease and definite ischemic pain preoperatively who has all grafts occluded postoperatively and yet maintains an active, vigorous life-style without any symptoms. Block et al. selected the 23 patients who were demonstrated to have all grafts occluded from among 1,082 patients who were operated in the Seattle heart watch.[52] Fifty percent of these were symptomatically improved. It is important to note, however, that severe disease was uncommon. Two patients had three-vessel disease, and the remainder were equally divided between single- and double-vessel disease. No significant increase in exercise performance could be documented for the group.

Increased Perfusion of Previously Ischemic Myocardium

Most investigators interested in the subject of coronary bypass surgery now feel that a major mechanism in the relief of angina pectoris is improved myocardial perfusion. McIntosh states that based on a review of the literature, "approximately 50 percent of patients operated will have objective evidence of increased blood flow."[7] The correlation between relief of angina and graft patency and complete revascularization previously noted would indicate that those patients who have adequately revascularized myocardium may have substantially greater objective evidence of increased blood flow.

Evidence for Increased Perfusion

Evidence for increased perfusion of the myocardium (see Chap. 3) is now available from a number of techniques, incuding electromagnetic flow probe measurements at surgery, xenon flow studies with and without exercise, postoperative exercise ECG testing, atrial pacing studies and evaluation of myocardial lactate production, hemodynamic response to exercise, myocardial perfusion scanning with exercise, and the relationship of completeness of revascularization to symptomatic improvement. Direct measurements of vein graft flow at the operating table using the electromagnetic flow probe demonstrate that 40 to 100 ml of flow occurs when grafting one of the major branches. Occlusion with release of the graft, which results in reactive hyperemia, or injection of papavarine into the graft produces a twofold to threefold increase in the flow. This was the first direct evidence that a greatly increased myocardial flow could be delivered immediately after coronary bypass surgery.

Angiographers performing postoperative studies on patients with coronary bypass surgery also see a graphic demonstration of increased flow through the bypass grafts. One need only contrast the slow filling and clearing of major occluded coronaries that are filled from collateral vessels from another coronary artery or from a Vineberg implant with the brisk filling and washout of contrast media seen when an unobstructed vein graft is connected distal to an obstructed artery. By injecting a small bolus of contrast media, transit time through the graft can be measured and flow calculated.

More precise measurements have been obtained with xenon washout techniques. Lichtlen et al. measured blood flow by xenon clearance techniques and found the same average flow for grafts to the anterior descending and right coronary arteries as they found in normal subjects through unobstructed left anterior descending and right coronary arteries.[53]

Myocardial perfusion scans have recently been applied to patients following coronary bypass surgery. Patients whose exercise thallium 201 scan shows perfusion defects that are not present on a resting scan uniformly show improvement in this exercise-induced defect following a successful bypass graft to the obstructed artery serving that segment. In a study by Ormand et al. thallium scanning was sensitive in identifying patients with three-vessel disease and somewhat less sensitive in patients with one- and two-vessel disease. When patients were studied postoperatively, reversal of previously positive thallium scans correlated closely with vein graft patency. Nine of 12 patients with abnormal thallium scans preoperatively demonstrated improved perfusion postoperatively.

Postoperative exercise testing has been performed

in patients with coronary bypass surgery (see Chap. 6). Siegel at el. reported 86 patients who had preoperative and postoperative exercise testing. Complete revascularization was accomplished in 33 patients. ST-segment changes were abolished in 89 percent postoperatively as compared to no change in exercise ST-segment changes in the 11 patients who had partial or complete graft failure. More recently, exercise data on the randomized clinical trials of medical and surgical therapy have been obtained. The Portland Veterans Administration study of chronic stable angina showed at 36 months mean follow-up that the surgical patients could achieve a significantly higher workload than the medical patients.[56] At 6 months, the work performed measured in killipound-meters decreased 15 percent in the medical group, while it increased 38 percent in the surgical group. Measurements during paced tachycardia also showed a significantly higher heart rate at angina in the operated versus the medically treated groups. Lactate extraction also improved in the surgical group but was unchanged in the medical group.

The Houston Veterans Administration prospective randomized study of chronic stable angina reported a mean follow-up period of 34 months.[31] Sixty-eight percent of the surgical group were asymptomatic as compared to 80 percent of the medical group. When objective exercise testing was done, 94 percent of the surgical patients had improved maximal exercise time as compared to 43 percent of the medical group. The pressure-rate product increased 19 percent in the surgical group but fell 10 percent in the medical group.

The Palo Alto Veterans Administration group evaluated their patients 5 years after entry into the chronic stable angina randomized trial.[57] The operated group had a significantly higher exercise tolerance time, maximum heart rate, and pressure-rate product than the medical patients.

The Mayo Clinic group showed that improvement in left ventricular and diastolic pressure to supine exercise was closely correlated with completeness of revascularization.[58] Eight of 11 patients who normalized their left ventricular end-diastolic pressure following supine bicycle exercise postoperatively had complete revascularization, while only 4 of 21 who failed to normalize the exercise left ventricular end-diastolic pressure had complete revascularization.

WILL THE RELIEF OF ANGINA PECTORIS BE SUSTAINED?

As we have seen, vein graft patency correlates well with both relief of angina and the demonstration of objective improvement. Studies that have shown a decline in symptomatic improvement show similar decline in vein graft patency.[59]

The primary questions remaining relate to the long-term fate of the bypass grafts and the native circulation. Many centers reported their early experience, with patency rates from 65 to 75 percent.[60-63] As more experience with the technique was obtained, the early patency rate improved. The two centers with the largest early experience have reported patency rates of 82 percent and 84 percent.[64,65] Early patency rates have been correlated with graft flows. Flows below 20 ml/min resulted in patency rates of 50 to 69 percent.[64,65] The Cleveland Clinic has the largest number of patients who have been restudied. Patency rates for the intervals between operation and postoperative angiography indicate little attrition in graft patency rates, being 86.8 percent at the end of the first year and 82.6 percent at the end of the fourth year.[66]

Most studies, such as the one just cited, have been performed at random times following surgery, making it difficult to establish whether or not late closure was actually occurring. One exception to this is the study from the Montreal Heart Institute. Their protocol was set up for studying grafts at 2 weeks, 1 year, and 3 years postoperatively. The first report from this group showed a high 1-year closure rate and little closure after this.[63] Following more experience with the technique, a study of 83 of a series of 100 consecutive patients demonstrated 2-week patency of 92 percent and 1-year patency of 86 percent.[67,68] After the first year, the entire group had an annual attrition rate of 2.1 percent. The second, more successful series had a late (after the first year) annual attrition rate of 0.7 percent. The time from surgery to recatheterization was 54 to 88 months in the entire group. The University of Alabama group also reported improving results with vein graft patency.[69] The 1-year patency rate was 76 percent for the years 1970–1973 but was 85 percent from 1974 to 1976. Of 116 grafts patent at 1 year, 5 closed in the follow-up period, producing an annual attrition rate of 1.7 percent for patients between 12 and 42 months postoperatively.

Lawrie et al. reported late (60 to 88 months) patency rates of 90.7 percent in 141 patients with 171 grafts.[70] This group found 87 percent patency during the first year and 82 percent patency during years 5 to 6.

Early changes in the vein grafts seemed to herald late closure. Campeau et al. found that grafts with early localized stenosis were more prone to occlusion, whereas no lesion was found in patients whose grafts appeared normal at 1 year.[68] Diffuse graft narrowing was seen frequently but did not seem to be progressive. The effect of early graft constriction was seen in another large Canadian series of restudies with a nearly complete 1-year follow-up. Fitzgibbon et al. studied a series of 409 consecutive survivors of bypass surgery at 2 weeks and again at 1 year.[71] In this series, 1,400 grafts were studied at 2 weeks and 1,032 grafts

TABLE 7-1
Patients most likely to be relieved of their angina

1. Those with angina of effort, with relief by rest and nitrites
2. Those having prolonged attacks of ischemic pain with classical characteristics
3. Those in whom there is objective evidence of ischemia on ECG stress testing and/or radionuclide stress imaging
4. Those with multiple high-grade proximal obstructions
5. Those with adequate left ventricular function
6. Those in whom there is an absence of congestive heart failure
7. Those who have decreased perfusion to viable myocardial segments
8. Those who have 2 mm smooth-walled distal arteries suitable for bypass
9. Those with all distal vessels suitable for bypass
10. Those who are psychologically motivated to improve
11. Those who are currently or recently employed

had been restudied at 1 year. Based on the initial study, grafts were graded ''A'' if there was no narrowing of the graft to more than 50 percent of the diameter of the grafted coronary artery and no new narrowing greater than 50 percent of the grafted coronary in a way that would impair blood supply to the segment of myocardium for which it was intended. Grafts were graded ''B'' if such narrowing existed, and ''O'' if totally occluded. The study at 2 weeks showed 89 percent patency and at 1 year, 81 percent patency. Seventy-nine percent of the 1-year patients were graded A. Of these grafts originally graded A, 90 percent remained so, 4 percent became grade B, and 6 percent occluded. Of grafts originally graded B, 37

TABLE 7-2
Patients least likely to be relieved of their angina

1. Those who have atypical or poorly defined chest pain without good effort relationship
2. Those who have multiple types of pain, including known or unknown noncardiac pain, i.e., chest wall, gallbladder, hiatal hernia, etc.
3. Those in whom there is no objective evidence of ischemia
4. Those who have single-vessel disease, especially if supplying a small amount of myocardium
5. Those with poor left ventricular function
6. Those with congestive heart failure
7. Those who have obstructed vessels serving mostly noncontractile myocardial segments
8. Those who have small and diseased distal arterial segments
9. Those with several distal vessels that cannot be bypassed
10. Those who are not motivated to improve
11. Those whose disability claims are being processed

percent became grade A, 39 percent remained grade B, and 24 percent occluded at 1-year follow-up.

Concern has been voiced about the fate of the grafted arteries. In 1973, Griffith et al. reported early experience from Johns Hopkins. Occlusive changes were found in a high percentage of the grafted coronary arteries.[60] Glassman et al. pointed out in 1974 that there are two types of intrinsic coronary changes seen on postoperative angiography.[61] One is progression of preexisting proximal obstructions owing to altered hemodynamics produced by the graft flow and the second are strictures at the anatomic site most likely induced at the time of surgery. The first type would represent the expected change with flow going through the bypass and little or no flow through a tight lesion, resulting in closure. This would be deleterious only if the graft closed as it did in 4 of the 80 grafts reported by Spencer. Strictures of the anatomic site would always be deleterious. The incidence of this type of change has decreased as operative experience has been gained.

Progression of preexisting stenoses in nongrafted arteries was recently studied by Bourassa.[72] Early 1-year progression was infrequent (9.5 percent), as had been seen in previous studies. When the patients were restudied at 6 years, however, progression was detected in 46 percent of the patients. New lesions in ungrafted arteries increased from 7.3 percent at 1 year to 41 percent at 6 years. Progression in the native coronary artery was not different at 6 years in the grafted versus the nongrafted arteries. The authors concluded that this is justification for bypassing all lesions including those previously thought to be borderline obstructive.

Long-term maintenance of adequate myocardial perfusion is a function of completeness of revascularization, surgical expertise in performing grafts, and late graft closure and progression rates in the native circulation. Fortunately, current patency rates seem to be about 90 percent. Late attrition of grafts has been reported from 0.7 percent to 1.7 percent per year. Long-term relief of angina is dependent on long-term maintenance of adequate myocardial perfusion. Current surgical results should make this a realistic expectation.

SUITABILITY FOR CORONARY BYPASS SURGERY TO IMPROVE ANGINA PECTORIS

Experience over the past 12 years has helped define certain characteristics of patients that are associated with improvement in or total relief from angina pectoris. The relief of angina correlates well with demonstrated increase in coronary blood flow to viable but previously ischemic myocardial segments. However, other factors influence the patient's clinical course following surgery. Tables 7-1 and 7-2 outline some of the characteristics of patients likely to be alleviated of their chest discomfort, as well as those patients likely to have persistent chest discomfort following surgery. Since coronary bypass surgery is applied in some very high risk subsets of patients who are mildly symptomatic or even asymptomatic, relief of angina cannot be expected. In these patients, postoperative chest wall discomfort and/or pericarditic pleuropericarditic symptoms may cause more discomfort postoperatively than they had preoperatively. This fact, of course, should be considered in context with the danger of the underlying lesion and the evidence for prolonged life in the subset being discussed.

For those patients suffering from angina pectoris, however, the available evidence would indicate that if they are suitable operative candidates, increased flow is the primary mechanism by which angina is relieved. Placebo effect is present in all cases, and the motivation of the patient is certainly important. If excellent complete revascularization can be achieved, the outlook for long-term angina relief is excellent. Current evidence would indicate that the expectancy for long-term graft patency is good if the patient is a suitable operative candidate and if an excellent complete grafting procedure is performed.

REFERENCES

1 Osler, W.: The Lumieian Lectures on Angina Pectoris, *Lancet*, 1910, pp. 697–702, 839–844, 973–977.

2 Willius, F. A., and Dry, T. J.: "A History of the Heart and Circulation," W. B. Saunders Company, Philadelphia, 1948, p. 15.

3 *Ibid*, p. 88.

4 *Ibid*, pp. 94, 95.

5 *Ibid*, p. 110.

6 *Ibid*, p. 234.

7 McIntosh, H. D., et al.: Indications for Saphenous Vein Aortocoronary Bypass Surgery, in R. Paoletti and A. M. Gotto, Jr. (eds.), "Atherosclerosis Reviews," Vol.1, Raven Press, New York, 1976, p. 185.

8 Beck, C. S.: Coronary Artery Disease. A Report to William Harvey 300 Years Later, *Am. J.Cardiol.*, January 1958, pp. 38–45.

9 Feil, H.: Clinical Appraisal of the Beck Operation, *Ann. Surg.*, 118(5):807–814, 1943.

10 Cobb, L. A., et al: An Evaluation of Internal-Mammary-Artery Ligation by a Double-Blind Technic, *N. Engl. J. Med.*, 260(22):1115-1118, 1959.

11 Dimond, E. G., et al.: Comparison of Internal Mammary Artery Ligation and Sham Operation for Angina Pectoris, *Am. J. Cardiol.*, April 1969, pp. 483–486.

12 Vineberg A.:"Revascularization by Unilateral-Bilateral Ventricular Mammary Artery Implants and Peri-Coronary Omental Grafts. Ten Year Follow-up," pp. 80–104.

13 Sewell, W. H.: Life Table Analysis of the Results of Coronary Surgery.

14 Dart, C. H., et al.: Direct Blood Flow Studies of Clinical Internal Thoracic (Mammary) Arterial Implants, *Circulation*, 2:64–71, 1970.

15 Langston M. F., et al. Evaluation of Internal Mammary Artery Implantation. *Am. J. Cardiol.*, 29:788–792, 1972.

16 Mundth, E. D., and Austen, W. G.: Surgical Measures for Coronary Heart Disease, *N. Engl. J. Med.*, 293:75–79, 124–129, 1975.

17 Sheldon, W. C., et al.: Surgical Treatment of Coronary Artery Disease: Pure Graft Operations, with a Study of 741 Patients Followed 3–7 years, *Prog. Cardiovasc. Dis.*, 18(3):237–252, 1975.

18 Logue, R. B., King, S. B., and Douglas, J. S.: A Practical Approach to Coronary Artery Disease, with Special Reference to Coronary Bypass Surgery, *Curr. Probl. Cardiol.*, 1(2), 1976.

19 Lawrie, G. M., et al.: Results of Coronary Bypass More Than 5 Years After Operation in 434 Patients. Clinical, Treadmill Exercise and Angiographic Correlations, *Am. J. Cardiol.*, 40(5):665–672, 1977.

20 Gott, V. L.: Outlook for Patients After Coronary Artery Revascularization, *Am. J. Cardiol.*, 33:431–436, 1974.

21 Ross, R. S.: Ischemic Heart Disease: An Overview, *Am. J. Cardiol.*, 40(5):665–672, 1977.

22 Laks, H., et al.: Coronary Revascularization Under Age 40 Years. Risk Factors and Results of Surgery, *Am. J. Cardiol.*, 41:584–589, 1978.

23 Anderson, R. P., et al.: The Prognosis of Patients with Coronary Artery Disease After Coronary Bypass Operations. Time-related Progress of 532 Patients with Disabling Angina Pectoris, *Circulation*, 50:274–281, 1974.

24 Wukasch, D. C., et al.: Reoperation Following Direct Myocardial Revascularization, *Circulation*, 56(3) (suppl. 2):3–11, 1977.

25 Hurst, J. W., King, S. B., III, et al.: Value of Coronary Bypass Surgery. Controversies in Cardiology: Part 1, *Am. J. Cardiol.*, 42:308–329, 1978.

26 Kannel, W. B., and Sorlie, P. D.: Remission of Clinical Angina Pectoris: The Framingham Study, *Am. J. Cardiol.*, 42:119–123, 1978.

82

27 Ayres, S. M., and Mueller, H. S.: Remission of Angina Pectoris, *Am. J. Cardiol.*, 42:520–521, 1978.

28 Douglas, I. S., and Hurst, J. W.: Limitations of Symptoms in the Recognition of Coronary Atherosclerotic Heart Disease, In J. W. Hurst (ed.), In "Update I: The Heart," McGraw-Hill Book Company, New York, in press.

29 Allison, R. B., Rodriguez, F. L., Higgins, E. A., Jr., et al.: Clinicopathologic Correlation in Coronary Atherosclerosis. Four Hundred Thirty Patients Studied with Post Mortem Coronary Arteriography, *Circulation*, 27:170–184, 1963.

30 Speikerman, R. E., Brandenburg, J. T., Achar, K. W. P., et al.: The Spectrum of Coronary Heart Disease in a Community of 30,000. A Clinicopathologic Study, *Circulation*, 25:57–65, 1962.

31 Guinn, G. A., and Mathur, V. S.: Surgical Versus Medical Treatment for Stable Angina Pectoris: Prospective Randomized Study with 1- to 4-Year Follow-up, *Ann. Thorac. Surg.*, 22:524–527, 1976.

32 Kloster, F. E., Kremkau, E. L., et al.: Prospective Randomized Study of Coronary Bypass Surgery for Chronic Stable Angina.

33 Pugh, B., Platt, M. R., et al.: Unstable Angina Pectoris: A Randomized Study of Patients Treated Medically and Surgically, *Am. J. Cardiol.*, 41:1291–1298, 1978.

34 McNeer, J. F., Starmer, C. F., et al.: The Nature of Treatment Selection in Coronary Artery Disease. Experience with Medical and Surgical Treatment of a Chronic Disease, *Circulation*, 49:606–614, 1974.

35 Murphy, M. L., Hultgren, H. N., et al.: Treatment of Chronic Stable Angina. A Preliminary Report of Survival Data of the Randomized Veterans Administration Cooperative Study, *N. Engl. J. Med.*, 297:621–626, 1977.

36 Hultgren, H., and the VA Study Participants: VA Cooperative Study of Stable Angina. Comparison of Medical Versus Surgical Treatment upon Symptoms, *Circulation*, 58:II-151, 1978. (Abstract.)

37 Conti, R., Becker, T., Biddle, A., et al.: Unstable Angina Pectoris. NHLBI Trial Effects of Early Non-fatal Myocardial Infarction on Subsequent Mortality and Symptoms, *Circulation*, 58(suppl. 2):152, 1978. (Abstract.)

38 King, S. B., Hurst, J. W., and Logue, R. B.: A debate on Coronary Bypass, *N. Engl. J. Med.*, 297:1468–1469, 1977.

39 Takaro, T., Hultgren, H. N., et al.: The VA Cooperative Randomized Study of Surgery for Coronary Arterial Occlusive Disease, *Circulation*, 54(suppl. 3) (6):107–116, 1976.

40 Buckley, B. H., and Ross, R. S.: Coronary-Artery Bypass Surgery: It Works, But Why?, *Ann. Intern. Med.*, 88:835–836, 1978.

41 Achuff, S. C., Lawrence, S. C., Conti, C. R., et al.: The Angina Producing Myocardial Segment: An Approach to the Interpretation of the Results of Coronary Bypass Surgery, *Am. J. Cardiol.*, 36:723–729, 1975.

42 Kannel, W. B., and Feinleib, M.: Natural History of Angina Pectoris in the Framingham Study, *Am. J. Cardiol.*, 29:154–162, 1972.

43 Amsterdam, E. A., Lee, G., et al.: Relationship of Myocardial Infarction to Presence of Angina Pectoris in Patients with Coronary Heart Disease: Lack of Abolition of Angina by Infarction, *Clin. Cardiol.*, 1:31–34, 1978.

44 Matthews, E., Amsterdam, E. A., et al.: Occurrence of Angina Pectoris in Relation to History of Myocardial Infarction: Lack of Abolition of Angina by Infarction, *Clin. Cardiol.*, III-5. (Abstract.)

45 Palmer, J. H.: The Prognosis Following Recovery from Coronary Thrombosis with Special Reference to the Influence of Hypertension and Cardiac Enlargement, *Q. J. Med.*, 6:49, 1937.

46 Wolf, S.: Effects of Suggestion and Conditioning on Action of Chemical Agents in Human Subjects—Pharmacology of Placebos, *J. Clin. Invest.*, 29:100–109, 1950.

47 Beecher, H. K.: Surgery as Placebo. A Quantitative Study of Bias, *J. A. M. A.*, July 1961, pp. 88–93.

48 Kitchell, J. R., Glover, R. P., et al.: Bilateral Internal Mammary Artery Ligation for Angina Pectoris; Preliminary Clinical Considerations, *Am. J. Cardiol.*, 1:46–50, 1958.

49 Brill, I. C., et al.: Internal Mammary Ligation, *Northwest Med.*, 57:483–486, 1958.

50 Ellis, L. G., et al.: Long-term Management of Patients with Coronary Artery Disease, *Circulation*, 17:945–952, 1958.

51 Kouchoukos, N. T., Kirklin, J. W., et al.: An Appraisal of Coronary Bypass Grafting, *Circulation*, 50:11, 1974.

52 Block, T., English, M., and Murray, J. A.: Changes in Exercise Performance Following Unsuccessful Coronary Artery Bypass Grafting, *Am. J. Cardiol.*, 37:122, 1976. (Abstract.)

53 Lichtlen, P., Mocetti, T., Halter, J., et al.: Postoperative Evaluation of Myocardial Blood Flow in Aorta-to-Coronary Artery Vein Bypass Grafting Using Xenon-Residue Detection Technique, *Circulation*, 46:445–455, 1972.

54 Ormand, J., Platt, M., Nels, L., et al.: Thallium 201 Syntography and Exercise Testing in Evaluating Patients Prior to and After Coronary Bypass Surgery, *Circulation*, 56 (suppl. 3):III-131.

55 Siegel, W., Lim, H. S., Proudfit, W. L., et al.: The Spectrum of Exercise Tests and Angiographic Correlation in Myocardial Revascularization Surgery, *Circulation*, 52 (suppl 1):56, 1975.

56 Kloster, F. , Kremkau, L., et al.: Prospective Randomized Study of Coronary Bypass Surgery for Chronic Stable Angina, *Am. J. Cardiol.*, 41, 1978. (Abstract.)

57 Fowles, R. E., Fitzgerald, J. W., et al.: Long-term Effects of Coronary Surgery Versus Medical Therapy on Exercise Performance, *Am. J. Cardiol.*, 41, 1978. (Abstract.)

58 Vlietstra, R. E., Chesebro, J. H., et al.: Exercise Hemo-

dynamic Improvement After Aorta-Coronary Artery Bypass Surgery, *Am. J. Cardiol.,* 41:410, 1978. (Abstract.)

59 Campeau, L., Hermann, J., et al.: Loss of Improvement of AP Between One and Six Years After Aorta-Coronary Bypass Surgery: Correlations with Changes in Vein Grafts and in Coronary Arteries, *Circulation,* 58(suppl. 2):16, 1978.

60 Griffith, L. S. C., Achuff, S. C., et al.: Changes in Intrinsic Coronary Circulation and Segmental Ventricular Motion After Saphenous Vein Coronary Bypass Graft Surgery, *N. Engl. J. Med.,* 288:589–594, 1973.

61 Glassman, E., Spencer, F. C., et al.: Changes in the Underlying Coronary Circulation Secondary to Bypass Grafting, *Circulation,* 49, 50 (suppl. 2), 1974.

62 Maurer, B. J., Oberman, A., et al.: Changes in Grafted and Nongrafted Coronary Arteries Following Saphenous Vein Bypass Grafting, *Circulation,* 50:293–299, 1974.

63 Grondin, C. M., Lesperance, J., et al.: Serial Angiographic Evaluation in 60 Consecutive Patients with Aortocoronary Artery Vein Grafts 2 Weeks, 1 Year, and 3 Years After Operation, *J. Thorac. Cardiovasc. Surg.,* 67:1–5, 1974.

64 Walker, J. A., Friedberg, H. D., et al.: Determinants of Angiographic Patency of Aortocoronary Vein Bypass Grafts, *Circulation,* 45, 46 (suppl. 1):86–90, 1972.

65 Sheldon, W. C., and Loop, F. D.: Direct Myocardial Revascularization—1976. Progress Report on the Cleveland Clinic Experience, *Cleve. Clin. Q.,* 43(3): Fall, 1976.

66 Sheldon, W. C.: Factors Influencing Patency of Coronary Bypass Grafts. The First Decade of Bypass Graft Surgery for Coronary Artery Disease; An International Symposium, *Syllabus,* September 1977, p. 77.

67 Campeau, L., Crochet, D., et al.: Postoperative Changes in Aortocoronary Saphenous Vein Grafts Revisited. Angiographic Studies at Two Weeks and at One Year in Two Series of Consecutive Patients, *Circulation,* 52:369–376, 1975.

68 Campeau, L., Lesperance, J., et al.: Aortocoronary Saphenous Vein Bypass Graft Changes 5 to 7 Years After Surgery, *Circulation,* 58(suppl. 1)(3):170–175, 1978.

69 Kouchoukos, N. T., Karp, R. B., et al.: Long-term Patency of Saphenous Veins for Coronary Bypass Grafting, *Circulation,* 58 (suppl. 1):96, 1978.

70 Lawrie, G. M., Lie, J. T., et al.: Vein Graft Patency and Intimal Proliferation After Aortocoronary Bypass: Early and Long-Term Angiopathologic Correlations, *Am. J. Cardiol.,* 38:856–862, 1976.

71 Fitzgibbon, G. M., Burton, J. R., and Leach, A. J.: Coronary Bypass Graft Fate. Angiographic Grading of 1400 Consecutive Grafts Early after Operation and of 1132 after One Year, *Circulation,* 57(6):1070–1074, 1978.

72 Bourassa, M. G., Lesperance, J., et al.: Progression of Obstructive Coronary Artery Disease 5 to 7 Years After Aortocoronary Bypass Surgery., *Circulation,* 58 (suppl. 1) (3):100–106, 1978.

Chapter 8

The Treatment of Prinzmetal's Variant Angina with Coronary Bypass Surgery*

ALBERT E. RAIZNER, M.D. and
ROBERT A. CHAHINE, M.D.

Variant angina is a form of ischemic heart disease characterized by attacks of chest pain, usually occurring at rest and accompanied by ST-segment elevation in the electrocardiographic lead corresponding to the ischemic area.[1,2] This syndrome was popularized and received its eponym when Myron Prinzmetal and co-workers described their first series in 1959.[1] In the original cases studied, the dominant postmortem finding was marked narrowing of a single large coronary artery.[1,2] The clinical presentation was believed to be a function of that type of anatomic pathology. Subsequent reports, however, recognized patients with variant angina and angiographically normal coronary arteries, and these patients were considered to represent a variant of the variant.[3] Many cases of Prinzmetal's variant angina have been described, and an intense interest has developed in the pathophysiology of the syndrome.

The management of patients with variant angina has undergone change, as has our understanding of the entity. In this chapter we will review the medical and surgical approaches that have been utilized and the results achieved by these therapeutic modalities.

CLINICAL CHARACTERISTICS

Patients with Prinzmetal's variant angina present with chest discomfort which is identical to that of classic angina pectoris.[4] It is usually retrosternal, constricting, pressing, aching, or burning and may radiate to the neck, arm, jaw, epigastrium, or back. It usually lasts for less than 15 min and subsides spontaneously. If nitroglycerin is administered, the discomfort will terminate in a shorter period of time. Thus the pain of variant angina cannot be readily distinguished from that of classic angina.

Several features, however, serve to distinguish the patient with Prinzmetal's variant angina:

1 The pain of variant angina occurs predominantly at rest and is not generally related to other known provoking

factors that increase the heart work, such as effort or emotion. Such patients may tolerate normal physical activity without developing anginal symptoms. Paradoxically, they may get the attack while sleeping, sitting, or being otherwise inactive. Although resting angina is the dominant feature in most patients, many will give a history of typical exertional angina as well.

2 Variant angina attacks tends to be cyclic. That is, the pain attacks may occur in clusters over a period of one to several hours. There may be several days or weeks when attacks are frequent, and the attacks may then subside with no further problems for several months.

3 There is a tendency for these attacks to occur at similar times on different days. That is, some patients may find that the attacks typically occur in the early morning hours, while others may say that the attacks generally occur in the late afternoon or at night.

4 The most typical feature of Prinzmetal's variant angina that has been the objective clinical marker separating it from classic angina pectoris is the presence of transient ST-segment elevation on the electrocardiogram during the anginal attack. (Fig. 8-1). This is in contradistinction to the classic angina patient, who characteristically manifests ST-segment depression during the ischemic episode. The onset of ST-segment elevation precedes changes in heart rate or blood pressure, indicating that the ischemia in this syndrome is related to diminished coronary blood flow rather than increased myocardial oxygen demand.[5]

Although the majority of patients diagnosed as having Prinzmetal's variant angina give a history of recurrent episodes of resting chest pain, patients with a single episode of chest pain associated with ST elevation that did not progress to acute myocardial infarction have also been included. Additionally, patients may have recurrent ST-segment elevation that is unassociated with chest pain.[6-8]

Attacks of Prinzmetal's variant angina are commonly associated with precarious arrhythmias. Serious arrhythmias that have been reported include ventricular premature beats, ventricular tachycardia, ventricular fibrillation, and various degrees of heart block, including complete atrioventricular heart block.[3,9-14] Sudden death can occur during an anginal attack in relation to these arrhythmias.[15]

The electrocardiogram may be helpful in the diagnosis of Prinzmetal's variant angina only if it is ob-

*From the Department of Medicine, Baylor College of Medicine, and the Cardiology Section of the Veterans Administration Hospital, Houston.

NO CHEST PAIN

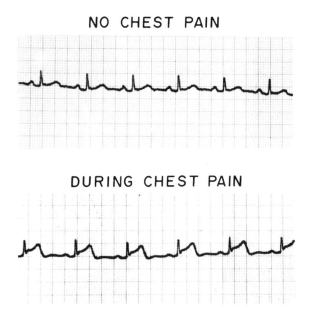

DURING CHEST PAIN

FIGURE 8-1 Electrocardiographic strip of a patient with Prinzmetal's variant angina. *Upper panel:* Before chest pain. *Lower panel:* During chest pain. There is marked ST-segment elevation during chest pain. ST-segment elevation in association with anginal pain is the electrocardiographic hallmark of Prinzmetal's variant angina.

tained during an episode of chest pain. If an electrocardiogram is performed after the pain subsides, it is likely to be normal or unchanged from the patient's previous electrocardiogram.[9] The electrocardiogram obtained during the ischemic phase may provide important information relative to the region of myocardium that is ischemic and, therefore, the coronary artery that is likely to be responsible[1,2] (Figs. 8-2a and b.)

The exercise stress test may offer some help in recognizing a patient with Prinzmetal's variant angina. MacAlpin and coworkers found no evidence of myocardial ischemia with good exercise tolerance during treadmill testing in the majority of their population of variant angina patients.[9] Approximately 15 percent of their patients developed ischemic ST-segment depression typical of classic angina pectoris, while an additional 15 percent developed ST-segment elevation during exercise. Consequently, two patterns may be suggestive of the diagnosis of Prinzmetal's variant angina: (1) the absence of ST-segment abnormality during stress testing with preservation of exercise capacity, despite the patient's history of severe resting angina; and (2) ST-segment elevation that occurs during the exercise test.

Perhaps the most significant data relative to the clinical diagnosis of Prinzmetal's variant angina are obtained from long-term electrocardiographic moni-

toring. As noted above, the characteristic ST-segment elevation in association with the chest pain will be observed in many patients. (Fig. 8-3). However, some patients with documented rest angina accompanied by ST-segment elevation may also have resting angina with ST-segment depression or T wave inversion.[16,17]

It should be emphasized that the syndrome of var-

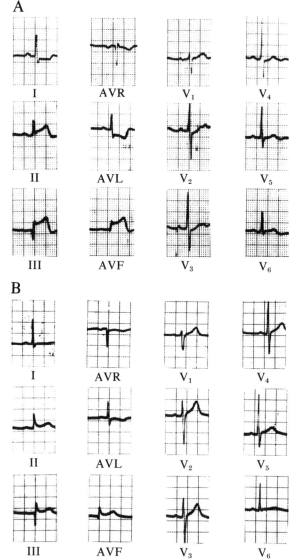

FIGURE 8-2 A 12-lead electrocardiogram in a patient who presented with recurrent resting angina. *a.* The electrocardiogram obtained during an anginal episode discloses ST-segment elevation in leads II, III, and aV$_F$. *b.* The electrocardiogram obtained after the pain subsided shows a return of the ST segments to normal. The electrocardiographic leads that manifest ST-segment elevation provide important information about the location of the pathologic abnormalities. In this patient, the ischemic process involved the inferior region of the myocardium and was attributable to disease in the right coronary artery.

iant angina and classic angina may coexist in the same individual.[16-20] A patient may have effort-related angina for months or years and enter a phase where resting pain develops or becomes more apparent. Similarly, a patient may appear with a clinical picture of variant angina; after medical treatment, the patient may continue to have angina that is predominantly effort-related. The reasons for this overlap of the syndrome of variant angina with classic angina are apparent if we consider the angiographic spectrum of Prinzmetal's variant angina and the pathophysiology of this syndrome.

NATURAL HISTORY OF PRINZMETAL'S VARIANT ANGINA

Several studies have directed attention to the natural course of the syndrome of variant angina. Bentivoglio et al. reviewed 90 cases reported between 1959 and 1972 where satisfactory follow-up information was available.[21] Since, in 1972, the pathophysiology of the syndrome was not clearly appreciated and appropriate therapy not yet applied, this group of cases is probably representative of the natural clinical course of the disease. In their review, these authors noted that 22 of 90 patients (24 percent) developed acute myocardial infarction within months after onset of attacks. Thirteen additional patients (14 percent) died suddenly. Thus, catastrophic events occurred in 39 percent of patients, often soon after the onset of symptoms.

Variant angina that develops following myocardial infarction (Fig. 8-4) is similarly associated with a high incidence of reinfarction and death. Stenson and coworkers noted a 33 percent mortality in 9 patients with postinfarction angina associated with ST-segment elevation.[22] The prognosis in these patients was significantly worse than that of patients with postinfarction

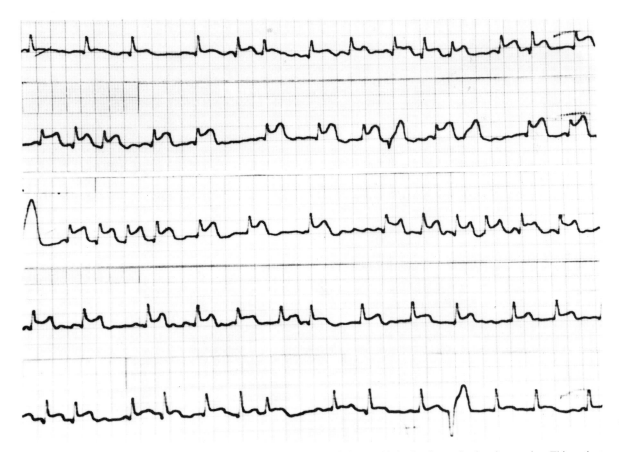

FIGURE 8-3 Ambulatory long-term electrocardiographic monitoring is invaluable in the diagnosis of variant angina. This patient with atrial fibrillation had multiple episodes of transient ST-segment elevation in a 24-h period. One episode is shown in this figure. Some of these episodes occurred in the absence of chest pain. Note the presence of ventricular ectopic beats during the ischemic phase. Long-term electrocardiographic monitoring should be routinely performed in the evaluation of patients with non-effort-related chest pain.

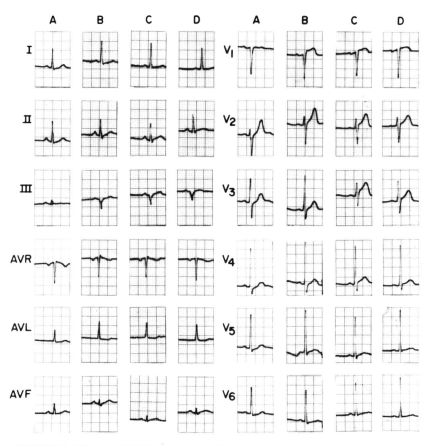

FIGURE 8-4 Sequential 12-lead electrocardiograms in a patient who was admitted with prolonged chest pain and diaphoresis. *a.* The initial admission electrocardiogram shows minimal nonspecific ST-segment depression. *b.* One day later, there is a loss of R wave in lead III compatible with inferior myocardial infarction. Cardiac enzymes confirmed the diagnosis of infarction. ST-segment elevation is seen in lead V₁. *c.* Subsequent electrocardiograms show transient ST-segment elevation in leads V₂ and V₃. This occurred on several occasions in the coronary care unit. During one of these episodes, he developed ventricular tachycardia which was successfully cardioverted. *d.* A later electrocardiogram shows return of ST segments. The pattern of transient ST-segment elevation in the post-myocardial infarction period has been associated with a more ominous prognosis[22] and may indicate disease in multiple vessels.

angina associated with ST-segment depression and those with no angina following infarction.[22]

While it is likely that the prognosis in an individual case may be more directly dependent on that patient's specific arteriographic and pathophysiologic findings, it is apparent that, as a group, patients with Prinzmetal's variant angina represent a high-risk subset within the spectrum of ischemic heart disease. As our knowledge of the coronary artery anatomy and our understanding of the pathophysiology of the syndrome have broadened, the approach to therapy has improved. The ominous natural course of Prinzmetal's variant angina may be favorably altered by rationally applied medical and surgical therapy.

ARTERIOGRAPHIC FINDINGS IN PRINZMETAL'S VARIANT ANGINA

Since the description by Prinzmetal in 1959, the prevailing opinion was that persons with the variant form of angina usually had a critical lesion involving a single major coronary artery. In the early 1970s, however, it became clear that variant angina could occur in patients with normal coronary arteriograms as well as in patients with multiple-vessel disease. A review of reports where adequately detailed coronary arteriographic information is available is shown in Table 8-1.[9,17,23-26]

Of 240 patients with Prinzmetal's variant angina,

TABLE 8-1
Coronary arteriographic findings in patients with Prinzmetal's variant angina

Author	No. of patients	Normal or minimal disease	One-vessel disease	Two-vessel disease	Three-vessel disease	Left main disease
MacAlpin et al., 1973[9]	19	2	14	0	1	2
Shubrooks et al., 1975[23]	20	3	5	9	2	1
Endo et al., 1975[24]	35	19	9	7	0	—
Higgins et al., 1976[25]	17	8	4	3	2	—
Johnson et al., 1978[26]	42	11	16	5	10	—
Maseri et al., 1978[17]	107	9	38	34	26	—
Totals	240	52	86	58	41	3
Percent		22%	36%	24%	17%	1%

(Table 8-1), critical atheromatous disease involving one or more coronary arteries was found in 188 patients, or 78 percent. Single-vessel involvement was noted in 36 percent, two-vessel disease in 24 percent, and three-vessel disease in 17 percent. Left main coronary stenosis was found in 1 percent. Thus, an overwhelming proportion of patients with Prinzmetal's variant angina have occlusive atheromatous disease, and the majority of these have multiple-vessel involvement.

Normal coronary arteriograms or minimal and insignificant atheromatous disease was noted in 22 percent of patients. Patients with normal or near normal coronary arteries may not be distinguished clinically from those with coronary atheromatous disease.[23]

Despite the rather diverse arteriographic spectrum seen in patients with Prinzmetal's variant angina, the unifying link appears to be the presence of coronary artery spasm.[5,10,18,24,25,27-37] Spontaneous spasm of a coronary artery has been documented in about 10 to 20 percent of patients studied and is associated with and responsible for the ischemic manifestations of anginal pain and ST-segment elevation seen in this syndrome[10] (Fig. 8-5). This relatively small percentage of spontaneously occurring spasm is understandable: the period of arteriographic observation is short; vasodilators, such as nitroglycerin, are often administered before arteriography; the angiographic contrast media are vasodilators; and angiographers are understandably hesitant to inject during chest pain when spasm is most likely to be observed.[28]

More recent studies have shown that spasm can be provoked in most patients with Prinzmetal's variant angina.[38-45] A variety of pharmacologic agents have been utilized. Ergonovine maleate is currently the most widely used provocative agent.[38-40] It has been said to be effective in inducing coronary artery spasm in over 90 percent of patients with a clinical picture of variant angina. Methacholine[41] and epinephrine in combination with propranolol[42] have also been em-

ployed, although experience with these agents has been rather limited.

Nonpharmacologic techniques for inducing coronary artery spasm have been studied. The cold pressor test, a sympathetic reflex activator, has been shown to induce coronary artery spasm.[43] Hyperventilation, in combination with TRIS buffer, may also induce spasm in some.[44] Additionally, coronary artery spasm has been induced by exercise during coronary arteriography.[45]

PATHOPHYSIOLOGY

It is now well accepted that Prinzmetal's variant angina results from recurrent transient narrowing of a major coronary artery.[46] The narrowing is the result of coronary artery spasm superimposed on various degrees of atheromatous disease (Fig. 8-5) or severe spasm occurring in angiographically normal segments. The common denominator appears to be coronary artery spasm with transient subtotal or total obstruction and consequent transmural ischemia. The clinically apparent pattern of pain and an injury pattern on the corresponding leads of the electrocardiogram reflect the transmural ischemia.[47,48]

The factors precipitating coronary artery spasm are largely unknown.[28,37,49,50] Because spasm tends to occur in areas of atheromatous disease, there is justifiable speculation that the atheromatous plaques may serve as a trigger for the spasm.[16] However, this hypothesis remains unproven. There is impressive evidence implicating the autonomic nervous system. The induction of spasm by simultaneous administration of epinephrine and propranolol[42] suggests a sympathetic interaction consisting of alpha sympathetic stimulation and beta sympathetic blockade. The ability of the cold pressor test to provoke coronary vasoconstriction[51] and spasm[43] further supports a sympathetic mecha-

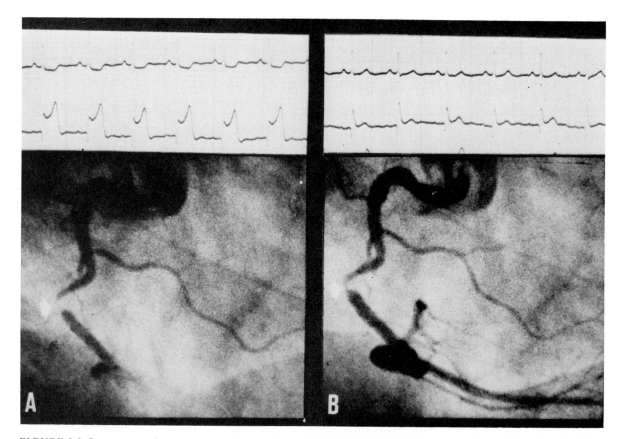

FIGURE 8-5 Coronary arteriogram and simultaneous electrocardiogram (leads I and III) in a patient with variant angina. *a.* The patient developed chest pain and marked elevation of the ST segment in lead III. Coronary arteriogram obtained during chest pain disclosed subtotal occlusion of the right coronary artery and virtually no distal filling of the artery. *b.* After the pain subsided and the ST segments returned to baseline, the lesion in the coronary is less stenosed (but still critical), and the artery fills well distally. Coronary artery spasm, often superimposed on an atheromatous lesion, is the pathophysiologic mechanism producing severe transient myocardial ischemia in patients with variant angina. (With the assistance of Dr. Tetsuo Ishimori, Mr. Tim Peasgood, and Mrs. Sherry Teeter). *(From R. A. Chahine and A. E. Raizner, Another Look at Prinzmetal's Variant Angina, Eur. J. Cardiol., 6:71, 1977. With the permission of the publisher.)*

nism. The demonstration of spasm production by the administration of methacholine[41] suggests participation by the parasympathetic nervous system. This agent may induce hypotension, and it is possible that its spasmogenic action may be explained by reflex sympathetic stimulation.

Nevertheless, despite the suggested role of the autonomic nervous system and, in particular, the sympathetic component, the most potent provocative agent currently used, ergonovine maleate, has a mechanism of action that may not be primarily related to autonomic stimulation. This agent seems to act by direct stimulation of vascular smooth muscle,[52] although some of this effect may be mediated by alpha-adrenergic receptors.[52,53] In addition, calcium release mechanisms have been implicated in the pathogenesis of coronary artery spasm.[44] Thus, other mechanisms

in addition to autonomic influences appear to be operative.

Of particular interest are the vasoactive substances released by platelets. These include serotonin, prostaglandins, endoperoxides, and thromboxanes.[37,54,55] The latter is one of the most potent vasoconstrictor substances known. Platelet aggregates are known to develop in areas of luminal irregularity,[56] such as at the site of an atheromatous plaque. The hypothesis that coronary artery plaques predispose to platelet aggregation and that platelet aggregates so formed release vasoactive substances which induce coronary vasospasm provides a potential explanation of the common association of coronary artery spasm with atheromatous coronary artery disease.

Since coronary artery spasm has been found in patients with classic angina pectoris,[20,57] unstable angina,[36] and myocardial infarction,[58,59] in addition to Prinzmetal's variant angina, the question arises of whether Prinzmetal's variant angina is a distinct syndrome or just another clinical presentation of atheromatous coronary artery disease.[60] The history of exertional chest pains in many patients with variant angina and the angiographic finding of critical lesions in over 75 percent of the patients studied clearly stress the importance of atherosclerosis in this syndrome. The link to atherosclerosis may turn out to be even greater when one considers the percentage of patients with angiographically normal or nearly normal coronary arteries who have apparent or occult plaques that may be playing a role in predisposing to, or triggering, the vasospastic phenomena. The salient clinical feature that makes Prinzmetal's angina a variant of classic angina is probably a tendency to be more prone to resting severe vasospasms.

The spectrum of ischemic heart disease therefore consists of a variety of clinical manifestations resulting from variable degrees of coronary obstruction secondary to a combination of fixed lesions and spasm. The clinical presentations may depend on the magnitude and duration of the resultant obstruction. In Prinzmetal's angina, it appears that the vasospasms are the dominant pathophysiologic elements responsible for the acute recurrent attacks, although in over 75 percent of the patients, these vasospasms are superimposed on significant critical atherosclerotic disease. These two elements should be carefully considered in order to offer rational management for these patients.

MEDICAL THERAPY

In view of the current understanding of the underlying pathophysiologic mechanisms, patients with variant angina who are demonstrated by arteriography to have critical atheromatous lesions of one or more coronary arteries should be considered to have a dual pathophysiologic condition: (1) coronary artery spasm and (2) atheromatous coronary artery disease. Treatment should be directed toward both of these factors.

During the acute phases of the disease when resting attacks of chest pain are frequent, the patients should be confined to bed rest in an intensive care or coronary care area where continuous monitoring is available. Since acute myocardial infarction can complicate the course of patients with Prinzmetal's variant angina, serial electrocardiograms and enzymes should be obtained to exclude that possibility.

The primary management of coronary artery spasm is medical. Sublingual nitroglycerin is highly effective in reversing the spasm and terminating the acute at-

tack. It should be taken at the very onset of symptoms. Occasionally, several nitroglycerin tablets are required to treat the acute attack. Since Prinzmetal's variant angina tends to be cyclic, with several attacks occurring in tandem, longer acting nitrate preparations, such as sublingual isosorbide dinitrate, should be given as soon as the nitroglycerin response occurs.

Maintenance medical therapy is aimed at preventing recurrent attacks of coronary artery spasm. Long-acting nitrates may be administered in several ways. Isosorbide dinitrate can be administered sublingually, 2.5 to 10 mg every 2 to 3 h, or orally, 5 to 40 mg every 4 h; topical or sustained release nitroglycerin preparations are required for nocturnal coverage. In view of the frequency of nocturnal attacks of variant angina, this aspect of medical treatment should not be overlooked.

Although nitroglycerin and nitrate preparations are effective in most patients, breakthrough attacks are common. The possibility should be considered that the dosage or frequency of administration of these medications is inadequate and should be adjusted accordingly.

Other groups of coronary vasodilators have been utilized in the management of variant angina. Alpha sympathetic blocking agents, such as phenoxybenzamine, have been tried with variable success.[42,57] Calcium antagonists, such as verapamil, nifedipine, and perhexiline, have been effectively used abroad[24,61,62] but have not yet been approved for use in the United States except in investigational programs. Our limited experience with verapamil has shown this drug to be most effective in preventing attacks of coronary spasm when used in conjunction with nitrates.[63]

The patient with Prinzmetal's variant angina should be cautioned about the possible provocation of coronary artery spasm by drugs or environmental influences. Cafergot, an ergot alkaloid used in migraine headache attacks, should be avoided. Propranolol may block the vasodilator effects of beta sympathetic stimulation and allow alpha sympathetic vasoconstriction effects to go unopposed.[42] We have consequently avoided its use in patients with variant angina, although some investigators have reported beneficial effects.[64] Sudden exposure to cold may precipitate arterial vasospasm,[43] and patients should be so informed.

In addition, since most patients with Prinzmetal's variant angina are found to have significant atherosclerotic disease, the usual measures against coronary disease risk factors utilized in the treatment of patients with atherosclerosis are also recommended, that is, programmed exercise, avoidance of smoking, control of hypertension, treatment of diabetes when present, and an appropriate diet.

RATIONALE FOR CORONARY ARTERY BYPASS SURGERY

As stated previously, most patients with the variant angina syndrome should be considered to have two functional disease states: (1) coronary artery spasm and (2) atheromatous coronary occlusive disease. In a given individual, a rational approach to therapy demands documentation of the existence and severity of each of these pathophysiologic factors.

The primary rationale for the use of coronary artery bypass procedures in patients with Prinzmetal's variant angina results from the observation that most patients with the syndrome have critical atheromatous narrowing of one or more major coronary arteries. Regardless of the effectiveness of medical management of the vasospastic component of their disease, these patients may continue to be limited by effort-related angina and may remain at risk of myocardial infarction and sudden death commensurate with the severity of the atheromatous occlusive coronary artery lesions.

Consequently, independent consideration must be given to the risks imposed by the presence of the atherosclerotic occlusive coronary artery disease. Although medical management of critical atheromatous coronary artery disease may lessen symptoms, it has become clear that the quality of life is significantly improved by coronary bypass surgery. Further, there is convincing evidence that survival in selected patients is significantly benefited by surgical intervention. These considerations are discussed at length in other chapters.

The following case illustrates the coexistence of coronary artery spasm and atheromatous coronary artery disease:

C. M., a 48-year-old male, presented with a 1-year history of substernal chest tightness. Initially, his chest discomfort was precipitated only by strenuous effort. Four months prior to admission he noticed that the chest discomfort began to occur at rest, in the absence of emotional or physical stimuli. During this period, he also had chest tightness during exertion. His risk factors for coronary artery disease included a strong family history and smoking two packs of cigarettes per day for 30 years.

His resting electrocardiogram was normal. During treadmill stress testing, he developed his characteristic chest discomfort. His exercise electrocardiogram revealed ST-segment depression in the anterior precordial leads.

During a spontaneous episode of chest pain, an electrocardiogram disclosed atrial flutter-fibrillation and ST-segment elevation in the anterior leads which resolved following sublingual nitroglycerin administration (Fig. 8-6).

Coronary arteriography disclosed a 95 percent stenosis in the proximal segment of the left anterior descending coronary artery. The right coronary and circumflex coronary arteries were patent. Coronary artery bypass was performed. Post-

operatively the patient had no effort or rest angina. Repeat coronary arteriogram disclosed a well-functioning bypass graft (Fig. 8-7).

An additional consideration supporting the rationale for coronary bypass surgery in patients with variant angina and severe atheromatous coronary artery disease is the limitation of choice of drug therapy. Propranolol, ordinarily an effective agent for symptomatic control of effort angina, may potentiate coronary artery spasm in certain individuals.[42] Therefore, its use in patients with vasospastic angina may be relatively contraindicated.

RESULTS OF CORONARY BYPASS SURGERY IN PATIENTS WITH PRINZMETAL'S VARIANT ANGINA

One of the earliest reports dealing with coronary artery bypass surgery in patients with variant angina was that of Silverman and Flamm.[65] These authors directed attention to Prinzmetal's observation of the association of variant angina with severe stenosis of a major coronary artery and suggested that the poor prognosis of such patients might be favorably altered by coronary artery bypass surgery. One of their 2 patients did well, but the other died of perioperative infarction. Subsequently, several isolated case reports appeared in which coronary bypass surgery was utilized with good results.[66-68] Dhurandar et al., however, reported 1 patient with coronary artery spasm but no critical atheromatous lesion who nevertheless underwent bypass surgery.[27] This patient died suddenly 2 weeks after surgery despite a patent graft.

Several larger series have since been published. MacAlpin et al. described 20 patients, 9 of whom underwent surgical treatment because of refractory symptoms.[9] Two of their patients had endarterectomy, and 1 had an internal thoracic artery implantation (Vineberg procedure). Of the 6 patients treated with saphenous vein bypass grafts (single in 5, double in 1), resting angina recurred postoperatively in 5. Three of these 5 had occluded grafts when restudied. Only 1 surgical patient was totally free of symptoms. No deaths were reported in this group, however. Eleven of the 20 patients were treated medically. One patient died suddenly 7 months later, and one other suffered a myocardial infarction with subsequent congestive heart failure. The course in the remaining patients was generally improved, although some continued to have effort angina. Despite the poor outcome in 2 of the 11 medically treated patients, these authors suggested that surgical treatment be reserved for patients with

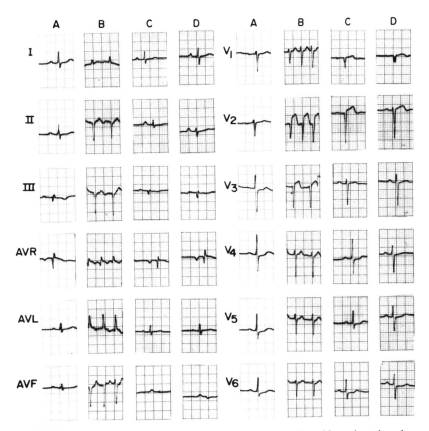

FIGURE 8-6 Sequential electrocardiograms of patient C. M. *a.* Normal resting electrocardiogram. *b.* During an episode of chest pain, the patient developed ST-segment elevation in leads V_2 and V_3 with atrial flutter-fibrillation, left anterior fascicular block, and development of Q waves in leads V_2 and V_3, suggesting a transmural infarction. *c.* ST segments subsided and anterior fascicular block resolved 30 min later. However, Q waves are still noted in leads V_1 and V_2. *d.* Several hours later, the ST segments have normalized. The ''infarct'' pattern is no longer present. This patient was subsequently found to have a critical stenosis in the proximal segment of the left anterior descending coronary artery.

incapacitating symptoms refractory to medical therapy.

Disappointing results of saphenous vein bypass grafting were reported by Gaasch et al. in 1974.[30] Their series consisted of 6 patients, 4 of whom had single- and 2 of whom had double-vessel grafts. One patient with coronary spasm but no fixed critical lesion underwent surgery after failure of medical therapy and died of refractory ventricular fibrillation. Two patients had perioperative infarction, 1 of whom was free of pain postoperatively despite an occluded graft. Two other patients were asymptomatic following surgery. One patient who had a graft placed in a spastic but non-occluded artery was improved but still symptomatic postoperatively.

A combined surgical and medical approach was utilized by Endo et al.[24] Of 35 patients with Prinzmetal's variant angina, 9 had single-vessel stenosis

that corresponded to the cardiac region manifesting ST-segment elevation. Coronary artery bypass was performed in these 9 with one operative death. Despite excellent graft patency in 7 of 8 survivors, symptoms were not permanently eliminated. The addition of the calcium antagonist, nifedipine, relieved symptoms in these surgically treated patients.

Favorable results with coronary artery bypass surgery were reported by Shubrooks et al.[23] These authors described 20 patients with variant angina, all but 1 presenting with progressive unstable angina. The anginal episodes were frequently associated with severe arrhythmias, including ventricular tachycardia and fibrillation and atrioventricular block. Medical therapy improved symptoms in some but was unsuccessful in relieving pain in the majority. Coronary arteriography disclosed critical coronary artery lesions in 17 of the 20 patients, including double-vessel dis-

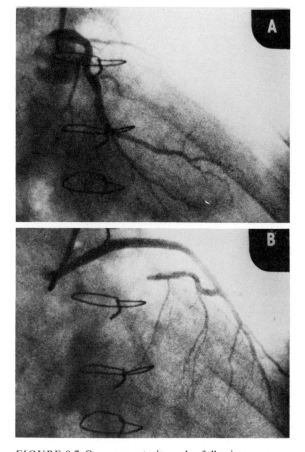

FIGURE 8-7 Coronary arteriography following coronary artery bypass surgery in patient C. M., whose electrocardiograms are shown in Figure 8-6. *a.* The native left coronary artery. The anterior descending is now completely stenosed near its origin. *b.* The bypass graft fills the anterior descending system antegrade and retrograde to the point of stenosis. The patient was totally free of resting and effort-related angina following bypass surgery.

ease in 9 and triple-vessel disease in 3. Coronary artery bypass grafting was performed in 15 patients with one in-hospital noncardiac death and one intraoperative infarction. All 14 patients surviving surgery were free of pain after an average follow-up of 17 months. Of the 3 patients with no significant coronary artery lesions who required medical treatment alone, 1 died suddenly, another had continued symptoms, and 1 became asymptomatic. Thus, in this series, a more favorable outcome was achieved in those patients with significant atheromatous lesions who underwent bypass surgery than in patients with no significant organic lesions who were treated medically.

Higgins et al. reported the results of coronary bypass surgery in 7 patients, 1 of whom did not have significant coronary artery lesions.[25] Of 6 patients with critical lesions treated with coronary bypass surgery, there were no operative or late deaths. Three patients were completely asymptomatic postoperatively. One patient without significant lesions was also treated surgically. Her postoperative course was stormy, with multiple episodes of ventricular tachycardia and fibrillation requiring the administration of intravenous nitroglycerin. Postoperatively, she remained symptomatic and required long-acting vasodilators. Ten patients were treated medically, including 3 patients with fixed obstructive lesions. One of these 3 patients infarcted 2 years later with subsequent relief of angina. One patient with normal coronaries died suddenly several months later. The remaining patients were improved but had continued symptoms. Thus, in this series, the only patients to achieve an uncomplicated asymptomatic status were those who underwent revascularization.

An interesting and obviously frustrating series of 29 patients was reported by Weiner et al.[14] Coronary artery spasm was documented in all 29 patients. The patients were initially treated medically. Only 3 patients had a completely satisfactory response to nitrates, while 5 others showed partial improvement. The remaining 21 patients were judged to be intractable to medical management. One patient died, and 2 suffered myocardial infarction while receiving medical therapy. Coronary artery bypass surgery was performed in 18 medically refractory patients who had atheromatous occlusive coronary artery disease. Nine of these patients were asymptomatic postoperatively. Unfortunately, there were 4 operative deaths, and 4 patients had perioperative infarctions. Despite a discouragingly high operative mortality and perioperative infarct rate, these investigators stressed the poor results achieved medically and advocated coronary bypass surgery as the only therapeutic alternative when medical therapy fails.

The largest series reported to date of patients with Prinzmetal's variant angina who underwent coronary artery bypass surgery is that of Johnson et al.[26] Twenty-seven of 42 patients with variant angina were treated surgically; 25 had significant atherosclerotic lesions, and 2 had insignificant plaques with superimposed spasm. Of the 25 patients with critical disease, there was 1 operative death and 2 perioperative infarctions. Eighteen of the 24 survivors were asymptomatic at an average follow-up of 14 months; 5 were improved, and only 1 continued to have effort-induced symptoms. Of 2 patients without significant lesions who were treated surgically for documented coronary artery spasm, 1 had a perioperative infarction, but both were improved postoperatively. Importantly, none of the patients who underwent coronary artery bypass had subsequent documented episodes of variant angina. Medical therapy alone was utilized in 15 patients with variant angina. Of these, 6 had critical atherosclerotic lesions, and 2 of 6 subsequently suffered myocardial infarction, while 3 became asymptomatic. Nine patients with no significant lesions were treated medically. One of these 9 had a myocardial infarction, and 3 others remained symptomatic. The results of this study are in agreement with those of Shubrooks et al.[23] and Higgins et al.,[25] supporting the beneficial results of coronary bypass surgery in patients with Prinzmetal's variant angina.

In order to place the role of medical and surgical therapy for Prinzmetal's variant angina in proper perspective, the results of these modes of management are listed and tabulated in Tables 8-2 through 8-5. These results are graphically displayed in Figs. 8-8 and 8-9.

The results of medical therapy of Prinzmetal's variant angina in 275 patients reported in eight studies,[9,14,23,25,26,69,70] are shown in Table 8-2. These include patients with (78 percent) and without (22 percent) critical obstructive coronary artery disease. Although the specific regimen of medical management differed from one series to another, the general approach relied principally on nitrates. Other medications included calcium antagonists, alpha-adrenergic blocking agents, and other vasodilators. Beta-adrenergic blocking agents were utilized in some series. Bed rest and tranquilizers were often prescribed.

The early mortality in all medically treated patients was 6 percent (Table 8-2 and Fig. 8-8). Myocardial infarction developed during hospitalization or within several months of discharge in 23 percent. An asymptomatic or improved clinical state was achieved in 47 percent, while an equal percentage of patients (47 percent) were unimproved or worse on medical management. Some of this latter group of patients who were considered to be refractory to medical management subsequently underwent coronary artery bypass surgery.

Bentivoglio et al. described the natural course of variant angina in patients reported between 1959 and 1972, an era when the pathophysiology of the syndrome was not yet understood, and noted a mortality of 14 percent.[21] Current medical treatment may represent an improvement in mortality (6 percent). However, the incidence of myocardial infarction is remarkably similar during both eras (23 percent versus 24 percent). This would certainly support the concept that Prinzmetal's variant angina represents a particularly unstable subgroup of patients within the spectrum of ischemic heart disease. Vigorous medical management alone may reduce early mortality, but these patients are still prone to develop myocardial infarction. A satisfactory clinical outcome, that is, an asymptomatic or improved state without myocardial infarction, can be anticipated in only one-half of the

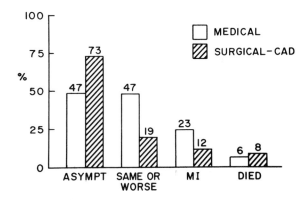

FIGURE 8-8 The results of medical and surgical treatment of Prinzmetal's variant angina. The medical group (clear bars) consists of cumulative patients from eight studies shown in Table 8-2. The surgical group (shaded bars) consists of patients with critical stenosis of one or more coronary arteries who received bypass grafts, as reported in 11 studies shown in Table 8-3. The percentages are shown above each bar. In this comparison, the results of surgical therapy are favorable, with more patients becoming asymptomatic and fewer developing myocardial infarction. The mortality is comparable in both groups.

patients in this group utilizing currently prescribed medical regimens alone. It is quite possible that these results may be improved as additional modalities of medical therapy become available.

The results of coronary artery bypass surgery in patients with variant angina are shown in Tables 8-3 and 8-4 and are compared to medical management in Figs. 8-8 and 8-9. The data are divided into those patients who had obstructive coronary atherosclerotic

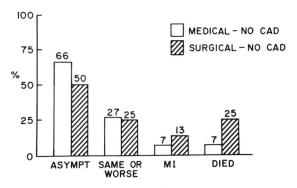

FIGURE 8-9 The results of medical (*n* = 41) and surgical (coronary bypass) (*N* = 8) treatment of variant angina in patients with normal coronary arteries or nonhemodynamically significant disease, from studies shown in Tables 8-4 and 8-5. Coronary bypass in this small group of patients was not favorable. Medical therapy gives beneficial results in most patients with no significant coronary artery disease. Myocardial infarction and death can occur, but their incidence is relatively small in medically treated patients.

TABLE 8-2
Results of medical therapy of Prinzmetal's variant angina

Author	No. of patients	Critical CAD		Asymptomatic or improved	Same or worse	MI	Died
		None	1 or more				
MacAlpin et al., 1973[9]	11[a]	2	8	7	3	1	1
Shubrooks et al., 1975[23]	20[b]	3	17	7	12	0	1
Higgins et al., 1976[25]	10	7	3	6	3	1	1
Selzer et al., 1976[69]	29[c]	9	20	12	14	4	3
Weiner et al., 1976[14]	29[d]	11	18	8	20	2	1
Clark et al., 1977[70]	23[e]	—	—	15	8	9	0
Johnson et al., 1978[26]	15	9	6	10	5	3	0
Maseri et al., 1978[17]	138[f]	8	98	—	—	28	5
Totals	275	49/219	170/219	65/137	65/137	48*/211*	12*/211*
Percent		22%	78%	47%	47%	23%	6%

[a]Coronary arteriography was done in 10 patients.

[b]Fifteen of these patients subsequently underwent surgery.

[c]Thirteen of these patients subsequently underwent surgery.

[d]Eighteen of these patients subsequently underwent surgery.

[e]Eight of these patients subsequently underwent surgery.

[f]Ten of these patients subsequently underwent surgery. Coronary arteriography was done in 106 patients.

*Sixty-four patients who subsequently underwent surgery are excluded in the tabulation. Their data regarding death and MI are listed in surgical results.

CAD, coronary artery disease; MI, myocardial infarction; —, not specified in articles.

disease (Table 8-3) and those who had arteriographically normal coronary arteries or hemodynamically insignificant lesions (Table 8-4). Data from earlier case studies are included along with more recent larger series. Single-vessel bypass was performed in 53 percent, double-vessel in 31 percent, and triple-vessel grafts were placed in 16 percent. Many of these patients were initially treated medically and were unresponsive. Thus, they may represent a more seriously ill group of variant angina patients.

The operative mortality in patients with obstructive coronary atherosclerotic disease (Table 8-3 and Fig. 8-8) was 8 percent, with 7 of 90 patients succumbing during surgery or during the postoperative hospitalization period. This operative mortality is high in relation to current operative standards. It is similar to the 6 percent mortality in the medically treated patients despite the fact that the surgical group consisted of sicker patients. In one series, 4 of 18 patients died at surgery, an operative mortality of 22 percent.[14] It

TABLE 8-3
Results of coronary artery bypass in patients with Prinzmetal's variant angina with obstructive coronary artery disease

Author	No. of patients	No. of bypasses			Asymptomatic or improved	Same or worse	MI	Died
		1	2	3				
Silverman et al., 1971[65]	2	2	0	0	1	0	1	1
Linhart et al., 1972[66]	1	0	1	0	1	0	0	0
Bolooki et al., 1972[67]	1	0	1	0	1	0	0	0
Buonanno et al., 1972[68]	2	1	1	0	2	0	0	0
MacAlpin et al., 1973[9]	6	5	1	0	1	5	0	0
Gaasch et al., 1974[30]	4	3	1	0	3	1	2	0
Shubrooks et al., 1975[23]	15	6	7	2	14	0	1	1
Higgins et al., 1976[25]	6	4	1	1	4	2	1	0
Weiner et al., 1976[14]	18	—	—	—	9	5	4	4
Johnson et al., 1978[26]	25	12	6	7	23	1	2	1
Maseri et al., 1978[17]	10	—	—	—	7	3	0	0
Total	90	33/62	19/62	10/62	66	17	11	7
Percent		53%	31%	16%	73%	19%	12%	8%

MI, myocardial infarction; —, not specified in article.

is not clear why the mortality was so high in this particular series. The surgical mortality in the remaining series included in Table 8-3 was 4 percent.

The incidence of myocardial infarction in the perioperative period or in the early months following surgery was 12 percent (Table 8-3). This finding compares favorably with the 23 percent myocardial infarction rate in the medically treated patients (Table 8-2). Of additional note, an asymptomatic or improved state was achieved in 73 percent of surgically treated patients. These results support the use of coronary bypass surgery in patients with Prinzmetal's variant angina who have critical obstructive coronary artery lesions.

Coronary bypass surgery has not been as successful in patients with variant angina who do not have critically occlusive atherosclerotic disease. Table 8-4 shows the results in 8 patients described in five studies.[25-27,30,32] The operative mortality was 25 percent. Myocardial infarction developed in 13 percent, and 25 percent were unchanged or worse following surgery. Only 50 percent achieved an asymptomatic or improved state (Fig. 8-9).

The reasons for the poor surgical results seem apparent. The predominant pathophysiologic condition in these patients is coronary artery spasm, which may involve the vessel diffusely rather than focally or may occur at variable locations. The bypass graft would be of no benefit when the spasm occurs distal to its insertion. Further, long-term patency of the graft may be jeopardized, since there is competition between flow in the graft and the native coronary artery when spasm is not present.

In contrast, medical management of this subgroup of variant angina patients has been more encouraging (Table 8-5 and Fig. 8-9). Of 41 patients without obstructive atherosclerotic disease receiving medical therapy, 7 percent died. Myocardial infarction developed in 7 percent. Sixty-six percent of patients were improved or became asymptomatic on medical management. Thus, while this group of patients should not be considered to have a benign course, as has been stated,[69] coronary artery bypass surgery does not appear to be beneficial and may be detrimental. Vigorous medical management is clearly the treatment of choice in this select group of patients.

OTHER SURGICAL APPROACHES TO THE TREATMENT OF PRINZMETAL'S VARIANT ANGINA

Investigation of possible mechanisms of coronary artery spasm has suggested an important role of the autonomic nervous system. Coronary vasoconstric-

TABLE 8-4

Results of coronary artery bypass in patients with Prinzmetal's variant angina without obstructive coronary artery disease

Author	No. of patients	Asymptomatic or improved	Same or worse	MI	Died
Dhurandar et al., 1972[27]	1	0	0	0	1
Gaasch et al., 1974[30]	2	1	0	0	1
Hart et al., 1974[32]	1	0	1	0	0
Higgins et al., 1976[25]	1	0	1	0	0
Johnson et al., 1978[26]	3	3	0	1	0
Totals	8	4	2	1	2
Percent		50%	25%	13%	25%

MI, myocardial infarction.

tion has been induced by electrical stimulation of the stellate ganglion.[71] This response can be blocked by alpha-adrenergic antagonists.[71] Reflex coronary vasoconstriction by cold pressor stimulation[51] and angiographic demonstration of coronary artery spasm following cold pressor stimulation[43] lend support to the hypothesis that neurogenic alpha-adrenergic stimulation may be an operative mechanism in some individuals with coronary artery spasm. The ability to provoke coronary spasm with epinephrine combined with propranolol[42] further demonstrates that activa-

TABLE 8-5

Results of medical therapy of Prinzmetal's variant angina without obstructive coronary artery disease

Author	No. of patients	Asymptomatic or improved	Same or worse	MI	Died
MacAlpin et al., 1973[9]	2	0	1	0	1
Shubrooks et al., 1975[23]	3	1	1	0	1
Higgins et al., 1976[25]	7	3	3	0	1
Selzer et al., 1976[69]	9	9	0	0	0
Weiner et al., 1976[14]	11	8	3	2	0
Johnson et al., 1978[26]	9	6	3	1	0
Totals	41	27	11	3	3
Percent		66%	27%	7%	7%

MI, myocardial infarction.

tion of alpha-adrenergic receptors, with blockade of vasodilating beta receptors, provides a plausible mechanism.

Brachfield et al. have shown that coronary blood flow increases following pericoronary denervation.[72] Additionally, ablation of coronary nerves prevents the vasoconstrictor response to stellate ganglion stimulation.[73] Thus the possibility must be entertained that denervation of cardiac sympathetic nerves might offer potential therapeutic benefits to some patients with coronary artery spasm.

Cardiac denervation has been utilized by Clark et al. in the treatment of variant angina.[70] Of 23 patients with variant angina, 8 were refractory to vigorous medical management with vasodilators. Each of these 8 patients was shown to have coronary artery spasm involving one or more vessels. In most instances in this series, there were no hemodynamically significant coronary atherosclerotic lesions in the spastic coronary arteries. Coronary artery bypasses were placed to the spastic arteries in all 8 medically refractory patients. Total cardiac denervation was performed in 2 of these 8 patients by transecting and reanastamosing the great vessels and both atria. Subtotal cardiac denervation was achieved in 3 patients by transection and reanastomosis of the great vessels, while the atria were left intact. In the 3 remaining patients, coronary artery bypass was done without a denervation procedure. Two of the 5 patients with denervation procedures died at or shortly after surgery, resulting in a surgical (denervation procedure) mortality of 40 percent. Three survivors of the denervation plus bypass operations and the 3 patients receiving bypass surgery alone were alive and well 2 years after surgery.

Of great interest is 1 patient who survived complete cardiac denervation and was restudied following surgery. Surprisingly, she still developed coronary artery spasm when provoked by ergonovine.

Firm conclusions cannot be drawn regarding the efficacy of cardiac denervation from this one study. Certainly, the high mortality in this small group warrants caution in this approach. Further, the observation that coronary artery spasm was still present despite autotransplantation raises serious doubts about a primary role of neurogenically induced vasospasm as the sole mechanism in the production of coronary artery spasm.

Thus the serious problem of the management of the patient with diffuse coronary artery spasm and no focal bypassable lesion who continues to have severe ischemic symptoms despite intense medical management remains unsolved. Hopefully the introduction of additional coronary vasodilator drugs, such as the calcium antagonists, will provide additional means of treating this difficult subgroup of variant angina patients.

SUMMARY AND RECOMMENDATIONS

Prinzmetal's variant angina represents an important subgroup of patients within the broad spectrum of ischemic heart disease in whom coronary artery spasm and atherosclerotic occlusive coronary artery disease contribute to the production of myocardial ischemia. The primary clinical manifestation of this condition is angina pectoris, occurring at rest and generally, although not universally, associated with ST-segment elevation. The importance of recognition of these individuals lies in their identification as an unstable group of patients with a high incidence of subsequent myocardial infarction and death.

Coronary arteriography should be performed in all patients with this syndrome in order to determine the nature and extent of underlying atherosclerotic occlusive disease. Coronary artery spasm should be sought and provocative maneuvers utilized when necessary. This is of particular importance in patients who are noted to have normal or nearly normal coronary arteriograms, since the demonstration of coronary artery spasm is needed to provide an explanation for the ischemic manifestations. The information so obtained is necessary to decide on a rational course of therapy. Both medical and surgical modalities play important roles in the management of these patients.

The patient who is found to have no hemodynamically significant atherosclerotic disease, in whom coronary artery spasm is the primary and possibly the sole cause of myocardial ischemia, is best treated with a vigorous medical program, as outlined earlier in the chapter. Coronary artery bypass surgery is not of demonstrated benefit and may worsen the course of such patients. Too little experience is available regarding surgical denervation procedures to assess its value to patients in this subset who are truly refractory to exhaustive medical therapy. Certainly, until greater knowledge and understanding of the pathophysiology of coronary artery spasm is achieved, the rationale for surgical denervation can only be speculative.

The patient who is found to have critical occlusive atherosclerotic disease should be considered for both medical and *surgical therapy.* Medical management is aimed at treating and preventing coronary artery spasm. Additionally, coronary artery bypass surgery is indicated if the location and severity of the occlusive disease justify this approach. Patients with proximal double- or triple-vessel disease or left main stenosis are prime surgical candidates if the distal vessels are suitable for grafting. Patients with single-vessel disease are treated surgically if the magnitude of the lesion and its location suggest that a significant portion of myocardium is precariously jeopardized. The surgical results in these patients have been gratifying.

Medical therapy with vasodilators is vigorously used postoperatively and is continued for several months to prevent recurrence of coronary artery spasm. These agents may then be gradually withdrawn if no further anginal episodes occur.

Therapeutic recommendations for the management of Prinzmetal's variant angina may change in the future. As knowledge of mechanisms is enhanced, as our experiences expand, and as improvements in medical modalities and surgical techniques occur, we must be prepared to readjust our approach.

REFERENCES

1 Prinzmetal, M., Kennamer, R., Merliss, R., Wada, T., and Bor, N.: Angina Pectoris. I. A. Variant Form of Angina Pectoris, *Am. J. Med.,* 27:375, 1959.

2 Prinzmetal, M., Ekmekci, A., Kennamer, R., Kwoczynski, J. K., Shubin, H., and Toyoshima, H.: Variant Form of Angina Pectoris. Previously Undelineated Syndrome, *J.A.M.A.,* 174:1794, 1960.

3 Cheng, T. O., Bashour, T., Kelser, G. A., Weiss, L., and Bacos, J.: Variant Angina of Prinzmetal with Normal Coronary Arteriograms. A Variant of the Variant, *Circulation,* 47:476, 1973.

4 Heberden, W.: Pectoris Dolor, in R. H. Major (ed.), "Classic Descriptions of Disease," 3d ed., Charles C Thomas, Publisher, Springfield, Ill., 1948, p. 420.

5 Maseri, A., Mimmo, R., Chierchia, S., Marchesi, C., Pesola, A., and L'Abbate, A.: Coronary Artery Spasm as a Cause of Myocardial Ischemia in Man, *Chest,* 68:625, 1975.

6 Kossowsky, W. A., Mohr, B. D., Summers, D. M., and Lyon, A. F.: Further Variant Patterns Within Prinzmetal Angina Pectoris, *Chest,* 66:622, 1974.

7 Guazzi, M., Olivari, M. T., Polese, A., Fiorentini, C., and Magrini, F.: Repetitive Myocardial Ischemia of Prinzmetal Type Without Angina Pectoris, *Am. J. Cardiol.,* 37:923, 1976.

8 Gorfinkel, H. J., Inglesby, T. V., Lansing, A. M., and Goodin, R. R.: ST-Segment Elevation, Transient Left-Posterior Hemiblock, and Recurrent Ventricular Arrhythmias Unassociated with Pain. A Variant of Prinzmetal's Anginal Syndrome, *Ann. Intern. Med.,* 79:795, 1973.

9 MacAlpin, R. N., Kattus, A. A., and Alvaro, A. B.: Angina Pectoris at Rest with Preservation of Exercuse Capacity: Prinzmetal's Variant Angina, *Circulation,* 47:946, 1973.

10 Oliva, P. B., Potts, D. E., and Pluss, R. G.: Coronary Arterial Spasm in Prinzmetal Angina. Documentation by Coronary Arteriography, *N. Engl. J. Med.,* 288:745, 1973.

11 Schroeder, J. S., Silverman, J. F., and Harrison, D. C.: Right Coronary Arterial Spasm Causing Prinzmetal's Variant Angina, *Chest,* 65:573, 1974.

12 Rose, F. J., Johnson, A. D., and Carleton, R. A.: Spasm of the Left Anterior Descending Coronary Artery, *Chest,* 66:719, 1974.

13 Marsh, C. A., Benchimol, A., and Desser, K. B.: Variant Angina Pectoris: Pain and Arrhythmias Controlled after Postoperative Myocardial Infarction, *J.A.M.A.,* 235:833, 1976.

14 Wiener, L., Kasparian, H., Duca, P. R., Walinsky, P., Gottlieb, R. S., Hanckel, F., and Brest, A. N.: Spectrum of Coronary Arterial Spasm. Clinical, Angiographic and Myocardial Metabolic Experience in 29 Cases, *Am. J. Cardiol.,* 38:945, 1976.

15 Prchkov, V. K., Mookherjee, S., Schiess, W., and Obeid, A. L.: Variant Anginal Syndrome, Coronary Artery Spasm and Ventricular Fibrillation in Absence of Chest Pain, *Ann. Intern. Med.,* 81:858, 1974.

16 Chahine, R. A., and Raizner, A. E.: Another Look at Prinzmetal's Variant Angina, *Eur. J. Cardiol.,* 6:71, 1977.

17 Maseri, A., Severi, S., DeNes, M., L'Abbate, A., Chierchia, S., Marzilli, M., Ballestra, A. M., Parodi, A., and Distante, A.: "Variant" Angina. One Aspect of a Continuous Spectrum of Vasospastic Myocardial Ischemia. Pathogenetic Mechanisms, Estimated Incidence and Clinical and Coronary Arteriographic Findings in 138 Patients, *Am. J. Cardiol.,* 42:1019, 1978.

18 Raizner, A. E., Chahine, R. A., Ishimori, T., and Luchi, R. J.: Coronary Artery Spasm. An Expanding Role in Ischemic Heart Disease, *Texas Med.,* 74:46, 1978.

19 Heupler, F. A.: Current Concepts of Prinzmetal's Variant Form of Angina Pectoris, *Clev. Clin. Q.,* 43:131, 1976.

20 Chahine, R. A., Raizner, A. E., and Luchi, R. J.: Coronary Arterial Spasm in Classic Angina Pectoris, *Cathet. Cardiovasc. Diagn.,* 1:337, 1975.

21 Bentivoglio, L. G., Ablaza, S. G. G., and Greenberg, L. F.: Bypass Surgery for Prinzmetal Angina, *Arch. Intern. Med.,* 134:313, 1974.

22 Stenson, R. E., Flamm, M. D., Zaret, B. L., and McGowan, R. L.: Transient ST-Segment Elevation with Postmyocardial Infarction Angina: Prognostic Significance, *Am. Heart J.,* 89:449, 1975.

23 Shubrooks, S. J., Bete, J. M., Hutter, A. M., Block, P. C., Buckley, M. H., Daggett, W. M., and Mundth, E. D.: Variant Angina Pectoris: Clinical and Anatomic Spectrum and Results of Coronary Bypass Surgery, *Am. J. Cardiol.,* 36:142, 1975.

24 Endo, M., Kanda, I., Hosoda, S., Hayashi, H., Hirosawa, K., and Konna, S.: Prinzmetal's Variant Form of

Angina Pectoris. Re-evaluation of Mechanisms, *Circulation,* 52:33, 1975.

25 Higgins, C. B., Wexler, L., Silverman, J. F., and Schroeder, J. S.: Clinical and Arteriographic Features of Prinzmetal's Variant Angina: Documentation of Etiologic Factors, *Am. J. Cardiol.,* 37:831, 1976.

26 Johnson, A. D., Stroud, H. A., Vieweg, V. R., and Ross, J.: Variant Angina Pectoris: Clinical Presentations, Coronary Angiographic Patterns, and the Results of Medical and Surgical Management in 42 Consecutive Patients, *Chest,* 73:786, 1978.

27 Dhurandar, R. W., Watt, D. L., Silver, M. D., Trimble, A. S., and Adelman, A. G.: Prinzmetal's Variant Form of Angina with Arteriographic Evidence of Coronary Arterial Spasm, *Am. J. Cardiol.,* 30:902, 1972.

28 Chahine, R. A., Raizner, A. E., Ishimori, T., Luchi, R., and McIntosh, H.: The Incidence and Clinical Implications of Coronary Artery Spasm, *Circulation,* 52:972, 1975.

29 King, M. J., Zir, L. M., Kaltman, A. J., and Fox, A. C.: Variant Angina Associated with Angiographically Demonstrated Coronary Artery Spasm and REM Sleep, *Am. J. Med. Sci.,* 265:419, 1973.

30 Gaasch, W. H., Lufschanowski, R., Leachman, R. D., and Alexander, J. K.: Surgical Management of Prinzmetal's Variant Angina, *Chest,* 66:614, 1974.

31 Kerin N., and MacLeod, C. A.: Coronary Artery Spasm Associated with Variant Angina Pectoris, *Br. Heart J.,* 36:224, 1974.

32 Hart, N. J., Silverman, M. E., and King, S. B.: Variant Angina Pectoris Caused by Coronary Artery Spasm, *Am. J. Med.,* 56:269, 1974.

33 Rose, F. J., Johnson, A. D., and Carleton, R. A.: Spasm of the Left Anterior Descending Coronary Artery, *Chest,* 66:719, 1974.

34 Applefield M. M., and Ronan, J. A.: Prinzmetal's Angina with Extensive Spasm of the Right Coronary Artery, *Chest,* 66:721, 1974.

35 Maseri, A., Parodi, O., Severi, S., and Pesola, A.: Transient Transmural Reduction of Myocardial Blood Flow, Demonstrated by Thallium-201 Scintigraphy, as a Cause of Variant Angina, *Circulation,* 54:280, 1976.

36 Maseri, A., Pesola, A., Marzelli, M., Severi, S., Parodi, O., L'Abbate, A., Ballestra, A. M., Maltini, G., Denes, D. M., and Biagini, A.: Coronary Vasospasm in Angina Pectoris, *Lancet,* 1:713, 1977.

37 Luchi, R. J., Chahine, R. A., and Raizner, A. E.: Coronary Artery Spasm, *Ann. Intern. Med.,* in press.

38 Heupler, F. A., Proudfit, W. L., Razavi, M., Shirey, E. K., Greenstreet, R., and Sheldon, W. C.: Ergonovine Maleate Provocative Test for Coronary Arterial Spasm, *Am. J. Cardiol.,* 41:631, 1978.

39 Schroeder, J. S., Bolen, J. L., Quint, R. A., Clark, D.

A., Hayden, W. G., Higgins, C. B., and Wexler, L.: Provocation of Coronary Spasm with Ergonovine Maleate. New Test with Results in 57 Patients Undergoing Coronary Arteriography, *Am. J. Cardiol.,* 40:487, 1977.

40 Curry, R. C., Pepine, C. J., Sabom, H. B., Feldman, R. L., Christie, L. G., and Conti, C. R.: Effects of Ergonovine in Patients With and Without Coronary Artery Disease, *Circulation,* 56:803, 1977.

41 Endo, M., Hirosawa, K., Kaneko, N., Hase, K., Inoue, Y., and Konno, S.: Prinzmetal's Variant Angina. Coronary Arteriogram and Left Ventriculogram During Angina Attack Induced by Methacholine, *N. Engl. J. Med.,* 294:252, 1976.

42 Yasue, H., Touyama, M., Kato, H., Tanaka, S., and Akiyama, F.: Prinzmetal's Variant Form of Angina as a Manifestation of Alpha-Adrenergic Receptor Medicated Coronary Artery Spasm: Documentation by Coronary Arteriography, *Am. Heart J.,* 91:148, 1976.

43 Raizner, A. E., Ishimori, T., Chahine, R. A., Jamal, N., and Luchi, R. J.: The Provocation of Coronary Artery Spasm by the Cold Pressor Test, *Am. J. Cardiol.,* 41:358, 1978.

44 Yasue, H., Nagao, M., Omote, S., Takizawa, A., Miwa, K., and Tanaka, S.: Coronary Arterial Spasm and Prinzmetal's Variant Form of Angina Induced by Hyperventilation and TRIS-buffer Infusion, *Circulation,* 58:56, 1978.

45 Fuller, C., Chahine, R. A., Raizner, A. E., Ishimori, T., Nahormek, P., and Mokotoff, D.: Coronary Artery Spasm Induced by Exercise in a Patient with Exercise-induced ST Segment Elevation, unpublished data.

46 Meller, J., Pichard, A., and Dack, S.: Coronary Arterial Spasm in Prinzmetal's Angina: A Proved Hypothesis, *Am. J. Cardiol.,* 37:938, 1976.

47 Ekmekci, A., Toyoshima, H., Kwoczynski, J. K., Nagaya, T., and Prinzmetal, M.: Angina Pectoris. IV. Clinical and Experimental Difference Between Ischemia with ST Elevation and Ischemia with ST Depression, *Am. J. Cardiol.,* 7:412, 1961.

48 Guazzi, M., Polese, A., Fiorentini, C., Magrini, F., Olivari, M. T., and Bartorelli, C.: Left and Right Hemodynamics During Spontaneous Angina Pectoris. Comparison Between Angina with ST Segment Depression and Angina with ST Segment Elevation, *Br. Heart J.,* 37:401, 1974.

49 Gensini, G. G.: Coronary Artery Spasm and Angina Pectoris, *Chest,* 68:709, 1975.

50 Hellstrom, H. R.: The Advantages of a Vasospastic Cause of Myocardial Infarction, *Am. Heart J.,* 90:545, 1975.

51 Mudge, G. H., Grossman, W., Mills, R. M., Jr., Lesch, M., and Braunwald, E.: Reflex Increase in Coronary Vascular Resistance in Patients With Ischemic Heart Disease, *N. Engl. J. Med.,* 295:1333, 1976.

52 Cipriano, P. R., Guthaner, D. F., Orlick, A. E., Ricci, D. R., Wexler, L., and Silverman, J. F.: The Effects of Er-

gonovine Maleate on Coronary Arterial Size, *Circulation,* 59:82, 1979.

53 Linegar, C. R.: The Modification of the Hemodynamic Effects of Acetylcholine by Ergotamine, *Am. J. Physiol.,* 129:53, 1940.

54 Ellis, E. F., Oelz, O., Roberts, L. J. I. I., Payne, N. A., Swetman, B. J., Nies, A. S., and Oates, J. A.: Coronary Arterial Smooth Muscle Contraction by a Substance Released from Platelets: Evidence That It Is Thromboxane A₂, *Science,* 193:1135, 1976.

55 Needleman, P., Kulkarni, P., and Raz, A.: Coronary Tone Modulation: Formation and Actions of Prostaglandins, Endoperoxides and Thromboxanes, *Science,* 195:409, 1977.

56 Folts, J. D., Crowell, E. B., and Rowe, G. G.: Platelet Aggregation in Partially Obstructed Vessels and Its Elimination with Aspirin, *Circulation,* 54:365, 1976.

57 Levene, D. A., and Freeman, M. R.: Alpha-Adrenoreceptor-Mediated Coronary Artery Spasm, *J.A.M.A.,* 236:1018, 1976.

58 Johnson, A. D., and Detwiler, J. H.: Coronary Spasm, Variant Angina, and Recurrent Myocardial Infarctions, *Circulation,* 55:947, 1977.

59 Oliva, P. B., and Breckinridge, J. C.: Arteriographic Evidence of Coronary Arterial Spasm in Acute Myocardial Infarction, *Circulation,* 56:366, 1977.

60 Chahine, R. A.: Prinzmetal's Variant Angina: A Syndrome Apart or Another Clinical Presentation of Atheromatous Heart Disease, *Arch. Intern. Med.,* 139:26, 1979.

61 Hosoda, S., and Kimura, E.: Efficacy of Nifedipine in the Variant Form of Angina Pectoris. Excerpta Medica International Congress Series, No. 388:195, 1976.

62 Parodi, O., Simonetti, I., and Maseri, A.: Management of "Crescendo" Angina by Verapamil. A Double Blind Cross-over Study in CCU, *Circulation,* 56 (suppl. 3):224, 1977.

63 Raizner, A. E., Gaston, W., Chahine, R. A., Luchi, R. J., Ishimoro, T., and Fulweber, R.: Unpublished observations.

64 Guazzi, M., Magrini, F., Fiorentini, C., and Polese, A.: Clinical, Electrocardiographic, and Hemodynamic Effects of Long-term Use of Propranolol in Prinzmetal's Variant Angina Pectoris, *Br. Heart J.,* 33:889, 1971.

65 Silverman, M. D., and Flamm, M. D.: Variant Angina Pectoris. Anatomic Findings and Prognostic Implications, *Ann. Intern. Med.,* 75:339, 1971.

66 Linhart, J. W., Beller, B. M., and Talley, R. C.: Preinfarction Angina: Clinical, Hemodynamic and Angiographic Evaluation, *Chest,* 61:312, 1972.

67 Bolooki, H., Vargas, A., Gharamani, A., Sommer, L., Orvald, T., Jude, J., and Baccabella K.: Aortocoronary Bypass Graft for Preinfarction Angina, *Chest,* 61:247, 1972.

68 Buonanno, C., Manucuso, M., Zanini, S., et al.: Diagnosi e Triattamento dell 'Inficienza Coronarica Acuta. A Proposito di Sei Casi, *G. Ital. Cardiol.,* 2:893, 1972.

69 Selzer, A., Langston, M., Ruggeroli, C., and Cohn, K.: Clinical Syndrome of Variant Angina with Normal Coronary Arteriogram, *N. Engl. J. Med.,* 295:1343, 1976.

70 Clark, D. A., Quint, R. A., Mitchell, R. L., and Angell, W. W.: Coronary Artery Spasm. Medical Management, Surgical Denervation, and Autotransplantation, *J. Thorac. Cardiovasc. Surg.,* 73:332, 1977.

71 Feigl, E. O.: Sympathetic Control of Coronary Circulation, *Cir. Res.,* 20:262, 1967.

72 Brachfield, N.: Effect of Pericoronary Denervation on Coronary Hemodynamics, *Am. J., Physiol.,* 199:174, 1960.

73 Kaye, M.: Localization and Surgical Section of Coronary Vasconstrictor Nerve, *Circulation,* 51 (suppl. 2):125, 1975.

Chapter 9

The Prevention of Myocardial Infarction by Coronary Bypass Surgery*

DEAN T. MASON, M.D., EZRA A. AMSTERDAM, M.D.,
ANTHONY N. De MARIA, M.D., JOAN L. SMITH, M.A.,
GARRETT LEE, M.D., JAMES A. JOYE, M.D.,
ZAKAUDDIN VERA, M.D., and NAJAM A. AWAN, M.D.

Extensive clinical investigations during the past decade have clearly documented that properly performed aortocoronary bypass is an effective and reliable surgical modality for providing a new source of blood supply to obstructed native arteries of the heart.[1-4] That this operative procedure improves diminished myocardial perfusion and thereby also relieves angina pectoris in appropriately selected patients is now well acknowledged by enthusiasts[1-10] and antagonists[11-20] alike. Furthermore, it is now well established that properly performed coronary bypass of diseased vessels effectively relieves severe drug-resistant myocardial ischemic pain in the various angina syndromes (stable, unstable, and variant types).[1-8,21-27] The potential importance of such direct revascularization surgery is emphasized by the treacherous consequences of coronary atherosclerosis which are often unrelated to the presence or degree of symptoms; this dangerous disorder of ubiquitous prevalence constitutes the predominant cause of disability and death nationally[28] and worldwide.[29]

EXTENSION OF CORONARY BYPASS INDICATIONS

Enhanced delivery of blood flow to previously ischemic myocardium can be accomplished in atherosclerotic diseased vessels via coronary bypass with low mortality by skilled surgeons utilizing modern methods for myocardial protection.[1-10] In addition to the generally accepted indications for the procedure in patients with chronic stable, incapacitating, maximal, drug-refractory angina with suitably operable

major vessel stenosis (in whom it was initially carried out) and in patients with high-grade obstruction in the left main coronary artery,[1-4] several outstanding referral institutions are now extending the operation to a number of relative indications on an individual patient basis.[1-10] These relative indications include a history of one of the conditions that make up the spectrum of unstable angina pectoris; a history of having been successfully resuscitated from ventricular fibrillation even without subsequent angina; individuals who have healed myocardial infarction with or without angina pectoris;[10,30] angina with left ventricular dysfunction; patients with obstructed coronary arteries in whom valvular disease is the primary indication for surgery; relatively young adults (usually less than 60 years of age) with severe coronary artery pathoanatomic subsets (three- or two-vessel proximal stenoses); and patients with single-vessel obstruction (left anterior descending proximal stenosis) without previous infarction who are at high risk for early mortality and in whom angina is not responsive to medical therapy or who otherwise have objective evidence of active myocardial ischemia. In these additional patient groups with relative indications for coronary bypass, the procedure is recommended only for ideally operable vessels as defined by selective arteriography (discrete proximal stenosis beneath which the distal segment is entirely patent), in contrast to coronary surgery applied to patients with incapacitating angina unaffected by optimal medical therapy in whom arteriography may reveal more diffuse disease less suited for ease of revascularization.[3,7,10,31,32]

The rationale for the above additional applications of coronary bypass surgery in patients with less than disabling chronic stable angina refractory or poorly responsive to intensive medical therapy, including propranolol, requires that the operative intervention must be performed with minimal risk (surgical mortality less than 2 percent, perioperative infarction less than 6 percent, all obstructive lesions in suitable major coronary vessels bypassed, one-year bypass graft patency rate greater than 90 percent, and amelioration of

*From the Section of Cardiovascular Medicine, Departments of Medicine and Physiology, University of California School of Medicine and Sacramento Medical Center, Davis and Sacramento.

Supported in part by Research Program Project Grant HL-14780 from the National Heart, Lung and Blood Institute, National Institutes of Health, Bethesda, Maryland.

myocardial ischemia) in these particular individuals, utilizing appropriate medical therapy postoperatively when necessary and instituting coronary risk factor reduction measures, including a program of exercise rehabilitation.[1-4,7] These comments are predicated on excellent surgical experience in specialized centers[2,33] to justify the recommendation that the characteristics of coronary obstruction and left ventricular performance (rather than the degree of symptoms alone) constitute the primary hallmarks upon which management is formulated in overt ischemic heart disease. Thus the location and extent of major vessel obstruction determine the indication for revascularization, and the integrity of ventricular function defines the risk.[10]

RATIONALE FOR PROPHYLACTIC CORONARY BYPASS

In considering the merits of elective coronary bypass principally carried out for prophylactic reasons in patients with minimal angina,[1-10] besides the essential requirement that the procedure be carried out in excellent fashion,[2,33] it is of paramount importance to assess the operation relative to the incidence of morbidity and mortality of the natural history of ischemic heart disease and to the value of modern medical therapeutics.[7,10] Therefore, although coronary bypass surgery plays an important role in the management of ischemic heart disease, in addition to pursuing the technical skills necessary for high success, it is also necessary to recognize that revascularization should only be undertaken on an individual patient basis when the mortality or morbidity risk with medical therapy appears greater than that expected with surgery. An unselective attitude of aggressive surgical management is imprudent and hazardous. The influence of coronary bypass on the incidence of late postoperative myocardial infarction is the primary subject of this chapter. In this regard, the salutary effects of properly performed coronary bypass on the reduction of the degree and presence of angina pectoris[1-10] and the apparent benefits of the procedure on life-span[1-10,34,35] favor the probability that myocardial revascularization also reduces the frequency and mortality of late postoperative acute myocardial infarction.

NATURAL HISTORY OF STABLE ANGINA PECTORIS

The advent of selective coronary angiography has provided a means for evaluating the relation of coronary artery pathoanatomy to the clinical manifestations and prognosis of ischemic heart disease. It is now established that the majority of patients with clinically evident coronary disease indicated by angina pectoris, myocardial infarction, or sudden death have severe and extensive obstruction of the coronary arteries. Approximately three-fourths of these patients have major stenoses in two or three coronary arteries.[36,37] Patients with clinically overt atherosclerotic heart disease and involvement of only one major vessel are less common, accounting for less than 30 percent of the coronary population. Data from our institution (University of California Davis Medical Center, Sacramento), shown in Fig. 9-1, exemplify these findings.[37] Angiographic studies have further demonstrated that clinically manifested myocardial ischemia is usually associated with compromise of more than 75 percent of the cross-sectional area (greater than 50 percent luminal diameter narrowing) of one or more coronary arteries.[38] Abnormalities of ventricular function in coronary heart disease, whether transient (angina) or permanent (infarction), are characteristically segmental in location[39] and distributed according to the regional perfusion deficits in the myocardium as determined by the sites of coronary obstruction. Although restricted coronary blood flow is principally caused by atherosclerotic vascular narrowing, it is now also appreciated that, in addition to its chief role in variant angina,[23] coronary spasm can occasionally result in further compromise of flow and produce myocardial ischemia and infarction in the common coronary syndromes.[40]

The clinical presentation of coronary heart disease has been demonstrated by the classic epidemiologic Framingham study of over 5,000 persons followed for more than 20 years.[41] In the male population that developed clinical coronary disease, the most common initial presentation was myocardial infarction (45 percent). Angina pectoris was next in frequency (32 percent), and sudden death was the initial manifestation in 9 percent of cases. Angina was frequently preceded by myocardial infarction in men. In women, angina accounted for 56 percent of the presenting events. Coronary heart disease resulted in considerable immediate mortality (33 percent), and long-term survival was impaired.

Meaningful analysis of long-term prognosis in coronary heart disease is predicated on appreciation of the heterogeneity of this population with respect to the variables influencing survival. The presence and degree of ischemic pain poorly relate to occurrence of disastrous events, and although progression of coronary atherosclerosis and development of life-threatening complications are relatively unpredictable, mortality and morbidity can be considerably better judged from knowledge of the number of obstructed major vessels and the status of left ventricular function.[42,43]

Although the annual mortality is 4 to 6 percent in patients with suggestive clinical evidence of coronary heart disease without angiographic confirmation,[41,44] recent studies based on coronary angiography demonstrated significant differences in survival relating to the extent of coronary artery involvement. These investigations have consistently shown that annual mortality is directly proportional to the number of obstructed coronary arteries. In two separate surveys involving a total of 832 stable angina patients,[45,46] annual mortality was compared to angiographically documented coronary artery obstruction and revealed similar data within vascular disease groups: one-vessel disease (3 to 4 percent), two-vessel disease (6 to 7 percent) and three-vessel disease (12 to 13 percent); the overall annual mortality in the 832 patients was 8 percent. In regard to single-vessel obstruction,[42] the yearly death rate is highest in left anterior descending coronary disease (4 to 6 percent); the rate in left circumflex disease is 3 to 4 percent, and that in right coronary disease, 2 to 3 percent. With obstruction of the left main coronary artery,[42-46] the death rate is highest within the first year (22 to 32 percent), with a subsequent annual mortality of 13 percent.

The adverse affects of healed myocardial infarction (segmental dyssynergy) and generalized left ventricular dysfunction in coronary heart disease are well documented.[46] Thus, over a 10-year course of nonsurgical intervention in patients with single-vessel coronary obstruction in whom coronary bypass was feasible, annual mortality of only 3 percent with normal cardiac performance (ejection fraction of > 50 percent) increases to 8 percent with significantly impaired left ventricular function (ejection fraction of < 30 percent). Similarly, the annual mortality of two-vessel coronary obstruction amenable to revascularization is increased from 5 percent to 8 percent, and the yearly death rate of 6 percent in three-vessel obstruction with normal heart performance that is amenable to revascularization is raised to nearly 10 percent annually with severely abnormal left ventricular function. From these data the general statement can be made that the frequency of sudden death and fatal myocardial infarction is greater in severe multivessel disease and that life-threatening dysrhythmias and acute necrosis are more often fatal with left ventricular dysfunction.

MYOCARDIAL INFARCTION INCIDENCE IN STABLE ANGINA

Although considerable information exists on mortality in chronic stable angina pectoris, there is a surprising lack of meaningful data concerning the incidence of acute myocardial infarction (fatal and nonfatal) in sta-

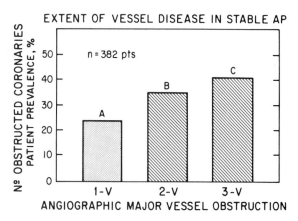

FIGURE 9-1 Proportion of stable angina pectoris (AP) coronary patients with one (1)-vessel (V) (bar A), two (2)-V (bar B), and three (3)-V (bar C) major coronary artery obstruction. Data based on coronary angiography of 382 coronary patients carried out at the University of California Davis Medical Center, Sacramento.

ble angina[47,48] to provide the necessary frame of reference for comparison with the expected benefit of coronary bypass on subsequent myocardial infarction—the main purpose of this report and a principal objective of direct revascularization itself. In view of the dearth of such data, one approach is to derive myocardial infarction incidence from mortality statistics. Since at least three-fourths of prehospital sudden cardiac deaths appear unrelated to new necrosis,[49,50] a conservative figure is that 40 percent of acute infarctions in stable angina patients are fatal within 1 month of the sudden necrotic process (at least one-half having died prior to hospitalization).[51] Furthermore, given that approximately 50 percent of sudden deaths are the result of dysrhythmias (ventricular fibrillation) without acute infarction[52] and that nearly 10 percent of mortality is related to causes other than such dysrhythmias of infarction, the 40 percent incidence of fatality resulting from acute myocardial infarction in previously stable angina is also substantiated. In hospitalized patients surviving acute infarction, the postdischarge mortality is 10 percent within the subsequent year,[53] of which one-half are judged to result from reinfarction. From these observations in stable angina patients (Fig. 9-2*A*), the annual rate of myocardial infarction is calculated at 8 percent (3.4 percent deaths and 4.6 percent survivors).

In recognition of the paucity of rigorously obtained data concerning the incidence of myocardial infarction in the medically treated coronary population without surgical intervention, we evaluated the rate of spontaneous occurrence and fate of acute infarction in 269 consecutive patients with stable angina pectoris in

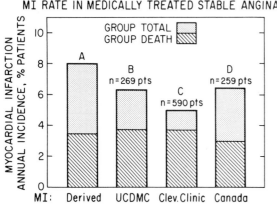

MI RATE IN MEDICALLY TREATED STABLE ANGINA

FIGURE 9-2 Annual incidence of myocardial infarction (MI) in medically treated stable angina patients (pts). Total percentage of patients who developed acute infarction per year is indicated by the full height (dotted plus diagonal areas) of each bar, and fatal infarctions are shown by the height of the diagonal-lined area within each bar. Bar A: derived from reported statistics as explained in text. Bar B: determined from angiographically defined coronary patients (*n*) at the University of California Davis Medical Center, Sacramento (UCDMC). Bar C: determined from angiographically defined coronary patients at the Cleveland Clinic.[46] Bar D: determined from angiographically defined coronary patients at the Queen's University Hospital in Ontario, Canada.[56]

whom the presence and extent of coronary disease was defined angiographically at the University of California Davis Medical Center, Sacramento (UCDMC). Multivessel obstruction was documented in 170 of these patients, and single-vessel obstruction was found in the remainder; the average duration of follow-up was 25 months. Infarction developed in a total of 34 patients, and the event was fatal in 20 of these patients. As shown in Fig. 9-2*B*, the annual incidence of total (6.3 percent) and fatal (3.7 percent) infarctions were similar to the derived rate of infarctions (Fig. 9-2*A*). In our UCDMC series (Fig. 9-2*B*), diagnosis of acute infarction was confined to inhospital ECG documentation and prehospital sudden deaths, and other causes of death were not counted as infarctions.

Consistent with the derived and UCDMC documented incidences of myocardial infarction in stable angina treated medically are the limited observations reported by others. Of the 590 nonsurgical coronary patients studied angiographically by the Cleveland Clinic from 1963 to 1965 and followed for 5 years, in the 327 survivors, infarction occurred in 42 patients (3 percent nonfatal infarctions annually), but data on fatal infarctions were not available at that time.[54,55] Recently, a 10-year follow-up report has been provided for these 590 Cleveland Clinic patients in which it was possible to ascertain fatal as well as nonfatal infarctions;[46] on a yearly basis over this extended pe-

riod, the total patient infarction rate was 5.0 percent, 3.7 percent of which were fatal (Fig. 9-2*C*). At the Queen's University Hospital in Ontario,[56] infarctions developed in 69 of 259 angiographically documented coronary patients treated medically for an average of 51 months (annual total infarction rate, 6.4 percent, and lethal infarctions, 3.0 percent annually) (Fig. 9-2*D*). As in our UCDMC study, none of the prehospital sudden deaths was considered as resulting from acute necrosis in the Cleveland Clinic and Canadian reports.

MODERN MEDICAL THERAPY OF STABLE ANGINA

The relatively recent introduction of propranolol and other beta-adrenergic blockers to medical treatment programs of coronary disease is believed by some clinicians to have considerably benefited life expectancy in patients with stable angina pectoris.[57,58] There are no scientifically valid data available to support this contention. These agents do represent the most important pharmacologic advancement in the medical relief of antianginal symptoms, but they provide less anginal relief than properly performed coronary bypass surgery.[1-10,34,35,59,60] Although a recent report implies that propranolol may reduce the frequency of completed necrosis in the intermediate syndrome of unstable angina,[61] a large body of data has shown that properly performed coronary bypass surgery is more effective in this regard.[1-4,21,22,24-27] The finding that propranolol appears to diminish ischemic injury in patients with acute myocardial infarction[62] has not been translated to improved subsequent morbidity and mortality. The preliminary aborted study[63] suggesting that long-term practolol administration in patients who have recovered from myocardial infarction might enhance prognosis requires substantiation and is oblique to the present discussion.

In the ongoing Veterans Administration multicenter prospective randomized study on the effectiveness of bypass surgery versus modern medical therapy in the treatment of chronic stable angina,[58] only the results on longevity have been reported. Despite a number of acknowledged imperfections inherent in the protocol and methods possible for statistical analysis,[17] overall cumulative survival in the surgical group (86 percent of patients) now exceeds that in the medical group (83 percent) at 4 years.[64] Disturbingly, the investigators consider their medical group survival (mortality 4.3 percent annually) to be enhanced[64] (a principal factor in preventing their surgical group survival from being significantly greater than medical survival) and largely attribute the improved medical longevity to the use of propranolol.[33,58] However, taking into account that their medical group comprises only selected good-risk patients, with 16 percent having just single-vessel stenosis (eliminated were 13 percent of the patient population because of left main coronary obstruction, as well as others because of unstable angina, recent healed infarction, or depressed left ventricular function), and that 17 percent of the original medical group were lost to follow-up (the majority of such nonadherers being medical treatment failures), the VA medical group survival rate is no better and probably even worse than in comparable coronary patients treated medically prior to propranolol and in such patients reported from epidemiologic studies without angiographic proof of coronary disease.[65,66]

In a potentially operable group of 352 arteriographically and ventriculographically documented comparable patients with one-, two- or three-vessel disease treated medically without beta blockers at the Cleveland Clinic for 4 years (1963 to 1966), the annual mortality was less than 5 percent.[46] Furthermore, in the VA prospective randomized trial of patients with left main coronary artery obstruction,[67] the annual mortality of propranolol-treated medical patients was 13 percent, in marked contrast to only 5 percent in the surgical group (including operative deaths) for the 3-year period of observation. Moreover, at the University of Alabama,[68] revascularization of three-vessel obstruction enhanced survival more than threefold at 3 years as compared concurrently to comparable patients receiving optimal medical therapy who were suitable candidates for grafting; surgery in two-vessel obstruction improved longevity twofold at 2 years versus potentially graftable patients given modern medical treatment. Recently, similar results in prospectively matched patients have been reported at the University of Washington Medical Center in Seattle[43] and at our institution (UCDMC).[34] It is also important to emphasize the hazards of procrastination[2] in allowing angina patients who are controlled by modern medical therapy to sustain nonfatal infarctions, with the result that such patients may change from revascularizable candidates to an inoperable status. It seems that proof is lacking that propranolol effectively prevents infarction and extends longevity in patients with angina pectoris.

PERIOPERATIVE MYOCARDIAL INFARCTION IN STABLE ANGINA

The merits of an operation in which a principal objective is prevention of a specific complication must necessarily be considered in relation to the incidence and consequences of that complication resulting from the procedure itself. Paradoxically, the most common potentially serious complication of pure coronary bypass is perioperative infarction, most reliably indicated as

transmural with the appearance of new and persistent pathologic Q waves on the body surface ECG within a few hours to several days postoperatively.[1,4,38,47,69-75] Since the infarction may not result in such diagnostic ECG changes, detection is aided by radionuclide cardiac hot-spot scintigraphy in which there is accumulation of intravenously injected technetium-99m-pyrophosphate within the area of fresh myocardial necrosis (Fig. 9-3).[76]

In addition, significant elevations of myocardial enzymes in the peripheral blood may help in the identification of perioperative infarction. Since myocardial injury of some degree nearly always occurs with direct revascularization surgery, transient ST-T wave changes and myocardial enzyme rises are commonly observed without necrosis. Myocardial enzyme alterations usu-

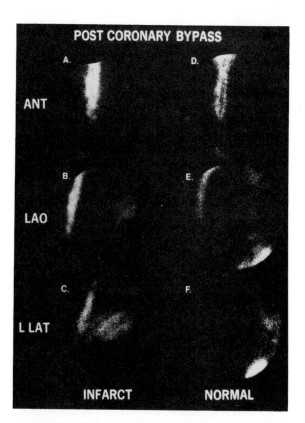

FIGURE 9-3 Technetium-99m-pyrophosphate (Tc-99m-PYP) scintigrams in the period immediately following coronary artery bypass in a patient with intraoperative posterolateral myocardial infarction (MI) (left column) and in a patient without intraoperative MI (right column). The perioperative MI is observed by the increased myocardial uptake of Tc-99m-PYP within the cardiac region in images A, B, and C comprising the left column, particularly image *C*. In contrast, there is no cardiac accumulation of Tc-99m-PYP in the noninfarction patient (images D, E, F). ANT, anterior view; LAO, left anterior oblique view; LLAT, left lateral view. Note the vertical line of decreased radioactivity in the anterior views (top panel) signifying the area of sternotomy.

ally associated with intraoperative infarction[71-75] include first-postoperative-day elevations of serum glutamic oxaloacetic transaminase (SGOT) levels of > 100 units per liter, creatine phosphokinase (CPK) levels of > 1,000 units per liter, lactic acid dehydrogenase (LDH) levels of > 900 units per liter, and myocardial-specific isoenzyme of creatine phosphokinase (CPK-MB) levels of > 30 units ml^{-1} kg cumulative release (delayed peak > 6 h and disappearance > 48 h).

The incidence of perioperative infarction depends principally on patient selection, anesthetic management, operative technique, myocardial protection, and postoperative management.[1] In general, increased hazard of infarction is related to previous infarction and left ventricular dysfunction; multivessel disease with poor distal patency; hypertension,[77] hypotension, and tachyarrhythmias during induction of anesthesia from intubation until institution of cardiopulmonary bypass; increased duration of cardiopulmonary bypass time and decreased mean arterial perfusion pressure; extended period of anoxic arrest and ventricular fibrillation; associated aortic valve replacement; postoperative hypotension, dysrhythmias and excessive use of intravenous dopamine-like cardiotonic agents; and bypass graft closure.

Postoperative angiographic studies have shown that there is an inconsistent relationship between the site of graft occlusion and the region of infarction.[1,38,47,74,78-82] Thus, 25 percent of perioperative infarctions are unassociated with the graft and occur in other areas supplied by a diseased but ungrafted native coronary. While 70 percent of infarctions occur in the area supplied by the graft, only one-half of these grafts are occluded. Approximately 20 percent of patients without infarction have closure of one graft. However, postoperative left ventricular dysfunction in patients with infarction is related to graft occlusion or progression of disease in ungrafted vessels. In addition, frequency of graft occlusions was four times greater in patients (50 percent) with transmural infarction than in patients without perioperative infarction.

Graft patency is now approximately 90 percent after 1 year, and subsequent occlusion occurs in less than 2 percent per year.[1-4,47,79-82] Five to 10 percent of grafts close early (within 2 weeks) as a result of thrombosis, and nearly an additional 10 percent occlude between 2 weeks and 1 year because of intimal fibrosis. Graft closure resulting from intimal proliferation is now unusual. Rare primary closure after 1 year appears to be the result of atherosclerotic disease.[82] Saphenous vein grafts with intraoperative flows of > 40 ml/min rarely occlude,[3] and those with flows of < 40 ml/min commonly thrombose. Although somewhat difficult to use technically, internal thoracic artery grafts (flows of > 20 ml/min) maintain 95 to 100 percent long-term patency.[3]

In regard to perioperative infarction, its initial incidence in 10 to 20 percent of patients has steadily declined in the past few years as a result of improvements in operative methodology, with the present rate being only 2 to 6 percent in most experienced institutions.[2-4,75] despite more grafts inserted per patient and an increase in the number of patients with multivessel disease undergoing direct complete revascularization. The factors most responsible for fewer perioperative infarctions of less serious consequence have been newer surgical techniques, improved anesthesiology, and in particular, better measures combined with total body cooling for myocardial protection from ischemia during induced cardiac arrest necessary for distal anastomosis. Currently, a variety of methods are used for improved myocardial preservation during saphenous vein aortocoronary bypass surgery,[83] including topical hypothermia with intermittent aortic cross-clamping for transient ischemic fibrillation and arrest for distal vein attachment alternating with satisfactory reperfusion of the beating heart during proximal anastomosis; uninterrupted aortic cross-clamping with cold hyperkalemic cardioplegia for placement of all grafts distally followed by aortic clamp release and performance of proximal anastomoses; and repeated cycles of initial attachment of the vein bypass to the aorta, followed by brief hypoxic arrest induced by aortic cross-clamping with topical hypothermia, during which time the distal anastomosis is accomplished. In addition, intraaortic balloon pump assist is valuable in enhancing coronary perfusion preoperatively, intraoperatively, and postoperatively.

Although perioperative infarction does not appear to be associated with decreased (or increased) relief of late postoperative angina,[75] the infarction is related to increased subsequent mortality and pump dysfunction symptoms.[47,74,75] In addition, operative transmural necrosis is accompanied by increased hospital and late mortality, greater subsequent infarction, and increased late occurrence of congestive heart failure. Thus, perioperative infarction is clearly a deleterious event. *However, it causes less mortality and morbidity than does late postoperative myocardial infarction occurring spontaneously remote from the revascularization procedure or spontaneous myocardial infarction in coronary patients who have not had coronary bypass surgery.*

LATE POSTOPERATIVE MYOCARDIAL INFARCTION IN STABLE ANGINA

The abundant reports on the results of coronary revascularization in chronic stable angina pectoris with single-vessel or multivessel disease have analyzed long-term effectiveness almost exclusively in terms of antianginal benefit and patient survival. Although perioperative infarction is usually described, information is sparse and rarely complete concerning the important complication of subsequent infarction occurring over several postoperative years following recovery from coronary bypass. Nevertheless, extensive evaluation carried out by the present authors revealed a total of eight institutions[32,84-90] that provided satisfactory data on the rate and fate of late infarctions in addition to the incidence and consequences of perioperative infarctions.

These accumulated data obtained from the combined total of 2,224 patients, displayed in Fig. 9-4, afford valuable insight on the efficacy of coronary artery bypass in protecting coronary patients from future and fatal infarctions. The periods of postoperative follow-up extended up to 7 years and averaged 2.6 years per study. Approximately 80 percent of patients had multivessel obstruction, and 20 percent had single-vessel obstruction. Figure 9-4B shows that late infarctions occurred yearly in only 2.1 percent of patients and that just 29 percent of late infarctions were fatal (0.6 percent annual rate of fatal late infarctions).

Since the annual rate of total and fatal late postoperative infarctions was relatively constant throughout the course of follow-up years, these results (including perioperative infarctions) indicate that in patients recovering from the revascularization procedure, the 5-year postoperative cumulative risk of infarction is only approximately 18 percent. Since the incidence of total perioperative infarctions was 7.7 percent, of which only 15 percent were fatal (Fig. 9-4A), at 1 year postoperatively, total perioperative or late infarctions develop in 9.8 percent of patients and account for 1.7 percent of first-year deaths (Fig. 9-4C). At 5 years postoperatively, the cumulative patient mortality is only 4.1 percent. These findings of a low mortality resulting from postoperative infarction are quite consistent with other clinical investigations carried out at our institution,[34] demonstrating that the vast majority of late postoperative deaths following coronary artery surgery in multivessel disease are the result of sudden cardiac death and that late postrevascularization mortality caused by congestive heart failure is relatively infrequent.

Consistent with these observations of reduced frequency and diminished lethal consequences of late infarction following coronary bypass surgery in stable angina patients with multivessel obstruction are three additional long-term follow-up studies.[8,91,92] At the University of Oregon Veterans Administration Hospital, there were no fatal infarctions among the 13 late postoperative cardiac deaths in 532 revascularized patients evaluated postoperatively for 4 years.[91] Of 1,453 patients who underwent coronary bypass surgery up to 6 years previously at the Good Samaritan Hospital

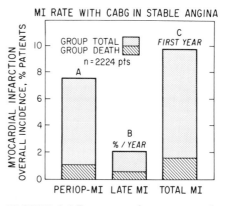

FIGURE 9-4 Frequency of occurrence of myocardial infarction (MI) during and following coronary artery bypass grafting (CABG) in 2,224 stable angina patients. Data obtained from eight referral institutions.[32,84-90] Bar A = percent incidence of patients with perioperative (Periop) MI (occurring within 30 days of CABG). Bar B = percentage of patients who developed MI per year subsequent to the first 30 days following CABG (late MI). Bar C = total incidence of patients who developed MI (Periop-MI plus Late MI) during the first postoperative year. Incidences of total and fatal MI are shown in each of the three bars.

in Los Angeles, postoperative yearly mortality of < 2 percent was attributed to late myocardial infarction in only about 30 percent of cases.[92] Finally, late myocardial infarction accounted for < 1 percent annual mortality in 846 patients evaluated for more than 5 years following coronary bypass performed at the Texas Heart Institute.[8]

CONCLUSIONS

In addition to the relief of myocardial ischemic pain in coronary patients with chronic stable angina pectoris are the more important long-term considerations of the influence of coronary bypass surgery on extending longevity and on protecting against acute myocardial infarction. That properly performed coronary revascularization is more effective than modern medical therapy in relieving angina and prolonging life in such patients is discussed in other chapters of this book and elsewhere.[1-4,34] The more difficult question of the benefit of coronary artery bypass on the prevention of myocardial infarction has not been assessed previously and is the principal subject evaluated in this chapter.

From careful examination of currently available

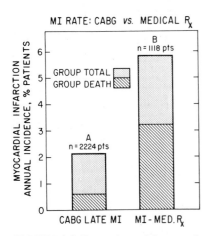

MI RATE: CABG vs. MEDICAL R$_x$

FIGURE 9-5 Comparison of the annual incidences of total and fatal myocardial infarctions (MI) in the surgically treated stable angina patients (Late-MI data representing Fig. 9-4*B*) to those in the medically treated (MED. Rx) stable angina patients (MI data obtained from Fig. 9-2*B*, *C*, and *D*).

data concerning the incidence and severity of acute myocardial infarction in matched coronary patients receiving medical versus surgical management, comparative analysis dictates that properly performed coronary bypass grafting is more effective than modern medical therapy in reducing both the incidence and the fatal outcome of subsequent acute myocardial infarction in patients with stable angina. This conclusion is provided by inspection of Fig. 9-5, which depicts the compiled and averaged data given in Fig. 9-4 (late postcoronary bypass infarction rate and fate) relative to that given in Fig. 9-2 (medical treatment–infarction rate and fate) in similar groups of coronary patients with stable angina pectoris. Fig. 9-5*A* (Fig. 9-4*B*) illustrates that the late postoperative annual incidences of total (2.1 percent) and fatal (0.6 percent) infarctions are significantly less than modern medical therapy annual incidences of total (5.9 percent) and fatal (3.5 percent) infarctions (Fig. 9-5*B*, averaged from Figs. 9-2*B*, *C*, and *D*) in equivalent surgical and medical groups with essentially similar extents of coronary obstructive disease, left ventricular function, and clinical symptoms prior to management.

Additional support for these views is afforded by the data recently reported from the University of Washington Veterans Administration Hospital in Seattle on the prospective comparison of medically versus surgically treated coronary cohorts with stable angina.[43] The incidence of myocardial infarction was significantly reduced by direct revascularization in single-vessel coronary obstruction, and the frequency of unstable angina was significantly decreased by coro-

nary bypass in patients with two-vessel obstruction and increased left ventricular end-diastolic volume. Furthermore, during the first 2 years of the prospective randomized trial of coronary bypass for stable angina being conducted at the University of Oregon Medical Center,[89] out of a total of 49 medically treated patients, unstable angina developed in 15 and acute myocardial infarction occurred in 9 (3 fatal), in contrast to the 51 surgically treated patients in whom unstable angina occurred in 6, 4 experienced perioperative infarction, and 6 experienced late postoperative infarctions. Likewise, surgically treated patients have had fewer serious complications of these types in the Houston Veterans Administration Hospital prospective randomized study of coronary bypass efficacy during an average follow-up of over 5 years.[90,93,94] Of the 56 patients in the surgical group, unstable angina has developed in 11, perioperative infarction in 4 (2 fatal), and late postoperative infarction in 7 patients; in contrast, unstable angina has occurred in 33 patients (2 fatal) and acute myocardial infarction in 13 (3 fatal) of the 60-patient medical group.

Since the annual incidence of late postoperative myocardial infarction remains at a relatively reduced frequency for at least several years following coronary bypass surgery, while the majority of bypass closures take place within the first postoperative year and thereafter are quite rare, it is suggested that late postoperative myocardial infarction after the initial year is usually related to progression of native coronary atherosclerosis often in ungrafted vessels.[80,81,95] The same mechanism appears to be responsible for deterioration of anginal symptoms; after the first postoperative year, approximately 10 percent of patients per year who were completely relieved of anginal pain by revascularization have return of some symptoms.[95] Stenoses of grafted vessels proximal to the site of anastomosis may develop accelerated obstruction.[96] However, there is no evidence that the bypass induces greater than natural progression of atherosclerosis in the distal segment of the native grafted vessel.[96] Although return of symptoms after the first postoperative year may be associated with late graft closure,[97] such bypass occlusion is usually secondary to progression of atherosclerotic disease downstream to the graft anastomosis, causing obstruction of flow in the distal segment and above.

Finally, medical and surgical treatment of the complications of coronary artery disease, including angina pectoris, as well as the objectives of extending life and preventing myocardial infarction, should not be viewed competitively but rather are complementary in management. The definitive solution of these complications requires the continued vigorous quest for effective means to prevent and reverse the disease process of coronary atherogenesis itself.

REFERENCES

1 Mundth, E. D., and Austen, G. W.: Surgical Measures for Coronary Heart Disease, *N. Engl. J. Med.,* 293:13, 75, 124, 1975.

2 Hurst, J. W., King, S. B., III, Logue, R. B., Hatcher, C. R., Jr., Jones, E. L., Craver, J. M., Douglas, J. S., Jr., Franch, R. H., Dorney, E. R., Cobbs, B. W., Jr., Robinson, P. H., Clements, S. D., Jr., Kaplan, J. A., and Bradford, J. M.: Value of Coronary Bypass Surgery, *Am. J. Cardiol.,* 42:308, 1978.

3 Johnson, W. D., and Shore, R: Coronary Bypass Surgery: Early and Long-term Results, in J. I. Haft and C. P. Bailey (eds.), "Advances in Management of Clinical Heart Disease," Futura Publishing Co., Mount Kisco, N.Y., 1978, p. 265.

4 Favaloro, R. G.: Direct Myocardial Revascularization: A Ten Year Journey, *Am. J. Cardiol.,* 43:109, 1979.

5 Kouchoukos, N. T., Kirklin, J. W., and Oberman, A.: An Appraisal of Coronary Bypass Grafting, *Circulation,* 50:11, 1974.

6 Sheldon, W. C., Rincon, G., Pichard, A. D., Razavi, M., Cheanvechai, C., and Loop, F. D.: Surgical Treatment of Coronary Artery Disease: Pure Graft Operations, with a Study of 741 Patients Followed 3-7 Years, *Prog. Cardiovasc. Dis.,* 18:237, 1975.

7 Mason, D. T., Miller, R. R., Amsterdam, E. A., DeMaria, A. N., and Vismara, L. A.: The Role of Elective Aortocoronary Bypass Surgery: Effects on Symptomatology and Longevity in Chronic Ischemic Heart Disease, in D. T. Mason (ed.), "Advances in Heart Disease," Vol. 1, Grune & Stratton, Inc., New York, 1977, p. 269.

8 Hall, R. J., Garcia, E., Mathur, V. S., Busch, U., Cooley, D. A., Gold, K. A., and Gray, A. G.: Longterm Follow-up After Coronary Artery Bypass, *Cleve. Clin. Q.,* 162, 1978.

9 Lawrie, G. M., Morris, G. C., Jr., Howell, J. F., Tredici, T. D., and Chapman, D. W.: Improved Survival After 5 Years in 1,144 Patients After Coronary Bypass Surgery, *Am. J. Cardiol.,* 42:709, 1978.

10 Collins, J. J., Jr.: Indications for Coronary Bypass Surgery, *Am. J. Cardiol.,* 43:129, 1979.

11 Russek, H. I.: Medical vs. Surgical Therapy—the Natural History of Coronary Heart Disease, *Chest,* 66:606, 1974.

12 Aronow, W. S., and Stemmer, E. A.: Two-Year Follow-up of Angina Pectoris: Medical or Surgical Therapy, *Ann. Intern. Med.,* 82:208, 1975.

13 Ross, R. S.: Ischemic Heart Disease: An Overview, *Am. J. Cardiol.,* 36:496, 1975.

14 Selzer, A., and Cohn, K.: Asymptomatic Coronary Artery Disease and Coronary Bypass Surgery, *Am. J. Cardiol.,* 39:614, 1977.

15 Braunwald, E.: Evaluation of the Efficacy of Coronary Bypass Surgery, *Am. J. Cardiol.,* 42:161, 1978.

16 Conti, C. R.: Influence of Myocardial Revascularization on Survival, *Am. J. Cardiol.,* 42:330, 1978.

17 Hultgren, H. M., Takaro, T., Detre, K. M., and Murphy, M. L.: Evaluation of the Efficacy of Coronary Bypass Surgery, *Am. J. Cardiol.,* 42:157, 1978.

18 McIntosh, H. D., and Garcia, J.: Aortocoronary Bypass Grafting, *Circulation,* 58:575, 1978.

19 Preston, T. A.: Pros and Cons of Surgery for Aortocoronary Bypass, *Chest,* 74:481, 1978.

20 Spodick, D. H.: Controlled Clinical Trials of Cardiac Surgery, *Cardiovasc. Med.,* 3(9):871, 1978.

21 Selden, R., Neill, W. A., Ritzmann, L. W., Okies, J. E., and Anderson, R. P.: Medical Versus Surgical Therapy for Acute Coronary Insufficiency, *N. Engl. J. Med.,* 293(26):1329, 1975.

22 Miller, R. R., Amsterdam, E. A., DeMaria, A. N., and Mason, D. T.: Preinfarction Angina: Evaluation, Treatment, and Prognosis, in D. T. Mason (ed.), "Advances in Heart Disease," Vol. 1, Grune & Stratton, Inc., New York, 1977, p. 169.

23 Kattus, A. A.: Prinzmetal Angina: Mechanisms, Evaluation, and Management, in D. T. Mason (ed.), "Advances in Heart Disease," Vol. 1, Grune & Stratton, Inc. New York, 1977, p. 245.

24 Langou, R. A., Wiles, J. C., and Cohen, L. S.: Coronary Surgery for Unstable Angina Pectoris—Incidence and Mortality of Perioperative Myocardial Infarction, *Br. Heart J.,* 40:767, 1978.

25 Matloff, J. M., Chaux, A., and Sustaita, H.: Unstable Angina—Experience with Surgical Therapy in the Subset of Patients Having Preinfarction Angina, *Cleve. Clin. Q.,* 184, 1978.

26 Russell, R. O., Resnekov, L., Wolk, M., Rosati, R. A., Conti, C. R., Becker, L. C., Hutter, A. M., Biddle, T. L., Schroeder, J., Kaplan, E. M., and Frommer, P. L.: Unstable Angina Pectoris: National Cooperative Study Group to Compare Surgical and Medical Therapy: In-hospital Experience and Initial Follow-up Results in Patients with One, Two and Three Vessel Disease, *Am. J. Cardiol.,* 42:839, 1978.

27 Kolibash, A. J., Goodenow, J. S., Bush, C. A., Tetalman, M. R., and Lewis, R. P.: Improvement of Myocardial Perfusion and Left Ventricular Function After Coronary Artery Bypass Grafting in Patients with Unstable Angina, *Circulation,* 59(1):66, 1979.

28 Levy, R. I.: Fourth Report of the Director of the National Heart, Lung and Blood Institute (DHEW Publication (NIH) 77-1170), March 1977.

29 Myocardial Infarction Community Registers: Public Health in Europe (WHO Report No. 5), 1976.

30 Miller, R. R., DeMaria, A. N., Vismara, L. A., Salel, A. F., Maxwell, K. S., Amsterdam, E. A., and Mason, D.

T.: Chronic Stable Inferior Myocardial Infarction: Unsuspected Harbinger of High-Risk Proximal Left Coronary Arterial Obstruction Amenable to Surgical Revascularization, *Am. J. Cardiol.*, 39:954, 1977.

31 Johnson, W. D., Hoffman, J. F., Jr., and Shore, R. T.: Myocardial Revascularization in the Absence of Cardiac Symptoms, *Am. J. Cardiol.*, 39:268, 1977.

32 Wynne, J., Cohn, L. H., Collins, J. J., Jr., and Cohn, P. F.: Myocardial Revascularization in Patients with Multivessel Coronary Artery Disease and Minimal Angina Pectoris, *Circulation*, 58 (suppl. 1):92, 1978.

33 Loop, F. D., Proudfit, W. L., and Sheldon, W. C.: Coronary Bypass Surgery Weighed in the Balance, *Am. J. Cardiol.*, 42:154, 1978.

34 Vismara, L. A., Miller, R. R., Price, J. E., Karem, R., DeMaria, A. N., and Mason, D. T.: Improved Longevity Due to Reduction of Sudden Death by Aortocoronary Bypass in Coronary Atherosclerosis: Prospective Evaluation of Medical Versus Surgical Therapy in Matched Patients with Multivessel Disease, *Am. J. Cardiol.*, 39:919, 1977.

35 Collins, J. J., Cohn, L. H., Koster, J. K., Jr., and Mee, R. B. B.: The Influence of Coronary Bypass Surgery on Longevity in Patients with Angina Pectoris, in D. T. Mason (ed.), "Advances in Heart Disease," Vol. 3, Grune & Stratton, Inc., New York, in press.

36 Proudfit, W. L., Shirey, E. K., and Sones, F. M.: Distribution of Arterial Lesions Demonstrated by Selective Cinecoronary Arteriography, *Circulation*, 36:54, 1967.

37 Amsterdam, E. A., and Mason, D. T.: Current Medical Management of Angina Pectoris, in J. I. Haft and C. P. Bailey (eds.), "Advances in Management of Clinical Heart Disease," Futura Publishing Co., Mount Kisco, N.Y., 1978, p. 237.

38 Logue, R. B., King, S. B., and Douglas, I. S.: A Practical Approach to Coronary Artery Disease with Special Reference to Coronary Bypass Surgery, in "Current Problems in Cardiology," Year Book Medical Publishers, Chicago, 1976.

39 Herman, M. V., Heinle, R. A., Klein, M. D., and Gorlin, R.: Localized Disorders in Myocardial Contraction. Asynergy and Its Role in Congestive Heart Failure, *N. Engl. J. Med.*, 277:222, 1967.

40 Masseri, A., Klassen, G. A., and Lesch, M.: "Primary and Secondary Angina Pectoris," Grune & Stratton, Inc., New York, 1978.

41 Kannel, W. B.: Some Lessons in Cardiovascular Epidemiology from Framingham, *Am. J. Cardiol.*, 37:269, 1976.

42 Farinha, J. B., Kaplan, M. A., Harris, C. N., Dunne, E. F., Carlish, R. A., Kay, J. H., and Brooks, S.: Disease of the Left Main Coronary Artery: Surgical Treatment and Long-term Follow-up in 267 Patients, *Am. J. Cardiol.*, 42:124, 1978.

43 Reeves, T. J., Oberman, A., Jones, W. B., and Sheffield, L. T.: Natural History of Angina Pectoris, *Am. J. Cardiol.*, 33:423, 1974.

44 Hammermeister, K. E., DeRouen, T. A., Murray, J. A., and Dodge, H. T.: Effect of Aortocoronary Saphenous Vein Bypass Grafting on Death and Sudden Death: Comparison of Nonrandomized Medically and Surgically Treated Cohorts with Comparable Coronary Disease and Left Ventricular Function, *Am. J. Cardiol.*, 39:925, 1977.

45 Amsterdam, E. A., and Mason, D. T.: Coronary Artery Disease: Pathophysiology and Clinical Correlations, in E. A. Amsterdam, J. H. Wilmore, and A. N. DeMaria (eds.), "Exercise in Cardiovascular Health and Disease," Yorke Medical Books, New York, 1977, p. 13.

46 Proudfit, W. L., Bruschke, A. V. G., and Sones, F. M., Jr.: Natural History of Obstructive Coronary Artery Disease: Ten-Year Study of 601 Nonsurgical Cases, *Prog. Cardiovasc. Dis.*, 21:53, 1978.

47 Litwak, R. S., Lukban, S. B., and Jurado, R. A.: Management of Angina Pectoris by Coronary Artery Bypass Grafts: A Status Report, in E. Donoso and R. Gorlin (eds.), "Angina Pectoris," Stratton Intercontinental Medical Book Corp., New York, 1977, p. 152.

48 Caves, P. K., and Stinson, E.: Surgical Treatment, in D. G. Julian (ed.), "Angina Pectoris," Churchill Livingstone, London, 1977, p. 227.

49 Baum, R. S., Alvarez, H., and Cobb, L. A.: Survival After Resuscitation from Out-of-Hospital Ventricular Defibrillation, *Circulation*, 50:1231, 1974.

50 Liberthson, R. R., Nagel, E. L., Hirschman, J. C., and Nusserfeld, S. R.: Prehospital Ventricular Fibrillation, *N. Engl. J. Med.*, 291:317, 1974.

51 Armstrong, A., Duncan, B., Oliver, M. F., Julian, D. G., Donald, K. W., Fulton, M., Lutz, W., and Morrison, S. L.: Natural History of Acute Coronary Heart Attacks: A Community Study, *Br. Heart J.*, 34:67, 1972.

52 Kuller, L.: Sudden Death in Arteriosclerotic Heart Disease: The Case for Preventive Medicine, *Am. J. Cardiol.*, 24:617, 1969.

53 Norris, R. M., Caughey, D. E., Mercer, C. J., and Scott, P. J.: Prognosis After Myocardial Infarction: Six-Year Follow-up, *Br. Heart J.*, 36:786, 1974.

54 Bruschke, A. V. G., Proudfit, W. L., and Sones, F. M., Jr.: Progress Study of 590 Consecutive Nonsurgical Cases of Coronary Disease Followed 5-9 Years. I. Arteriographic Correlations, *Circulation*, 47:1147, 1973.

55 Bruschke, A. V. G., Proudfit, W. L., and Sones, F. M., Jr.: Progress Study of 590 Consecutive Nonsurgical Cases of Coronary Disease Followed 5-9 Years. II. Ventriculographic and Other Correlations, *Circulation*, 47:1154, 1973.

56 Burggraf, G. W., and Parker, J. O.: Prognosis in Coronary Artery Disease—Angiographic, Hemodynamic and Clinical Factors, *Circulation*, 51:146, 1975.

57 Braunwald, E.: Coronary Artery Surgery at the Crossroads, *N. Engl. J. Med.*, 297:661, 1977.

58 Murphy, M. L., Hultgren, H. M., Detre, K., Thomsen, J., and Takaro, T.: Treatment of Chronic Stable Angina—

a Preliminary Report of Survival Data of the Randomized Veterans Administration Cooperative Study, *N. Engl. J. Med.,* 297:12:621, 1977.

59 Amsterdam, E. A., Hughes, J., Miller, R. R., Salel, A. F., Massumi, R. A., Zelis, R., and Mason, D. T.: Clinical Assessment of Saphenous Vein Bypass Graft in Coronary Artery Disease: Determination of Blood Flow to Ischemic Myocardium and Comparison with Beta-Adrenergic Blockade, in M. Kaltenbach, P. Lichtlen, and G. Friesinger (eds.), "Coronary Heart Disease" (Second International Symposium, at Frankfurt, 1972), George Thieme Verlag, Stuttgart, 1973, p. 301.

60 Lee, G., Kaku, R. F., Amsterdam, E. A., Harris, F. J., Mason, D. T., and DeMaria, A. N.: Greater Relief of Myocardial Ischemia in Coronary Patients by Aortocoronary Bypass Surgery Compared to Modern Medical Antianginal Therapy: Documentation by Exercise Stress Testing and Myocardial Oxygen Needs, *Am. J. Cardiol.,* 43:383, 1979.

61 Norris, R. M., Clarke, E. D., and Sammel, N. L.: Protective Effect of Propranolol in Threatened Myocardial Infarction, *Lancet,* 2:907, 1978.

62 Gold, H. K., Leinbach, R. C., and Maroko, P. R.: Propranolol-induced Reduction of Signs of Ischemic Injury During Acute Myocardial Infarction, *Am. J. Cardiol.,* 38:689, 1976.

63 Improvement in Prognosis of Myocardial Infarction by Long-term Beta-Adrenoreceptor Blockade Using Practolol: A Multicentre International Study, *Br. Med. J.,* 3:735, 1975.

64 Read, R. C., Murphy, M. L., Hultgren, H. N., and Takaro, T.: Survival of Men Treated for Chronic Stable Angina Pectoris—a Cooperative Randomized Study, *J. Thorac. Cardiovasc. Surg.,* 75:1, 1978.

65 Collins, J. J., Jr., Cohn, L. H., Koster, J. K., and Mee, R. B. B.: Debate on Coronary Bypass Surgery, *N. Engl. J. Med.,* 297:1464, 1977.

66 Mason, D. T., and Vismara, L. A.: Reduction of Sudden Death by Aortocoronary Bypass Surgery, *Am. J. Cardiol.,* 41:793, 1978.

67 Takaro, T., Hultgren, H. N., Lipton, M. J., and Detre, K. M.: The VA Cooperative Randomized Study of Surgery for Coronary Arterial Occlusive Disease: Subgroup with Significant Left Main Lesions, *Circulation,* 54 (6, suppl. 3):107, 1976.

68 Kouchoukos, N. T., Oberman, A., and Karp, R. B.: Results of Surgery for Disabling Angina Pectoris, in A. N. Brest and S. H. Rahimtoola (eds.), *Coronary Bypass Surgery,* F. A. Davis Company, Philadelphia, 1977, p. 157.

69 Brewer, D. L., Bilbrow, R. H., and Bartel, A. G.: Myocardial Infarction as a Complication of Coronary Bypass Surgery, *Circulation,* 47:58, 1973.

70 Espinoza, J., Lipski, J., Litwak, R., Donoso, E., and Dack, S.: New Q Waves After Coronary Artery Bypass Surgery for Angina Pectoris, *Am. J. Cardiol.,* 33:221, 1974.

71 Rose, M. R., Glassman, E., Ison, O. W., and Spencer, F. C.: Electrocardiographic and Serum Enzyme Changes of Myocardial Infarction After Coronary Artery Bypass Surgery, *Am. J. Cardiol.,* 33:215, 1974.

72 Delva, E., Maille, J. G., Solymoss, B. C., Chabot, M., Grondin, C. M., and Bourassa, M. G.: Evaluation of Myocardial Damage During Coronary Artery Grafting with Serial Determinations of Serum CPK MB Isoenzyme, *J. Thorac. Cardiovasc. Surg.,* 75:467, 1978.

73 Gray, R. J., Shell, W. E., Conklin, C., Ganz, W., Shah, P. K., Miyamoto, A. T., Matloff, J. M., and Swan, H. J. C.: Quantification of Myocardial Injury During Coronary Artery Bypass Graft, *Circulation,* 58 (3, suppl. 1):38, 1978.

74 Lim, J. S., Proudfit, W. L., Sheldon, W. C., Alosilla, C., Phillips, D. F., and Loop, F. D.: Perioperative Myocardial Infarction Related to Coronary Bypass Surgery, *Am. Heart J.,* 96(4):463, 1978.

75 Oberman, A., Kouchoukos, N. T., Makar, Y. N., Russell, R. O., Jr., Sheffield, L. T., Ray, M., Allen, R. E., and Kitts, Jr.: Perioperative Myocardial Infarction After Coronary Bypass Surgery, *Cleve. Clin. Q.,* 45:172, 1978.

76 Berman, D. S., Amsterdam, E. A., Hines, H. H., Salel, A. F., Bailey, G. J., DeNardo, G. L., and Mason, D. T.: New Approach to Interpretation of Technetium-99m Pyrophosphate Scintigraphy in Detection of Acute Myocardial Infarction: Clinical Assessment of Diagnostic Accuracy, *Am. J. Cardiol.,* 39:341, 1977.

77 Stengert, K. B., Wilsey, B. L., Hurley, E. J., Grehl, T. M., Lurie, A. J., Klein, R. C., and Upjohn, L. R.: Incremental Intravenous Nitroglycerin for Control of Afterload During Anesthesia in Patients Undergoing Myocardial Revascularization, *Anaesthesist,* 27:223, 1978.

78 Assad-Morell, J. L., Frye, R. L., Connolly, D. C., Gau, G. T., Pluth, J. R., Barnhorst, D. A., Wallace, R. B., Davis, G. D., Elveback, L. R., and Danielson, G. K.: Relation of Intraoperative or Early Postoperative Transmural Myocardial Infarction to Patency of Aortocoronary Bypass Grafts and to Diseased Ungrafted Coronary Arteries, *Am. J. Cardiol.,* 35(6):767, 1975.

79 Kouchoukos, N. T., Karp, R. B., Oberman, A., Russell, R. O., Jr., Alison, H. W., Holt, J. H., Jr.: Long-term Patency of Saphenous Veins for Coronary Bypass Grafting, *Circulation,* 58 (suppl. 1):96, 1978.

80 Robert, E. W., Guthaner, D. F., Wexler, L., and Alderman, E. L.: Six-Year Clinical and Angiographic Follow-up of Patients with Previously Documented Complete Revascularization, *Circulation,* 58 (suppl.1):194, 1978.

81 Seides, S. F., Borer, J. S., Kent, K. M., Rosing, D. R., McIntosh, C. L., and Epstein, S. E.: Long-term Anatomic Fate of Coronary-Artery Bypass Grafts and Functional Status of Patients Five Years After Operation, *N. Engl. J. Med.,* 298:1213, 1978.

82 Uricchio, J. F., and Bentivoglio, L. G.: Patency of Saphenous Vein Grafts Five or More Years After Coronary Bypass Surgery, *Am. J. Med.,* 65:619, 1978.

114

83 Adappa, M. G., Jacobson, L. B., Hetzer, R., Hill, J. D., Kamm, B., and Kerth, W. J.: Cold Hyperkalemic Cardiac Arrest Versus Intermittent Aortic Cross-clamping and Topical Hypothermia for Coronary Bypass Surgery, *J. Thorac. Cardiovasc. Surg.*, 75:171, 1978.

84 Bolooki, H., Thurer, R. J., Ghahramani, A., Vargas, A., Williams, W., and Kaiser, G.: Objective Assessment of Late Results of Aortocoronary Bypass Operation, *Surgery*, 76(6):925, 1974.

85 Techlenberg, P. L., Alderman, E. L., Miller, D. C., Shumway, N. E., and Harrison, D. C.: Changes in Survival and Symptom Relief in a Longitudinal Study of Patients After Bypass Surgery, *Circulation*, 52 (suppl. 1):98, 1975.

86 Aintablian, A., Hamby, R. I., Weisz, D., Hoffman, I., Voleti, C., and Wisoff, B. G.: Results of Aortocoronary Bypass Grafting in Patients with Subendocardial Infarction: Late Follow-up, *Am. J. Cardiol.*, 42:183, 1978.

87 Donaldson, R. M., Honey, M., Sturridge, M. F., Wright, J. E. C., and Balcon, R.: Results of Aortocoronary Bypass Operations—Follow-up in 343 Patients, *Br. Heart J.*, 40:1200, 1978.

88 Ison, O. W., Spencer, F. C., Glassman, E., Cunningham, J. N., Teiko, P., Reed, G. E., and Boyd, A. D.: Does Coronary Bypass Increase Longevity? *J. Thorac. Cardiovasc. Surg.*, 75:28, 1978.

89 Kloster, F. E., Kremkau, E. L., Ritzmann, L. W., Rahimtoola, S. H., Rosch, J., and Kanarek, P. H.: Coronary Bypass for Stable Angina—a Prospective Randomized Study, *N. Engl. J. Med.*, 300(4):149, 1979.

90 Mathur, V. S., and Guinn, G. A.: Long-term Follow-up (4-7 Years) of a Prospective Randomized Study to Evaluate Surgical vs. Medical Treatment for Stable Angina Pectoris: Clinical Status, Exercise Performance and Survival, *Am. J. Cardiol.*, 43:382, 1979.

91 Anderson, R. P., Rahimtoola, S. H., Bonchek, L. I., and Starr, A.: The Prognosis of Patients with Coronary Artery Disease After Coronary Bypass Operations, *Circulation*, 50:274, 1974.

92 Stiles, Q. R., Lindesmith, G. G., Tucker, B. L., Hughes, R. K., and Meyer, B. W.: Long-term Follow-up of Patients with Coronary Bypass Grafts., *Circulation*, 52 (suppl. 2):143, 1975.

93 Mathur, V. S., Guinn, G. A., Anastassiades, L. C., Chahine, R. A., Korompai, F.L., Montero, A. C., and Luchi, R. J.: Surgical Treatment for Stable Angina Pectoris—Prospective Randomized Study, *N. Engl. J. Med.*, 292(14):709, 1975.

94 Mathur, V. S., and Guinn, G. A.: Prospective Randomized Study of the Surgical Therapy of Stable Angina, in S. H. Rahimtoola and A. N. Brest (eds.), "Coronary Bypass Surgery," F. A. Davis Company, Philadelphia, 1977, p. 136.

95 Winkle, R. A. Alderman, E. L., Shumway, N. E., and Harrison, D. C.: Results of Reoperation for Unsuccessful Coronary Artery Bypass Surgery, *Circulation*, 52 (suppl. 1):61, 1975.

96 Bourassa, M. G., Lesperance, J., Corbara, F., Saltiel, J., and Campeau, L.: Progression of Obstructive Coronary Artery Disease 5 to 7 Years After Aortocoronary Bypass Surgery, *Circulation*, 58 (suppl 1):100, 1978.

97 Allen, R. H., Stinson, E. B., Oyer, P. E., and Shumway, N. E.: Predictive Variables in Reoperation for Coronary Artery Disease, *J. Thorac. Cardiovasc. Surg.*, 75(186):192, 1978.

The authors gratefully acknowledge the technical assistance of Robert Klickner, Linda Hunter, and Leslie Silvernail.

Chapter 10

Use of the Coronary Bypass Operation in the Treatment of Selected Patients with Myocardial Infarction*

ELLIS L. JONES, M.D.

The coronary artery bypass operation is applicable to patients following acute myocardial infarction in two entirely different clinical situations. In the first situation are those patients who have had acute myocardial infarction but have minimal or no symptoms of angina pectoris following the ischemic event. These patients are in a stable clinical state, and assuming that left ventricular function is good, prognosis is related to the presence or absence of associated multivessel coronary artery disease. In the second situation are those patients who have had recent myocardial infarction but continue to demonstrate clinical instability manifested by medically uncontrollable rest pain, ventricular arrhythmias, or evidence of reduced cardiac output.

MYOCARDIAL INFARCTION FOLLOWED BY A STABLE CLINICAL COURSE

Several studies have noted the frequency of significant multivessel disease in patients with uncomplicated isolated inferior myocardial infarction.[1,2] The incidence of isolated right coronary artery disease was 20 percent; double-vessel disease, 35 percent; and triple-vessel disease, 45 percent in these select groups of patients. Approximately two-thirds of these same patients had significant stenosis of the proximal left anterior descending coronary artery, even when symptoms after infarction were minimal. Our experience has not been so revealing, and in the majority of patients with inferior infarction, isolated disease of the right coronary artery only has been found. However, before assuming that series are comparable, the ages of the groups must be carefully defined, as the incidence of multivessel disease increases with the age of the population under discussion. Our experience may underestimate the incidence of multivessel disease,

since we tend to be more diagnostically aggressive with younger patients.

Because mortality from ischemic heart disease is related to the number and distribution of significantly involved coronary vessels, and because the presence of inferior myocardial infarction is frequently associated with a significant incidence of double- and triple-vessel disease, it has been argued that mortality in patients with uncomplicated inferior myocardial infarction can be anticipated to be significant over a 5-year period.[1,3,4] For this reason, every effort should be made to avoid damage to the anterior left ventricular wall in order to prevent the dreaded occurrence of sudden death or left ventricular pump failure and cardiogenic shock. Patients with inferior myocardial infarction should therefore be considered carefully for the possible association of significant left-sided arterial disease.

With the decline in operative risk and the improvement in technical factors in recent years for patients undergoing coronary artery bypass surgery, we believe that long-term survival has been improved in patients with both double- and triple-vessel disease (Fig. 10-1). However, once left ventricular damage has occurred, as manifested by repeated myocardial infarction or abnormal left ventricular contractility, survival is much less satisfactory, even following coronary artery bypass grafting (Fig. 10-2).

Realizing that there are definite dangers in procrastination, our present approach in management of asymptomatic or minimally symptomatic patients with recent isolated uncomplicated inferior myocardial infarction is to perform cardiac catheterization 5 to 6 weeks after infarction in order to exclude the possibility of significant anterior descending, double- or triple-vessel disease. The age of the patient is important in determining the aggressiveness of the diagnostic procedures, and we have been very aggressive with younger patients. Individuals with anterior ST-T changes following myocardial infarction should be studied in anticipation of a high incidence of proximal left anterior descending (LAD) disease. Patients found to have significant multivessel or proximal LAD disease in this clinical setting are offered coronary bypass surgery.

*From the Department of Surgery, Emory University School of Medicine, Atlanta.

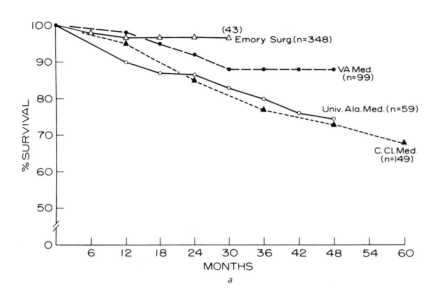

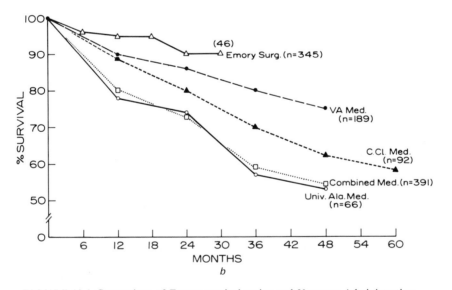

FIGURE 10-1 Comparison of Emory surgical series and Veterans Administration medical centers,* University of Alabama medical series,† and Cleveland Clinic medical series‡ for patients with (*a*) double- and (*b*) triple-vessel disease. (*Reprinted by permission of R. C. Read et al., Survival of Men Treated for Chronic Stable Angina Pectoris: A Cooperative Randomized Study, J. Thorac. Cardiovasc. Surg., 75:1, 1978. †Reprinted from N. T. Kouchoukos et al., Results of Surgery for Disabling Angina Pectoris, in A. N. Brest and S. H. Rahimtoola (eds.), "Cardiovascular Clinics (Coronary Bypass Surgery)," F. A. Davis Company, Philadelphia, 1977, p. 157, with permission. ‡Reprinted from A. V. Bruschke, Ten Year Follow-up of 601 Nonsurgical Cases of Angiographically Documented Coronary Disease. Angiographic Correlations, in "The First Decade of Bypass Graft Surgery for Coronary Artery Disease." (International symposium, Cleveland Clinic Foundation, 1977, p. 77), with permission.)*

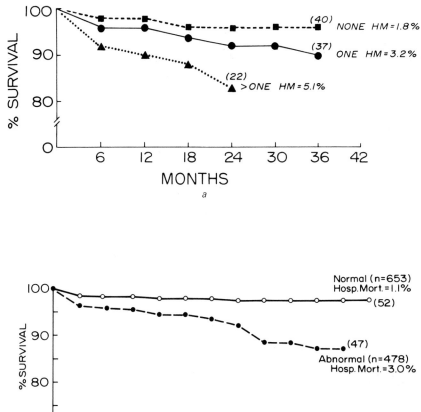

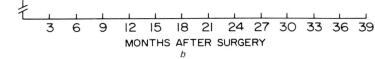

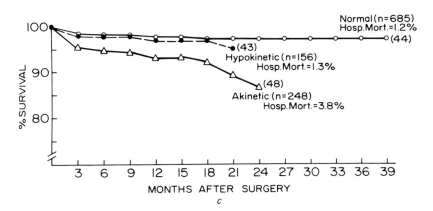

FIGURE 10-2 Effect of (*a*) the number of previous myocardial infarctions (AMI), (*b*) left ventricular (LV) contractility, and (*c*) LV segmental wall motion on hospital mortality (HM) and survival.

MYOCARDIAL INFARCTION FOLLOWED BY AN UNSTABLE CLINICAL COURSE

Some investigators believe that the resting ECG, exercise stress testing, age, and functional classification are poor predictors of the number and location of stenotic vessels.[1] Others believe these clinical descriptors are important in predicting lesions and thus patient survival.[2] Humphries,[5] Moss,[6] and others[7] have stated that in a select group of survivors of myocardial infarction, it was possible to identify a high-risk group characterized by angina at ordinary levels of activity or rest, hypotension in the coronary care unit, frequent premature ventricular contractions or ventricular tachycardia, ST-segment depression, and cardiomegaly on chest x-ray. Medical mortality in this group was 38.5 percent in 3 years.[7] The risk of dying in these patients was relatively high in the first several months or first year after acute infarction, regardless of location of the myocardial infarction; but in subsequent years, mortality returned to an estimated 4 to 5 percent per year, which was similar to the overall mortality for patients with chronic stable angina. Other studies also have documented the unstable course of some patients following acute myocardial infarction.[8,9] Although immediate prognosis was good after subendocardial myocardial infarction, Madigan and coworkers found the incidence of unstable angina or later transmural infarction to be 46 and 21 percent, respectively.[8] When left ventricular power failure and cardiogenic shock occur as a complication of acute myocardial infarction, medical mortality is high and approaches 80 to 90 percent in most series.[10-14] Recently, Stenson et al. have identified a group of postinfarction patients with persistent or recurrent pain and ST-segment elevation who had a very high mortality on medical therapy and observation alone.[15] Medical therapy using beta blockade in the face of recent acute myocardial infarction and low output may even be dangerous, especially in a clinical setting of cardiogenic shock.[15,16]

In recent years, major emphasis has been placed on reducing or limiting infarct size either pharmacologically, mechanically (by reducing afterload and oxygen requirements), or by increasing blood supply with myocardial revascularization. The goal of salvaging recently damaged myocardium is based on evidence that a marginal or border zone of ischemic tissue exists around an area of infarction. Since the fate of ischemic myocardium depends on oxygen supply and energy utilization, attempts have been made primarily to alter these two factors.[17,18] There has not been complete agreement as to the efficacy of myocardial revascularization in the clinical setting of acute myocardial infarction because of the historically high operative risk and theoretical and experimental objections regarding the effect that reperfusion may have on infarct extension. Dawson et al. have reported a mortality of 38 percent in patients who underwent coronary bypass within the first 7 days after acute infarction.[19] This rate was more than six times greater than their mortality in patients who were operated on 31 to 60 days after infarction (5.8 percent).

The controversy over the possible deleterious effects of reperfusion following acute myocardial ischemia began when it was demonstrated that reperfusion following arterial ligation in experimental animals produced myocardial hemorrhage in the border zones of the necrotic area, with evidence of actual infarct extension.[20,21] Kloner and coworkers demonstrated that after 90 min of ischemia, a no-reflow phenomenon occurs with endothelial swelling, cellular edema, and fibrin thrombi.[22] The no-reflow phenomenon may contribute to the reperfusion injury and thus create a vicious cycle of increasing cell swelling and more severe ischemia. Because of these experimental studies, it was felt that revascularization shortly after myocardial infarction might be extremely hazardous and might convert a previously ischemic infarct into a hemorrhagic one with extension of myocardial necrosis. The no-reflow phenomenon and the finding of hemorrhagic infarction were used to explain the extremely poor prognosis of previous patients undergoing myocardial revascularization soon after acute myocardial infarction.

Accurate assessment of the real risks and results of coronary artery bypass grafting following acute myocardial infarction has been difficult to ascertain, primarily because of the imprecise definition of acute infarction, but also because of the inclusion in some series of a large number of patients in cardiogenic shock who had little chance of survival regardless of the form of therapy.[16-28] In general, however, the operative mortality has ranged from 5 to 35 percent, depending on the state of ventricular function at the time of operation. Medical mortality has been universally high in patients with persistent or recurrent chest pain following infarction, and such patients should be placed in a high-risk category for developing immediate or late complications of ischemia, consisting of ventricular arrhythmias, reinfarction, cardiogenic shock, or death. Identification of such patients at risk allows time for surgical intervention, provided the latter can be accomplished with acceptable mortality and morbidity. In recent years, we have become impressed with the dangers of infarct extension in patients with persistent rest pain following recent myocardial infarction. For this reason, in selected patients, we have developed an aggressive attitude involving myocardial revascularization at some time in the postinfarction period. At Emory University Hospital, we have operated upon 35 patients having clinical instability within 30 days of acute myocardial infarction, and much of the discussion that follows has been based on our experience with these patients.

Infarction was defined as prolonged ischemic pain accompanied by ECG presence of new 0.04-s waves or acute ST depression and/or T wave inversion associated with creatinine phosphokinase (CPK) elevation to at least twice normal levels. No patient was operated upon as an emergency secondary to a complication of cardiac catheterization. In 4 patients, cardiac catheterization was performed prior to development of acute myocardial infarction. Patients were arbitrarily divided into three groups defined by the interval between infarction and revascularization. Group I ($n = 10$ patients) underwent operation within 24 h of acute myocardial infarction; Group II ($n = 9$ patients) had revascularization 2 to 7 days following infarction, and Group III ($n = 16$ patients) had revascularization 8 to 30 days after infarction. Clinical instability was manifested as persistent pain in spite of maximal therapy with vasodilator drugs, narcotics, and propranolol; persistent or recurrent pain associated with ventricular arrhythmias (premature ventricular contractions, ventricular tachycardia, ventricular fibrillation); or persistent or recurrent pain associated with objective signs of reduced cardiac output. Of the 35 patients, there were 34 men and 1 woman. Mean age was 53 years. There was no age difference among the groups.

Special Techniques for Cardiac Catheterization

Because of the unstable clinical state of patients with recent infarction, the technique of catheterization and arteriography becomes important in assuring that there is no deterioration of cardiac function during or following the procedure. All patients undergo selective coronary arteriography and left ventriculography by the single-catheter femoral percutaneous technique.[29,30] Medical therapy is not interrupted prior to catheterization. Sublingual nitroglycerin is administered prior to and following left ventricular injection when ischemic pain occurs or when left ventricular end-diastolic pressure becomes greater than 20 mm Hg. In patients with recent infarction and markedly impaired left ventricular wall motion, a separate postnitroglycerin ventriculogram is performed. Sublingual nitroglycerin is used to enhance distal opacification of totally occluded vessels and to exclude coronary spasm. Treatment of ischemic pain during the catheterization is directed at cautious reduction of the heart rate–blood pressure product and left ventricular wall tension by administration of sublingual nitroglycerin, intravenous

meperidine, elevation of the upper trunk, and 1-mg increments of propranolol intravenously. Sufficient time is allowed between coronary injections for relief of pain and return of ST segments, heart rate, and left ventricular end-diastolic pressure to prestress values. Transient hypotension after coronary injections is common but is effectively treated by having the patient cough to momentarily increase aortic pressure and enhance clearing of contrast media from the coronary circulation. The number of coronary injections is minimized to reduce cardiac stress but without compromising the objective of obtaining clear definition of coronary anatomy. Although it is our policy to utilize the intraaortic balloon whenever necessary to support patients who are hemodynamically unstable, none of our patients required the balloon pump prior to coronary arteriography.

Clinical Profile

Indications for operation included medically uncontrollable pain following infarction in all 35 patients, pain with persistent ventricular arrhythmias in 10 patients (29 percent), and pain with evidence of reduced cardiac output (3 requiring pharmacologic support) in 5 patients (14 percent) (Table 10-1).

Of the 10 patients undergoing myocardial revascularization within 24 h of infarction (Group I), 2 required preoperative cardioversion for ventricular fibrillation, 2 received inotropic support to increase cardiac output prior to operation, and 2 demonstrated transient ST-segment elevation associated with anginal pain. Of the 16 patients in Group III (revascularization 8 to 30 days after infarction), 2 developed ventricular tachycardia, and 1 required inotropic drugs for acute hemodynamic deterioration just prior to operation. Four patients in the series had symptoms of congestive heart failure (paroxysmal nocturnal dysp-

TABLE 10-1

Indications for operation in 35 patients following acute myocardial infarction (ventricular arrhythmias = premature ventricular contraction, ventricular tachycardia, or ventricular fibrillation)

	Series*	Group I†	Group II	Group III
Pain alone	22	5	7	10
Pain + ventricular arrhythmias	10	3	2	5
Pain + poor peripheral perfusion	5	3	None	2

*Two patients had pain, arrhythmias, and poor peripheral perfusion.

†See discussion for definitions of groups I, II, and III.

nea and/or orthopnea) prior to cardiac catheterization or operation. It must be emphasized that our criteria for patient selection is very rigid, and no patient is considered a candidate for myocardial revascularization if pain disappears following infarction or if there is cardiogenic shock requiring mechanical circulatory assistance for survival.

In our patients, there was an almost equal incidence of transmural (46 percent) and subendocardial (54 percent) infarction (16 of 35 and 19 of 35, respectively). If the infarction was transmural, it was most often inferior in location, whereas if it was subendocardial, there was an equal incidence of anterior and inferior location (Fig. 10-3). Of the 3 patients in the series with anterior transmural myocardial infarction, 2 were in Group I. ECG evidence of prior myocardial infarction (q wave) was present in 6 of the 35 patients.

Mean CPK for groups I, II, and III at the time of infarction was 455 μU/ml, 536 μU/ml, and 1067 μU/ml, respectively. The mean interval between infarction and revascularization was 5.7 days for Group II and 18 days for Group III.

Cardiac Catheterization

LEFT VENTRICULAR FUNCTION

Ejection fraction for the patients selected for operation was surprisingly good ($\overline{m}$ = 0.43). Ejection fraction was approximately the same for those operated on within 24 h and those operated on 8 to 30 days after infarction; however, ejection fraction was significantly better for Group II patients (Table 10-2). Resting left ventricular end-diastolic pressure (LVEDP) was within normal limits ($\leq$15 mm Hg) in 71 percent (25 of 35 patients) of the series, and slightly better in Group II patients (Table 10-2). Four of the 16 patients in our Group III had resting LVEDP $\geq$ 20 mm Hg. Angiographic wall segment motion was essentially normal

TABLE 10-2
Preoperative left ventricular function in patients with recent myocardial infarction

	Group I* (n=10)	Group II (n=9)	Group III (n=16)
$\overline{m}$ EF	0.38	0.53	0.40
$\geq$ 0.40	5 patients	7 patients	8 patients
$\leq$ 0.35	5 patients	1 patient	8 patients
$\overline{m}$ LVEDP	13 mm Hg	8 mm Hg	13 mm Hg
$\leq$ 15 mm Hg	5 patients	9 patients	11 patients
$\geq$ 20 mm Hg	1 patient	None	4 patients

*See discussion for definitions of groups I, II, and III.

in 8 patients, hypokinetic in 20 patients, and akinetic in at least one segment in 7 patients in the series (Fig. 10-4).

CORONARY ARTERY DISEASE

Left main coronary artery obstruction of at least 50 percent of the lumenal area was present in 4 patients in the series, 3 in Group II, and 1 in Group III. Single-vessel disease occurred only in Group III patients (4 of 16). Triple-vessel disease occurred in 18 patients in the series (51 percent) and with equal frequency among the groups. The left anterior descending coronary artery was significantly diseased in 80 percent of patients (28 of 35) and was totally occluded in 37 percent patients (13 of 35). There was total occlusion of both left anterior descending and right coronary arteries in 7 patients (20 percent) (see Fig. 10-5). The mean diameter of arteries proposed for bypass, determined at the time of cardiac catheterization, was 2 mm for the series, with no significant difference among the groups. Mitral regurgitation was not present in any patient.

Operation

To maintain stability in the critical prebypass period, precise monitoring of the rate–pressure product, inferior and V_5 precordial ECG changes, pulmonary capillary wedge pressure, and cardiac output should be performed. However, Swan-Ganz catheters may be dangerous if routinely employed in patients demonstrating ventricular arrhythmias in the preoperative period. Anesthesia is maintained primarily by frequent doses of morphine sulfate, with diazepam and nitrous oxide as indicated to control blood pressure or heart rate. For most patients (except those with evidence of reduced cardiac output), propranolol therapy should be continued until the time of anesthetic induction. We have found the routine preoperative use of beta

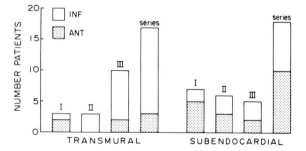

FIGURE 10-3 Type and location of myocardial infarction (AMI, acute myocardial infarction). See discussion for definitions of groups I, II, and III.

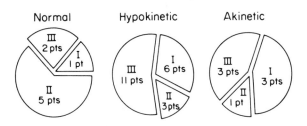

FIGURE 10-4 Preoperative angiographic wall segment motion in 35 patients undergoing revascularization after acute myocardial infarction. See discussion for definitions of groups I, II, and III.

blocking drugs to be extremely helpful in preventing prebypass hemodynamic instability as manifested by acute hypertension, tachycardia, ischemic ECG changes, and ventricular arrhythmias. Patients with clinical signs of reduced cardiac output and poor perfusion are generally not candidates for beta blockade therapy. If tachycardia or hypertension occurs prior to bypass, it is promptly treated with small doses of intravenous propranolol or a trinitroglycerin drip, respectively. Since employing this aggressive pharmacologic approach during the critical prebypass period, evidence of myocardial ischemia has been surprisingly rare prior to the actual operation. The operative technique in these patients is no different from that used in other coronary artery bypass patients and, at our institution, consists of moderate systemic hypothermia and minimizing left ventricular depressive factors, such as ventricular distension and fibrillation. Combined coronary bypass and infarctectomy is rarely indicated and may be considered only when there is impending cardiac rupture or perhaps for ventricular tachycardia. Myocardial preservation is accomplished with either a cold (4°C) hyperkalemic,* or hyperkalemic hyperosmolar† solution injected into the aorta at the time of aortic cross-clamping. A single aortic cross-clamp period is used for all distal anastomoses, regardless of the degree of ventricular dysfunction or the number of bypass grafts to be performed.

In our experience, single coronary bypass grafting was infrequently performed (6 of 35 patients), whereas three or more coronary artery bypass grafts were performed in 51 percent (18 of 35 patients). The incidence of multiple grafting was approximately the same for all groups, although Group II had more grafts per patient (3.3) than did Group I (2.6) or Group III (2.3) (see Fig. 10-6).

---

*KCl solution (20 mEq/liter) buffered to pH 7.40.

†KCl-mannitol solution: 4 parts KCl solution (35 mEq/liter) plus 1 part mannitol (15% solution); pH 8.1, osmol = 400–430 mOsm; K+ = 27 mEq/liter (final concentration).

Hospital Mortality and Morbidity

There were no operative deaths in this group of 35 patients. Inotropic drugs were required in the postbypass period in 5 patients (14 percent). All were in Group I or Group III and, as a group, represented those patients with the worst preoperative left ventricular function. Intraaortic balloon pumping was required in 7 patients (20 percent), 2 of whom did not need inotropic support postoperatively. In 5 of the 7 patients requiring balloon support, preoperative ejection fraction was ≤ 0.20. Intraaortic balloon pumping was initiated preoperatively in 4 of the 7 patients for control of either ventricular arrhythmias or marginal cardiac output. Lidocaine was necessary for treatment of postbypass ventricular arrhythmias in 5 patients (14 percent) (see Fig. 10-7). However, these were not necessarily the patients who had ventricular arrhythmias preoperatively.

Perioperative infarction (new *q* wave) occurred in one patient (3 percent). Mean total CPK on the day of surgery was 810 μU/ml for the series, but significantly higher in Group I patients (1405 μU/ml) than in groups II and III (633 μU/ml and 393 μU/ml, respectively). CPK isoenzymes were not routinely measured postoperatively during the interval of this study, but in 13 patients in which they were obtained, they were negative in 1, trace in 9, and only 1+ in 3.

Late Follow-up

There have been no late deaths during an admittedly short follow-up period of 9.8 months. Sixty-nine percent of patients (24 of 35) are presently free of pain, and 31 percent (11 of 35), although improved, do complain of some degree of residual chest discomfort, thought to represent angina pectoris. Only 6 percent of patients are worse or unchanged following revascularization (Fig. 10-8).

Repeat cardiac catheterization was performed 1 to 19 months following operation in 17 of the 35 patients.

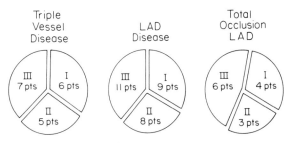

FIGURE 10-5 Distribution of coronary disease in patients with recent myocardial infarction. See discussion for definitions of groups I, II, and III.

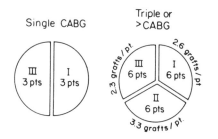

FIGURE 10-6 Frequency of bypass grafting in patients with recent infarction. See discussion for definitions of groups I, II, and III.

Graft patency was 84 percent (36 of 43) for the series, and 76 percent of patients (13 of 17) had all grafts patent. In 14 of the 17 patients, grafts placed into the area of myocardial infarction were patent at the time of restudy; this is in agreement with findings of others.[31] Mean ejection fraction following revascularization increased slightly (0.44 to 0.50) for the series. Normal wall motion by angiography was present in 47 percent patients (8 of 17) after operation, as compared to 23 percent of patients (8 of 35) at the time of original catheterization. Changes in ejection fraction are demonstrated in Fig. 10-9. Most patients demonstrated either an improvement in ejection fraction when this value was depressed preoperatively or very little deterioration when ejection fraction was high preoperatively. Only 1 patient demonstrated severe deterioration in ejection fraction, and this patient had a myocardial infarction after catheterization and just prior to surgery. Improvement in segmental wall motion following revascularization occurred in 7 patients, whereas no change or deterioration of movement occurred in 6 and 2 patients, respectively.

DISCUSSION

Persistent or recurrent pain following infarction, as we have defined it in our patients, is interpreted as incomplete myocardial infarction distal to an obstructed artery or reduction of collateral blood flow to the peri-infarction ischemic zones supplied by another significantly obstructed major coronary artery. This interpretation has been corroborated by autopsy studies of patients with transient ST-segment elevation and persistent pain following myocardial infarction.[15] In our experience, persistent postinfarction pain has also meant a very high incidence of multivessel disease and especially high grades of stenosis in the proximal left anterior descending coronary artery.

As mentioned previously, the goal of salvaging is-

chemic but not yet irreversibly damaged myocardial tissue is based on evidence that a marginal or border zone of unknown size exists around the area of infarction, and for an unknown period after acute infarction, the fate of the jeopardized area remains uncertain.[32] Past attempts at surgically reducing loss of muscle in this setting have been fraught with increased risk. Mills et al. reported 20 patients having myocardial revascularization within 2 days of infarction.[33] Hospital mortality was 15 percent, and late mortality was 10 percent. Loop et al. operated on 37 patients shortly after myocardial infarction.[31] Hospital mortality was 14 percent, but 4 of the 5 deaths occurred in patients who were in shock before operation. Cheanvechai and coworkers reported 29 patients operated on less than 12 h after the onset of chest pain (8 others were operated on more than 3 days after infarction and had recurring angina) with an overall mortality of 5.4 percent.[27] A subsequent report with additional patients from this group describes seven deaths in 66 patients, a mortality of 10.6 percent.[34] In another series reported by Dawson et al., 11 patients were subjected to coronary bypass within 1 to 21 h after acute myocardial infarction, 9 of whom had life-threatening complications of shock or recurrent cardiac arrest.[19] The overall mortality was 38 percent. Keon and coworkers successfully performed myocardial revascularization operation in 3 patients, 3, 4, and 12 h after the onset of chest pain and infarction.[35,36] Of particular interest was a subgroup of 43 patients without shock who were operated upon within 12 h of the onset of chest pain and myocardial infarction, and the mortality was 4.6 percent.

The use of intraaortic balloon pumping has been envisioned by some investigators in the past to increase surgical salvage and reduce operative risks in unstable patients following myocardial infarction. This feeling has experimental basis in the fact that intraaortic balloon pumping in dogs undergoing experimental acute infarction produced a significant delay in quantitative CPK loss and onset of necrosis, suggesting a delay in the ischemic process.[37] Intraaortic balloon pumping also was shown to improve blood flow to the

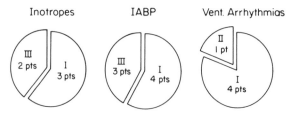

FIGURE 10-7 Complications following myocardial revascularization and recent infarction. IABP, intraaortic balloon pump. See discussion for definitions of groups I, II, and III.

Hospital deaths - None
Late deaths - None (m̄ follow-up 9.8 mos.)

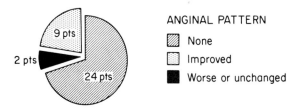

ANGINAL PATTERN

▨ None
▢ Improved
■ Worse or unchanged

FIGURE 10-8 Mortality and residual anginal pattern in 35 patients following revascularization soon after infarction.

ischemic and marginal zones during both acute ischemia and reperfusion, suggesting that it might be useful for myocardial protection prior to reperfusion and for overcoming the no-reflow phenomenon after coronary reperfusion.[38] Mundth and coworkers reported 52 patients with complicated myocardial infarction or shock who could not be weaned from the intraaortic balloon pump after 2 to 10 days.[25] If patients with ventricular septal rupture or mitral regurgitation were excluded, the survival rate was only 22 percent. These patients had emergency coronary artery bypass grafting, but in spite of revascularization, survival in this particularly ill group of patients was not good. In another series of patients with anterior myocardial infarction less than 6 h old, Leinbach et al. used the intraaortic balloon pump in an attempt to control injury.[39] There were no cases of shock. Five patients responded with a fall in ST-segment elevation in 1 h, with preservation of precordial R waves and good ventricular function. In contrast, 6 patients responded poorly, with a poor response in reducing ST-segment elevation in 1 h, *q* wave development, and poor residual left ventricular function. Their conclusions were that benefit could be obtained from intraaortic balloon pumping in cases of anterior myocardial infarction only as long as there was residual left anterior descending artery patency following the proximal occlusion. Others have reported use of preoperative intraaortic balloon pumping in a more select group of patients. Bardet et al. describe 21 patients with postinfarction angina (2 to 15 days after acute myocardial infarction) unresponsive to medical therapy.[16] They were treated by preoperative intraaortic balloon pumping, and both anginal pain and ECG ST-segment changes were prevented with the intraaortic balloon pump in all patients. Sixteen of 17 patients undergoing coronary revascularization survived the operation; all survivors were in clinically improved condition, and 14 were free of pain. Although limited, our experience with intraaortic balloon pumping in this clinical setting has not been nearly so encouraging,

and we have noted extension of infarction with anterior *q* wave development in spite of circulatory assistance. At our institution, a patient is not considered a surgical candidate if mechanical circulatory assistance is required for the treatment of cardiogenic shock. Patients in cardiogenic shock requiring mechanical circulatory assistance usually have too great a loss of myocardial muscle mass for this technique to be routinely used or practical at the present time. Although there may be dramatic instances where patients requiring such circulatory assistance survive operation, long-term results in the overwhelming majority are extremely poor. We have also felt that once committed to intraaortic balloon pumping following myocardial infarction, valuable time is lost in attempts to stabilize the patient prior to revascularization.

In our series, three groups of patients were arbitrarily defined according to the infarction-revascularization interval to discern if hospital morbidity or mortality could be correlated with the temporal relationship between myocardial necrosis and revascularization. Hemodynamic instability in the postoperative period, however, was related more to preoperative left ventricular function than to the interval between infarction and revascularization. Left ventricular function, as measured by ejection fraction, left ventricular end-diastolic pressure, and segmental wall motion, were better for patients in Group II than for those in groups I or III, and all patients requiring either inotropic or balloon support in the postoperative period were in these latter two groups.

Besides careful selection, we attribute the low hospital and late mortality in our patients to advances in many areas of patient care. When operating on individuals with recent myocardial infarction and marginal

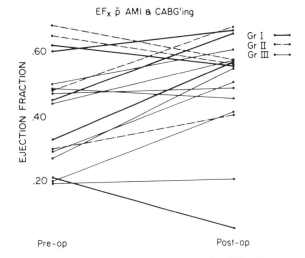

FIGURE 10-9 Change in ejection fraction following myocardial revascularization.

myocardial reserve, certain factors in the perioperative period become extremely important. Precise anesthetic management is critical in assuring a stable condition prior to cardiopulmonary bypass. During this period, any increase in oxygen demand or decrease in oxygen supply must be avoided. We have found good correlation between the rate–pressure product and ischemic V_5 precordial ECG changes prior to bypass (J. A. Kaplan, unpublished data). Therefore, factors that increase heart rate, left ventricular contractility, or wall tension must be avoided or recognized early and treated promptly. In order to avoid tachycardia and hypertension during the prebypass period, we have insisted that patients receiving propranolol have this drug continued and that the last dose be administered 12 h prior to anesthetic induction. Episodes of hypertension or increases in pulmonary wedge pressure (both of which increase oxygen demand) are promptly treated with intravenous nitroglycerin. In order to prevent reduction in coronary perfusion pressure, hypotension is treated by administration of small, and sometimes frequent, doses of peripheral vasoconstrictors. The importance of prebypass monitoring is demonstrated by the positive correlation between a rate–pressure product greater than 12,000 and appearance of ischemic ECG changes (J. A. Kaplan, unpublished data). Elevation of the rate–pressure product in the prebypass period is usually a result of increase in heart rate above 90 beats per minute.

The operative technique used in these patients is no different from that used in other coronary bypass patients. Although not substantiated by this study, we believe that use of a single cross-clamp technique, combined with potassium cardioplegia, may minimize ventricular distension and maintain a hypothermic hypometabolic flaccid myocardium until rewarming begins. Use of a hyperosmolar solution may reduce any endothelial or myocardial cellular swelling present in these acutely ischemic ventricles and may enhance reperfusion once bypass grafting has been accomplished.[40,41] Technical emphasis has been placed on performing anastomoses distal to disease whenever possible, even if the caliber of the vessel is significantly smaller than the more proximal diseased arteries.

As stressed previously, we have tried to avoid operating on patients in cardiogenic shock, who require mechanical support for maintenance of adequate cardiac output. These patients continue to represent a formidable therapeutic challenge and are associated with too great an operative risk to be routinely practical at the present time. However, intraaortic balloon pumping has been used judiciously in patients prior to cardiopulmonary bypass to reduce or terminate refractory ventricular arrhythmias, minimize ischemic trauma associated with anesthetic induction, and reduce left ventricular work associated with the return of cardiac function at the conclusion of an operative procedure. The low incidence of preoperative cardiogenic shock in our patients can probably be attributed to patient selection and the infrequent finding of recent anterior transmural infarction. The latter finding has been associated with a high incidence of cardiogenic shock and death.[8,25] Although intraaortic balloon support may be advantageous in stabilizing the patient prior to cardiac catheterization, it was not used in any of our patients. We would agree with others[27,42,43] that cardiac catheterization can be performed safely in patients soon after myocardial infarction.

The satisfactory perioperative myocardial infarction rate demonstrated in our series may be related to the technique of myocardial preservation, although the presence of transmural myocardial infarction in some of the patients may have "masked" the appearance of new q waves. In one patient undergoing coronary artery bypass grafting following an acute transmural anterior myocardial infarction, regeneration of R wave forces occurred on the day after surgery. The interesting subject of regeneration of anterior QRS forces following revascularization has been discussed by Helfant.[44] Helfant has stated that Q waves may not actually be synonymous with transmural myocardial infarction. He feels that transient Q waves may be produced by myocardial ischemia alone. Although these patients undoubtedly represent a small group, the finding supports the concept that chronically ischemic myocardium may, in certain instances, produce Q waves that may be reversible upon reestablishment of adequate perfusion.

We attribute high early postoperative creatinine phosphokinase enzyme levels in Group I patients to the extremely labile course of patients in the first 24 h after myocardial infarction, resulting in more perioperative myocardial damage. Isoenzymes, when measured, were indicative of minimal perioperative injury in the majority of patients.

By operating on selected patients soon after acute myocardial infarction, we feel major objectives of therapy have been realized: there has been no early or late mortality, only a small percentage of patients had an unfavorable result, and the graft patency rate for most patients was gratifying. Our findings of a high patency rate in grafts performed to the area of infarction agrees with the clinical studies of others.[28,45] Left ventricular function was preserved and frequently improved, as demonstrated by postoperative changes in ejection fraction and left ventricular segmental wall function.

Although conclusive data regarding the best mode

of therapy in this particular patient population would best be achieved by a medical and surgical randomized study, we have attempted to show that adequate revascularization can now be accomplished safely and effectively in a group of patients previously deemed at very high operative risk. It might be argued that more persistent medical therapy would be effective in temporarily controlling ventricular arrhythmias, pain, or even reduced cardiac output; however, our feeling is that revascularization of the ischemic and injured myocardium can be accomplished effectively with low operative risk and offers the best chance of minimizing left ventricular muscle damage and patient mortality.

REFERENCES

1 Miller, R. R., DeMaria, A. N., Vismara, L. A., Salel, A. F., Maxwell, K. S., Amsterdam, E. A., and Mason, D. T.: Chronic Stable Inferior Myocardial Infarction: Unsuspected Harbinger of High Risk Proximal Left Coronary Arterial Obstruction Amenable to Surgical Revascularization, *Am. J. Cardiol.*, 39:954, 1977.

2 Chaitman, B. R., Waters, D. D., Corbara, F., and Bourassa, M. G.: Prediction of Multivessel Disease After Inferior Myocardial Infarction, *Circulation*, 57:1085, 1978.

3 Oberman, A., Jones, W. B., Riley, C. P., et al.: Natural History of Coronary Artery Disease, *Bull. N.Y. Acad. Med.*, 48:1109, 1972.

4 Bruschke, A. V. G., Proudfit, W. L., and Sones, F. M.: Progress in the Study of 590 Consecutive Non-surgical Cases of Coronary Disease Followed 5.9 Years. I—Arteriographic Correlation, *Circulation*, 47:1147, 1973.

5 Humphries, J. O.: Expected Course of Patients with Coronary Artery Disease, *Cardiovasc. Clin.*, 8(2):41, 1977.

6 Moss, A. J., DeCamilla, J., David, H., et al.: The Early Posthospital Phase of Myocardial Infarction: Prognostic Stratification, *Circulation*, 54:58, 1976.

7 Coronary Drug Project Research Group: Prognostic Importance of Premature Beats Following Myocardial Infarction, *J.A.M.A.*, 223:1116, 1973.

8 Madigan, N. P., Rutherford, B. D., and Frye, R. L.: The Clinical Course, Early Prognosis and Coronary Anatomy of Subendocardial Infarction, *Am. J. Med.*, 60:634, 1976.

9 Levy, W. K., and Cannom, L. S.: Prognosis of Subendocardial Myocardial Infarction, *Circulation*, 51, 52 (suppl. 2):107, 1975.

10 Cronin, R. G. P., and Moore, S., and Marpole, D. G.: Shock Following Myocardial Infarction: A Clinical Survey of 140 Cases, *Can. Med. Assoc. J.*, 93:57, 1965.

11 Killip, J., and Kimball, J. J.: Treatment of Myocardial Infarction in a Coronary Care Unit. A Two-Year Experience with 250 Patients, *Am. J. Cardiol.*, 20:457, 1967.

12 Nielsen, B. L., and Marner, I. L.: Shock in Acute Myocardial Infarction, *Acta Med. Scand.*, 175:65, 1964.

13 Scheibt, S., Ascheim, R., and Killip, T.: Cardiogenic Shock After Acute Myocardial Infarction, *Am. J. Cardiol.*, 26:556, 1970.

14 Lown, B., Vassaux, G., Hoop, W. B., Fakhro, A. M., Kaplinsky, E., and Roberge, G.: Unresolved Problems in Coronary Care, *Am. J. Cardiol.*, 20:494, 1967.

15 Stenson, R. E., Flamm, M. D., Jr., Zaret, B. L., and McGowan, R. L.: Transient ST-Segment Elevation with Postmyocardial Infarction Angina: Prognostic Significance, *Am. Heart J.*, 89:449, 1975.

16 Bardet, J., Rigaud, M., Kahn, J. C., Huret, J. F., Gandjbakhch, I., and Bourdarias, J. P.: Treatment of Post-myocardial Infarction Angina by Intra-aortic Balloon Pumping and Emergency Revascularization, *J. Thorac. Cardiovasc. Surg.*, 74:299, 1977.

17 Maroko, P. R., Kjeksus, J. K., Sobel, B. E., et al.: Factors Influencing Infarct Size Following Experimental Coronary Artery Occlusion, *Circulation*, 43:67, 1971.

18 Maroko, P. R., and Braunwald, E.: Modification of Myocardial Infarction Size After Coronary Occlusion, *Ann. Intern. Med.*, 79:720, 1973.

19 Dawson, J. T., Hall, R. J., Hallman, G. L., and Cooley, D. A.: Mortality in Patients Undergoing Coronary Artery Bypass Surgery After Myocardial Infarction, *Am. J. Cardiol.*, 33:483, 1974.

20 Costantini, C., Corday, E., Lang, T. W., et al.: Revascularization After Three Hours of Coronary Arterial Occlusion: Effects on Regional Cardiac Metabolic Function and Infarct Size, *Am. J. Cardiol.*, 37:368, 1975.

21 Bresnahan, G. F., Roberts, R., Schell, W. E., et al.: Deleterious Effects Due to Hemorrhage After Myocardial Reperfusion, *Am. J. Cardiol.*, 33:82, 1974.

22 Kloner, B. A., Ganote, C. E., and Jennings, R. B.: The "No Reflow" Phenomenon After Temporary Coronary Occlusion in Dogs, *J. Clin. Invest.*, 54:1496, 1974.

23 Hill, J. D., Kerth, W. J., Kelly, J. J., Selzer, A., Armstrong, W., Popper, R. W., Langston, M. F., and Cohn, K. E.: Emergency Aortocoronary Bypass for Impending or Extending Myocardial Infarction, *Circulation*, 43, 44 (suppl. 1):105, 1971.

24 Kongtahworn, C., Zeff, R. H., Iannone, L., Gordon, D., Brown, T., and Phillips, S. J.: Emergency Myocardial Revascularization During Acute Evolving Myocardial Infarction, *Chest*, 72:403, 1977.

25 Mundth, E. D., Buckley, M. J., Leinbach, R. C., DeSantis, R. W., Sanders, C. A., Kantrowitz, A., and Austen, W. G.: Myocardial Revascularization for the Treat-

ment of Cardiogenic Shock Complicating Acute Myocardial Infarction, *Surgery,* 70:78, 1971.

26 Madigan, N. P., Rutherford, B. D., Barnhorst, D. A., and Danielson, G. K.: Early Saphenous Vein Grafting After Subendocardial Infarction. Immediate Surgical Results and Late Prognosis, *Circulation,* 56 (suppl. 2):1, 1977.

27 Cheanvechai, C., Effler, D. B., Loop, F. D., Groves, L. K., Sheldon, W. C., Razavi, M., and Sones, F. M., Jr.: Emergency Myocardial Revascularization, *Am. J. Cardiol.,* 32:901, 1973.

28 Berg, R., Jr., Kendall, R. W., Duvoisin, G. E., Ganji, J. H., Rudy, L. W., and Everhart, F. J.: Acute Myocardial Infarction: A Surgical Emergency, *J. Thorac. Cardiovasc. Surg.,* 70:432, 1975.

29 Schoonmaker, F.W., and King, S. B., III: Coronary Arteriography by the Single Catheter Percutaneous Femoral Technique. Experience with 6,800 Cases, *Circulation,* 50:735, 1974.

30 King, S. B., III, and Douglas, J. S., Jr.: Coronary Arteriography and Left Ventriculography, in J. W. Hurst, R. B. Logue, R. C. Schlant, and N. K. Wenger (eds.), "The Heart," 4th ed., McGraw-Hill Book Company, New York, 1978.

31 Loop, F. D., Cheanvechai, C., Sheldon, W. C., Taylor, P. C., and Effler, D. B.: Early Myocardial Revascularization During Acute Myocardial Infarction, *Chest,* 66:478, 1974.

32 Engler, R. L., and Ross, J. R.: Is There a Role for Surgery in Acute Myocardial Infarction? *Cardiovasc. Clin.,* 8(2):213, 1977.

33 Mills, N. L., Ochsner, J. L., Bower, P. J., Patton, R. M., and Moore, C. B.: Coronary Artery Bypass for Acute Myocardial Infarction, *South. Med. J.,* 68:1475, 1975.

34 Sheldon, W. C., Rincon, G., Pichard, A. D., et al.: Surgical Treatment for Coronary Artery Disease, *Prog. Cardiovasc. Dis.,* 18:237, 1975.

35 Keon, W. J., Abbas, S. Z., Shankar, K. R., et al.: Emergency Aortocoronary Venous Bypass Grafting: Cardiogenic Shock, *Can. Med. Assoc. J.,* 105:1292, 1971.

36 Keon, W. J., Bedard, P., Shankar, K. R., Ayurekli, Y., Nino, A., and Berkman, F.: Experience with Emergency Aortocoronary Bypass Grafts in the Presence of Acute Myocardial Infarction, *Circulation,* 47, 48 (suppl. 3):151, 1973.

37 DeLaria, G. A., Johansen, K. H., Sobel, B. E., et al.: Delayed Evolution of Myocardial Ischemic Injury After Intraaortic Balloon Counter Pulsation, *Circulation,* 49, 50 (suppl. 2):242, 1974.

38 Saini, V. K., Hood, W. B., Heckman, H. B., et al.: Nutrient Myocardial Blood Flow in Experimental Myocardial Ischemia, *Circulation,* 52:1085, 1975.

39 Leinbach, R. C., Gold, H. K., Harper, R. W., Buckley, M. J., and Austen, W. G.: Early Intraaortic Balloon Pumping for Anterior Myocardial Infarction Without Shock, *Circulation,* 58:204, 1978.

40 Willerson, J. T., Curry, G. C., Atkins, J. M., Parkey, R., and Horwitz, L. D.: Influence of Hypertonic Mannitol on Ventricular Performance and Coronary Blood Flow in Patients, *Circulation,* 51:1095, 1975.

41 Jones, E. L., Tyras, D. H., King, S. B., III, Logue, R. B., and Hatcher, C. R., Jr.: Myocardial Revascularization Combined with Intracoronary Infusion of Hyperosmolar Solution in the Early Management of Postinfarction Ventricular Septal Defect. Report of a Case, *Circulation,* 52:170, 1975.

42 Cohn, L. H., Gorlin, R., Herman, M. V., and Collins, J. J., Jr.: Aorto-coronary Bypass for Acute Coronary Occlusion, *J. Thorac. Cardiovasc. Surg.,* 64:503, 1972.

43 Begg, F. R., Kooros, M. A., Magovern, G. J., Kent, E. M., Brent, L. B., and Cushing, W. B.: The Hemodynamics and Coronary Arteriography Patterns During Acute Myocardial Infarction, *J. Thorac. Cardiovasc. Surg.,* 58:647, 1969.

44 Helfant, R. H.: Q Waves in Coronary Heart Disease: Newer Understanding of Their Clinical Implications, *Am. J. Cardiol.,* 38:662, 1976.

45 Cheanvechai, C., Effler, D. B., Loop, F. D., Groves, L. K., Sheldon, W. C., and Sones, F. M., Jr.: Aortocoronary Artery Graft During Early and Late Phases of Acute Myocardial Infarction, *Ann. Thorac. Surg.,* 16:249, 1973.

46 Read, R. C., Murphy, M. L., Hultgren, H. N., et al.: Survival of Men Treated for Chronic Stable Angina Pectoris: A Cooperative Randomized Study, *J. Thorac. Cardiovasc. Surg.,* 75:1, 1978.

47 Kouchoukos, N. T., Oberman, A., and Karp, R. B.: Results of Surgery for Disabling Angina Pectoris, in A. N. Brest and S. H. Rahimtoola (eds.)., "Cardiovascular Clinics (Coronary Bypass Surgery)," F. A. Davis Company, Philadelphia, p. 157.

48 Bruschke, A. V.: Ten Year Follow-up of 601 Nonsurgical Cases of Angiographically Documented Coronary Disease. Angiographic Correlations, in "The First Decade of Bypass Graft Surgery for Coronary Artery Disease." (International symposium, Cleveland Clinic Foundation, 1977), p. 77.

Chapter 11

Prevention of Sudden Death by Coronary Bypass Surgery*

DEAN T. MASON, M.D., ANTHONY N. De MARIA, M.D., GARRETT LEE, M.D., and EZRA A. AMSTERDAM, M.D.

Despite the impressive inroads during the past three decades in which the death rate from heart and vascular diseases declined by 30 percent, cardiovascular diseases still account for more deaths (51 percent of annual national mortality) than all other causes combined.[1] Nearly every adult American is afflicted by atherosclerosis, and the various complications of atherosclerosis produce more than four-fifths (800,000 deaths annually) of all cardiovascular mortality. Coronary artery disease represents the most prevalent cause of death, being responsible for more than one-third (600,000 deaths each year) of all national mortality. Moreover, 60 percent of coronary mortality occurs suddenly,[2] and even surviving patients with acute myocardial infarction who are fortunate enough to receive modern in-hospital coronary care are at increased risk of subsequent acute fatal coronary events.[3] These alarming epidemiologic observations emphasize that immediate, unexpected, premature death occurring outside the hospital as a complication of coronary artery disease is the gravest health problem in our country,[4] claiming 400,000 lives annually, and at least 100,000 of these fatalities take place in the prime of life of persons (greatest prevalence in young adult men) less than 65 years of age.

PATHOPHYSIOLOGY

Postmortem studies have shown that most persons who die suddenly have extensive coronary atherosclerosis accompanied by old myocardial infarction but are usually without evidence of new necrosis or acute thrombosis.[5] These findings of the lack of acute myocardial infarction suggest that sudden coronary death is due to ventricular fibrillation of reentrant mechanism triggered by deterioration of aerobic metabolism in ischemic areas of heart muscle.[6] Furthermore, recent advances in neurochemistry and psychodynamics indicate that the fibrillation threshold is lowered in ischemic myocardium by adrenergic stimulation via sympathetic pathways emanating from the hypothalamus.[4,7]

SUDDEN CORONARY DEATH RISK FACTORS

Besides the precursors of coronary atherosclerosis and the presence of multivessel coronary disease, specific risk factors for sudden death have been identified in coronary patients.[8] Especially relevant is the presence of ventricular ectopy which is best detected and evaluated by dynamic ambulatory electrocardiography,[9] particularly the serious forms of premature contractions (multifocal, paired, R-on-T phenomenon, frequency greater than 5 per minute) and episodic ventricular tachycardia,[4] in clinically stable coronary disease (Fig. 11-1)[8] or persisting after convalescence from acute myocardial infarction (Fig. 11-2).[3,10] In addition, other factors have been correlated with the occurrence of unexpected lethal dysrhythmias in the coronary disease population, including recent (within 6 months) myocardial infarction;[11] ventricular dysfunction;[8] segmental dyssynergy;[8] myocardial ischemia (angina pectoris, persistent ST depression on resting electrocardiogram, exercise-induced ST depression, positive exercise cold-spot myocardial scintigraphy, and abnormal exercise radionuclide ventriculography);[3,8,12,13] ventricular hypertrophy (Fig. 11-3);[8] treadmill exercise-induced hypotension;[14,15] premature beats of left ventricular origin (ectopic right bundle branch block);[8] and environmental stress (undue anxiety and bereavement).[4] Although there has only been limited evaluation of the prophylactic efficacy of ambulatory medical therapy in the prevention of sudden coronary death, long-term trials with certain antiarrhythmics,[4,16,17] platelet antiaggregants,[18] and antianginal drugs[19] have provided preliminary evidence of effectiveness.

*From the Section of Cardiovascular Medicine, Departments of Medicine and Physiology, University of California, School of Medicine and Sacramento Medical Center, Davis and Sacramento.

Supported in part by Research Program Project Grant HL-14780 from the National Heart, Lung and Blood Institute, National Institutes of Health, Bethesda, Maryland.

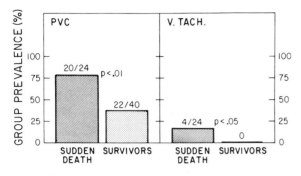

FIGURE 11-1 Frequency of premature ventricular contractions (PVC) (left panel) and ventricular tachycardia (V. tach.) obtained by ambulatory ECG monitoring in 64 patients with chronic coronary artery disease who were matched for equal extent of multivessel coronary disease and ventricular dysfunction assessed by cardiac catheterization and then followed up prospectively for 30 months. Twenty-four of the patients died suddenly (left bar in each panel), and 40 patients survived (right bar in each panel). Serious ventricular tachyarrhythmias were more frequent and the extent of ST-segment depression was greater in the group who died suddenly. *(From L. A. Vismara et al., Identification of Sudden Death Risk Factors in Acute and Chronic Coronary Artery Disease, Am. J. Cardiol., 39:821, 1977.)*

IMPROVED LONGEVITY FOLLOWING REVASCULARIZATION

Since it is now well established that properly performed elective coronary bypass surgery in appropriately selected coronary patients increases regional perfusion of ischemic myocardium (Fig. 11-4)[20] and is more effective than modern medical therapy in the symptomatic management of chronic stable angina pectoris (surgery: angina was decreased in 90 percent of patients and abolished in 67 percent of patients versus medical therapy: 75 percent decreased and 33 percent abolished),[21] logic clearly dictates that such a revascularization procedure can also prolong life.[22] It is also perfectly rational to expect that for a disorder (coronary atherosclerosis) in which diminished coronary blood flow represents the basic pathophysiologic deficiency, restoration of normal coronary blood flow (coronary bypass surgery) constitutes a more sound approach than reduction of cardiac oxygen requirements (modern medical therapy)[23] in the relief of ischemic pain and extension of life-span.

Indeed, there now exists an overwhelming body of scientifically valid evidence[21,22,24-32] that leads to the conclusion that properly performed elective coronary bypass, carried out in appropriately selected subgroups of coronary patients with chronic stable angina pectoris, more effectively extends longevity than currently available medical therapy. These appropriate subsets include those who are at high risk of dying

from advanced native ischemic heart disease with obstruction of the left main coronary artery or with triple- or double-vessel obstruction of the major coronary arteries[21,22] and perhaps certain individuals with single-vessel proximal stenosis of the left anterior descending coronary artery.[31]

This rationale concerning improved life-span pertains to patients with incapacitating angina (stable, unstable, or variant in type) receiving adequate medical treatment in whom coronary bypass is considered feasible despite less than ideally operable vessels even with depressed left ventricular function.[21,22] Furthermore, on an individual basis, this reasoning about revascularization-enhanced longevity can usually be extended to young and middle-aged adult coronary patients (generally less than 65 years of age) who have the same high-risk pathoanatomic subsets with chronic stable angina responsive to medical management (or objective evidence of active myocardial ischemia or remote myocardial infarction),[21,22,33] provided that operation can be achieved with negligible mortality and complications, i.e., that the diseased vessels are optimal for successful bypass (proximal stenosis with

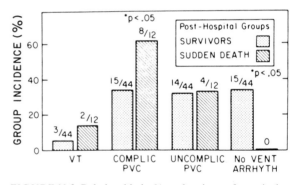

FIGURE 11-2 Relationship in 64 total patients of ventricular dysrhythmias (PVC) obtained by ambulatory ECG monitoring late in the course of hospitalization for acute myocardial infarction to sudden death after hospital discharge. All patients who died suddenly had ventricular ectopy late during their hospitalization (but not necessarily early in the coronary care unit), whereas those without ventricular dysrhythmias in the hospital prior to discharge subsequently survived (average follow-up period 26 months). Sudden death occurred an average of only 8 months after hospitalization, and most were young adult males less than 50 years of age. In addition, sudden death patients were distinguished by their increased prevalence of complicated (complic) PVCs (67 percent) as compared to survivors (only 34 percent). VT, ventricular tachycardia; uncomplic, uncomplicated; vent. arrhyth, ventricular dysrhythmias: VT, complic PVC, or uncomplic PVC; PVC, premature ventricular contraction. *(From L. A. Vismara et al., Relation of Ventricular Arrhythmias in the Late Hospital Phase of Acute Myocardial Infarction to Sudden Death After Hospital Discharge, Am. J. Med., 56:6, 1975.)*

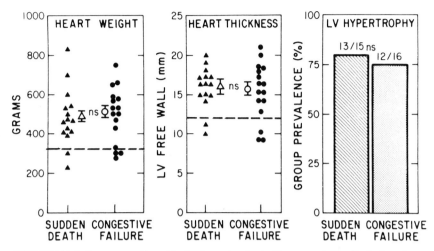

FIGURE 11-3 Frequency of ventricular hypertrophy in 31 young adult patients (less than 50 years of age) who died of premature coronary artery disease with cardinal coronary atherogenic risk factors. Fifteen patients died suddenly (left column of each panel), and 16 patients died with congestive heart failure (right column of each panel). The left panel indicates total heart weight at necropsy, the middle panel shows left ventricular free wall thickness at necropsy, and the right panel depicts electrocardiographic left ventricular (LV) hypertrophy before death. In each panel, 13 of the 15 patients who died suddenly demonstrated evidence of left ventricular hypertrophy. The horizontal broken line in the left and middle panels indicates the upper limit of normal. ns = $p > .05$. *(From L. A. Vismara et al., Identification of Sudden Death Risk Factors in Acute and Chronic Coronary Artery Disease, Am. J. Cardiol., 39:821, 1977.)*

excellent to good distal patency demonstrated by no or less than 20 percent luminal narrowing below the obstruction, good opacification, and rapid runoff of contrast dye in the distal segment), that normal ventricular function is present and that the patient is in otherwise excellent health. Relevant to the above comments, we have recently shown that chronic stable inferior myocardial infarction serves as a highly reliable harbinger indicating the presence of high-risk proximal left coronary artery obstruction amenable to surgical revascularization[34] (Fig. 11-5).

Cardiac ischemia is implicated in the pathogenesis of unexpected lethal dysrhythmias causing sudden coronary death.[35] Thus, it is reasonable to anticipate that interventions that improve the imbalanced relationship between myocardial oxygen supply and demand should provide a rational therapeutic approach to the problem of sudden death. It has been shown in a few instances that refractory life-threatening ventricular tachyarrhythmias can be terminated with aortocoronary bypass surgery.[36-38] However, the relation of elective myocardial revascularization in general to improved survival has been speculative, and the salutary mechanism responsible for enhanced longevity requires elucidation. The principal purpose of this chapter is the assessment of the influence of coronary bypass surgery on the incidence of sudden cardiac death.

PROSPECTIVE STUDY OF REVASCULARIZATION ON SUDDEN DEATH IN CHRONIC STABLE ANGINA

To examine the efficacy of coronary bypass surgery on the overall improvement of longevity and specifically on the mode of subsequent mortality which allows such enhanced life-span, prospective evaluation was carried out at our institution (University of California Davis Medical Center, Sacramento) in patients with similar multivessel coronary artery disease managed with either modern medical therapy or aortocoronary bypass surgery.[39] The study population consisted of 247 consecutive patients with significant stenosis (75 percent or more cross-sectional luminal narrowing) of two or three major coronary arteries documented by angiography. The surgically treated group comprised 135 consecutive patients undergoing elective saphenous vein myocardial revascularization within 1 month of cardiac catheterization; the remaining 112 patients were those consecutively treated medically during the entire study period.

Since there existed differences of opinion regarding indications for surgery among our senior cardiology faculty during the time of the study entry period (1970 to 1973), the proper circumstances pertained that allowed coronary patients with similar anatomic vessel disease (Fig. 11-6), ventricular function (Fig. 11-7), coronary risk factors (Fig. 11-8), and symptoms (Fig. 11-9A and C) to be equally matched for appropriate assessment of surgical versus medical therapy including administration of propranolol. Furthermore, all patients remained throughout the study period within the therapeutic group (surgical versus medical) to which they were initially assigned. Thus, although therapy was not randomized as such, both groups included patients with a comparable broad range of clinical manifestations and similar multivessel coronary disease, cardiac performance, and coronary atherogenic precursors. In addition, at the onset of the study the surgical and medical groups were similar in age (average 52 years) and in male/female ratio (3.3). Furthermore, the duration of clinically evident coronary

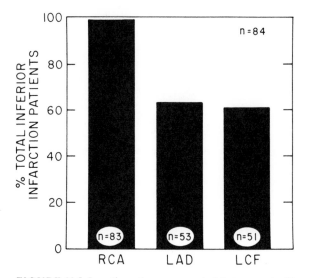

FIGURE 11-5 Location of coronary arterial stenoses in 84 patients with uncomplicated inferior myocardial infarction. LAD, proximal left anterior descending coronary artery; LCF, proximal left circumflex artery; RCA, right coronary artery; *n*, number of patients. In 80 percent of LAD stenoses and in 70 percent of LCF stenoses, these vessels were ideally suitable for coronary bypass. In 45 of these patients with proximal left coronary artery stenosis followed up for 18 months, 14 who underwent coronary bypass surgery were compared with 31 medically treated patients with similar cardiac function (ejection fraction: surgery 0.47; medical 0.52) and coronary pathoanatomy. Ten surgically treated patients (71 percent) had reduced angina compared with only 9 medically treated patients (29 percent). There were no operative or subsequent deaths in the surgery group, whereas 2 medical patients died. Thus, serious proximal left coronary artery disease is highly prevalent as well as operable in patients with chronic inferior myocardial infarction. The latter condition thereby provides a clinically useful and sensitive marker of high-risk coronary arterial stenoses. *(From R. R. Miller et al., Chronic Stable Inferior Myocardial Infarction: Unsuspected Harbinger of High-Risk Proximal Left Coronary Arterial Obstruction Amenable to Surgical Revascularization, Am. J. Cardiol., 39:954, 1977.)*

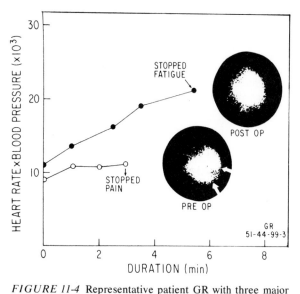

FIGURE 11-4 Representative patient GR with three major vessel coronary stenoses showing improvement in myocardial perfusion following triple aortocoronary bypass grafts. Preoperatively (preop) the exercise myocardial scintigram demonstrated apical ischemia (white arrows). Postoperatively (postop) scintigraphy revealed normal apical myocardial perfusion. Also consistent with the improvement in diminished coronary blood flow to the ischemic area after bypass are the findings depicted graphically with respect to exercise performance. Open circles represent the preoperative study, and the solid circles document the postoperative improved performance. Thus, external workload was enhanced by the increases in both the duration and intensity of exercise performed after surgery (horizontal axis) and in the heart rate–blood pressure product (bpm·mm Hg) (index of myocardial oxygen consumption) after coronary revascularization (vertical axis). *(From A. J. Lurie et al., Determination of Improved Myocardial Perfusion After Aortocoronary Bypass Surgery by Exercise Rubidium-81 Scintigraphy, Circulation, 54 (suppl. 3):20, 1976.)*

disease before entry into the study averaged 3.9 years in the surgical and medical groups and included prior myocardial infarction in 75 percent for both groups.

The duration of evaluation was similar and concurrent in the surgical and medical groups and averaged 39 months (range 24 to 62 months). Drug therapy was also similar in the medical and surgical groups during the evaluation period for digitalis (50 percent of patients), diuretics (48 percent), and non-beta blocking antiarrhythmics, (43 percent) with the exception that more medically treated (30 percent) than surgically treated (12 percent) patients required propranolol. Sudden death, established by interviews with witnesses, was defined as death occurring within 6 h of symptoms, clinically attributable to unexpected dysrhythmias, and unrelated to congestive heart failure, shock, or systemic illness.

The final clinical status for patients in both groups was obtained at the completion of the follow-up period.[39] This information was derived either at completion of the study (39 months) or at the outpatient clinic evaluation before the occurrence of death. Angina pectoris was completely absent in 60 percent of surgically treated patients, whereas only 30 percent of medically treated patients were free of angina (Fig. 11-9B and D). In addition, functional status according to the New York Heart Association classification was considerably improved by coronary bypass (Fig. 11-9B). In contrast, medical therapy only minimally abated angina and did not result in significant improvement in functional status (Fig. 11-9D). The group incidence of congestive heart failure symptoms was not significantly altered in the two patient groups (Fig. 11-9B and D).

In the total group of 135 surgically treated patients, operative mortality was 3 percent, and perioperative infarction as evidenced by new pathologic Q waves occurred in 5 percent of patients. Including the surgical mortality, overall longevity was significantly extended by coronary bypass (82 percent patient survival) in comparison to medical management (58 percent survival) after 39 months of evaluation. Interestingly, comparison of surgical to medical treatment revealed that death rates from congestive heart failure (4 percent versus 7 percent) and noncardiac causes (3 percent versus 7 percent) did not differ significantly between the two therapeutic modalities.

Most important, however, is that the incidence of sudden death was markedly reduced by surgery as compared to medical therapy.[39] Thus, assessed relative to the total surgical group of 135 patients versus the total medical group of 112 patients at 39 months, in the surgical group the incidence of postoperative sudden death was only 5 percent (7 patients), and the incidence of sudden death including operative mortality was only 8 percent, which was in striking contrast to the group incidence of sudden death of 21 percent (23 patients) in the medical patients.

Furthermore, analysis of sudden death without congestive heart failure and noncardiac mortality showed that postoperative sudden death frequency was only 6 percent (7 of 121 patients) as compared to the 24 percent (23 of 96 patients) sudden death incidence in the medical group (Fig. 11-10). Moreover, even the addition of intraoperative mortality to subsequent evaluation period sudden deaths provided only a 9 percent incidence of sudden death in the 121 coronary bypass patients in whom follow-up deaths were not due to congestive heart failure or noncardiac causes. The average interval from the onset of the

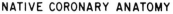

NATIVE CORONARY ANATOMY

| CORONARY DISEASE ≥ 75% | CAD GROUP PREVALENCE (%) | | p value |
	SURGERY n = 121	MEDICAL n = 96	
3 - VESSEL	67	68	ns
2 - VESSEL	33	32	ns
L. MAIN	12	6	ns
LAD	88	86	ns
LCF	79	88	ns
RCA	91	93	ns

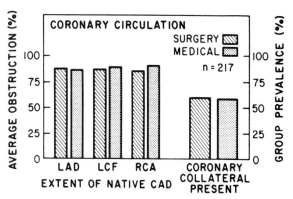

FIGURE 11-6 Coronary pathoanatomy in the medically and surgically treated patient groups at study entry. The two groups were closely matched (difference not significant) in the number of major coronary vessels obstructed (75 percent or more stenosis) and in specific vessels obstructed (top panel) (all patients had multivessel disease). CAD, coronary artery disease; L. main, left mainstem coronary artery; LAD, left anterior descending coronary artery; LCF, left circumflex coronary artery; *n*, number of patients; ns, not significant; *p*, probability; RCA, right coronary artery. In addition (bottom panel), the average obstruction (percentage of luminal narrowing) of each major coronary artery (ns) and the presence of coronary collateral channels (ns) were equally matched in the medical and surgical groups. *(From L. A. Vismara et al., Improved Longevity Due to Reduction of Sudden Death by Aortocoronary Bypass in Coronary Atherosclerosis: Prospective Evaluation of Medical Versus Surgical Therapy in Matched Patients with Multivessel Disease, Am. J. Cardiol., 39:919, 1977.)*

study to sudden death was 1.2 months. The accuracy of determining sudden deaths is established by the high frequency of this mode of fatality occurring instantaneously in both treatment groups (4 of 7 patients, 57 percent, and 15 of 23, 65 percent, of surgically and medically managed patients, respectively).

Therefore, these data indicate that properly performed coronary bypass surgery is capable of prolonging life in angina patients with double- or triple-vessel coronary obstruction[39] and provide insight

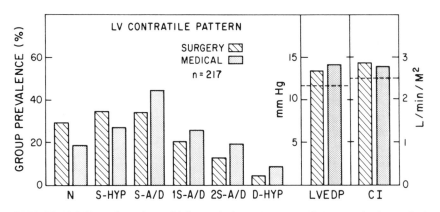

FIGURE 11-7 Hemodynamics and left ventricular (LV) contractile patterns in the medical and surgical group at study entry. N, normal; S-HYP, segmental hypokinesis; S-A/D, segmental akinesis (A) or dyskinesis (D); 1S-A/D, one area of A or D; 2S-A/D, two or more areas of A or D; D-HYP, diffuse hypokinesis; LVEDP, left ventricular end-diastolic pressure; CI, cardiac index; horizontal broken line for LVEDP indicates upper limit of normal; horizontal broken line for CI indicates lower limit of normal. There was no statistical difference in any of these variables, including ejection fraction, between medical and surgical groups. *(From L. A. Vismara et al., Improved Longevity Due to Reduction of Sudden Death by Aortocoronary Bypass in Coronary Atherosclerosis: Prospective Evaluation of Medical Versus Surgical Therapy in Matched Patients with Multivessel Disease, Am. J. Cardiol., 39:919, 1977.)*

concerning the mechanism (reduction of sudden death) by which life is extended after the operative procedure.[39] In regard to the degree of diminution of sudden death frequency afforded by successful revascularization in multivessel coronary disease, our prospective investigation found that the incidence rate of sudden death in surgically treated patients was about one-third that in carefully matched medically treated patients.

It is also important to point out that the overall cardiac mortality for our medical group was 10 percent per year.[39] Because all of our medically treated patients (as well as our surgically treated patients) had two or three major vessel obstruction, the prognosis of our medically treated patients is quite consistent with previously reported data. The annual mortality of medically treated patients with angina pectoris and multivessel stenoses has been established to range

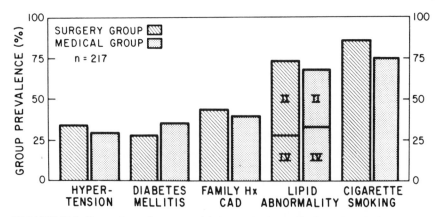

FIGURE 11-8 Comparison of coronary risk factors in the medically and surgically treated groups of patients at study entry. There was an equal prevalence of these factors in both groups on entry into the prospective study. CAD, coronary artery disease; Hx, history; *n*, number of patients; II and IV, type II and type IV hyperlipoproteinemia. *(From L. A. Vismara et al., Improved Longevity Due to Reduction of Sudden Death by Aortocoronary Bypass in Coronary Atherosclerosis: Prospective Evaluation of Medical Versus Surgical Therapy in Matched Patients with Multivessel Disease, Am. J. Cardiol., 39:919, 1977.)*

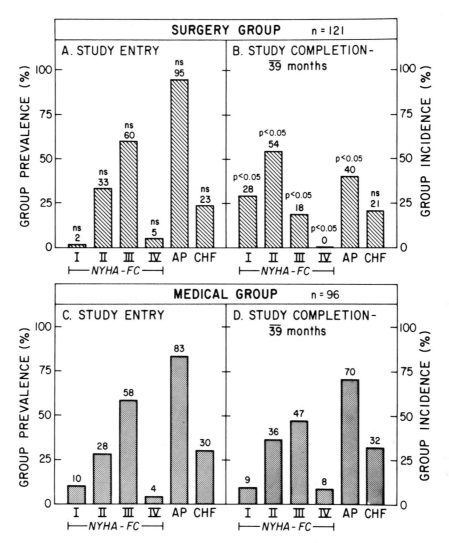

FIGURE 11-9 Symptoms in the medically and surgically treated groups at study entry (A and C) and at study completion (B and D) (average follow-up, 39 months = $\overline{39}$). New York Heart Association (NYHA) functional classification (FC) is indicated by classes I, II, III, and IV. AP, presence of angina pectoris; CHF, congestive heart failure symptoms. Statistical comparisons in panel A are related to panel C, and those in panel B are related to panel D (ns = $p > .05$). *(From L. A. Vismara et al., Improved Longevity Due to Reduction of Sudden Death by Aortocoronary Bypass in Coronary Atherosclerosis: Prospective Evaluation of Medical Versus Surgical Therapy in Matched Patients with Multivessel Disease, Am. J. Cardiol., 39:919, 1977.)*

from 7 to 13 percent for two-vessel disease and from 10 to 16 percent for three-vessel disease.[40-42] Furthermore, because more than two-thirds of our medically treated patients manifested triple-vessel coronary obstruction, our annual death rate was within the lower range for medical therapy alone.[22,30] Thus, it is evident that the more favorable prognosis achieved by coronary bypass grafting in our surgical patients with multivessel disease (mortality only 5 percent per year including the initial operative deaths) was not the result of excessive mortality in the medical group.

ADDITIONAL SUPPORTIVE STUDIES

Reports by other investigators on the results of coronary bypass surgery are in agreement that the revascularization procedure can reduce the incidence of sudden cardiac death in patients with multiple high-risk coronary lesions. Thus Hammermeister, Dodge, and colleagues recently evaluated sudden death prospectively for 4 years in medically and surgically treated patients angiographically matched for coro-

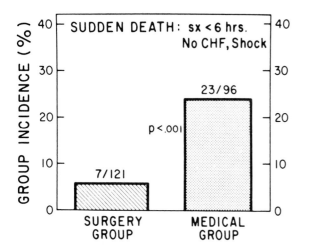

FIGURE 11-10 Comparison of the occurrence of sudden death from coronary disease in the medically and surgically treated groups during the average 39-month period of prospective evaluation. Only 7 of the 121 (6 percent) surgical patients died suddenly in contrast to 23 of the 96 (24 percent) medically treated patients. CHF, congestive heart failure; hrs, hours; mos, months; sx, symptoms. *(From L. A. Vismara et al., Improved Longevity Due to Reduction of Sudden Death by Aortocoronary Bypass in Coronary Atherosclerosis: Prospective Evaluation of Medical Versus Surgical Therapy in Matched Patients with Multivessel Disease, Am. J. Cardiol., 39:919, 1977.)*

nary pathoanatomy and ventricular function.[43] In their examination of three different categories of ejection fraction in patients with one-, two-, and three-vessel obstruction, the percentage of patients who died suddenly was less in each category of surgically treated patients than in matched medical groups. For each subgroup the rate of sudden death was 2 to 11 times higher in the medical than in the surgical cohort; revascularization indicated greatest benefit in reducing such fatalities in patients having multivessel disease with low ejection fractions.

In addition, Favaloro has also recently reported his findings concerning the influence of myocardial revascularization on sudden cardiac death rate.[44] In coronary patients with multivessel disease evaluated prospectively, a striking reduction of sudden death incidence was clearly evident in surgical versus medical management. Thus, in 206 surgical patients compared to 196 angiographically matched medical patients followed for a period of 40 months, the cumulative sudden death mortality of 2 percent in patients who underwent coronary bypass surgery was significantly less than that of 11 percent in the medically treated group.

Finally, further confirmation that coronary artery bypass reduces the incidence of sudden cardiac death has very recently been reported by Greene in a prospective study demonstrating that surgical revascularization improves long-term survival as compared to medical treatment in angiographically matched patients.[45] In 875 surgically treated patients at the Buffalo General Hospital observed for 1 to 9 years (average 32 months), there were only five incidents of sudden death among a total of 71 fatalities. The remaining deaths resulted from congestive heart failure or noncardiac causes.

MECHANISM OF REDUCED SUDDEN DEATH RATE

At present, the physiologic process by which myocardial revascularization appears to reduce the incidence of subsequent sudden death from coronary artery disease requires clarification. However, there is abundant clinical and experimental evidence that myocardial ischemia is a potent stimulus in the initiation and perpetuation of ventricular dysrhythmias. Thus, a reduction in ischemic myocardium as the result of an improved oxygen supply and demand relationship postoperatively provides a rational explanation for the reduced incidence of sudden death. Although lessened myocardial ischemia could have resulted from postoperative myocardial fibrosis, this explanation appears unlikely because of the low rate of clinically apparent perioperative infarction observed in our study described herein,[39] as well as in the reports of others.[22,43-45]

Recent studies carried out by our group[46,47] indicate that a high incidence of ventricular ectopy (55 to 69 percent of patients) is detected with continuous ambulatory electrocardiographic monitoring after bypass surgery. Nevertheless, these preliminary results suggest that effective myocardial revascularization may reduce the frequency not only of ventricular tachycardia but also of potentially life-threatening forms of ventricular ectopic beats that are frequent (more than 20 per hour), multifocal, or paired or that interrupt the preceding T wave. Because these serious types of ventricular dysrhythmias are implicated as independent risk factors for sudden death,[3,4,8] revascularization may favorably alter the clinical significance of ventricular ectopy by suppressing these serious forms of ventricular tachyarrhythmias despite persistent uncomplicated premature ventricular contractions in the postoperative state.

REFERENCES

1 Levy, R. I.: Fourth Report of the Director of the National Heart, Lung and Blood Institute. (DHEW Publication (NIH) 77-1170), March 1977.

2 Kuller, L.: Sudden Death in Arteriosclerotic Heart Disease: The Case for Preventive Medicine, *Am. J. Cardiol.*, 24:617, 1969.

3 Vismara, L. A., Amsterdam, E. A., and Mason, D. T.: Relation of Ventricular Arrhythmias in the Late Hospital Phase of Acute Myocardial Infarction to Sudden Death After Hospital Discharge, *Am. J. Med.*, 59:6, 1975.

4 Lown, B.: Sudden Cardiac Death: The Major Challenge Confronting Contemporary Cardiology, *Am. J. Cardiol.*, 43:313, 1979.

5 Reichenbach, D. D., Moss, N. S., and Meyer, E.: Pathology of the Heart in Sudden Cardiac Death, *Am. J. Cardiol.*, 39:865, 1977.

6 Corday, E., Heng, M. K., Meerbaum, S., Lang, T., Farcot, J., Osher, J., and Hashimoto, K.: Derangements of Myocardial Metabolism Preceding Onset of Ventricular Fibrillation After Coronary Occlusion, *Am. J. Cardiol.*, 39:880, 1977.

7 Lown, B., Verrier, R. L., and Rabinowitz, S. H.: Neural and Psychologic Mechanisms and the Problem of Sudden Cardiac Death, *Am. J. Cardiol.*, 39:890, 1977.

8 Vismara, L. A., Vera, Z., Foerster, J. M., Amsterdam, E. A., and Mason, D. T.: Identification of Sudden Death Risk Factors in Acute and Chronic Coronary Artery Disease, *Am. J. Cardiol.*, 39:821, 1977.

9 Vismara, L. A., Pratt, C., Price, J. E., Miller, R. R., Amsterdam, E. A., and Mason, D. T.: Correlation of the Standard Electrocardiogram and Continuous Ambulatory Monitoring in the Detection of Ventricular Arrhythmias in Coronary Patients, *J. Elect.*, 10:299, 1977.

10 Vismara, L. A., DeMaria, A. N., Hughes, J. L., Mason, D. T., and Amsterdam, E. A.: Evaluation of Arrhythmias in the Late Hospital Phase of Acute Myocardial Infarction Compared to Coronary Care Unit Ectopy, *Br. Heart J.*, 37:598, 1975.

11 Moss, A. J., DeCamilla, J., and Davis, H.: Cardiac Death in the First 6 Months After Myocardial Infarction: Potential for Mortality Reduction in the Early Posthospital Period, *Am. J. Cardiol.*, 39:816, 1977.

12 Bruce, R. A., DeRouen, T., Peterson, D. R., Irving, J. B., Chinn, N., Blake, B., and Hofer, V.: Noninvasive Predictors of Sudden Cardiac Death in Men with Coronary Heart Disease: Predictive Value of Maximal Stress Testing, *Am. J. Cardiol.*, 39:833, 1977.

13 Ritchie, J. L., Hamilton, G. W., Trobaugh, G. B., Weaver, W. D., Williams, D. L., and Cobb, L. A.: Myocardial Imaging and Radionuclide Angiography in Sur-

vivors of Sudden Cardiac Death Due to Ventricular Fibrillation, *Am. J. Cardiol.*, 39:852, 1977.

14 Irving, J. B., and Bruce, R. A.: Exertional Hypotension and Postexertional Ventricular Fibrillation in Stress Testing, *Am. J. Cardiol.*, 39:849, 1977.

15 Irving, J. B., Bruce, R. A., and DeRouen, T. A.: Variations in and Significance of Systolic Pressure During Maximal Exercise (Treadmill) Testing: Relation to Severity of Coronary Artery Disease and Cardiac Mortality, *Am. J. Cardiol.*, 39:841, 1977.

16 Vismara, L. A., Mason, D. T., and Amsterdam, E. A.: Disopyramide Phosphate: Clinical Efficacy of a New Oral Antiarrhythmic Agent, *Clin. Pharmacol. Ther.*, 16:330, 1974.

17 Lown, B., and Graboys, T. B.: Management of Patients with Malignant Ventricular Arrhythmias, *Am. J. Cardiol.*, 39:910, 1977.

18 Sherry, S.: Sulfinpyrazone in the Prevention of Cardiac Sudden Death After Myocardial Infarction, *N. Engl. J. Med.*, 298:289, 1978.

19 Multicentre International Study: Improvement in Prognosis of Myocardial Infarction by Long-term Beta-adrenoreceptor Blockade Using Practolol, *Br. Med. J.*, 3:735, 1975.

20 Lurie, A. J., Salel, A. F., Berman, D. S., DeNardo, G. L., Hurley, E. J., and Mason, D. T.: Determination of Improved Myocardial Perfusion After Aortocoronary Bypass Surgery by Exercise Rubidium-81 Scintigraphy, *Circulation*, 54 (suppl. 3):20, 1976.

21 Mason, D. T., Miller, R. R., Amsterdam, E. A., DeMaria, A. N., and Vismara, L. A.: The Role of Elective Aortocoronary Bypass Surgery: Effects on Symptomatology and Longevity in Chronic Ischemic Heart Disease, in D. T. Mason (ed.), "Advances in Heart Disease," Vol. 1, Grune & Stratton, Inc., New York, 1977, p. 269.

22 Hurst, J. W., King, S. B., III, Logue, R. B., Hatcher, C. R., Jr., Jones, E. L., Craver, J. M., Douglas, J. S., Jr., Franch, R. H., Dorney, E. R., Cobbs, B. W., Jr., Robinson, P. H., Clements, S. D., Jr., Kaplan, J. A., and Bradford, J. M.: Value of Coronary Bypass Surgery, *Am. J. Cardiol.*, 42:308, 1978.

23 Lee, G., Kaku, R. F., Amsterdam, E. A., Harris, F. J., Mason, D. T., and DeMaria, A. N.: Greater Relief of Myocardial Ischemia in Coronary Patients by Aortocoronary Bypass Surgery Compared to Modern Medical Antianginal Therapy: Documentation by Exercise Stress Testing and Myocardial Oxygen Needs, *Am. J. Cardiol.*, 43:383, 1979.

24 Cohn, L. H., Boyden, C. M., and Collins, J. J.: Improved Long-term Survival After Aortocoronary Bypass for Advanced Coronary Artery Disease, *Am. J. Surg.*, 129:380, 1975.

25 Reul, G. J., Jr., Cooley, D. A., Wukasch, D. C., Kyger, E. R., III, Sandiford, F. M., Hallman, G. L., and Norman, J. C.: Long-term Survival Following Coronary Artery Bypass. Analysis of 4,522 Consecutive Patients, *Arch. Surg.*, 110:1419, 1975.

26 Farinha, J.B., Kaplan, M. A., Harris, C. N., Dunne, E. F., Carlish, R. A., Kay, J. H., and Brooks, S.: Disease of the Left Main Coronary Artery: Surgical Treatment and Long-term Follow-up in 267 Patients, *Am. J. Cardiol.*, 42:124, 1978.

27 Gunnar, R.: Improved Survival Following Surgical Therapy in Patients with Chronic Angina Pectoris. A Single Hospital's Experience in a Randomized Trial. Presented at the Annual Meeting of the Association of University Cardiologists, Phoenix, Arizona, January 19, 1978.

28 Johnson, W. D., and Shore, R. T.: Coronary Artery Bypass Surgery—Early and Long-term Results, in J. I. Haft and C. P. Bailey (eds.), "Advances in Management of Clinical Heart Disease," Futura Publishing Co., Mount Kisco, N. Y., 1978, p. 265.

29 Lawrie, G. M., Morris, G. C., Jr., Howell, J. F., Tredici, T. D., and Chapman, D. W.: Improved Survival After 5 Years in 1,144 Patients After Coronary Bypass Surgery, *Am. J. Cardiol.*, 42:709, 1978.

30 Mason, D. T., and Vismara, L. A.: Reduction of Sudden Death by Aortocoronary Bypass Surgery, *Am. J. Cardiol.*, 41:795, 1978.

31 Sheldon, W. C.: Effect of Bypass Graft Surgery on Survival. A 6- to 10-year Follow-up Study of 741 Patients, *Cleve. Clin. Q.*, 45:166, 1978.

32 Collins, J. J., Jr., Cohn, L. H., Koster, J. K., Jr., and Mee, R. B. B.: The Influence of Coronary Bypass Surgery on Longevity in Patients with Angina Pectoris, in D. T. Mason (ed.), "Advances in Heart Disease," Vol. 3, Grune & Stratton, Inc., New York, in press.

33 Wynne, J., Cohn, L. H., Collins, J. J., Jr., and Cohn, P. F.: Myocardial Revascularization in Patients with Multivessel Coronary Artery Disease and Minimal Angina Pectoris, *Circulation*, 58 (suppl. 1):92, 1978.

34 Miller, R. R., DeMaria, A. N., Vismara, L. A., Salel, A. F., Maxwell, K. S., Amsterdam, E. A., and Mason, D. T.: Chronic Stable Inferior Myocardial Infarction: Unsuspected Harbinger of High-Risk Proximals Left Coronary Arterial Obstruction Amenable to Surgical Revascularization, *Am. J. Cardiol.*, 39:954, 1977.

35 Han, J.: Mechanism of Ventricular Arrhythmias Associated with Myocardial Infarction, *Am. J. Cardiol.*, 24:800, 1969.

36 Ecker, R. R., Mullins, C. B., and Grammer, J. C.: Control of Intractable Ventricular Tachycardia by Coronary Revascularization, *Circulation*, 44:666, 1971.

37 Amsterdam, E. A., Miller, R. R., Hughes, J. L., Bogren, H., Hurley, E., and Mason, D. T.: Emergency Surgical Therapy of Complicated Acute Myocardial Infarction: Indications and Results in Cardiogenic Shock, Intractable Ventricular Tachycardia and Extending Infarction, in H. I. Russek (ed.), "Cardiovascular Problems: Perspective and Progress," University Park Press, Baltimore, 1976, p. 445.

38 Tabry, I. F., Geha, A. S., Hammond, G. L., and Baue, A. E.: Effect of Surgery on Ventricular Tachyarrhythmias Associated with Coronary Arterial Occlusive Disease, *Circulation*, 58 (suppl. 1):166, 1978.

39 Vismara, L. A., Miller, R. R., Price, J. E., Karem, R., DeMaria, A. N., and Mason, D. T.: Improved Longevity Due to Reduction of Sudden Death by Aortocoronary Bypass in Coronary Atherosclerosis: Prospective Evaluation of Medical Versus Surgical Therapy in Matched Patients with Multivessel Disease, *Am. J. Cardiol.*, 39:919, 1977.

40 Oberman, A., Jones, W. B., and Riley, C. P.: Natural History of Coronary Artery Disease, *Bull. N.Y. Acad. Med.*, 48:1109, 1972.

41 Bruschke, A. V. G., Proudfit, W. L., and Sones, F. M., Jr.: Progress Study of 590 Consecutive Nonsurgical Cases of Coronary Disease Followed 5-9 Years, *Circulation*, 47:1147, 1973.

42 Reeves, T. J., Oberman, A., and Jones, W. B.: Natural History of Angina Pectoris, *Am. J. Cardiol.*, 33:423, 1974.

43 Hammermeister, K. E., DeRouen, T. A., Murray, J. A., and Dodge, H. T.: Effect of Aortocoronary Saphenous Vein Bypass Grafting on Death and Sudden Death: Comparison of Nonrandomized Medically and Surgically Treated Cohorts with Comparable Coronary Disease and Left Ventricular Function, *Am. J. Cardiol.*, 39:925, 1977.

44 Favaloro, R. G.: Direct Myocardial Revascularization: A Ten-Year Journey, *Am. J. Cardiol.*, 43:109, 1979.

45 Greene, D. G.: Long-term Survival After Coronary Bypass Surgery. Buffalo General Hospital, State University of New York (brochure for exhibit at American Medical Association meeting, St. Louis, 1978).

46 Price, J. E., Vismara, L. A., Amsterdam, E. A., DeMaria, A. N., and Mason, D. T.: Evaluation of Ventricular Arrhythmias Post-coronary Bypass Surgery: Decreased Prevalence Following Hospital Discharge Determined by Ambulatory ECG Monitoring, *Am. J. Cardiol.*, 39:269, 1977.

47 Pratt, C. M., Price, J. E., Vismara, L. A., Amsterdam, E. A., DeMaria, A. N., and Mason, D. T.: Importance of Myocardial Segmental Dyssynergy as a Determinant of Ventricular Arrhythmias Post-aortocoronary Bypass, *Clin. Res.*, 25:245, 1977.

We gratefully acknowledge the technical assistance of Robert Kleckner and Leslie Silvernail.

Chapter 13

The Prolongation of Life by Coronary Bypass Surgery– The Emory University Hospital Experience*

J. WILLIS HURST, M.D., and SPENCER B. KING III, M.D.

INTRODUCTION

Several years ago, it became evident that properly performed coronary bypass surgery would increase coronary blood flow in patients with fixed obstruction of the proximal coronary arteries resulting from atherosclerosis (see Chap. 3). It also became increasingly obvious that coronary bypass surgery would relieve angina pectoris in 90 percent of patients. Complete relief could be expected in 60 to 70 percent of patients (see Chap. 7). At that point in history, the patient had to be virtually disabled from angina pectoris despite every type of medication before he or she was considered for coronary bypass surgery.

The overall operative mortality then decreased from 5 percent to 1 percent as surgeons, anesthesiologists, pump technicians, intensive care nurses, and medical cardiologists refined their techniques and procedures. When this occurred the definition of unacceptable stable angina pectoris changed. Unacceptable stable angina pectoris was redefined as discomfort that interfered with the desired life-style of the patient despite the use of propranolol (Inderal) in a dosage that achieved a heart rate of 50 to 60 beats per minute and isosorbide dinitrate (Isordil) in a dosage that was a little less than the amount that produces a headache. The problem of unstable angina pectoris was not considered a few years ago because the physician treating the patient would "wait for collaterals" to develop and would take time to try every medication that was available. As time passed, often more than 60 days, some of the patients shifted to stable angina pectoris or had no angina. It then became apparent that a considerable number of patients with unstable angina continued to have difficulty and had to have surgery because of unacceptable angina pectoris. (This was later

*From the Emory University School of Medicine, Atlanta.

proven to occur in one-third of the patients with unstable angina reported by the National Institutes of Health).[1] Then, too, it became evident that patients with unstable angina were at greater risk of infarction and sudden death than were patients who had stable angina pectoris.[2] Accordingly, unstable angina pectoris is now considered to be unacceptable angina pectoris because its consequences are so grave.

Physicians began to wonder if a procedure that relieved one type of ischemic event—angina pectoris—by increasing coronary blood flow might not prevent other ischemic events such as sudden death and myocardial infarction with its associated shock or heart failure (see Chap. 3). Patients began to ask whether the procedure would prolong life or prevent a heart attack in addition to relieving angina pectoris. Common sense dictated that it was reasonable to assume that a procedure that would increase coronary blood flow in patients with obstructive coronary disease might prolong life. Such thinking was an acceptable extension of the concepts laid down by our predecessors, who taught us that the clinical problems related to obstructive coronary disease result from a decrease in coronary blood flow.[3] Although the logic seems sound, it was necessary to obtain new scientific data to clarify the debate that was developing in this area. The first scientific evidence that bypass surgery might prolong the life of certain patients was presented by the Veterans Administration and resulted from their study of stable angina caused by obstruction of the left main coronary artery. This was known in 1974 and appeared in print in 1976.[4]

The data used by our group to support the view that bypass surgery prolongs the life of certain subsets of patients with obstructive coronary disease when the operative risk of 0.5 to 2 percent were provided by the Veterans Administration, from many medical centers, and our own institution. These data are presented in the discussion that follows.

RÉCENT SCIENTIFIC DATA

Data Provided by the Veterans Administration Which Indicate That Life Is Prolonged by Bypass Surgery

The results of *prospective randomized* studies performed by the Veterans Administration hospitals indicate that certain subsets of patients with obstructive coronary disease live longer when they have coronary bypass surgery. Three aspects of these studies will be presented here.

1 The results of the 3-year follow-up of patients with stable angina pectoris who had obstruction of the left main coronary artery were published in 1976.[4] The results were conclusive (Fig. 13-1). The patients who were randomized to the surgical treatment group had a 3-year cumulative survival rate of about 85 percent. The patients who were randomized to the medical treatment group had a 3-year cumulative survival rate of about 60 percent. As will be discussed later, the initial operative mortality is much

lower now than it was then, and the survival curve for this subset of patients who have surgery is even better now than it was then.

2 The results of the 36-month follow-up of patients with stable angina pectoris (excluding obstruction of the left main coronary artery) were published in September 1977.[5] The study purported to show no difference in survival between those patients who were treated medically and those who were treated surgically. The results of the study were immediately misinterpreted by many newspaper reports and many physicians. Many observers indicated that the operative mortality of 5.6 percent, the graft patency rate of 69 percent, the high perioperative infarction rate, and the failure to accomplsh complete revascularization in the surgical group does not reflect the surgical situation as it exists today. The fact that the group of patients with left main coronary artery obstruction were excluded from the study group was often lost sight of by many casual readers. The fact that the Veterans Administration recommended surgery for patients with unacceptable angina pectoris was missed in the newspaper reporting, which often displayed the headline—*coronary bypass surgery of no value*. Despite the operative mortality of 5.6 percent, the study indicated that patients

LEFT MAIN CORONARY ARTERY OBSTRUCTION (CUMULATIVE) VA RANDOMIZED STUDY

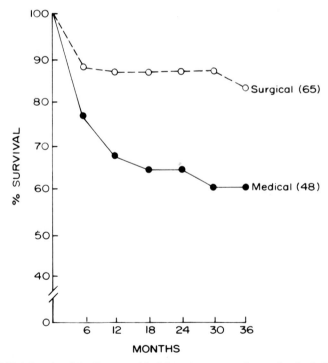

FIGURE 13-1 Results of the Veterans Administration prospective randomized clinical trial of patients with obstruction of the left main coronary artery. (*Reproduced from T. Takaro et al., The VA Cooperative Randomized Study of Surgery for Coronary Arterial Occlusive Disease. II. Subgroup with Significant Left Main Lesions, Circulation, 54 (suppl. 3):107-117, 1976, the American Heart Association, Inc.*)

with triple-vessel obstruction and poor left ventricular function who had been randomized to surgery were surviving longer than those who were randomized to medical therapy. The crossover of survival curves took place at about 36 months. Later, Read published the 54-month follow-up of the same patients, which showed a more definite shift toward improved survival rates for the surgical group (Fig. 13-2).[6] Still later, Hultgren stated, "In patients with three-vessel disease and poor left ventricular function, four-year follow-up data suggest a possible favorable effect of surgery."[7]

3 The Hines Veterans Administration Hospital contributed 20 percent of the total patients with stable angina pectoris (excluding left main coronary obstruction) who were reported by Murphy et al. in September 1977. The results of the patients studied at the Hines Veterans Administration Hospital differed from the results of the larger study of which the Hines patients were a part. The 5-year cumulative survival rate of patients with stable angina pectoris (excluding those with left main coronary artery obstruction) who had bypass surgery at the Hines Veterans Administration Hospital was about 90 percent, as compared to the cumulative survival rate of about 70 percent for the medically treated group. The experience at the Hines Veterans Administration Hospital is presented in Chap. 17 of this book.

Data from Other Medical Centers

The data from other medical centers, for the most part, are derived from *nonrandomized studies*.[8] Theoretically, prospective randomized studies should reveal the best data regarding the value of coronary bypass surgery. Unfortunately, coronary atherosclerotic heart disease is so complex that there can be no appropriate guarantees that the patients are properly matched or that similar treatment is offered to each patient in the study groups. The pitfalls of each of the study methods is discussed by Proudfit in Chap. 2 of this book. Those who discard all the data derived from nonrandomized studies are probably wrong. If such critics demand a prospective randomized study for all medical and surgical therapy, then we must discontinue using a great deal of treatment that has gradually earned its proper place in modern medicine. We do not believe that certain nonrandomized studies should be discarded. We emphasize again, as we have emphasized repeatedly, that there are no perfect studies on the subject. The report of each study can be faulted, but each report teaches us something useful.

The famous Bruschke curves reveal the best data we have on the natural history of coronary atherosclerotic heart disease.[9] Sones "discovered" coronary arteriography in 1958 (see Chap. 1). Accordingly, it followed that the workers at the Cleveland Clinic were able to study patients earlier than was possible elsewhere. They began their study of the natural history

of the illness at a time when the profession used nitroglycerin for angina pectoris but offered little else except for ineffective long-acting nitrites, advice regarding life-style and activity, and better coronary care in hospitalized patients. Later, propranolol was probably used in some patients. The workers at the Cleveland Clinic deserve the credit for performing coronary arteriograms on a large number of patients and, having proven they had obstructive coronary disease, obtaining follow-up data on them for 10 years.[9] They wisely separated their patients into those with left main coronary obstruction, those with triple-vessel obstruction, those with double-vessel obstruction, and those with single-vessel obstruction (Fig. 13-3). They showed that the patients who had left main obstruction or triple-vessel obstruction had a poor cumulative survival rate at 5 years and at 10 years (Fig. 13-3). Patients with double-vessel disease fared better, and patients with single-vessel disease had the best 5- and 10-year survival curves (Fig. 13-3). They led the way to the creation of subsets based on symptoms and coronary arteriographic data. The workers at the Cleveland Clinic and others recognized that the contractility of the left ventricle noted at the time of the arteriogram and left ventriculogram also determined the prognosis of the patient. Now it would appear that it is important to use the contractility of the left ventricle, the extent and degree of coronary artery obstruction, and the symptoms and age of the patient to estimate the prognosis of an individual patient who has coronary atherosclerotic heart disease. The workers at the Cleveland Clinic taught us that the prognosis of a patient

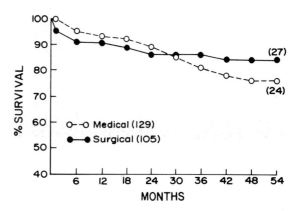

FIGURE 13-2 Survival curves of 129 medically and 105 surgically treated patients with triple-vessel obstruction who had an abnormal left ventricle (from the Veterans Administration prospective randomized study of patients with chronic stable angina pectoris). *(Reproduced from R. C. Read et al., Survival of Men Treated for Chronic Stable Angina Pectoris: A Cooperative Randomized Study, J. Thorac. Cardiovasc. Surg. 75:1-16, 1978, with permission of the authors and the Journal of Thoracic and Cardiovascular Surgery.)*

MEDICAL TREATMENT

CANDIDATES FOR PARTIAL
OR COMPLETE REVASCULARIZATION

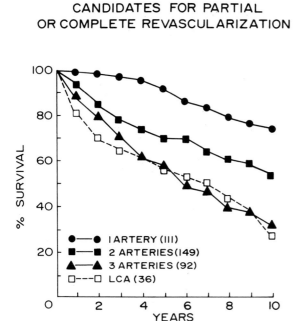

FIGURE 13-3 Survival curves of medically treated candidates for partial or complete revascularization (see text). LCA, left main coronary artery. *(Reprinted from A. V. Bruschke, Ten Year Follow-up of 601 Nonsurgical Cases of Angiographically Documented Coronary Disease. Angiographic Correlation, Syllabus—the First Decade of Bypass Graft Surgery for Coronary Artery Disease (International symposium, Cleveland Clinic Foundation, September 15-17, 1977), with permission of the authors and the Cleveland Clinic.)*

cannot be accurately determined by the symptoms expressed by the patient.[10] They also taught us that a diagnosis, based on symptoms, is commonly wrong. Our own work confirms their observations.[11] Later, the workers at the Cleveland Clinic showed that bypass surgery improved the survival of patients in comparison to the survival of similar patients treated medically[12] (see Chap. 20). The similarity of the two groups was determined by coronary arteriography and ventriculography. Some observers fault these studies because the results of the surgical group are compared to a medical group that was treated at an earlier time (presumably before propranolol was used routinely for angina pectoris). The claim is then made that medical therapy has gradually improved and that it has improved the survival of patients treated medically. The implication is that the improvement in survival claimed for bypass surgery would not be apparent today because medical management has improved. Although this is a valid criticism, it should not be accepted with-

out carefully looking at the available data. First, surgical treatment has also improved during the last 2 years. Second, it is not possible to prove that modern medical therapy has improved the survival curves of patients with left main obstruction, and the difference in survival curves for patients with triple-vessel and double-vessel disease treated recently as compared to similar patients treated at an earlier time is not great.[8] The following discussion deals with this subject.

The survival curves for patients treated medically followed at an earlier time and reported by the Cleveland Clinic can be compared to the survival curves of patients treated during a more recent period and reported by the Veterans Administration,[4,6] and both of these can be compared to the survival of similar patients treated surgically and reported by the Cleveland Clinic.[12] One should keep in mind that it is not possible to determine the exact medical management of individual patients who are reported in study groups, and remember, too, that surgery is better at the Cleveland Clinic now (as it is in many centers) than it was when the 5-year follow-up studies were reported.

Figure 13-4 shows a cumulative survival curve of 61 percent of the Veterans Administration's medically treated group of patients with *left main coronary artery obstruction.*[4] The follow-up period was 3 years. The 3-year cumulative survival curve for the medically treated patients reported by the Cleveland Clinic was about 63 percent.[9] The difference in survival between the Veterans Administration's medically treated group and the medically treated group reported by the Cleve-

LEFT MAIN DISEASE

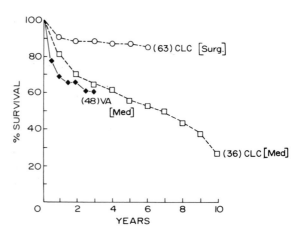

FIGURE 13-4 Survival curve of patients with obstruction of the left main coronary artery treated with coronary bypass surgery (Surg.) at the Cleveland Clinic (CLC) (upper curve)[12] and treated medically (Med.) at the Cleveland Clinic (middle curve)[9] or by the Veterans Administration (VA) groups (lower curve).[4]

land Clinic is not significant. Although it is not possible to determine what medications each individual received in the study groups, it is highly likely that the Cleveland Clinic group of patients received less propranolol than did the Veterans' group, since the Cleveland Clinic study was started at an earlier time. This would suggest that modern medical treatment does not differ from other medical treatment in improving the survival curves for patients with left main coronary artery obstruction. Figure 13-4 also shows that patients with left main obstruction who had bypass surgery at the Cleveland Clinic had a cumulative survival rate of about 86 percent at 6 years,[12] as compared to a 6-year cumulative survival rate of 52 percent for the medically treated patients reported by the Cleveland Clinic.[9]

Figure 13-5 shows a cumulative survival rate of about 75 percent (at 4 years) for the Veterans Administration's medically treated group of patients with *triple-vessel coronary obstruction*.[6] The 4-year survival rate for patients treated medically and reported by the Cleveland Clinic was 63 percent.[9] The difference (12 percent) between the two medically treated groups may reflect an improvement in medical management (the use of propranolol) that occurred in the Veterans' group as compared to the treatment that was available at the time the Cleveland Clinic study began. On the other hand, the patients in the Veterans' study had

stable angina pectoris, and it is highly likely that some of the patients reported by the Cleveland Clinic had unstable angina pectoris as well as stable angina pectoris. It is disappointing that the difference in survival between the two medically treated groups is not greater. The cumulative survival rate for patients treated surgically at the Cleveland Clinic was about 82 percent at 6 years of follow-up[12] as compared to the cumulative survival rate of about 50 percent for patients treated medically and reported at 6 years by the Cleveland Clinic.[9]

Figure 13-6 shows a cumulative survival rate of about 89 percent (at 4 years) for the Veterans Administration's medically treated group of patients with *double-vessel obstruction*.[6] The cumulative survival rate at 4 years for patients treated medically and reported by the Cleveland Clinic was 76 percent.[9] The difference between the two medically treated groups may reflect an improvement in medical management (the use of propranolol) that occurred in the Veterans' group as compared to the treatment that was available at the time the Cleveland Clinic study began. On the other hand, the patients in the Veterans' study had stable angina pectoris, and it is highly likely that some of the patients reported by the Cleveland Clinic had unstable angina pectoris as well as stable angina pectoris. Again, it is disappointing that the difference in survival between the two medically treated groups is

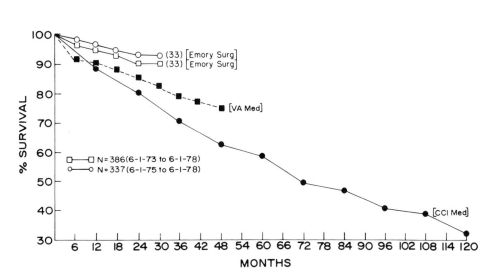

TRIPLE VESSEL DISEASE

FIGURE 13-5 Survival curves of patients with triple-vessel obstruction who were treated medically at the Cleveland Clinic (CCl Med)[9] (lower curve) and by the Veterans Administration group[6] (VA Med) (black squares) and treated with coronary bypass surgery (Surg) at Emory University Hospital from June 1, 1973 to June 1, 1978 (open squares) and from June 1, 1978 (open circles). *N* = number of patients.

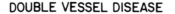

DOUBLE VESSEL DISEASE

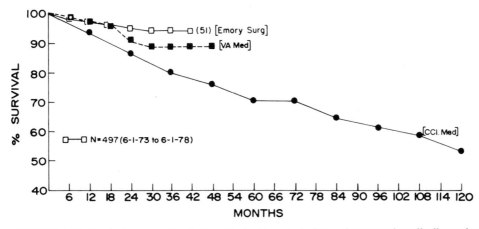

FIGURE 13-6 Survival curves of patients with double-vessel obstruction treated medically at the Cleveland Clinic[9] (CCl Med) (lower curve) and by the Veterans Administration group[6] (VA Med) (black squares) and treated with bypass surgery (Surg) at Emory University Hospital between June 1, 1973 and June 1, 1978 (open squares). *N* = number of patients.

not greater. The cumulative survival rate for patients treated surgically at the Cleveland Clinic was about 83 percent at 6 years of follow-up[12] as compared to the cumulative survival rate of about 70 percent for the patients treated medically and reported by the Cleveland Clinic.[9]

Figure 13-7 shows a cumulative survival curve of about 97 percent (at 4 years) for the Veterans Administration's group of medically treated patients with *single-vessel obstruction.*[6] The cumulative survival rate for patients treated medically and reported by the Cleveland Clinic after 4 years of follow-up was about 95 percent.[9] There is no significant difference between the two groups. This implies that the survival curves of patients with single-vessel disease has not been changed with modern medical management. This occurs because patients with single-vessel disease do well, as far as survival is concerned, regardless of

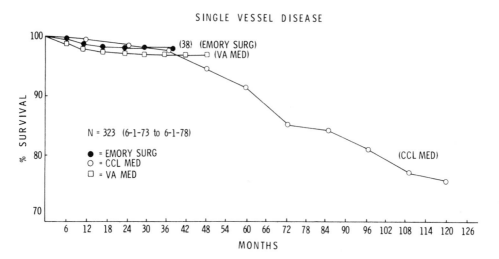

FIGURE 13-7 Survival curves of patients with single-vessel obstruction treated medically at the Cleveland Clinic[9] (CCl Med) (lower curve) and by the Veterans Administration group (VA Med) (open squares), and treated with bypass surgery (Emory surgery) (black circles) at Emory University Hospital from June 1, 1973 to June 1, 1978. *N* = number of patients.

treatment. The cumulative survival rate for patients treated surgically at the Cleveland Clinic was about 90 percent at 6 years of follow-up[12] as compared to the cumulative survival rate of about 83 percent for patients treated medically and reported by the Cleveland Clinic.[9]

Kouchoukos et al. reported findings similar to those discussed above.[13] Kouchoukos divided his patients into three groups: those with triple-, double-, and single-vessel disease who were operated on, those who were operable but were not operated on, and those who were inoperable. The patients were not randomized but were studied during the same time frame. The patients with triple-vessel and double-vessel disease had survival curves that were superior to those patients who were operable but were not operated on (Figs. 13-8 and 13-9). The patients who were inoperable had the poorest survival curves. The manner in which the three survival curves split apart for triple-vessel disease and double-vessel disease is, we believe, important.

Several groups of investigators have compared the survival rates of their operated patients with the survival rates of patients who have been matched for age and sex in the general population. The general population is composed of a mixture of truly well persons, persons who have disease and do not know it (including persons who may have an accident), and sick persons. The patients in the study groups have known coronary atherosclerotic heart disease. The work of Kirklin,[14] Greene,[15] Lawrie,[16] and Austen[17] persuade us to point out that with modern surgery (operative risk of about 1 percent), one can predict that the 5-year survival rates will be as follows.

When the operative risk is about 1 percent, one can determine that the 5-year cumulative survival rate for patients with left main coronary artery obstruction will be about 87 percent, as compared to the cumulative survival rate of about 94 percent for individuals who are matched for age and sex in the general population. The patients treated medically by the Veterans Administration had a 5-year survival rate of about 63 percent, whereas the survival rate for the individuals matched for age and sex in the general population was about 96 percent.

When the operative risk is about 1 percent, one can determine that the 5-year cumulative survival rate for patients with triple-vessel disease will be about 89 percent as compared to the cumulative survival rate of 95 percent for individuals who are matched for age and sex in the general population. The 5-year survival rate for patients treated medically by the Veterans Administration was about 74 percent, whereas the survival rate for the individuals matched for age and sex in the general population was about 94 percent.

When the operative risk is 1 percent, one can de-

termine that the 5-year cumulative survival rate for patients with double-vessel disease will be about 93 percent, which is the same as that for individuals who are matched for age and sex in the general population. The patients treated medically by the Veterans Administration had a 5-year survival rate of about 87 percent, whereas the survival rate for the individuals matched for age and sex in the general population was about 94 percent.

At this time, it is not possible to show improved survival of surgically treated patients with triple-vessel disease over medically treated patients with single-vessel disease. In fact, the surgically treated group, the medically treated group, and the group of individuals who are matched for age and sex in the general population have similar survival curves. The 5-year cumulative survival rate for each group is about 94 to 96 percent.

Vismara et al. found that sudden death occurred in 23 of 96 patients treated medically and in 7 of 121 patients treated surgically[18] (Fig. 13-10). The patients

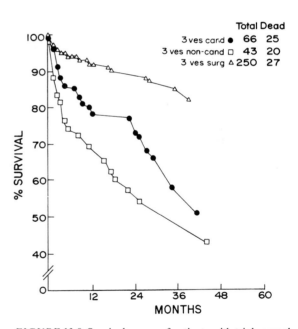

FIGURE 13-8 .Survival curves of patients with triple-vessel obstruction who were treated and followed up at the University of Alabama. The upper curve shows the survival curve of the patients who had bypass surgery (surg). The middle curve shows the survival curve of the patients who could have been operated on but were not (3 ves cand). The lower curve shows the survival curve for the patients who could not be operated on (non-cand). *(Reproduced from N. T. Kouchoukos et al., Results of Surgery for Disabling Angina Pectoris, in A. N. Brest and S. H. Rahimtoola (eds.), "Cardiovascular Clinics (Coronary Bypass Surgery)," F. A. Davis Company, Philadelphia, 1977, with permission of the authors and publisher.)*

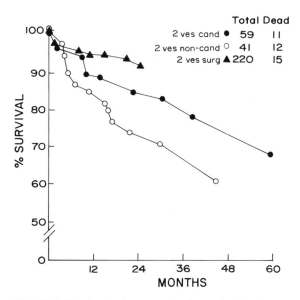

FIGURE 13-9 Survival curves of patients with double-vessel obstruction who were treated and followed up at the University of Alabama. Upper curve, patients who had bypass surgery (surg); middle curve, patients who could have been operated on but were not (2 ves cand); lower curve, patients who could not be operated on (2 ves non-cand). *(Reproduced from N. T. Kouchoukos et al., Results of Surgery for Disabling Angina Pectoris, in A. N. Brest and S. H. Rahimtoola (eds.), "Cardiovascular Clinics (Coronary Bypass Surgery)," F. A. Davis Company, Philadelphia, 1977, with permission of the authors.)*

had double- and triple-vessel disease and were followed for 39 months. The study was prospective, using angiographically matched patients. Hammermeister et al. found that sudden death rates for subgroups of medically treated patients was 1.8 to 10.9 times higher than the rates in subgroups of surgically treated patients with a comparable extent of coronary disease and ejection fraction.[19]

Data from Emory University Hospital

The survival curves for patients with left main coronary obstruction, triple-vessel disease, double-vessel disease, and single-vessel disease who had coronary bypass surgery at Emory University Hospital have been published previously.[8] A recent update of the results has now become available. The follow-up period is longer now, and our results are, we believe, even more meaningful. Most of the patients who are operated on at Emory University Hospital have unstable angina pectoris. The survival curves of these patients can be compared with the survival curves of patients with stable angina pectoris treated medically

by the Veterans Administration. The fact that many of the Emory University Hospital surgically treated patients had unstable angina pectoris and the Veterans Administration medically treated patients had stable angina pectoris should favor the medically treated group. However, despite this obstacle, the Emory surgically treated group fared much better than the medically treated group reported by the Veterans Administration. The cumulative survival rate at 30 months for the Emory patients who were operated on with left main coronary artery obstruction was about 89 percent, whereas the cumulative survival rate at that time of the patients treated medically by the Veterans Administration was about 61 percent[3] (Fig. 13-11). The cumulative survival rate for patients operated on at Emory during the last 3 years and followed for 24 months is even better (93 percent survival rate). The cumulative survival rate at 30 months for the Emory University Hospital patients who were operated on with triple-vessel disease was about 93 percent, whereas the cumulative survival rate at the same time for the patients treated medically by the Veterans Administration was about 83 percent[6] (Fig. 13-5). The cumulative survival rate at 42 months for the Emory patients who were operated on with double-vessel disease was about 94.5 percent, whereas the cumulative survival rate at the same time for the patients treated medically by the Veterans Administration was about 89 percent[6] (Fig. 13-6). The cumulative survival rate at 36 months for Emory patients who were operated

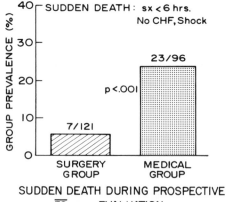
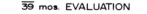

FIGURE 13-10 Prevalence of sudden death in patients with double- and triple-vessel obstruction. CHF, congestive heart failure; *p*, probability; sx, symptoms. *(Reproduced from L. A. Vismara et al., Improved Longevity Due to Reduction of Sudden Death by Aortocoronary Bypass in Coronary Atherosclerosis. Prospective Evaluation of Medical Versus Surgical Therapy in Matched Patients with Multi-vessel Disease, Am. J. Cardiol., 39:919-924, 1977, with permission.)*

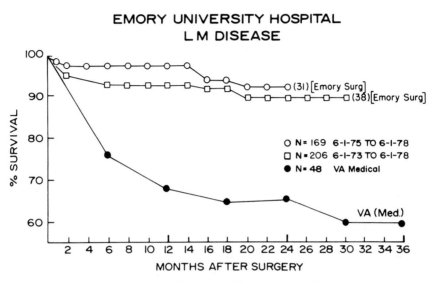

FIGURE 13-11 Survival curves of patients with obstruction of the left main coronary artery treated medically (Med.) by the Veterans Administration (VA) groups (lower curve)[4] and treated with bypass surgery (Surg.) at Emory University Hospital between June 1, 1973 and June 1, 1978 (middle curve) and between June 1, 1975 and June 1, 1978 (upper curve). *N* = number of patients.

on with single-vessel disease was about 98 percent, whereas the cumulative survival rate at the same time for the patients treated medically by the Veterans Administration was about 97 percent.[6] The cumulative survival rate of patients treated medically and reported by the Cleveland Clinic was about 98 percent at 36 months' follow-up. (Fig. 13-7). There is no difference in survival of patients with single-vessel disease treated medically by the Veterans Administration, in those treated medically and reported by the Cleveland Clinic, and in those treated surgically. It may be, however, that the period of follow-up is not long enough to detect a difference. It could be that 5 to 7 years of follow-up may be needed for the survival curves to separate.

These data support the view that coronary bypass surgery at Emory Hospital improves the survival rate of patients who have left main coronary artery obstruction, triple-vessel obstruction, and double-vessel obstruction when compared to similar patients treated medically in the Veterans Administration.

INDICATIONS FOR CORONARY BYPASS SURGERY

The current average operative risk for patients operated on at Emory University Hospital is about 1 percent.[8] Certain subsets of patients have an operative risk of 2 to 3 percent, and other subsets have an operative risk of 0 to 0.5 percent. The perioperative infarction rate at Emory is 4 to 6 percent, and 90 percent

of the grafts are patent at 1 year following surgery.[8] These results have led us to recommend the following indications for coronary bypass surgery. Please note that the indications are determined by considering age, symptoms, location of obstructive lesions, and ejection fraction. Coronary bypass surgery is recommended* for the following[10,18]:

Patients who have stable angina pectoris that interferes with their desired life-style. (This indication will be especially applicable to patients under 65 years of age.)

Young patients with minimal angina pectoris who have left main coronary artery obstruction, triple-vessel obstruction, double-vessel obstruction, or obstruction of the proximal portion of the left anterior descending artery.

Patients who have unstable angina pectoris or episodes of prolonged myocardial ischemia without objective signs of infarction. (This indication will be especially applicable to patients under 65 years of age.)

Patients 65 to 70 years of age or older who have unacceptable angina pectoris despite modern medical therapy. Under these circumstances, patients with left main coronary obstruction, triple-vessel obstruction, double-vessel obstruction, or single-vessel obstruction (especially if the left anterior descending artery is obstructed) may be candidates for surgery. When mild symptoms are present in this age group and the condition is stable, surgery may be reserved for those with left main coronary

---

*These recommendations are predicated on the basis that the surgical team has demonstrated an overall operative mortality of about 1 percent. The indications are reproduced with some modification by permission of J. Willis Hurst, M.D., and the publisher of *Primary Cardiology*.[20]

artery obstruction, triple-vessel obstruction, and double-vessel obstruction when one of the vessels is the left anterior descending artery.

Patients with myocardial infarction who continue to have repeated episodes of myocardial ischemia despite medical management.

Patients with Prinzmetal's angina, when the coronary arteriogram shows the syndrome is caused by persistent obstruction of the coronary arteries.

Patients without symptoms who undergo coronary arteriography because of a very positive exercise ECG and whose arteriograms show high-grade obstruction in the left main coronary artery or triple- or double-vessel obstruction (especially when one of the obstructed vessels is the left anterior descending artery). This indication is especially applicable to patients under 65 years of age.

Patients with compelling coronary anatomy who are candidates for aortic or mitral valve surgery.

REFERENCES

1 Hutter, A. M., Jr., Russell, R. O., Jr., Resnekov, L., et al.: Unstable Angina Pectoris. National Randomized Study of Surgical vs. Medical Therapy: Results in 1, 2, and 3 Vessel Disease, *Circulation,* 55, 56 (suppl. 3):60, 1977.

2 Plotnick, G. D., and Conti, C. R.: Unstable Angina: Angiography, Short- and Long-term Morbidity, Mortality and Symptomatic Status of Medically Treated Patients, *Am. J. Med.,* 63:870–873, 1977.

3 Hurst, J. W.: From Harvey to Coronary Bypass Surgery, in J. W. Hurst (ed.), *Update I: The Heart,* McGraw-Hill Book Company, New York, in press.

4 Takaro, T., Hultgren, H. N., Lipton, M. J., et al.: The VA Cooperative Randomized Study of Surgery for Coronary Arterial Occlusive Disease. II. Subgroup with Significant Left Main Lesions, *Circulation,* 54 (suppl. 3): 107–117, 1976.

5 Murphy, M. L., Hultgren, H. N., Detre, K., et al.: Treatment of Chronic Stable Angina: A Preliminary Report of Survival Data of the Randomized Veterans Administration Cooperative Study, *N. Engl. J. Med.,* 297:621–627, 1977.

6 Read, R. C., Murphy, M. L., Hultgren, H. N., et al.: Survival of Men Treated for Chronic Stable Angina Pectoris: A Cooperative Randomized Study, *J. Thorac. Cardiovasc. Surg.,* 75:1–16, 1978.

7 Hultgren, H. N., Takaro, T., Detre, K. M., et al.: Evaluation of the Efficacy of Coronary Bypass Surgery—1, *Am. J. Cardiol.,* 42:157, 1978.

8 Hurst, J. W., King, S. B. III, Logue, R. B., et al.: Value of Coronary Bypass Surgery: Controversies in Cardiology: Part I, *Am. J. Cardiol.,* 42:308–329, 1978.

9 Bruschke, A. V.: Ten Year Follow-up of 601 Nonsurgical Cases of Angiographically Documented Coronary Disease. Angiographic Correlations, Syllabus—the First Decade of Bypass Graft Surgery for Coronary Artery Disease. (International symposium, Cleveland Clinic Foundation, September 15-17, 1977.)

10 Proudfit, W. L., Shirey, E. K., and Sones, F. M., Jr.: Selective Cine Coronary Arteriography: Correlation with Clinical Findings in 1,000 Patients, *Circulation,* 33:901, 1966.

11 Douglas, J. S., Jr., and Hurst, J. W.: Limitations of Symptoms in the Recognition of Coronary Atherosclerotic Heart Disease, in J. W. Hurst (ed.), *Update I: The Heart,* McGraw-Hill Book Company, New York, in press.

12 Sheldon, W. C.: Effect of Bypass Graft Surgery on Survival. A Six to 10 Year Follow-up Study of 741 Patients, Syllabus—the First Decade of Bypass Graft Surgery for Coronary Artery Disease. (International symposium, Cleveland Clinic Foundation, September 15-17, 1977.)

13 Kouchoukos, N. T., Oberman, A., and Karp, R. B.: Results of Surgery for Disabling Angina Pectoris, in A. N. Brest and S. H. Rahimtoola (eds.), "Cardiovascular Clinics (Coronary Bypass Surgery)," F. A. Davis Company, Philadelphia, 1977, p. 157.

14 Kirklin, J. W.: Research Related to Surgical Treatment in Coronary Artery Disease. Presented at the 30th Anniversary of the American Heart Association and National Heart, Lung and Blood Institute Scientific Symposium: Current Horizons in Atherosclerosis and Hypertension, Washington, D. C., February 9, 1978.

15 Greene, D. G., Bunnell, I. L., Arani, D. T., et al.: Long-term Survival After Coronary Bypass Surgery. Buffalo General Hospital, State University of New York (brochure for exhibit at American Heart Association Meeting, Miami, 1977).

16 Lawrie, G. M., Morris, G. C., Jr., Howell, J. F., et al.: Improved Survival After 5 Years in 1,144 Patients After Coronary Bypass Surgery, *Am. J. Cardiol.,* 42(5):709–715, 1978.

17 Austen, W. G.: Personal communication, April 1978.

18 Vismara, L. A., Miller, R. R., Price, J. E., et al.: Improved Longevity Due to Reduction of Sudden Death by Aortocoronary Bypass in Coronary Atherosclerosis: Prospective Evaluation of Medical Versus Surgical Therapy in Matched Patients with Multi-vessel Disease, *Am. J. Cardiol.,*39:919–924, 1977.

19 Hammermeister, K. E., DeRouen, T. A., Murray, J. A., et al.: Effect of Aortocoronary Saphenous Vein Bypass Grafting on Death and Sudden Death: Comparison of Nonrandomized Medically and Surgically Treated Cohorts with Comparable Coronary Disease and Left Ventricular Function, *Am. J. Cardiol.,* 39:925–934, 1977.

20 Hurst, J. W.: Coronary Bypass Surgery: The Evolution of a Point of View, *Primary Cardiology,* 5:19, 1979.

Chapter 14

Prolongation of Life After Coronary Artery Bypass Surgery at the University of Alabama Medical Center*

CHARLES E. RACKLEY, M.D.

INTRODUCTION

Coronary artery bypass grafting has become an important form of treatment for coronary artery disease. Earlier reports documented the clinical benefit in terms of relief of ischemic pain in the year following coronary surgery. In addition to the relief of ischemic pain and improvement in life-style, another important consideration has been the prolongation of the patient's life. Several studies have reported increased longevity in selected patients undergoing coronary artery bypass grafting. This review will discuss the reported surgical experience with coronary artery bypass grafting at the University of Alabama Medical Center.

PATIENT SELECTION

Coronary arteriography has been performed at this institution since 1967. Oberman and associates have maintained follow-up at yearly intervals of all patients who have undergone the procedure.[1] Initially, coronary arteriography was performed by the Sones technique, but in recent years the femoral approach of Judkins has been employed for visualization of the coronary arteries. Ventricular function has been evaluated with biplane angiocardiography and determination of ejection fraction.[2] Wall motion abnormalities have also been quantitated by the technique of Field and colleagues with superimposition of diastolic and systolic ventriculograms.[3] In addition to the quantitation of global ventricular function and akinetic ventricular wall motion abnormalities, more recent modifications have permitted segmental analysis of left ventricular wall motion in terms of segmental ejection fraction. The coronary arteriograms have traditionally been reviewed independently by the cardiologists, radiologists, and cardiovascular surgeons.

Since 1970, Kouchoukos and colleagues have also maintained a file on patients undergoing coronary artery bypass grafting.[4] In this manner, patients are followed at yearly intervals after coronary arteriography and/or coronary artery surgery in this institution. The indications for cardiac catheterization, coronary arteriography, and angiocardiography are (1) diagnostic evaluation for the origin of chest pain, (2) documentation of the anatomic extent of coronary artery disease, and (3) assessment of left ventricular function in patients with clinical manifestations of coronary artery disease. Patients are usually referred for refractoriness to medical management of ischemic pain, for progressive or unstable angina, and for the assessment of possible coexisting coronary artery disease in conjunction with recognized valvular heart disease. In recent years, patients less than 60 years of age with a recent myocardial infarction have been studied 3 or more weeks after the acute event.[5] Individually selected patients with positive graded exercise test results also are evaluated for the possibility of underlying coronary artery disease. Finally, patients are often referred to the cardiovascular surgeons from other hospitals in which cardiac catheterization and coronary arteriography have already been performed.

SURGICAL EXPERIENCE IN CORONARY ARTERY BYPASS GRAFTING

Since the first coronary artery bypass procedure performed at the University of Alabama Medical Center in 1970, Drs. Kouchoukos, Oberman, and associates have carefully tabulated statistics on this procedure each year. The 30-day hospital mortality for coronary bypass grafting from 1970 through 1976 is shown in Table 14-1.[6] These statistics include those for bypass grafting alone, as well as the experience with bypass grafting plus excision of scar or aneurysm of the left ventricle. In 1970, the first year of coronary artery bypass grafting, 29 patients underwent the procedure

*From the Division of Cardiology, Department of Medicine, University of Alabama Medical Center, University Station, Birmingham.

and 4 died in the hospital (13.8 percent mortality). The 30-day hospital mortality rapidly declined in the following year in which 134 operations were performed and 2 deaths occurred, resulting in a 1.5 percent hospital mortality. During the last year, 1976, that statistics were tabulated in this series, 739 patients were operated on, with a 1.5 percent mortality. During this 7-year period from 1970 through 1976, 2,300 patients underwent bypass grafting alone; there were 39 deaths, resulting in a 30-day hospital mortality of 1.7 percent. More recent figures of Kirklin and associates in the year 1977 revealed that 757 patients underwent coronary artery bypass grafting with 7 hospital deaths and a 0.9 percent mortality.[7] Kouchoukos has recently compared the 30-day hospital mortality for coronary bypass grafting for the years 1970 through 1973 to the years 1974 to 1977.[8] During the period 1970–1973, 590 patients underwent isolated bypass grafting, with 16 hospital deaths and a mortality of 2.7 percent. For the period 1974–1977, 2,467 patients underwent the procedure, with 30 hospital deaths and a mortality of 1.2 percent.

Also illustrated in Table 14-1 is the gradual increase in number of patients undergoing both coronary bypass grafting and excision of myocardial scar or ventricular aneurysm. During the early years in 1970 and 1971 the mortality was 33.3 percent and 50 percent, respectively. There has been a significant decline in the mortality attending this procedure, and in 1976, 28 patients underwent bypass grafting plus excision of ventricular scar without a hospital death. In Kouchoukos' recent comparison of the periods 1970–1973 and 1974–1977, bypass grafting and excision of scar during the former period was associated with 5 deaths in 30 patients for a 16.7 percent mortality. During the period 1974–1977, 111 patients had the combined procedure of bypass grafting and excision of scar with 3 deaths and a mortality of 2.7 percent.

In addition to the reduction in 30-day hospital mortality of coronary artery bypass grafting, the number of vein grafts per patient has steadily increased from 1970 through 1976. As shown in Figure 14-1, in 1970, the first year of the operation, the mean number of grafts was 1.4 per patient, and by 1976, this had increased to 2.9 grafts per patient. The increased number of grafts per patient was attended by a steady decline in 30-day hospital mortality. As shown in Table 14-2, Kirklin and colleagues have reviewed the number of distal anastomoses in coronary artery bypass grafting for the year 1977.[7] In the total of 757 patients, 36 (5 percent) underwent a single anastomosis, 245 (32 percent) underwent three anastomoses, and 354 (47 percent) underwent a total of four to seven distal anastomoses. The average number of grafts per patient was 3.4, and the hospital mortality 0.9 percent.

With the increased recognition of anatomic coronary artery disease and the reduction in operative mortality, the use of this surgical procedure has increased in both younger and older patients. In Table 14-3 the age range for patients and the hospital mortality are shown for the year 1977 at the University of Alabama Medical Center.[7] Although the majority of the patients were 40 to 70 years old, ages ranged from 20 to 40 years and above 70 years of age. Mortality increased significantly in patients above the age of 70 undergoing coronary artery bypass surgery.

In addition to the increased number of anastomoses per patient undergoing coronary artery bypass grafting, the incidence of perioperative myocardial infarction has steadily declined since 1970. Perioperative infarction is based on electrocardiographic and enzymatic abnormalities during the course of the procedure. Ta-

TABLE 14-1

Thirty-day mortality rates for coronary bypass grafting procedures at the University of Alabama Medical Center, 1970–1976

| Year of operation | Bypass grafting alone | | | Bypass grafting plus excision of scar or aneurysm | | |
| | No. of patients | 30-day mortality | | No. of patients | 30-day mortality | |
		No.	%		No.	%
1970	29	4	13.8	3	1	33.3
1971	134	2	1.5	6	3	50.0
1972	163	5	3.1	6	0	0
1973	264	5	1.9	15	1	6.7
1974	434	5	1.2	17	1	5.9
1975	537	7	1.3	30	1	3.3
1976	739	11	1.5	28	0	0
Totals	2,300	39	1.7	105	7	6.6

TABLE 14-2
Primary coronary artery bypass grafting* UAB, 1977

No. of distal anastomoses	% of total patients	No. of patients			Hospital deaths		
					No.	%	70% CL†
1	5%	36	0.6%‡		—	0 %	0–5.4%
2		122	(CL 0.1–2.1%)		1	0.8%	0.1–2.8%
3	32%	245			1	0.4%	0.1–1.4%
4		214			2	0.9%	0.3–2.2%
5	47%	113	1.4%‡		3	2.7%	1.2–5.3%
6		22	(CL 0.8–2.4%)		—	0 %	0–8.4%
7		5			—	0 %	
Total		757			7	0.9%	0.6–1.4%

*Exclusive of those with concomitant valve surgery, left ventricular resection, or extracardiac vascular surgery.

†CL, 70% confidence limits.

‡p for difference = 0.45

ble 14-4 shows Kouchoukos' analysis of the incidence of definite and probable perioperative infarctions for the years 1970 to 1975 with coronary bypass grafting.[6] In 1972, 10 out of 111 patients (9.0 percent) undergoing the procedure had a definite perioperative infarction. In 1975, 6 of 489 patients being operated on had a definite perioperative infarction for a 1.2 percent incidence. Kouchoukos has examined the frequency of perioperative myocardial infarction from 1970 to 1977. In the period 1970–1973, there were 45 patients with perioperative infarctions in 395 operations, resulting in a 11.4 percent incidence. For 1974–1976, 23 patients exhibited evidence of perioperative myocardial infarction in 987 operations for a 2.3 percent incidence. A variety of modifications during extracorporeal bypass has been evaluated in an effort to preserve myocardium. The current surgical technique of hypothermic cardioplegia arrest has been found superior to hypothermic ischemic arrest. A recent report by McDaniel, Kouchoukos, and colleagues, using the enzymatic assay of CK-MB isoenzyme for evidence of myocardial damage, demonstrated a statistically significant reduction in enzyme release in hypothermic cardioplegia as compared to hypothermic ischemic arrest.[9]

Kouchoukos has recently reviewed the 30-day hospital mortality for coronary artery bypass grafting over the period 1970–1977 and compared the earlier period 1970–1973 to the later period 1974–1977. Surgery for single-vessel coronary disease was examined in 228 patients. During the period 1970–1973, there was 1 death in 61 patients for a 1.6 percent mortality, whereas in the period 1974–1977, 1 death occurred in 167 patients for a 0.6 percent mortality. The overall surgical mortality during this period was 0.9 percent for single-vessel coronary artery disease. There were 807 patients operated with two-vessel coronary artery disease. For the period 1970–1973, there were 3 deaths

in 197 patients, resulting in a 1.5 percent mortality, and this compared to 3 deaths in 610 patients in the period 1974–1977 for a 0.5 percent mortality. Thus the overall surgical mortality for two-vessel coronary disease was 0.7 percent. There were 1,580 patients in the three-vessel coronary artery disease group. For 1970–1973, there were 9 deaths in 250 patients for a 3.6 mortality, which compared to 18 deaths in 1,330 patients for 1.4 percent mortality in the period 1974–1977. The overall mortality for coronary bypass grafting in three-vessel disease was 1.7 percent. Finally, in 442 patients with left main coronary artery disease, in the period 1970–1973, there were 5 deaths in 82 procedures, resulting in a 6.1 percent mortality. This compared to 6 deaths in 360 patients for a 1.7

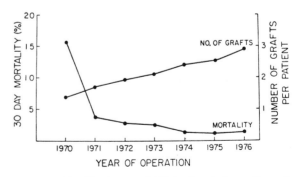

FIGURE 14-1 The decrease in 30-day hospital mortality and the increase in the number of vein grafts per patient for coronary artery bypass surgery at the University of Alabama Medical Center are shown for the years 1970 through 1976. *(Reprinted with permission from N. T. Kouchoukos et al., Coronary Artery Bypass Grafting, in C. E. Rackley and R. O. Russell, Jr. (eds.), "Coronary Artery Disease: Recognition and Management," Futura Publishing Company, Mt. Kisco, N.Y., 1979.)*

TABLE 14-3
Primary coronary artery bypass grafting* UAB, 1977

Age (years)	No. of patients		Hospital deaths		
			No.	%	70% CL†
< 20	—		—		
20 < 30	3		—	0 %	0–47%
30 < 40	26		1	3.8%	0.5–12%
40 < 50	157	0.4%‡	1	0.6%	0.1–2.2%
50 < 60	361	(CL 0.2–0.8%)	1	0.3%	0.04–0.9%
60 < 70	190		0	0 %	0–1.0%
70 < 80	19	20.0%‡	4	21.1%	11.0–35.0%
> 80	1	(CL 10.4–33.4%)	—	0 %	0–86%
Total	757		7	0.9%	

*Exclusive of those with concomitant valve surgery, left ventricular resection, or extracardiac vascular surgery.

†CL, 70% confidence limits.

‡p for difference < 0.0001.

percent mortality in the period 1974–1977. The overall mortality for left main disease was 2.5 percent.

Therefore, the experience of the cardiovascular surgeons at the University of Alabama Medical Center from 1970 to 1977 has demonstrated a decrease in operative mortality for coronary artery bypass grafting, an increased number of vein grafts per patient, and a decreased incidence of perioperative myocardial infarction.

SURVIVAL WITH SINGLE-VESSEL DISEASE

Follow-up studies on patients with single-vessel coronary artery disease at the Cleveland Clinic revealed an average mortality of 2.3 percent per year during the first 4 years.[10] Kouchoukos and colleagues at this in-

TABLE 14-4
Perioperative myocardial infarction associated with coronary bypass grafting procedures, 1970–1975

Year of operation	No. of patients	Perioperative infarction					
		Definite		Probable		Total	
		No.	%	No.	%	No.	%
1970	10	0	—	1	10	1	10
1971	67	5	7.5	4	5.8	9	13
1972	111	10	9.0	4	3.6	14	13
1973	207	15	7.2	6	2.9	21	10
1974	315	6	1.9	4	0.9	9	3
1975	489	6	1.2	2	0.4	8	1.6
Totals	1,199	42	3.5	20	1.7	62	5.2

stitution followed 24 medically treated patients with left anterior descending coronary artery involvement for 54 months, and only a single death occurred, which was noncardiac.[11] All patients in Kouchoukos' study exhibited 75 to 100 percent proximal stenotic lesions in the left anterior descending coronary with normal or minimally impaired left ventricular function.

The 5-year follow-up experience in patients undergoing coronary artery bypass surgery for single-vessel disease has been examined by Kirklin and colleagues and is shown in Fig. 14-2. Surgical survival statistics for 182 patients are compared to the curve of a matched population taken as a whole from life tables. An age-, sex-, and race-matched survival curve was constructed from the 1974 U. S. Life Tables generated by the Department of Health, Education and Welfare.[12] The number of patients followed and surviving at 1, 2, 3, 4, and 5 years was 167, 101, 67, 42, and 19, respectively. Thus the experience at this institution demonstrates that patients with single-vessel coronary artery disease undergoing bypass surgery and surviving hospitalization have a 5-year life expectancy, which is not significantly different from a matched population.

SURVIVAL WITH TWO-VESSEL CORONARY ARTERY DISEASE

In the natural history follow-up of the annual and 5-year accumulative mortality of patients with significant two-vessel coronary artery disease (greater than

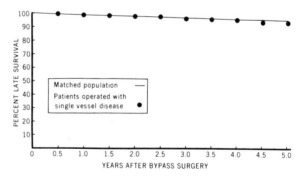

FIGURE 14-2 The percentage of late survival for 5 years after bypass surgery in patients operated with single-vessel coronary disease (solid circles) is compared to the survival curve of a matched population (solid line) from life tables. For patients undergoing surgery at the University of Alabama Medical Center, the 5-year life expectancy was not significantly different from that of the matched population. (*Reprinted with permission from J. W. Kirklin et al., Research Related to Surgical Treatment in Coronary Artery Disease, Circulation, in press.*)

50 percent stenosis), Oberman and associates at this institution calculated an annual mortality of 5.9 percent. An earlier report by Kouchoukos and associates revealed a significantly lower survival rate in the surgical candidate group as compared to operated patients, as shown in Figure 14-3. Also illustrated are the survival curves of 41 patients who, because of diffuse anatomic disease or severe impairment of left ventricular function, were not considered suitable surgical candidates. In this study, patients who underwent bypass surgery and candidates for the procedure were similar in age, sex, history of hypertension, cholesterol levels, symptoms of failure, and electrocardiographic evidence of previous myocardial infarction. Although the difference at 24 months was not statistically significant, the long-term survival appeared better for the surgically treated patients than for the medically managed individuals considered candidates for operation.

Kirklin and associates recently reported 508 patients surviving coronary artery bypass grafting for two-vessel coronary artery disease. The number of patients traced and surviving at 1, 2, 3, 4, and 5 years was 467, 347, 226, 135, and 75, respectively, as shown in Fig. 14-4. A comparison of survival of the surgically treated coronary artery disease patients to a matched

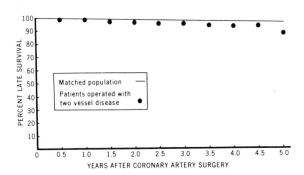

FIGURE 14-4 The percentage of late survival for 5 years after coronary artery surgery in patients with two-vessel disease at the University of Alabama Medical Center is compared to a matched population. At 5 years, 87.6 percent of the surgically treated patients survived as compared to 95 percent of the matched population. *(Reprinted with permission from J. W. Kirklin et al., Research Related to Surgical Treatment in Coronary Artery Disease, Circulation, in press.)*

population at 5 years revealed 87.6 percent survival of the surgically treated individuals as compared to 95 percent for the matched population.

SURVIVAL WITH THREE-VESSEL CORONARY ARTERY DISEASE

Several natural history follow-up studies of three-vessel coronary artery disease have consistently documented a substantially increased annual mortality in these individuals. Oberman and associates reported from 1970 to 1977 an annual mortality for three-vessel coronary disease (greater than 50 percent stenosis), excluding left main coronary artery disease, of 8.8 percent and a 5-year cumulative mortality of 44.3 percent. Thus the 5-year survival rate in these patients was 55.8 percent.

Kouchoukos and associates earlier reported survival curves for 359 patients with severe occlusive disease of all three major coronary arteries without disease in the left main coronary artery, as shown in Fig. 14-5. In comparing the 250 patients surgically treated with the 66 patients considered surgical candidates, one can see that the statistics were significantly different at and beyond 6 months. Kirklin, Kouchoukos, and associates recently evaluated 863 patients surviving coronary artery bypass grafting with three-vessel coronary artery disease, as shown in Fig. 14-6. The number of patients traced and surviving at 1, 2, 3, 4, and 5 years was 776, 511, 282, 141 and 73, respectively. Survival of the surgically treated coronary artery disease patients at 5 years was 88.9 percent, compared to 95 percent in the matched population.

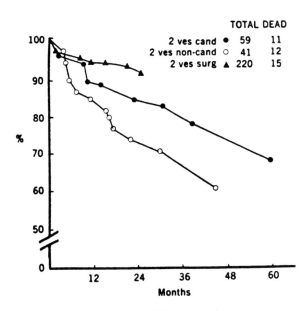

FIGURE 14-3 In patients with two-vessel coronary artery disease, both candidates for surgery and noncandidates for surgery demonstrated a lower survival than did patients undergoing the operation. *(Reprinted with permission from N. T. Kouchoukos, et al., Results of Surgery for Disabling Angina Pectoris, in A. N. Brest and S. H. Rahimtoola (eds.), "Cardiovascular Clinics (Coronary Bypass Surgery)," F. A. Davis Company, Philadelphia, 1977.)*

156

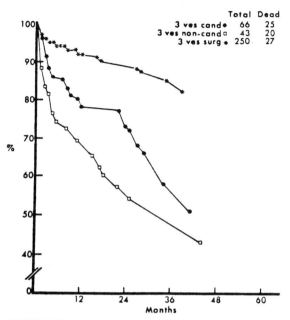

FIGURE 14-5 In patients with three-vessel coronary artery disease, the surgical candidates and noncandidates demonstrated reduced survival at and beyond 6 months as compared to the surgically treated patients at the University of Alabama Medical Center. *(Reprinted with permission from N. T. Kouchoukos et al., Results of Surgery for Disabling Angina Pectoris, in A. N. Brest and S. H. Rahimtoola (eds.), "Cardiovascular Clinics (Coronary Bypass Surgery)," F. A. Davis Company, Philadelphia, 1977.)*

SURVIVAL WITH LEFT MAIN CORONARY ARTERY DISEASE

Significant stenoses of greater than 50 percent of the left main coronary artery are usually associated with multivessel coronary disease and render a particularly high mortality to the patient. Experience at the University of Alabama Medical Center has been similar to that of other institutions in that these patients demonstrate reduced survival rates for 2 years after coronary arteriography. Oberman and associates reported 2-year survival statistics in patients with left main coronary disease and documented a significant increase in survival for those undergoing surgery versus the medically managed patients.[13] Kirklin, Kouchoukos, and associates compared 247 patients after bypass grafting for left main coronary disease to a matched population, as shown in Fig. 14-7. The number of patients traced and surviving at 1, 2, 3, 4, and 5 years was 226, 156, 93, 52 and 24, respectively. Again, the survival at 5 years for the operated patient was slightly less than that for the matched population. The 5-year survival of the surgically treated patients with left main disease was 86.7 percent as compared to 94.4 percent for the matched population.

SURVIVAL WITH TWO- AND THREE-VESSEL CORONARY DISEASE WITH LEFT VENTRICULAR DYSFUNCTION

With improved operative techniques and enhanced myocardial preservation during coronary bypass surgery, increasing numbers of patients with multivessel coronary disease and impaired left ventricular function are undergoing bypass grafting. Kouchoukos and colleagues reported on patients with multivessel coronary disease and generalized hypokinesis and cardiomegaly, as shown in Fig. 14-8. The 24-month survival rate was 85 percent for the 59 patients surgically treated, as compared to 67 percent survival for the 89 patients managed medically. In the 16 surgically treated patients followed longer than 24 months, there were no recorded deaths.

DISCUSSION

A number of factors have to be considered and assessed in the evaluation of patient survival after coronary artery bypass surgery. Patient selection for coronary arteriography reflects an increased suspicion by the physician for underlying coronary artery disease, as well as improved noninvasive methods of evaluation. Improved techniques for cardiac catheterization, as well as technical advances in fluorographic equipment, have contributed to enhanced delineation of the coronary anatomy and better assessment of ventricular function. Recognized risk factors in the genesis of

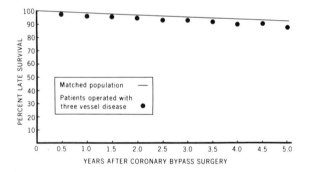

FIGURE 14-6 Patients operated on with three-vessel coronary artery disease at the University of Alabama Medical Center are compared to a matched population. At 5 years, 88.9 percent of surgically treated patients survived, as compared to 95 percent of the matched population. *(Reprinted with permission from J. W. Kirklin et al., Research Related to Surgical Treatment in Coronary Artery Disease, Circulation, in press.)*

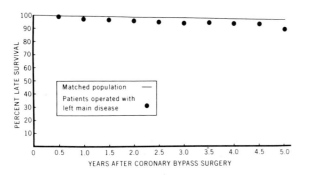

FIGURE 14-7 The percentage of late survival for patients operated with left main coronary artery disease at the University of Alabama Medical Center is compared to a matched population (solid line) for 5 years. At 5 years, 88.9 percent of the surgically treated patients survived, as compared to 95 percent of the matched population. *(Reprinted with permission from J. W. Kirklin et al., Research Related to Surgical Treatment in Coronary Artery Disease, Circulation, in press.)*

coronary artery disease are being modified in medical as well as surgical forms of treatment. Finally, important contributions to coronary artery bypss grafting include more complete revascularization, better preservation of ischemic myocardium during surgery, and a reduced incidence of myocardial necrosis during surgery.

Physicians have become increasingly aware of the prevalence of underlying coronary artery disease and the lack of correlation between a patient's symptoms, clinical manifestations, and abnormalities on coronary arteriography. Therefore, noninvasive tools such as exercise testing and the recent addition of thallium perfusion studies during exercise and rest have significantly increased the number of candidates for coronary arteriography. The addition of thallium myocardial scanning to standard exercise testing has increased the detection of ischemic myocardium. The improved fluoroscopic equipment and power sources now provide clearer delineation of coronary arterial anatomy from a wider range of views than previously available during coronary arteriography. Refinements in cardiac catheterization and reduced morbidity in studying patients have resulted in broad clinical indications for the use of this diagnostic technique in the detection of coronary artery disease. An increasing number of patients with positive exercise test results, as well as patients recovered from a recent acute myocardial infarction, are now advised to undergo coronary arteriography. These clinical considerations must then contribute to an increased recognition of anatomic coronary artery disease and provision of a larger number of patients for coronary artery bypass grafting.

Risk factors such as smoking, hypertension, and

lipid abnormalities warrant clinical consideration in both the medical and the surgical management of patients with coronary artery disease. Control of risk factors is important for patients who undergo coronary artery bypass grafting as well as for those treated medically. Uncontrolled risk factors, particularly cigarette smoking, have been shown to correlate with progressive anatomic coronary artery disease in patients managed either medically or surgically. Even though risk factors have been aggressively treated, clinical trials have suggested that medical management alone will not consistently control ischemic chest pain. This has been evidenced by the number of medically treated patients with unstable angina in randomized medical studies who cross over to surgery during the follow-up period.

Besides the increased detection and diagnostic accuracy of noninvasive and invasive studies for the recognition of coronary artery disease, major factors responsible for the improved surgical survival in patients with coronary artery disease include more complete revascularization of the myocardium with an increased

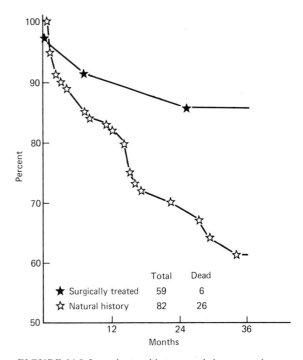

FIGURE 14-8 In patients with two- and three-vessel coronary artery disease and generalized hypokinesis and cardiomegaly, the 24-month survival rate was 85 percent for patients surgically treated, as compared to 67 percent for medically managed individuals. *(Reprinted with permission from N. T. Kouchoukos et al., Results of Surgery for Disabling Angina Pectoris, in A. N. Brest and S. H. Rahimtoola, "Cardiovascular Clinics (Coronary Bypass Surgery)," F. A. Davis Company, Philadelphia, 1977.)*

number of vein grafts and preservation of the myocardium during the operative procedure. Surgical expertise now permits bypass grafting not only to the major coronary arteries but also to the branch vessels. Even with a high percentage of graft patency demonstrated at 1 and 5 years in patients with previous coronary surgery, total revascularization at the time of surgery physiologically affords additional protection for future impairment of myocardial flow. These surgical advances have permitted coronary artery bypass grafting to be performed in conjunction with aneurysm resection and, in some instances, replacement of diseased cardiac valves. The reduction of perioperative myocardial infarction must be attributed to improved surgical techniques and methods for protecting the ischemic myocardium. The use of sensitive cardiac isoenzymes to detect myocardial injury will not only increase the sensitivity for detection but also confirm the improvement in surgical techniques. The current surgical technique for cold cardioplegic arrest has contributed significantly to the preservation of the myocardium during the procedure and reduction of perioperative myocardial infarction.

Thus, surgical statistics during the hospitalization and late follow-up periods indicate improved survival for patients with single-, double- and triple-vessel coronary disease, including involvement of the left main coronary artery. Although continued acquisition and analysis of clinical experience remain important, as does the contribution of randomized medical and surgical studies, coronary artery bypass grafting has contributed significantly to the prolongation of life in patients with coronary artery disease. Finally, continued compilation of statistics in terms of hospital mortality, perioperative myocardial necrosis, and long-term follow-up should be maintained and constantly updated in every institution performing coronary artery bypass grafting. This information should be accessible to cardiac surgeons, cardiologists, physicians, and finally patients.

REFERENCES

1 Oberman, A., Jones, W. B., Riley, E. P., Reeves, T. J., Sheffield, L. T., and Turner, M. E.: Natural History of Coronary Artery Disease, *Bull. N.Y. Acad. Med.*, 48:1109, 1972.

2 Rackley, C. E.: Quantitative Evaluation of Left Ventricular Function by Radiographic Techniques, *Circulation*, 54:862, 1977.

3 Field, B. J., Russell, R. O., Jr., Dowling, J. T., and Rackley, C. E.: Regional Left Ventricular Performance in the Year Following Myocardial Infarction, *Circulation*, 46:679, 1972.

4 Kouchoukos, N. T., Oberman, A., and Karp, T. B.: Results of Surgery for Disabling Angina Pectoris, in A. N. Brest and S. H. Rahimtoola (eds.), "Cardiovascular Clinics (Coronary Bypass Surgery)," F. A. Davis Company, Philadelphia, 1977, p. 157.

5 Russell, R. O., Jr., Rogers, W. J., Mantle, J. A., Kouchoukos, N. T., and Rackley, C. E.: Coronary Arteriography within Two Months After Acute Myocardial Infarction. Preliminary Report, *Cardiovasc. Med.*, 2:679, 1977.

6 Kouchoukos, N. T., and Oberman, A.: Coronary Artery Bypass Grafting, in C. E. Rackley and R. O. Russell, Jr. (eds.), "Coronary Artery Disease: Recognition and Management," Futura Publishing Company, Mount Kisco, N.Y., 1979, p.299.

7 Kirklin, J. W., Kouchoukos, N. T., Blackstone, E. H., and Oberman, A.: Research Related to Surgical Treatment in Coronary Artery Disease, *Circulation*, in press.

8 Kouchoukos, N. T.: Personal communication, 1979.

9 McDaniel, H. G., Reeves, J. G., Kouchoukos, H. T., Smith, L. R., Rogers, W. J., Lell, W. A., and Samuelson, P. N.: Myocardial Preservation: Detection of Cardiac Injury After Coronary Bypass with Hypothermic Cardioplegic Arrest, *Am. J. Cardiol.*, in press.

10 Bruschke, A. V. G., Proudfit, W. L., and Sones, F. M., Jr.: Progress Study of 590 Consecutive Nonsurgical Cases of Coronary Disease Followed 5-9 Years. 1. Arteriographic Correlations, *Circulation*, 47:1147, 1973.

11 Kouchoukos, N. T., Oberman, A., Russell, R. O., Jr., and Jones, W. B.: Comparison of Surgical and Medical Treatment for Occlusive Disease Confined to the Anterior Descending Artery, *Am. J. Cardiol.*, 35:836, 1975.

12 "Vital Statistics of the United States," Vol. 11, Sect. 5, "Life Tables," Department of Health, Education and Welfare, Rockville, Md., 1976.

13 Oberman, A., Kouchoukos, N. T., Harrell, R. R., Holt, J. H., Jr., Russell, R. O., Jr., and Rackley, C. E.: Surgical Versus Medical Treatment in Disease of the Left Main Coronary Artery, *Lancet*, 2:591, 1976.

The author would like to express appreciation to Dr. Nicholas T. Kouchoukos and Dr. John W. Kirklin and their surgical colleagues for the use of their surgical data, to Dr. Al Oberman for his extensive follow-up information on medically and surgically treated patients, finally, to Dr. Richard O. Russell, Jr. and his associates for cardiac catheterization findings. Mrs. Juanita Kilgore has provided excellent illustrations, and I am grateful to Mrs. Sylvia Bell for typing the manuscript.

Chapter 15

Preservation of the Myocardium by Coronary Bypass Surgery: The Effect on Survival*

DAVID G. GREENE, M.D., IVAN L. BUNNELL, M.D.,
DJAVAD T. ARANI, M.D., GEORGE SCHIMERT, M.D.,
THOMAS Z. LAJOS, M.D., ARTHUR B. LEE, M.D.,
RAVINDER N. TANDON, M.D., M.R.C.P. (Edinburgh),
WALTER T. ZIMDAHL, M.D., JOHN M. BOZER, M.D.,
ROBERT M. KOHN, M.D., JOHN P. VISCO, M.D.,
and GRETCHEN L. SMITH, R.N., M.S.

Coronary artery bypass surgery in patients with ischemic heart disease has three objectives: diminution of symptoms, increase in capacity for physical activity, and prolongation of life. It achieves these objectives by increasing the blood flow to parts of the myocardium threatened by lesions in the coronary arteries supplying them. Its aim is to preserve viable areas of the myocardium of the left ventricular free wall and septum.

Preservation of myocardium lends itself poorly to easy clinical evaluation after surgery either by symptoms or by simple clinical tests. But if myocardium is preserved, survival after surgery should reflect the improvement. This chapter, like those preceding and following it, will attempt to assemble and evaluate the data presently available concerning the effect of coronary bypass surgery on life expectancy.

HISTORICAL COMPARISONS

Although the symptom that causes most patients to consider coronary bypass surgery is angina pectoris, the surgery is performed only for demonstrated coronary arteriosclerosis. This distinction is important when evaluating survival after surgery in comparison with medically treated groups of patients. Approximately 1 patient in 5 with angina pectoris is shown on coronary arteriography to have normal coronary arteries and an excellent prognosis as to survival. However, when the diagnosis depends on the history, electrocardiogram, and other clinical data alone without arteriography, these patients will be included and will bias the results in favor of medical management.

Studies of the natural history of angina pectoris diagnosed clinically (without angiographic confirmation) show 5-year survival rates that vary considerably (see Table 15-1). The variability lies largely with the selection of cases. Feil's series reflects the fact that he reported patients with myocardial infarction separately.[4] The series of Zukel et al. was taken from a young healthy military population, and 52 percent of their patients were under 40 years of age when first diagnosed.[5] Two more recent series come from surveys of general populations and reflect survival after the first appearance of symptoms, not after the first visit to a physician.[6,7] The 5-year survival for men was 87 and 83 percent in the two series. Probably any extrapolations from these data should take these figures as about the best that can be expected from medical treatment.

The comparison with present-day surgical results becomes tenuous because of differences in the populations from which these patients are drawn, differences in age, differences in diagnosis, differences in sex, differences in stage and extent of disease, and differences in era of observation. The series of Richards et al. is limited to patients first seen in 1920 to 1931.[1] The medical management of coronary artery disease has changed tremendously in the past 50 years, and new antianginal drugs, beta blocking drugs, antiarrhythmic drugs, coronary care units, and cardiopulmonary resuscitation methods have all contributed to improved survival under medical management.

*From the Departments of Medicine and Surgery, SUNY at Buffalo and the Buffalo General Hospital, Buffalo.

Supported in part by Program Project Grant No. HL 15194 from the National Heart, Lung and Blood Institute and by gifts in memory of Cecil Kisiel.

159

TABLE 15-1
**Five-year survival for patients with clinically
diagnosed angina pectoris**

| Authors | Five-year survival, percent | | |
	Males	Females	Combined
Richards et al.[1]	69	76	70
Parker et al.[2]			53
Block et al.[3]	56	69	58
Feil[4]	82	86	83
Zukel et al.[5]	90		
Population studies			
Kannel et al.[6]	87	92	89
Frank et al.[7]	83		

ANGIOGRAPHICALLY DOCUMENTED SERIES

The same differences affect attempts to compare groups of patients with angiographically diagnosed coronary artery disease from different centers, but the hazards are less serious. To begin with, the diagnosis of coronary arteriosclerosis can be made with great precision angiographically. Experience has shown that the number of vessels involved with critical narrowing affects the prognosis more than most other identifiable characteristics.[8] Coronary arteriography allows one to categorize patients in this regard and to match only those groups in which the severity of the disease is equivalent. Good coronary arteriography always includes ventriculography. The contractile state of the left ventricular wall so measured also greatly affects the prognosis and must be considered in comparing groups of cases. Coronary arteriography became a generally used clinical test only in the 1960s, and so the time differences between series are a decade or less. Nonetheless, an important reservation must be noted about any comparison between series from different centers collected by different workers at different times.[9]

In this chapter, we will be referring frequently to the series of patients evaluated angiographically and treated surgically at the Buffalo General Hospital. Since these data have not been previously reported except in abstract form,[9a] we will describe them more fully than would otherwise be necessary. We will also be forced, because of space limitations, to treat similar reports from other centers more briefly than would otherwise be appropriate. Most of our data refer to the first 875 uncomplicated cases to have coronary bypass surgery in our hospital. These patients had one to eight grafts between 1969 and September 30, 1976 and were all followed through October 1, 1977. In our series, the term "uncomplicated" means no associated valve replacement, no ventricular resection, no

Vineberg operation, no congenital heart disease, no reoperation, and no unplanned salvage procedure. The average age was 52.4 years with a range of 29 to 73 years. The series included 736 males (84 percent); 52 percent of all patients had unstable angina, and 49 percent had a history of a myocardial infarction. Ninety-two patients (11 percent) had critical narrowing of the main left coronary artery, critical narrowing being defined as 75 percent of the cross section, which in a cylinder equals 50 percent of the diameter. Of the remainder, 372 patients (43 percent) had critical narrowing of three main arteries, 258 (29 percent) had two-vessel disease, and 153 (17 percent) had critical narrowing of only one vessel. No patient had surgery who did not have critical narrowing of at least one vessel supplying a contractile segment of the left ventricular free wall or septum.

Because the idea of bringing a new blood supply to an area lacking blood seemed so reasonable, we have always had high hopes for coronary bypass surgery and have treated few operable patients medically once surgery became available. We therefore have no matched groups of patients treated medically with which we can compare our surgical results. We have

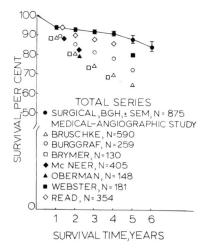

FIGURE 15-1 Survival calculated by the actuarial method of the first 875 uncomplicated patients to have coronary bypass surgery at the Buffalo General Hospital is compared with survival with medical management of seven large series[10-16] reported completely enough so that survival by number of vessels involved was calculable. In this and subsequent figures, the ordinate scale indicates the percentage of cases surviving, and the abscissa gives the time following surgery or coronary arteriography if no surgery was performed.

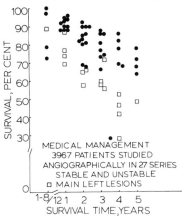

FIGURE 15-2 Survival with medical management in 27 series[10-36,45] of patients diagnosed angiographically and reported in enough detail so that actuarial analysis of at least one point was possible. Small series with fewer than 30 patients were excluded. The first time interval includes data points from the first 8 months after diagnostic catheterization. Otherwise axes are as in Fig. 15-1.

had to turn to the large published series of patients studied angiographically, treated medically, and followed long enough so that actuarial analysis of the results could be obtained. The series picked to illustrate these comparisons were selected because they reported data suitable for actuarial analysis, and because they reported them according to the number of vessels involved. For Fig. 15-1 and subsequent figures, some of the data were read off published graphs, and errors of 1 or 2 percent may have been introduced in this way. Brymer and colleagues were kind enough to supply some of their raw data and actuarial analyses.[12] The data of Bruschke et al. and of Webster et al. are both from the Cleveland Clinic, but Webster's cases were specifically selected for their suitability for surgery by subsequent standards.[10,15] The series of Burggraf et al. excluded patients with lesions of the main left coronary artery.[11]

From Fig. 15-1 it is clear that surgery results in better survival than has been found in the selected series of similar patients treated medically. We have already cited the difficulties in drawing conclusions from comparisons between series collected by different workers in different institutions. Certainly, some differences in selection exist. On the other hand, the surgery probably has contributed to the difference, at least in part.

To get a firmer idea about the question, we have summarized all the large (over 30 patients) series of

angiographically diagnosed coronary arteriosclerosis treated medically with a significant follow-up period (over 2 years) where enough data were presented in written, tabular, or graphic form to permit actuarial analysis of survival. The data points are displayed in Fig. 15-2. Series that included only patients with lesions of the main left coronary artery are indicated by open squares. The results vary widely. In Fig. 15-3 the upper limit of the medically managed survival is plotted against our surgical survival. At 3 years, a difference in favor of surgery appears and grows wider at 4 years.

Figure 15-4 shows the results in survival of all the medical series, with survivals falling somewhere in the shaded area below the best survival curve. No angiographically diagnosed and medically treated series has been reported with better than an 80 percent 5-year survival. Against this area we have plotted the data on survival with surgical treatment in eight different series taken from the literature and from our own institution. The point of this illustration is to show that many different centers provide surgical treatment which after 5 years has a better survival rate than any reported survival on medical treatment.

When patients are categorized according to which vessels are critically narrowed, interesting differences appear. Probably no other single characteristic of a patient affects the prognosis more. Patients with lesions of the main left coronary artery survive less well than do other patients with coronary arteriosclerosis, as is shown in Fig. 15-2. When the survival with surgery is plotted on the same scale, as in Fig. 15-5, the prolongation of life by surgical treatment appears

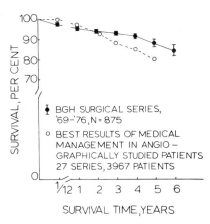

FIGURE 15-3 Survival in first 875 uncomplicated surgical cases at the Buffalo General Hospital is compared with the best results at each interval in the medically managed series plotted in Fig. 15-2. The time scale changes between 1 month and 1 year.

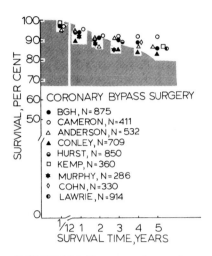

FIGURE 15-4 The area and upper border of the points plotted in Fig. 15-2 are indicated by the shading. The survivals in our surgical series and in eight other selected surgical series[27a,31,50,61-64] are plotted on the same scale. The overlap of medical treatment and surgery is complete at first, but by the third year, four surgical series are better than the best medical reports, and at 5 years, the overlap has disappeared. Many surgical services are reporting better results than have been reported with medical management alone.

likely, even though the various series come from different times, places, and authors.

Quite similar data concerning triple-vessel disease are shown in Fig. 15-6. Survival with medical treatment has not been good in any of the reported series, which are the only large series of medically managed patients in which actuarial analyses can be made from the available data. The surgical survival shows a sharp break in the curve, with decreasing survival after the fourth year following surgery. There are several possible causes for this break. The surgery may have simply postponed the survival curve by about 4 years, with the downward trend resuming at about its original rate as the disease progresses. Or, the fact that these data points reflect the survival of the patients operated on in the early years may indicate that the benefits of the early surgery were shorter lasting than those of more recent operations. Another factor is the smaller number of patients at risk in the fifth and sixth years, 68 and 26 respectively. This same change in the curve after the fourth year appears in several of the subsets in our series. We have not seen it in any reports of survival after surgery from other institutions.

The data on double-vessel disease in Fig. 15-7 show a similar pattern. The medically treated series are from

the same institutions as in the previous figure, and the survival is slightly better than with three-vessel disease. Survival of the surgical series fractionally tops 88 percent in the fifth year and 85 percent in the sixth year, with 64 and 36 patients at risk, respectively. The sharp change in direction noted in three-vessel disease survival does not appear in this graph.

A somewhat different picture appears in Fig. 15-8, which deals with single-vessel disease. Survival is good in the various medical series and is also good with surgery. The differences in the early years are negligible, but at the fifth year the differences between the surgical series and Bruschke's series attains significance at the 1 percent level.

Tukey has pointed out the pitfalls of comparisons such as these between different groups of patients from different institutions, times, and places diagnosed and treated by different physicians.[9] From a statistical point of view, he is correct. Attempts to obtain better data should be and are being made and will be presented later in this chapter. Nonetheless, these historical comparisons cannot be completely discounted, as some would suggest.[37-39] They are the way much medical progress has been made in the past.

With the exception of some forms of cancer treatment, we are unaware of any operations that have been validated by prospective randomized trials.[40] Most important in the claims for giving some weight to these data is our ability to categorize patients into subsets that most significantly affect survival by our angiographic assessment of the coronary circulation and ventricular function. When age and sex are added

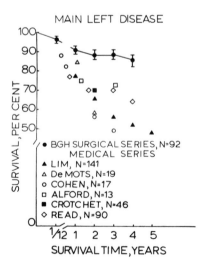

FIGURE 15-5 Survival of our surgical patients with critical narrowing of the left main coronary artery is plotted against reported series with medical management.[16,17,20,23,24,29]

to the angiographic assessment, we have two other patient characteristics that have been shown to have an important effect on survival. We therefore believe that these historical comparisons make a strong case for the addition of surgery to our best medical treatment for coronary arteriosclerosis.

RANDOMIZED PROSPECTIVE SERIES

A great contribution to our understanding of coronary arteriosclerosis and its surgical treatment has been made by the randomized prospective cooperative study of patients with stable angina pectoris (excluding left main coronary artery obstruction) by the Veterans Administration.[16,31] It is not a perfect study, and critics have pointed out that the surgical mortality was higher than in some more experienced institutions at the time of the study and higher than it has generally become since the study was made.[41] Also, a large number of patients dropped out of the medical series and have had surgery. But this study has focused our attention on the question of survival and, beyond that, on the elements of a good comparative series.

The Veterans Administration study has shown that those patients with 50 percent or greater narrowing in diameter of the left main coronary artery do better with surgery than with medical management alone. The difference between survivals of treatment groups

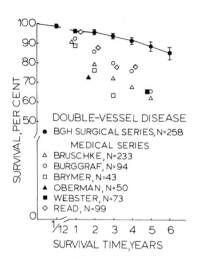

FIGURE 15-7 Survival rates of our surgical patients with double-vessel disease and of similar patients angiographically diagnosed and treated medically in six other series.[10-12,14-16]

is significant at the 5 percent level.[42] This finding has confirmed the conclusions reached by others on the basis of historical comparisons and has been widely accepted.

The remaining patients in the series, those with one-, two-, and three-vessel disease, fail to show a statistically significant difference in survival either when separated into groups by number of vessels involved or when taken as a whole.[16] The failure to demonstrate the superiority of surgery over medical treatment in these patients may have several explanations. The one most commonly cited is the high 30-day mortality (5.6 percent) in the surgical group. When it is compared with the present-day surgical mortality of less than 2 percent in many institutions and of 1 percent or less in several busy clinics,[43] it is easy to imagine that 3 or 4 percent could be added to the surgical survival were the series to be repeated now. The graft patency, which was less than acceptable by present-day standards, would also be improved now and could affect the surgical survival favorably. These data can even be interpreted as showing an advantage for surgical treatment.[44] Both groups started with 100 percent at zero time, but after 1 month, only 94.4 percent of the surgical group were alive. The number in the medical group alive at 1 month has not been published, but presumably was over 99 percent. If the two groups are indistinguishable at 36 months,[31] the surgical attrition curve must have been shallower in the intervening 35 months, and if projected as a straight line, it will ultimately become higher than the medical curve similarly projected. This sort of calculation is, of course, speculative. In one subset of patients in the

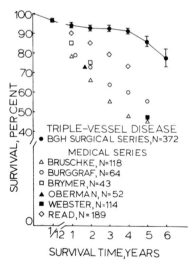

FIGURE 15-6 Survival rates of our surgical patients with three-vessel disease and of similar patients angiographically diagnosed and treated medically in six other series.[10-12,14-16]

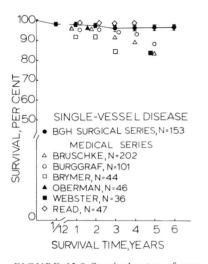

FIGURE 15-8 Survival rates of our surgical patients with one-vessel disease and of similar patients angiographically diagnosed and treated medically in six other series.[10-12,14-16]

Veterans Administration study, the data show exactly that pattern (Fig. 15-9). In patients with three-vessel disease and an angiographically demonstrated abnormality of left ventricular contraction, the surgical survival curve drops at 1 month and runs below the medical curve until 30 months.[16] Thereafter, it runs above the medical curve, but the differences are not statistically significant.

One of the difficult aspects of the cooperative study to evaluate is the low mortality in the medical group. Three possible explanations come to mind. The medical treatment may have been better than reported in other series, with more use of beta blockade and long-acting nitrates. The patients in the Veterans Administration study may have had less severe disease than patients in other studies. Or, finally and least likely because of the precautions taken to avoid it, bias may have crept into the selection of patients for the study.

The preliminary results of the European multicenter randomized prospective trial have been presented by Varnauskas.[45] These patients were males below 65 years of age with 50 percent or more narrowing of diameter in at least two major coronary arteries and left ventricular ejection fractions of at least 0.5. Because discretion was allowed in the enrollment of patients with left main disease, only 59 of the 768 patients randomized were so affected. At 2 years, 92.5 percent of 373 medical patients and 94.7 percent of 394 surgical patients were known to be alive, statistically an insignificant difference. The only significant difference (*p* < 0.05) was in three-vessel disease, with 89.9 percent survival of 188 patients randomized to medicine and

95.9 percent survival of 219 patients randomized to surgery. The actual results for the whole group were more in favor of surgery than these statistics suggest, because 6 patients randomized to surgery and counted in the surgical group died before surgery could be performed. Also 50 (13 percent) of the patients randomized to medicine have so far had surgery because of unresponsive symptoms.

Two other multicentric collaborative trials performed on a prospective randomized basis are currently being conducted in the United States. One, a study of stable angina, will be closely watched for its 30-day mortality, since the surgical achievements of the participating institutions are uneven in quality.[46] Surgery for chronic stable angina in males without lesions of the left main coronary artery should be performed with a mortality of less than 1 percent. Comparing medical treatment with less than excellent surgery is valueless. The other study, of unstable angina, is discussed later in the chapter.[35]

Because it takes so long to accumulate cases, randomized prospective trials in one institution tend to be small.[30,47] So far, no significant differences in survival have been demonstrated in such series.

In summary, the Veterans Administration cooperative study has demonstrated the superiority of surgical treatment over medical in prolonging survival in patients with left main coronary artery disease, and the European multicenter trial has demonstrated improved survival with surgery in three-vessel disease. No other statistically significant differences have appeared in randomized prospective trials of stable angina.

MATCHED HISTORICAL CONTROLS

By careful matching of such variables as number of vessels involved, ejection fraction, age, and sex, it is possible to assemble retrospectively series of patients given alternative treatments and to compare them with more assurance than when such factors are not carefully balanced. Hammermeister et al. compared the survival of patients treated medically and surgically.[48] They were selected from a large group and matched in two major prognostic variables, the ejection fraction and the number of major vessels narrowed by 70 percent of the lumen diameter. Left main coronary arteries were scored as two vessels. They found that survival improved with surgery in patients with two-vessel disease and ejection fractions above 50 percent or in the 30 to 50 percent range. In the group as a whole, surgical treatment did not appear better than medical treatment except that there were fewer sud-

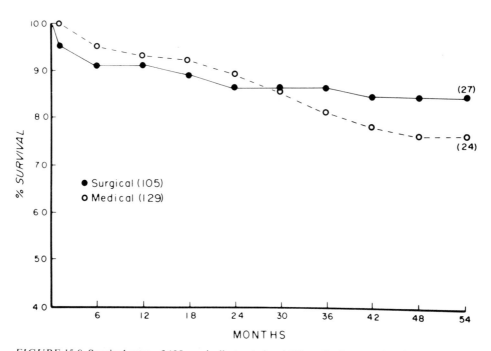

FIGURE 15-9 Survival rates of 105 surgically treated and 129 medically treated patients with triple-vessel disease and an abnormal left ventricle reported in the Veterans Administration Collaborative Trial. (*Reprinted from R. C. Read et al., Survival of Men Treated for Chronic Stable Angina Pectoris. A Cooperative Randomized Study, J. Thorac. Cardiovasc. Surg., 75:1, 1978, with permission of the author and the Journal of Thoracic and Cardiovascular Surgery.*)

den deaths in the surgically treated group ($p < 0.01$). This study was characterized by a high 30-day surgical mortality (5 percent) and by an attempt to eliminate bias in favor of surgery by not counting medical deaths occurring in the first 30 days after catheterization. This precaution may have been reasonable in the local circumstances. A more recent report of this series indicates prolongation of life by surgery in 97 matched pairs with two-vessel disease ($p = 0.0002$).[48a]

Vismara et al. matched patients for medical and surgical treatment in a prospective manner.[49] They failed to find a statistically significant difference between the two groups as a whole, but there was a 24 percent incidence of sudden death in the medical group as compared with 6 percent in the surgical group ($p < 0.05$).

COMPARISON WITH THE GENERAL POPULATION

Because of the difficulty in comparing a surgical survival curve with a medical curve from another institution, we have turned to the survival of a group of the general population selected to match our series by age and sex. This can be determined from the vital statistics obtained from the U.S. Public Health Service. We used the 1975 data to construct the curve and found that such a group had a 99 percent survival at 1 year and an annual attrition rate of 1 percent thereafter. As is shown in Fig. 15-10, our surgical series had a 97.6 percent survival at 1 month, a 95.2 percent survival at 1 year, and then ran parallel to the age- and sex- matched group of the general population for 3 years. In the fifth and sixth years, we again note the change in slope of our data.

Comparison with the general population has been used by others to demonstrate the good prognosis that results when good surgery is added to good medical management. Lawrie et al. reported on a consecutive group of 1,000 male patients and 144 females who had surgery for coronary artery disease in 1971 and 1972.[50] In analyzing their male patients with good left ventricular function (no akinetic area or ventricular aneurysm) and no main left coronary artery disease, they found that the 5-year survival exceeded that of the U.S. population matched for age. In analyzing the surgical series at Alabama, Kirklin found that in one-vessel disease, survival in the fifth year was 94.8 percent, as compared with survival of 94.9 percent in the U.S. population in 1974 matched for age, sex, and race.[51] In more severe disease, with more vessels involved, the differences were between 6 and 7 percent. The

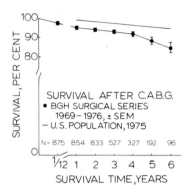

FIGURE 15-10 Survival rates of our surgical patients are compared with that of a cohort of the U.S. population matched by age and by sex. The figures at the bottom indicate the number of patients at risk at the beginning of each time interval.

differences were almost identical in two-vessel disease, three-vessel disease, and left main coronary artery disease.

The choice of general population as a comparative group has been criticized in that at the beginning of the survival curve it includes not only the healthy members of the population but also people in hospitals and elsewhere with terminal illnesses whose outlook is clearly limited and who bias the curve unfavorably. The criticism certainly is valid in the early part of the curve, but most of these acute problems must resolve in a few months. It seems unlikely that the curve will be much affected by such cases after the first year. Our own survival curves reported here include all deaths, not just those from cardiovascular disease.

SURVIVAL IN SUBSETS OF PATIENTS

Number of Vessels Diseased

The data presented so far have stressed differences in survival between medical and surgical treatment. We turn now to differences in survival in various subgroups of patients. When survival after surgery is plotted according to the number of vessels critically narrowed and compared with the survival of an age- and sex-matched group of the U.S. population, the results are as shown in Fig. 15-11. Several points stand out. Although there is little difference between the groups in survival at 30 days, at 1 year, patients with left main disease do less well than patients with three-vessel disease, who in turn are outlived by patients with one- and two-vessel disease. From 1 year until 4 years, the

survival in each group is roughly parallel to that of the general population. In the fifth and sixth years, a significant change in slope of the survival curve occurs in the two- and three-vessel groups, more marked in the latter. There are no further deaths in the single-vessel disease cohort, and their survival becomes indistinguishable from that of the U.S. population. There are too few patients with left main lesions at risk after 4 years to justify plotting those points. Although Fig. 15-12 shows a tendency for patients with more severe coronary arteriosclerosis to survive less well, statistically significant differences at the 5 percent level are found in only 4 of the 30 possible intergroup comparisons in the first 4 years. These are three-vessel versus two-vessel disease at 1 month ($p < 0.02$), left main disease versus two-vessel and one-vessel disease at 2 years ($p < 0.05$ and < 0.04), and left main disease versus one-vessel disease at 4 years ($p < 0.04$).

Ejection Fraction

As has been shown in many series, ventricular function has an important influence on survival. The most convenient and reliable approaches to ventricular function are the measurement of ejection fraction and the measurement of end-diastolic pressure in the left ventricle. Poor ventricular function is often signaled by elevation of the end-diastolic pressure, or by reduction of the ejection fraction, or by both. The end-diastolic pressure varies with the physiologic state of

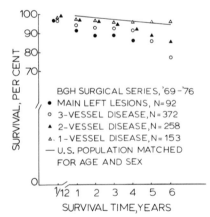

FIGURE 15-11 Survival rates of our surgical series by type of vessel involvement. The only statistically significant differences are between three-vessel and two-vessel disease at 1 month, between left main disease and two- and one-vessel disease at 2 years, and between left main disease and one-vessel disease at 4 years. The survival rate of the U.S. population matched by age and sex is also indicated.

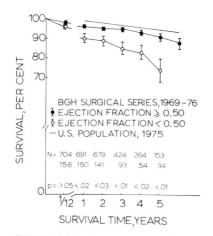

BGH SURGICAL SERIES,1969-76
EJECTION FRACTION ≥ 0.50
EJECTION FRACTION < 0.50
U.S. POPULATION, 1975

FIGURE 15-12 Survival rates in our surgical series, subdivided into those with ejection fractions below 0.50 and those 0.50 and above. The table gives the numbers at risk at each time interval, with the higher ejection fraction series above the lower. The p values at the bottom apply to the comparison between our two groups. The anticipated survival of a similar cohort of the U.S. population is drawn above.

the ventricle from normal to grossly abnormal values in many patients after an intervention such as left ventriculography or coronary arteriography[52] but reflects the basic contractility of the ventricle less well than does the ejection fraction. The ejection fraction has been shown by many investigators to influence survival after surgery. Vliestra et al.,[36] Murphy et al.,[31] and Lawrie et al.[50] have all found increased survival in those patients whose ejection fraction was over 0.5. Our own series demonstrates this phenomenon well (Fig. 15-12). At 1 year, survival is significantly different at the 2 percent level between the two groups and continues to be different for the first 5 years. Patients with the higher ejection fraction have a survival curve that runs just below that of the general public; it is 91 percent at 5 years and 88 percent at 6 years. In the group with ejection fractions of less than 0.5, the lower the ejection fraction, the poorer the survival curve. The numbers are small, and the differences do not attain statistical significance.

Manley et al. have published results of surgery on patients with ejection fractions of 0.3 and lower.[53] Such surgery entails a significant increase in 30-day mortality, and long-term results vary between 40 and 80 percent at 5 years, depending on the severity of the clinical symptoms. From the point of view of the individual patient, such surgery is probably reasonable. The economic burden appears less justifiable in a patient with a 50 percent 5-year survival than in one with a 90 percent 5-year survival.

Age

Among the characteristics of a patient that can be identified as affecting survival after surgery, age, number of vessels critically narrowed, and contractility as estimated by ejection fraction are the three most important. The survival of our own surgical series is illustrated in Fig. 15-13, which plots the survival of our patients under 40 years of age, of those in the fifth decade, of those in the sixth decade, and of those 60 years of age or more. In many forms of surgery the younger patient has a more favorable outlook than the older patient. This trend clearly appears in our material. Those under 40 survive more frequently than those in the fifth decade, who in turn do better than those in the sixth decade. The differences between the first and second groups and between these two groups and the third are statistically significant ($p < 0.05$) at the second, third, and fourth years after surgery.

Improved Survival After More Recent Operations

In the cooperative study of surgery for stable angina of the Veterans Administration, the 1972–1974 results have been criticized for having a high surgical mortality.[41] The response has been that the mortality was not out of line with the experience in several other

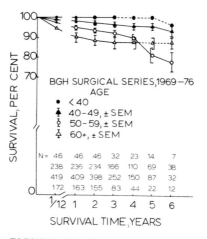

BGH SURGICAL SERIES,1969-76
AGE
< 40
40-49, ± SEM
50-59, ± SEM
60+, ± SEM

FIGURE 15-13 Survival rates of our surgical series by age in years. The numbers at the bottom indicate the number at risk in each subgroup entering each interval. From above downward, the table gives the numbers for those less than 40 years of age, for those in the fifth decade, for those in the sixth decade, and for those over 60 years of age. The dashed lines lead to points representing fewer than 25 patients at risk.

institutions in those same years and that it should not be compared with more recent surgical experience. At Emory University, the more recent surgical experience has been more successful than the series that includes earlier results.[27a]

At the Buffalo General Hospital, we have examined the immediate surgical mortality and 1-year survival of uncomplicated cases on an annual basis, as shown in Table 15-2. Through the years the number of cases has grown, the surgical mortality has fallen, and the 1-year survival has climbed. The curve of improvement has some irregularity, but a decided upward spurt occurs with the 1974–1975 data. Shortly after that came the introduction of improved techniques of myocardial preservation by the surgeons at our hospital along with continuous refinements in techniques, so the improvement may be more than fortuitous.[54] If our series is divided into two cohorts, those having surgery before 1973 and those having surgery between 1973 and 1976, the differences in long-term survival appear striking (see Fig. 15-14). The initial 30-day mortalities, 3.7 and 2.0 percent respectively, are not significantly different, but the survival rates at each of the next 4 years do differ statistically ($p < 0.02$). The difference between the 4-year survival rates of 86 and 94 percent reaches significance at the 0.005 level.

To a certain extent, surgical mortality and perhaps even long-term survival rates can be affected by the policy of selection of patients. We examined two important determinants of survival, ejection fraction and age, in the early and late cohorts in our series. As shown in Fig. 15-14, the mean ejection fractions in the two groups were identical, and the age was slightly younger in the earlier group. We therefore doubt that patient selection has much to do with the observed change in survival. The more recent group of patients had a 30-day mortality of 2 percent. At 4 years, their survival is 94 percent, just 2 percent below the antic-

ipated survival of an age- and sex-matched group of the general population. Data of this sort should be considered by those who advocate randomized trials of surgical treatment as soon as a new surgical procedure is proposed.[38,39,55] Another view of the recent series is seen in Fig. 15-15, where the group is broken down into number of vessels involved, and the survival is plotted against that of the matched U.S. population. Although the group with left main coronary artery disease appears to have a lower survival curve than the others, followed by triple-vessel disease, none of the possible comparisons of one subgroup with another at any one of five time intervals attains statistical significance at the 5 percent level.

Unstable Angina

The diagnosis of unstable angina has been made with a variety of criteria in many different clinics. We have tried to be inclusive, postulating that if we identified all possible cases, we could then look back to see which criteria were associated with an unfavorable outcome. We therefore have diagnosed as unstable angina all those patients with new angina in the previous 3 months, accelerating angina with increasing severity or frequency in the previous 3 months, angina at rest, angina that awakens the patient at night, or angina that requires observation in the hospital to rule out a myocardial infarction. With this definition, we have categorized 455 of our first 875 uncomplicated cases at the Buffalo General Hospital as unstable angina. Their survival is shown in Fig. 15-16, where it is compared with the few series that have been treated medically and reported in enough detail so that actuarial analysis can be done. In this figure we have included some medical cases in which the diagnosis has not been confirmed angiographically, particularly the

TABLE 15-2
Surgical experience at the Buffalo General Hospital, uncomplicated cases

Year	Number of cases	30-day mortality		Additional deaths, first year	One-year survival, percent
		No.	Percent		
1969–1970	19	1	5.3	3	79
1970–1971	35	2	5.7	1	91
1971–1972	64	2	3.1	3	92
1972–1973	99	3	3.0	3	94
1973–1974	144	6	4.2	4	93
1974–1975	199	1	0.5	3	98
1975–1976	317	6	1.9	4	97
1976–1977	391	5	1.3	—	—
1977–1978	401	3	0.8	—	—
Totals	1669	29	1.7	21	95

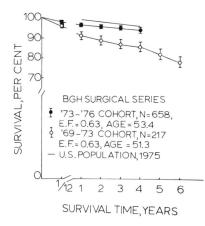

FIGURE 15-14 Survival rates in our surgical series, subdivided into those operated on up to and since October 1, 1973. The more recent series has a 2 percent mortality at 1 month and is 2 percent below the age- and sex-matched U.S. population at 4 years. The ejection fractions in the two groups have identical averages, and the more recent group averages 2 years older.

series of Gazes,[57] in which angiographic confirmation was lacking. It is clear that no medically treated series has achieved the long-term survival of our surgical series.

The Unstable Angina Pectoris Study Group has recently reported the results of a randomized prospective trial of medical and surgical treatment of unstable angina pectoris.[35] All 288 patients in their study had angiographically demonstrated narrowing of 70 percent of the diameter of at least one major vessel and narrowing of at least 50 percent of any other vessel counted as diseased. Patients with 50 percent or more narrowing of the left main coronary artery were excluded, as were patients with an infarct within the previous 3 months. Each of the patients had transient electrocardiographic changes with the angina. All patients had an ejection fraction of greater than 30 percent and an end-diastolic volume of the left ventricle of less than 125 ml/m² of body surface area. The medical and surgical groups had 1-year survival rates of 93 and 92 percent, respectively, and 2-year survivals of 91 and 90 percent. These differences were not statistically different from each other nor from the 1- and 2-year survivals in our series of 95 and 94 percent. Important differences between the Cooperative Study patients and ours include their insistence on 70 percent narrowing of diameter of one vessel, whereas we included patients with narrowing of 50 percent in diameter; their requiring electrocardiographic changes with the angina; and our inclusion of patients with left

main disease and a few with ejection fractions of less than 0.30. The crossover of 36 percent of their patients randomized to medicine because of intractable angina further complicates the interpretation of this randomized series. It is quite probable that these patients with intractable pain would have been the source of many deaths had they not had surgery. The crossover may have obscured a true benefit of surgery in this group.

In the Buffalo General Hospital series, the 455 patients with unstable angina differ little in their survival from the 420 patients with chronic stable angina. In the first 5 years after surgery, the differences are not significant and do not exceed 2 percent (see Fig. 15-17). In the sixth year the stable group has an 83 percent survival, the unstable 86 percent, and again the difference is not statistically significant. We have compared stable versus unstable angina in our series in left main disease; in one-, two-, and three-vessel disease; in males versus females; in ejection fractions above and below 0.5, and in age groups under 40 years and in the fifth, sixth, and seventh decades. In none of these subgroups does the survival of unstable angina differ significantly from that of stable angina, nor is there any suggestion of a trend that may be obscured by strict adherence to statistical criteria. We believe that these data justify our policy of prompt angiography of these patients as soon as we can be sure by electrocardiographic and enzyme criteria that we are not dealing with an acute myocardial infarct. The timing of surgery then depends not only on the symptoms but also on the angiographic findings. Where we find narrow channels, with only 10 to 30 percent of the lumen diameter remaining (10 percent or less in cross

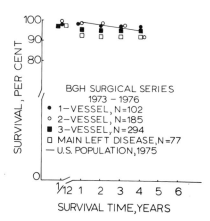

FIGURE 15-15 Survival rates in our more recent series by type of vessel involvement. None of the differences between groups at one time interval is statistically significant. The survival of the age- and sex-matched U.S. population is also shown.

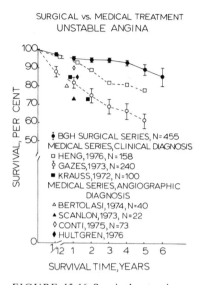

FIGURE 15-16 Survival rates in our surgical series of 455 patients with unstable angina and of patients in three series diagnosed clinically[56-58] and in four series diagnosed angiographically.[19,22,33,64]

section), and where the left main coronary artery is severely narrowed, we try to arrange surgery for the same day or within 24 h. The most severely symptomatic patients are sometimes studied with the surgical team and operating room in readiness so that they may have their bypass grafts within hours of the angiography. Another reason for proceeding promptly with angiography in these patients is the finding of angiographically normal coronary arteries in about one-fifth of the patients with this clinical presentation. Such patients have an excellent prognosis and can be treated on an ambulatory basis.

In a study of patients with unstable angina at the Cleveland Clinic, a higher than usual mortality associated with early surgery for unstable angina was noted.[59] The difference between the two experiences may have been that the Cleveland patients were operated on within 24 h of their admission and may have included more unrecognized myocardial infarctions. We agree with the recommendations that a period of longer than 24 h may be useful in stabilizing the patient and ruling out a fresh infarct.

Gazes' High-Risk Group

One subset of patients with unstable angina that we have distinguished is similar to the high-risk group described by Gazes et al.[57] They reviewed their 10-year follow-up of patients with unstable angina to detect the clinical characteristics associated with an unfavorable prognosis and found that persistent angina in

the hospital on medical treatment was a prominent feature of those who died during the period of observation. We have found 46 such patients in our 875 uncomplicated cases (5 percent). Two of them died within 30 days of surgery and 3 died in the next 11 months. The survival of 89 percent at 1 year has been maintained since, with 100 percent follow-up for 1 year longer than the rest of our follow-up data. Forty-one patients were at risk in the third year and 19 in the fourth. In Fig. 15-18 the contrast between survival after surgery and high-risk patients followed medically by Gazes is striking. It must be remembered, however, that the medical treatment was that of a decade ago and did not include long-acting nitrates and beta blockade.

Severity of Coronary Arterial Disease

The disparity in grading the severity of coronary arterial lesions leads to confusion in comparing the results in different centers. Some workers speak of a 50 percent narrowing and mean that the diameter is reduced by one-half. Others speak in terms of cross section, and the same narrowing would be called a 75 percent lesion. Clarity in definition of terms overcomes this problem. A more important difference arises when one group requires 70 percent narrowing in diameter (90 percent in cross section) to classify a vessel as diseased, while others accept 50 percent in diameter (75 percent in cross section), or when one group requires 70 percent diameter in one vessel but classifies the second and third vessels as involved if they are narrowed by 50 percent.[35] To test the effect of such classification on our data, we reviewed all of

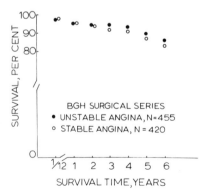

FIGURE 15-17 Survival rates in our surgical series of 455 patients with unstable angina and 420 patients, most of whom had stable angina. No statistically significant differences were found at any time interval.

our patients originally classified as having three-vessel disease because they had 75 percent or greater narrowing in cross section of three main arterial trunks. We separated out patients who had three-vessel disease by the most rigid criteria—90 percent or greater narrowing in cross section (70 percent in diameter) in all three vessels. As shown in Fig. 15-19, we compared their long-term survival with the rest of the group who had 75 percent or greater cross-sectional narrowing of all three vessels but who had, in at least one vessel, less than 90 percent narrowing. The patients who satisfied the more rigorous criteria had a higher mortality in the first 30 days, but after that, the survival curves of the two groups run parallel. After the initial 30 days then, our data fail to show any difference in survival between these two subgroups of patients.

Sex and Survival After Surgery

Some workers have reported that survival after coronary bypass surgery in men exceeds that in women. Reasons advanced have included the small size of the vessels in women. In our series, the 30-day mortality for women, 4.3 percent, is twice that for men, 2 percent. Thereafter, the annual survival rates for women runs about 2 percent below that for men until the fourth year, when the rates are 91.9 and 88.8 percent. In the fifth year the rates are 89.8 and 74.4 percent, but even so, the difference does not reach statistical significance at the 5 percent level.

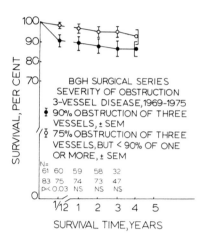

FIGURE 15-19 Survival rates in our surgical series of patients with three-vessel disease who had surgery between 1969 and 1975. One group had 90 percent narrowing in cross section of all three vessels. The other group had at least 75 percent narrowing of all three vessels but less than 90 percent narrowing of at least one. This distinguishes patients who fit strict criteria from those who fit less strict criteria. The group in which stricter criteria were used have a higher 30-day mortality, but after that the two groups run a parallel course. The figures at the bottom indicate the number at risk in each interval, with the group having stricter criteria shown above. Only at 1 month are the two groups significantly different statistically.

History of Myocardial Infarction

Of our 875 patients, 428 or 49 percent gave a history of at least one myocardial infarction in the past. The difference in survival between them and the 447 who gave no such history was not significant at 30 days nor at yearly intervals for 5 years. At 5 years, the patients with previous myocardial infarction had an 86 percent survival rate, while the others had an 89 percent survival rate, but the difference was not statistically significant.

The Ideal Candidate

If we take into consideration the era of surgery, the ejection fraction, and the sex, we can select from our series 441 males with ejection fractions of 0.5 or more who had surgery between 1973 and 1976. This group of ideal candidates made up 50.4 percent of our series and included left main disease and one-, two-, and

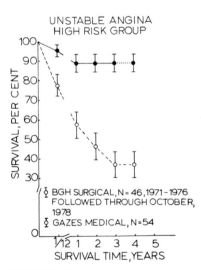

FIGURE 15-18 Survival rates in our surgical series of 46 patients with high-risk unstable angina and of a clinically similar group treated medically by Gazes 10 years earlier.[57] The dotted line leads to a point representing fewer than 25 patients at risk.

three-vessel disease. Although their ejection fractions were 0.5 or greater by the two-diameter method,[65] many had localized areas of hypokinesis. Their survival was 98.9 percent at 1 month, 98.0 percent at 1 year, 96.8 percent at 2 and 3 years, and 95.9 percent at 4 years. In the fourth year, 94 patients were at risk. This survival rate at 4 years is as good as that anticipated by a male cohort of similar age in the U.S. population (94.6 percent). We believe that in 1979, many patients who seek treatment for angina pectoris can be treated surgically with an acceptable mortality and a solid expectation that their long-term survival will be significantly prolonged beyond that to be anticipated from medical management alone.

SUMMARY

On the basis of the evidence available at this time, we believe that preservation of viable myocardium with threatened coronary arterial supply is best achieved by supplementing the best current medical therapy with coronary bypass grafts where they are anatomically possible. Such surgery certainly prolongs survival in left main coronary artery disease and almost as certainly in double- and triple-vessel disease. More data in these categories will be welcome. Patients with single-vessel disease survive well with either medical or surgical management, at least as determined from the first 5 years' follow-up. Both medical treatment and surgery on the coronary arteries in 1979 differ greatly from that of 5 years earlier, and the record now being written will undoubtedly show improvement in the long-term results over those now available. From this review, it appears likely that the superiority of combined medical-surgical treatment over medical treatment alone will be even more firmly established.

The factors favoring better long-term survival after surgery include youth, a normal ejection fraction, and the quality of modern (last 4 years) surgery. Once surgery has been performed, the influence of the extent of coronary artery disease (number of main trunks involved) lessens as compared with survival on medical management. Unstable angina can be successfully treated surgically as soon as a recent myocardial infarct has been ruled out.

REFERENCES

1 Richards, D. W., Bland, E. F., and White, P. D.: A Completed Twenty-five-year Follow-up Study of 456 Patients with Angina Pectoris, *J. Chron. Dis.*, 4:423, 1956.

2 Parker, R. L., Dry, T. J., Willius, F. A., and Gage, R. P.: Life Expectancy in Angina Pectoris, *J.A.M.A.*, 131:95, 1946.

3 Block, W. J., Jr., Crumpacker, E. L., Dry, T. J., and Gage. R. P.: Prognosis of Angina Pectoris. Observations in 6,882 Cases, *J.A.M.A.*, 150:259, 1952.

4 Feil, H.: "Coronary Heart Disease. A Personal Clinical Study," Charles C Thomas, Publisher, Springfield, Ill., 1964.

5 Zukel, W. J., Cohen, B. M., Mattingly, T. W., and Hrubec, Z.: Survival Following First Diagnosis of Coronary Heart Disease, *Am. Heart J.*, 78:159, 1969.

6 Kannel, W. B., and Feinleib, M.: Natural History of Angina Pectoris in the Framingham Study. Prognosis and Survival, *Am. J. Cardiol.*, 29:154, 1972.

7 Frank, C. W., Weinblatt, E., and Shapiro, S.: Angina Pectoris in Men. Prognostic Significance of Selected Medical Factors, *Circulation*, 47:509, 1973.

8 Friesinger, G. C., Page, E. E., and Ross, R. S.: Prognostic Significance of Coronary Arteriography, *Trans. Assoc. Am. Physicians*, 83:78, 1970.

9 Tukey, J. W.: Some Thoughts on Clinical Trials, Especially Problems of Multiplicity, *Science*, 198:679, 1977.

9a Greene, D. G., Bunnell, I. L., Arani, D. T., Schimert, G., Lajos, T. Z., Lee, A. B., Tandon, R. N., Zimdahl, W. T., Bozer, J. M., Kohn, R. M., Visco, J. P., and Smith, G. L.: Actuarial Analysis of Survival of 875 Cases of Coronary Bypass Surgery, *Abstracts*, 1:0487, VIII World Congress of Cardiology, September 17-23, 1978, Tokyo.

10 Bruschke, A. V. G., Proudfit, W. L., and Sones, F. M., Jr.: Progress Study of 590 Consecutive Nonsurgical Cases of Coronary Disease Followed 5-9 Years. I. Arteriographic Correlations, *Circulation*, 47:1147, 1973.

11 Burggraf, G. W., and Parker, J. O.: Prognosis in Coronary Artery Disease. Angiographic, Hemodynamic and Clinical Factors, *Circulation*, 51:146, 1975.

12 Brymer, J. F., Buter, T. H., Walton, J. A., Jr., and Willis, P. W., III: A Natural History Study of the Prognostic Role of Coronary Arteriography, *Am. Heart J.*, 88:139, 1974.

13 McNeer, J. F., Starmer, C. F., Bartel, A. G., Behar, V. S., Kong, Y., Peter, R. H., and Rosati, R. A.: The Nature of Treatment Selection in Coronary Artery Disease. Experience with Medical and Surgical Treatment of a Chronic Disease, *Circulation*, 49:606, 1974.

14 Oberman, A., Kouchoukos, N. T., Harrell, R. R., Holt, J. H., Jr., Russell, R. O., Jr., and Rackley, C. E.: Surgical Versus Medical Treatment in Disease of the Left Main Coronary Artery, *Lancet*, 2:591, 1976.

15 Webster, J. S., Moberg, C., and Rincon, G.: Natural History of Severe Proximal Coronary Artery Disease as Documented by Coronary Cineangiography, *Am. J. Cardiol.*, 33:195, 1974.

16 Read, R. C., Murphy, M. L., Hultgren, H. N., and Takaro, T.: Survival of Men Treated for Chronic Stable Angina Pectoris. A Cooperative Randomized Study, *J. Thorac. Cardiovasc. Surg.*, 75:1, 1978.

17 Alford, W. C., Jr., Shaker, I. J., Thomas, C. J., Jr., Stoney, W. S., Burrus, G. R., and Page, H. L.: Aorto-coronary Bypass in the Treatment of Left Main Coronary Artery Stenosis, *Ann. Thoracic Surg.*, 17:247, 1974.

18 Anderson, R. P., Rahimtoola, S. H., Boncheck, L. I., and Starr, A.: The Prognosis of Patients with Coronary Artery Disease After Coronary Bypass Operations. Time-related Progress of 532 Patients with Disabling Angina Pectoris, *Circulation*, 50:274, 1974.

19 Bertolasi, C. A., Trongé, J. E., Carreño, C. A., Jalon, J., and Vega, M. R.: Unstable Angina—Prospective and Randomized Study of Its Evolution, with and without Surgery, *Am. J. Cardiol.*, 33:201, 1974.

20 Cohen, M. V., and Gorlin, R.: Main Left Coronary Artery Disease. Clinical Experience from 1964-1974, *Circulation*, 52:275, 1975.

21 Conti, C. R., Brawley, R. K., Griffith, L. S. C., Pitt, B., Humphries, J. O'N., Gott, V. L., and Ross, R. S.: Unstable Angina Pectoris: Morbidity and Mortality in 57 Consecutive Patients Evaluated Angiographically, *Am. J. Cardiol.*, 32:745, 1973.

22 Conti, C. R., Gilbert, J. B., Hodges, M., Hutter, A. M., Jr., Kaplan, E. M., Newell, J. B., Resnekov, L., Rosati, R. A., Ross, R. S., Russell, R. O., Jr., Schroeder, J. S., and Wolk, M.: Unstable Angina Pectoris: Randomized Study of Surgical vs. Medical Therapy, *Am. J. Cardiol.*, 35:129, 1975. (Abstract.)

23 Crochet, D., Petitclerc, R., and Campeau, L.: Left Main Coronary Artery Stenosis: Significance of Degree of Obstruction, Associated Involvement of Other Coronary Arteries and of Status of Left Ventricular Contraction as Related to Surgery (147 Cases), *Circulation*, 49, 50: (suppl. 3):111, 1974.

24 DeMots, H., Bonchek, L. I., Rosch, J., Anderson, R. P., Starr, A., and Rahimtoola, S. H.: Left Main Coronary Artery Disease. Risks of Angiography, Importance of Coexisting Disease of Other Coronary Arteries and Effects of Revascularization, *Am. J. Cardiol.*, 36:136, 1975.

25 Fischl, S. J., Herman, M. V., and Gorlin, R.: The Intermediate Coronary Syndrome. Clinical, Angiographic and Therapeutic Aspects, *N. Engl. J. Med.*, 288:1193, 1973.

26 Gross, H., Vaid, A. K., and Cohen, M. V.: Prognosis in Patients Rejected for Coronary Revascularization Surgery, *Am. J. Med.*, 64:9, 1978.

27 Humphries, J. O'N., Kuller, L., Ross, R. S., Friesinger, G. C., and Page, E. E.: Natural History of Ischemic Heart Disease in Relation to Arteriographic Findings. A Twelve Year Study of 224 Patients, *Circulation*, 49:489, 1974.

27aHurst, J. W., King, S. B., III, Logue, R. B., Hatcher, C. R., Jones, E. L., Craver, J. M., Douglas, J. S., Jr., Franch, R. H., Dorney, E. R., Cobbs, B. W., Jr., Robinson, P. H., Clements, S. D., Jr., Kaplan, J. A., and Bradford, J. M.: Value of Coronary Bypass Surgery. Controversies in Cardiology: Part I, *Am. J. Cardiol.*, 42:308, 1978.

28 Kloster, F., Kremkau, L., Rahimtoola, S., Griswold, H., Ritzman, L., Neill, W., and Starr, A.: Prospective Randomized Study of Coronary Bypass Surgery for Chronic Stable Angina, *Circulation*, 52 (suppl. 2):90, 1975.

29 Lim, J. S., Proudfit, W. L., and Sones, F. M., Jr.: Left Main Coronary Arterial Obstruction: Long-term Follow-up of 141 Nonsurgical Cases, *Am. J. Cardiol.*, 36:131, 1975.

30 Mathur, V. S., Guinn, G. A., Anastassiades, L. C., Chahine, R. A., Korompai, F. L., Montero, A. C., and Luchi, R. J.: Surgical Treatment for Stable Angina Pectoris. Prospective Randomized Study, *N. Engl. J. Med.*, 292:709, 1975.

31 Murphy, M. L., Takaro, T., Hultgren, H. N., and Detre, K. M.: Surgical Versus Medical Therapy for Coronary Artery Disease—Survival Data—a Preliminary Report of the Randomized V.A. Cooperative Study, *Am. J. Cardiol.*, 39:286, 1977.

31aMurphy, M. L., Hultgren, H. N., Detre, K., Thomsen, J., Takaro, T., and Participants of the Veterans Administration Cooperative Study: Treatment of Chronic Stable Angina. A Preliminary Report of Survival Data of the Randomized Veterans Administration Cooperative Study, *N. Engl. J. Med.*, 297:621, 1977.

32 Oberman, A., Jones, W. B., Riley, C. P., Reeves, T. J., Sheffield, L. T., and Turner, M. E.: Natural History of Coronary Artery Disease, *Bull. N.Y. Acad. Med.*, 48:1109, 1972.

33 Scanlon, P. S., Nemickas, R., Moran, J. F., Talano, J. V., Amirparviz, F., and Pifarre, R.: Accelerated Angina Pectoris. Clinical, Hemodynamic, Arteriographic and Therapeutic Experience in 85 Patients, *Circulation*, 47:19, 1973.

34 Selden, R., Neill, W. A., Ritzmann, L. W., Okies, J. E., and Anderson, R. P.: Medical Versus Surgical Therapy for Acute Coronary Insufficiency. A Randomized Study, *N. Engl. J. Med.*, 293:1329, 1975.

35 Unstable Angina Pectoris Study Group: Unstable Angina Pectoris: National Cooperative Study Group to Compare Surgical and Medical Therapy. II. In-hospital Experience and Initial Follow-up Results in Patients with One, Two and Three Vessel Disease, *Am. J. Cardiol.*, 42:839, 1978.

36 Vlietstra, R. E., Assad-Morell, J. L., Frye, R. L., Elveback, L. R., Connolly, D. C., Ritman, E. L., Pluth, J. R., Barnhorst, D. A., Danielson, G. K., and Wallace, R. B.: Survival Predictors in Coronary Artery Disease: Medical and Surgical Comparisons, *Mayo Clin. Proc.*, 52:85, 1977.

37 Spodick, D. H.: The Surgical Mystique and the Double Standard. Controlled Trials of Medical and Surgical Therapy for Cardiac Disease: Analysis, Hypothesis, Proposal, *Am. Heart J.*, 85:579, 1973.

38 Preston, T. A.: "Coronary Artery Surgery. A Critical Review," Raven Press, New York, 1977.

39 Preston, T. A.: Editorial. The Hazard of Poorly Controlled Studies in the Evaluation of Coronary Artery Surgery, *Chest*, 73:441, 1978.

40 Baum, M.: Surgery and Radiotherapy in Breast Cancer, *Semin. Oncol.,* 1:101, 1974.

41 Special Correspondence. A Debate on Coronary Bypass, *N. Engl. J. Med.,* 297:1464, 1977.

42 Takaro, T., Hultgren, H. N., and Lipton, M. J.: The V. A. Cooperative Randomized Study of Surgery for Coronary Arterial Occlusive Disease. II. Subgroup with Significant Main Left Lesions, *Circulation,* 54:(suppl. 3):107, 1976.

43 Bennett, D. J., Loop, F. D., Sheldon, W. C., and Effler, D. B.: Direct Myocardial Revascularization. Operative Mortality in the Cleveland Clinic Experience, *Cleve. Clin. Q.,* 41:51, 1974.

44 Greene, D. G.: Special Correspondence. A Debate on Coronary Bypass, *N. Engl. J. Med.,* 297:1467, 1977.

45 Varnauskas, E.: Symposium, Long-term Results of Coronary Surgery. VIII World Congress of Cardiology, September 18, 1978, Tokyo.

46 Killip, T.: Symposium, Long-term Results of Coronary Surgery. VIII World Congress of Cardiology, September 18, 1978, Tokyo.

47 Aronow, W. S., and Stemmer, E. A.: Two-year Follow-up of Angina Pectoris: Medical or Surgical Therapy, *Ann. Intern. Med.,* 82:208, 1975.

48 Hammermeister, K. E., DeRouen, T. A., Murray, J. A., and Dodge, H. T.: Effect of Aortocoronary Saphenous Vein Bypass Grafting on Death and Sudden Death, *Am. J. Cardiol.,* 39:925, 1977.

48a Hammermeister, K. E., DeRouen, T. A., and Dodge, H. T.: The Effect of Surgical Versus Medical Therapy on Survival of Patients with Coronary Disease. A Matched Pair Analysis of Non-randomized Cohorts, *Am. J. Cardiol.,* 41:356, 1978. (Abstract.)

49 Vismara, L. A., Miller, R. R., Price, J. E., Karem, R., DeMaria, A. N., and Mason, D. T.: Improved Longevity Due to Reduction of Sudden Death by Aortocoronary Bypass in Coronary Atherosclerosis. Prospective Evaluation of Medical Versus Surgical Therapy in Matched Patients with Multivessel Disease, *Am. J. Cardiol.,* 39:919, 1977.

50 Lawrie, G. M., Morris, G. C., Jr., Howell, J. F., Tredici, T., and Chapman, D. W.: Improved Survival After 5 Years in 1144 Patients After Coronary Bypass, *Am. J. Cardiol.,* 42:709, 1978.

51 Kirklin, J. W.: Research Related to Surgical Treatment in Coronary Artery Disease. Address, 30th Anniversary of American Heart Association and National Heart, Lung and Blood Institute, Washington, D.C., February 9, 1978.

52 Das Gupta, R., Greene, D. G., and Bunnell, I. L., quoted in Greene, D. G., and Bunnell, I. L.: Quantitative Left Ventriculography; Structure and Function of the Adult Human Left Ventricle in Health and Disease, in P. N. Yu

and J. F. Goodwin (eds.), "Progress in Cardiology," Vol. 4, Lea & Febiger, Philadelphia, 1975, p. 71.

53 Manley, J. C., King, J. F., Zeft, H. J., and Johnson, W. D.: The "Bad" Left Ventricle. Results of Coronary Surgery and Effect on Late Survival, *J. Thorac. Cardiovasc. Surg.,* 72:841, 1976.

54 Lajos, T. Z., Levinsky, L., Lee, A. B., Schimert, G., Greene, D. G., Bunnell, I. L., Arani, D. T., Visco, J. P., Tandon, R. N., Zimdahl, W. T., Kohn, R. M., and Bozer, J. M.: Refinements in Coronary Artery Surgery Contributing to Improved Survival, *Abstracts,* 1:0458, VIII World Congress of Cardiology, September 17-23, 1978, Tokyo.

55 Chalmers, T. C.: Randomization and Coronary Artery Surgery, *Ann. Thorac. Surg.,* 14:323, 1972.

56 Heng, M-K., Norris, R. M., Singh, B. N., and Partridge, J. B.: Prognosis in Unstable Angina, *Br. Heart J.,* 38:921, 1976.

57 Gazes, P. C., Mobley, E. M., Jr., Fanis, H. M., Jr., Duncan, R. C., and Humphries, G. B.: Preinfarction (Unstable) Angina—a Prospective Study—Ten Year Follow-up, *Circulation,* 48:331, 1973.

58 Krauss, K. R., Hutter, A. M., Jr., and DeSanctis, R. W.: Acute Coronary Insufficiency. Course and Follow-up, *Circulation,* 45, 46(suppl. 1):66, 1972.

59 Golding, L. A. R., Loop, F. D., Sheldon, W. C., Taylor, P. C., Groves, L. K., and Cosgrove, D. M.: Emergency Revascularization for Unstable Angina, *Circulation,* 58:1163, 1978.

60 Anderson, R. P., Rahimtoola, S. H., Bonchek, L.I., and Starr, A.: The Prognosis of Patients with Coronary Artery Disease After Coronary Bypass Operations. Time-related Progress of 532 Patients with Disabling Angina Pectoris, *Circulation,* 50:274, 1974.

61 Cameron, A., Kemp, H. G., Shimomura, S., Santilli, E., Green, G. E., and Hutchinson, J. E., III: Coronary Artery Bypass Surgery. Long-term Follow-up, *N.Y. State J. Med.,* 77:27, 1977.

62 Cohn, L. H., Boyden, C. M., and Collins, J. J., Jr.: Improved Long-term Survival After Aortocoronary Bypass for Advanced Coronary Artery Disease, *Am. J. Surg.,* 129:380, 1975.

63 Kemp, V. E., Szentpetery, S., Levinson, H. J., Mammana, R. B., and Lower, R. R.: Safety and Effectiveness of Coronary Artery Bypass for Angina Pectoris Judged by Life Table Analysis, *Am. J. Cardiol.,* 39:267, 1977. (Abstract.)

64 Hultgren, H. N.: Medical Versus Surgical Treatment of Unstable Angina, *Am. J. Cardiol.,* 38:479, 1976.

65 Greene, D. G., Carlisle, R., Grant, C., and Bunnell, I. L.: Estimation of Left Ventricular Volume by One-Plane Cineangiography, *Circulation,* 35:61, 1967.

Chapter 16

The Prolongation of Life by Coronary Bypass Surgery*

ROBERT J. HALL, M.D., VIRENDRA S. MATHUR, M.D.,
EFRAIN GARCIA, M.D., and
CARLOS M. De CASTRO, M.D.

INTRODUCTION

The diagnostic and therapeutic modalities in cardio-vascular medicine have undergone a radical change in the last two decades. During the last 8 years the increasing popularity and success of coronary artery bypass in direct myocardial revascularization have opened new horizons for patients suffering from serious coronary artery disease. The decrease of angina is so dramatic in most patients that some of the earliest reports,[1-5] although based on uncontrolled, nonrandomized studies, resulted in widespread acceptance of the procedure. Within the first 4 years of use of this technique, several centers reported encouraging results in the form of acceptable mortality risk and good symptomatic relief.[6-11] The results of the first prospective randomized study were reported in 1973[12] and published in 1975.[13] Although a relatively small number of patients were studied, the report documented the superiority of coronary bypass surgery over vigorous medical therapy in regard to both subjective and objective improvement. The uniform results reported by multiple centers[14-19] have helped resolve the issue of symptomatic improvement following coronary bypass surgery. It is now widely accepted that anginal symptoms are completely relieved in 60 to 75 percent of patients and that partial relief is experienced by another 15 to 20 percent.[20-29] The results of two multicenter studies have added support to these observations.[30,31] The expected duration of such improvement is unknown at this time.

The question of prolonged life as a result of coronary artery bypass is more difficult to answer, and the controversial issue has not yet been resolved to the satisfaction of all concerned physicians. In judging the efficacy of symptomatic relief provided by any treatment modality, the patients serve as their own control. Such a simple method cannot be employed in studying prolongation of life. The most acceptable method of resolving this issue is a well-controlled randomized study, but this is difficult to implement and has its own problems.[32-37] The discussion[25,26,38-42] that has followed publication of the preliminary results of the Veterans Administration cooperative study[43-46] highlights the resistance to widespread acceptance of the results even when a careful randomized study is conducted. The controversy that followed the publication of the University Group Diabetes Program study[47] several years ago still continues after 10 years, and the conclusions based on the study have not yet been accepted. Another method of resolving the issue is to compare current results with ''historic'' controls. The problem with this approach is that the medical management of patients with coronary disease is itself undergoing change,[48-53] and there are suggestions that the natural history of patients with coronary disease has changed in the last decade.[54-59] An additional criticism of comparisons with historic controls is that some of the patients were unsuitable for surgery because of more diffuse disease and would have had a worse prognosis.[60] Some institutions have retrospectively reanalyzed the data of nonoperated patients, and separate survival curves have been presented for operable and inoperable patients.[61] Comparison of the results of surgically treated patients with matched controls is another approach, but the validity of results depends on the quality of matching. Although matching is easy for some readily identifiable parameters, the unrecognized factors and those more subtle or difficult to quantify invariably will remain ''unmatched'' in such attempts.

Our purpose in this chapter is to present long-term survival data from a large population of patients who underwent coronary artery bypass at our institution and to scrutinize the details in smaller subsets to determine if certain conclusions are self-evident. Since this is neither a randomized nor a matched study, we have selected for careful analysis those subsets of patients whose medical prognosis has been uniformly reported to be poor in the absence of coronary bypass surgery.

MATERIAL AND METHODS

During the period 1968–1978,† 15,119 patients underwent direct revascularization of the ischemic myocar-

---

*From St. Luke's Episcopal Hospital, Texas Heart Institute, and Clayton Foundation for Cardiovascular Research, Houston.

†The data for calendar year 1978 are incomplete at present.

dium with autologous saphenous vein grafts at our institution. Among these, 13,004 patients underwent coronary artery bypass alone, and 2,115 had associated cardiac procedures. The early and late mortalities of this group are presented in Figs. 16-1 and 16-2. The early mortality declined with increasing experience and ranged between 2.0 and 2.5 percent in the last 3 years (Table 16-1).

TABLE 16-1
Patients undergoing coronary artery bypass* surgery

Year	Total no.	Early deaths (30 day)	Mortality
1970	181	19	10.5%
1971	741	55	7.4%
1972	794	54	6.8%
1973	1033	54	5.2%
1974	1297	41	3.2%
1975	1809	65	3.6%
1976	2404	59	2.5%
1977	2496	51	2.0%
1978†	2239	56	2.5%

*No associated major cardiac surgery. Several patients underwent associated noncardiac surgery.

†Complete data for 1978 not yet available.

For a more detailed analysis, we selected 846 consecutive and personally managed patients from one cardiology section who underwent coronary artery bypass alone from January 1970 through June 1976.[62,63] The clinical, electrocardiographic, and angiographic characteristics of this *consecutive* series of 846 patients are presented in Tables 16-2 to 16-4. Follow-up information is available on 825 patients (97.5 percent). Survival curves of various subsets of this population have been generated using an actuarial method[64] and form the basis of this report. All deaths, both cardiac and noncardiac, have been included. Our patient population was further analyzed by division into two equal time periods of 39 months each: from January 1970 through March 1973 (Group I, 252 patients) and April 1973 through June 1976 (Group II, 594 patients). The indication for surgery in 96.1 percent (813 of 846) patients was the presence of angina (not satisfactorily controlled with medical therapy) with or without symptoms of heart failure. The other 3.9 percent (33 of 846) of patients did not complain of exertional angina at the time of surgery but were found to have severe coronary disease. Surgery was recommended because these patients had either experienced multiple clinical episodes of infarction or unstable angina in the past or evidence of severe ischemia was present during exercise tests or both were present.

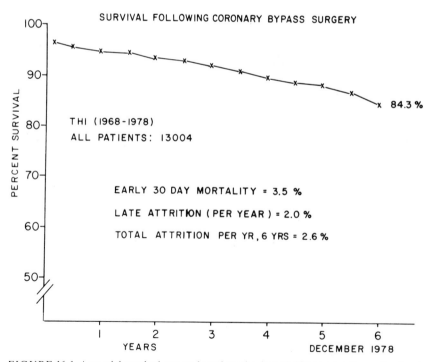

FIGURE 16-1 Actuarial survival curves based on the first 13,004 consecutive patients who underwent coronary bypass operation at Texas Heart Institute without associated cardiac operation. The data from 1978 is incomplete at present. Deaths from all causes (cardiac and noncardiac) have been included.

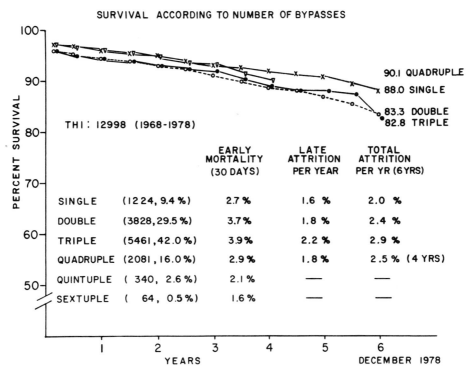

SURVIVAL ACCORDING TO NUMBER OF BYPASSES

		EARLY MORTALITY (30 DAYS)	LATE ATTRITION PER YEAR	TOTAL ATTRITION PER YR (6 YRS)
SINGLE	(1224, 9.4%)	2.7%	1.6%	2.0%
DOUBLE	(3828, 29.5%)	3.7%	1.8%	2.4%
TRIPLE	(5461, 42.0%)	3.9%	2.2%	2.9%
QUADRUPLE	(2081, 16.0%)	2.9%	1.8%	2.5% (4 YRS)
QUINTUPLE	(340, 2.6%)	2.1%	—	—
SEXTUPLE	(64, 0.5%)	1.6%	—	—

THI: 12998 (1968-1978)

90.1 QUADRUPLE
88.0 SINGLE
83.3 DOUBLE
82.8 TRIPLE

DECEMBER 1978

FIGURE 16-2 Actuarial curves of all Texas Heart Institute bypass patients according to the number of vessels bypassed. Survival curves reveal low early mortality for patients receiving four, five, or six bypasses and excellent long-term survival for patients receiving four bypasses. The number of patients with five or six bypasses available for follow-up is too small at this time to plot the survival curves.

TABLE 16-2
Clinical characteristics

	Total: 846 Jan. 1970–June 1976	Group I: 252 Jan. 1970–Mar. 1973	Group II: 594 Apr. 1973–June 1976
Males	87.5%	83.7%	89.1%
Females	12.5%	16.3%	10.9%
Average age	53		
Angina FC I*	3.9%	2.3%	4.5%
Angina FC II	14.7%	9.5%	16.8%
Angina FC III	62.3%	69.8%	59.1%
Angina FC IV	19.1%	18.2%	19.5%
Angina stable	39.1%	33.3%	41.6%
Angina unstable	60.9%	66.7%	58.4%
Angina unstable, FC IV	16.9%	15.9%	17.3%
History of MI	63.2%	62.7%	63.5%
History of CHF	15.4%	21.8%	12.6%
In past	11.2%	13.9%	10.1%
Current	4.2%	7.9%	2.5%
History of arrhythmia	1.3%	0.7%	1.5%
Associated risk factors			
Hypertension	34.2%	31.3%	35.4%
Diabetes	11.8%	12.3%	11.6%
Smoking	72.3%	74.6%	71.3%
Family history	57.3%	54.7%	58.5%
Cholesterol ≥ 300	26.2%	29.7%	24.6%
Triglycerides ≥ 150	51.2%	46.0%	53.4%

*FC, New York Heart Association functional class.

TABLE 16-3
Electrocardiographic features in 846 patients

Normal ECG	17.1%
Transmural myocardial infarction	69.5%
ST depression	46.6%
T wave abnormality	55.2%
Left ventricular hypertrophy	8.9%
1° AV block	4.7%
Right bundle branch block	0.8%
Left bundle branch block	1.2%
Arrhythmias	5.7%
Treadmill test*	
Positive	81.5%
Negative	4.5%
Borderline	5.5%
Indeterminate	8.4%

*Treadmill test performed in only 424 patients; severe or unstable symptoms prevented the test in majority of others.

Angiographic Methods

The angiograms were interpreted by at least three observers, and a consensus was obtained. A major vessel was considered critically diseased only if ≥ 75 percent reduction in diameter was present. The left ventriculograms were analyzed for ejection fraction as well as for wall motion abnormalities. The left ventricle was considered abnormal if global or regional contraction abnormality was present.

RESULTS

The early mortality (30-day) and 5- and 6-year actuarial survival for the total patient population and the early mortality and 4-year actuarial survival for Group II patients are presented in Tables 16-5 to 16-8. There were 25 early deaths within 30 days of surgery and 50 late deaths in 2- to 8-year follow-up. Twelve of the early deaths were among 252 patients in Group I, and 13 were among 594 patients in Group II (Table 16-5), with early mortality of 4.76 percent and 2.19 percent, respectively. There were 34 late deaths in Group I with 5- to 8-year follow-up, and 16 late deaths in Group II with 2- to 5-year follow-up. The 50 late deaths included 5 from malignancy, 1 from trauma, 5 from cerebrovascular accident, and 1 from renal failure. For actuarial survival, all deaths, both cardiac and noncardiac, have been included. The actuarial survival curves for the total population based on the number of vessels involved, the number of bypasses, the functional classification according to degree of angina, and the presence or absence of perioperative myocardial infarction are depicted in Figs. 16-3 to 16-7.

TABLE 16-4
Angiographic characteristics

	Total: 846 Jan. 1970–June 1976	Group I: 252 Jan. 1970–Mar. 1973	Group II: 594 Apr. 1973–June 1976
Major vessels (with stenosis ≥ 75%)			
One vessel	12.1%	14.3%	11.1%
Two vessels	33.5%	38.9%	31.1%
Three vessels	46.5%	35.3%	51.2%
Left main ± others	8.0%	11.5%	6.6%
Major vessels (with stenosis ≥ 50%)			
One vessel	6.0%	8.7%	4.9%
Two vessels	22.2%	26.6%	20.4%
Three vessels	56.9%	46.0%	61.5%
Left main ± others	14.9%	18.7%	13.3%
LV contraction abnormality	67.3%	54.0%	72.9%
Ejection fraction			
≥ 0.60	52.8%	52.8%	52.9%
≥ 0.45 to < 0.60	29.6%	29.0%	29.8%
≥ 0.30 to < 0.45	12.3%	11.1%	12.8%
< 0.30	5.2%	7.1%	4.4%
Bypasses performed			
One	7.8%	13.1%	5.6%
Two	38.8%	62.7%	28.6%
Three	45.2%	23.4%	54.4%
Four or more	8.2%	0.8%	11.3%

TABLE 16-5
Survival related to clinical characteristics

	Total: 846				Group II: 594		
	No. pts.	30-day mortality(%)	5-Year survival(%)	6-Year survival(%)	No. pts.	30-day mortality(%)	4-Year survival(%)
All patients	846	2.96	89.2	86.4	594	2.18	93.4
Males	740	2.57	89.6	87.1	529	1.89	93.5
Females	106	5.66	86.7	82.7	65	4.62	92.1
Angina FC*							
I	33	0.00	97.0	—	27	0.00	100.0
II	124	2.42	91.1	—	100	0.00	98.9
III	527	2.66	89.0	86.3	351	2.85	92.1
IV	162	4.94	87.5	87.5	116	2.59	91.8
I and II	157	1.91	91.4	—	127	0.00	—
III and IV	689	3.19	88.6	86.2	467	2.78	—
Angina patterns							
Stable	331	3.32	86.6	86.6	247	2.02	93.9
Progressive/unstable	515	2.72	90.2	86.0	347	2.31	92.8
Prolonged coronary insufficiency							
Single episode	169	1.78	92.5	92.5			
Recurrent episodes	128	3.91	85.9	82.6			
No episodes	549	3.10	89.1	85.8			
Severe, unstable FC IV	143	3.50	88.8	88.8	103	1.94	91.6
All others	703	2.84	89.1	85.8	491	2.24	93.9
History of myocardial infarction							
None		3.86	93.3	89.7	217	4.15	94.9
Yes	535	2.43	86.9	84.6	377	1.07	92.8
One episode	390	2.56	86.6	83.0			
Two episodes	115	1.74	92.4	92.4			
Three episodes	21	4.76	82.1	—			
Four episodes	9	0.00	—	—			
Time of myocardial infarction							
Within 1 month	27	0.00	76.5	76.5			
Between 1–2 months	30	6.66	93.3	93.3			
Between 2–6 months	126	0.79	86.8	86.8			
Within 6 months	183	1.64	86.2	86.2			
Beyond 6 months	352	2.84	86.2	84.3			
Congestive heart failure							
None	716	3.21	93.3	91.5	519	2.50	—
By history	95	1.05	79.9	72.1	60	0.00	86.4
Current congestive heart failure	35	2.85	53.6	53.6	15	0.00	80.1
By history or current	130	1.54	72.7	66.8	75	0.00	84.9
Risk factors							
Hypertension	289	3.46	90.8	88.4	210	2.38	94.6
No hypertension	557	2.69	88.6	85.6			
Diabetes	100	8.00	80.9	75.7	69	4.35	91.1
No diabetes	746	2.28	90.5	88.0	525	1.90	93.7
Smoking	612	2.61	88.7	85.0			
No smoking	234	3.85	91.0	91.0			
Cholesterol ≥ 300	222	1.80	87.3	87.3			
Cholesterol < 300	624	3.37	90.0	85.9			
Triglycerides ≥ 150	433	3.93	87.2	82.6			
Triglycerides < 150	413	1.94	91.1	89.8			
Family history +	485	2.68	90.0	87.5			
Family history −	361	3.32	88.4	85.0			
Associated diseases							
Pulmonary +	71	4.23	83.0	83.0			
Pulmonary −	775	2.84	89.8	86.6			
Cerebrovascular +	39	2.56	90.2	54.1			
Cerebrovascular −	807	2.97	89.2	87.0			
Renal +	19	10.53	71.6	71.6			
Renal −	827	2.78	89.6	86.7			

*FC, New York Heart Association function class.

TABLE 16-6
Survival related to electrocardiographic findings

	Total: 846				Group II: 594		
	No. pts.	30-day mortality(%)	5-Year survival(%)	6-Year survival(%)	No. pts.	30-day mortality(%)	4-Year survival(%)
Resting electrocardiogram							
Normal	145	2.76	96.5	92.1			
Abnormal	701	2.99	87.7	85.1			
Transmural myocardial infarction	588	2.55	88.9	85.8	416	1.45	93.8
LBBB (with myocardial infarction)	9	0.00	—	—			
Myocardial infarction (including LBBB)	597	2.51	88.8	85.9			
No transmural myocardial infarction	249	4.02	90.4	87.9	178	3.93	92.5
LVH +	75	4.00	80.6	74.8			
LVH −	625	2.88	88.5	86.5			
Treadmill test (TMT)							
Not done*	422	4.03	84.5	82.3			
Done preop	424	1.89	95.1	91.2			
Exercise duration							
< Bruce stage I	96	2.08	96.8	91.4			
< Bruce stage II	140	2.14	93.1	86.4			
< Bruce stage III	82	1.22	94.8	94.8			
< Bruce stage IV	33	0.00	100.0	—			
Heart rate achieved							
≤ 66% of PMHR†	167	2.99	93.4	90.4			
67–80%	130	0.77	94.4	86.5			
81–90%	73	2.74	97.3	97.3			
≥ 91%	54	0.00	100.0	—			
Ischemic response							
Positive	341	1.76	94.9	90.3			
Negative	19	0.00	100.0	—			
Borderline	23	0.00	100.0	—			
Indeterminate	35	5.71	90.9	—			

*In most instances, the patients were considered too symptomatic or unstable to perform a treadmill test.
†PMHR, predicted maximal heart rate.

TABLE 16-7
Survival related to angiographic data

	Total: 846				Group II: 594		
	No. pts.	30-day mortality(%)	5-Year survival(%)	6-Year survival(%)	No. pts.	30-day mortality(%)	4-Year survival(%)
Major vessels stenosed (≥ 75%)							
One vessel	102	1.96	95.0	90.9	66	1.52	96.9
Two vessels	283	2.47	91.2	91.2	185	2.16	93.0
Three vessels	393	3.82	86.5	81.9	304	2.63	93.8
Left main ± others	68	1.47	84.8	79.0	39	0.00	88.1
All pts. without LM	778	3.08	89.6	87.2	555	2.34	93.8
LV contraction							
Normal	277	4.33	93.1	89.0	161	4.35	94.3
Abnormal	569	2.28	86.4	85.0	433	1.39	93.1
Vessels and LV contraction							
One with normal	51	3.91	96.1	90.3	27	3.70	96.3
One with abnormal	51	0.00	93.8	93.8	39	0.00	97.3
Two with normal	106	3.77	92.7	92.7	59	5.08	93.2
Two with abnormal	177	1.69	89.8	89.8	126	0.79	92.4
Three with normal	101	5.94	90.6	79.6	66	4.55	93.7
Three with abnormal	292	3.08	84.0	84.0	238	2.10	93.7
Left main with normal	19	0.00	100.0	100.0	9	0.00	—
Left main with abnormal	49	2.04	77.9	69.2	30	0.00	84.3
Three vessels or LM, normal	120	5.00	92.1	83.8	75	4.00	94.4
Three vessels or LM, abnormal	341	2.93	83.4	80.6	268	1.87	92.6

TABLE 16-7 *Continued*
Survival related to angiographic data

	No. pts.	30-day mortality(%)	5-Year survival(%)	6-Year survival(%)	No. pts.	30-day mortality(%)	4-Year survival(%)
	Total: 846				**Group II: 594**		
All without LM, normal	258	4.65	92.5	88.0	152	4.60	94.0
All without LM, abnormal	520	2.31	87.3	87.3	403	1.49	93.7
Ejection fraction							
≥0.60	447	3.58	94.2	90.3	314	3.50	94.5
≥0.45 to <0.60	250	2.40	90.2	90.2	177	1.13	93.5
≥0.30 to <0.45	104	1.92	78.4	71.6	76	0.00	93.9
<0.30	44	2.27	60.2	60.2	26	0.00	76.6
≥0.45	697	3.16	92.8	90.3	491	2.65	94.1
<0.45	148	2.03	72.8	68.4	102	0.00	89.8
One vessel, EF ≥0.45	99	2.02	97.0	92.8	64	1.56	98.5
One vessel, EF <0.45	3	0.00	—	—	2	0.00	—
Two vessels, EF ≥0.45	246	2.44	93.6	93.6	162	2.47	93.2
Two vessels, EF <0.45	37	2.70	75.3	75.3	23	0.00	91.3
Three vessels, EF ≥0.45	298	4.36	91.1	84.9	233	3.43	93.9
Three vessels, EF <0.45	94	2.13	73.5	73.5	70	0.00	92.8
Left main, EF ≥0.45	54	1.85	90.2	90.2	32	0.00	91.7
Left main, EF <0.45	14	0.00	66.5	—	7	0.00	—
Functional class III (with EF ≥0.45)							
One vessel	50	0.00	100.0	94.5	26	0.00	100.0
Two vessels	153	2.61	93.4	93.4	93	3.23	93.4
Three vessels	189	4.23	89.3	85.2	144	4.86	91.7
Left main	36	0.00	91.4	91.4	20	0.00	92.0
(with EF ≤0.45)							
One vessel	—	—	—	—	—	—	—
Two vessels	23	0.00	83.1	83.1	16	0.00	93.8
Three vessels	65	3.08	72.0	72.0	46	0.00	87.6
Left main	9	0.00	—	—	5	0.00	—
Number of bypasses							
One	66	0.00	93.1	88.9	33	0.00	100.0
Two	328	2.13	89.1	87.0	170	1.18	94.6
Three	382	4.19	87.9	83.5	323	2.79	91.5
Four or more	69	2.90	97.0	—	67	2.99	96.9
Bypasses and ventricular abn.							
Single, normal	37	0.00	97.0	90.9	16	0.00	100.0
Single, abnormal	29	0.00	85.3	85.3	17	0.00	100.0
Double, normal	116	2.59	93.4	91.2	47	4.26	93.4
Double, abnormal	212	1.89	85.7	83.8	123	0.00	94.5
Triple, normal	108	7.41	91.6	81.9	83	4.82	93.9
Triple, abnormal	274	2.92	86.1	86.1	240	2.08	90.6
Quadruple, normal	16	6.25	—	—	15	6.66	—
Quadruple, abnormal	53	1.89	—	—	52	1.92	98.0
Periop myocardial infarction							
Yes	93	9.68	85.6	80.7	61	9.84	88.2
No	753	2.12	89.7	87.3	533	1.31	94.1
No preop or periop myocardial infarction	210	2.38	91.8	91.8	152	2.63	93.0

TABLE 16-8
Survival related to vessels involved if criterion for stenosis is ≥ 50% diameter reduction

	No. pts.	30-day mortality(%)	5-Year survival(%)	6-Year survival(%)	No. pts.	30-day mortality(%)	4-Year survival(%)
	Total: 846				**Group II: 594**		
One vessel (≥ 50%)	51	0.00	98.0	90.7	29	0.00	100.0
Two vessels	188	1.60	92.4	92.4	121	2.48	92.9
Three vessels	481	3.33	88.9	85.6	365	2.74	93.3
Left main ± others	126	4.76	81.7	77.2	79	0.00	92.0
All patients without left main disease	720	2.64	90.8	88.3	515	2.52	93.7

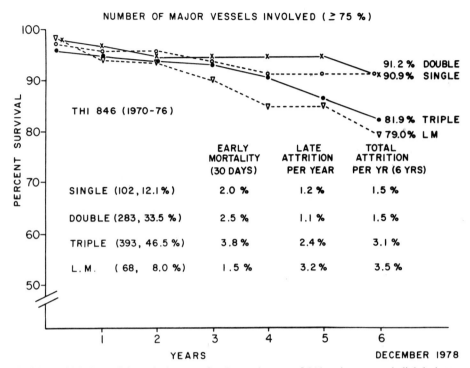

FIGURE 16-3 Actuarial survival curves for the total group of 846 patients reveal slightly better survival for patients with single- and double-vessel disease (≥ 75% diameter reduction). Early mortality includes the surgical mortality and all deaths within 30 days of surgery. Total attrition rate during follow-up has been derived on the basis of actuarial survival at 6 years. Late attrition has been calculated by subtracting early mortality from total mortality.

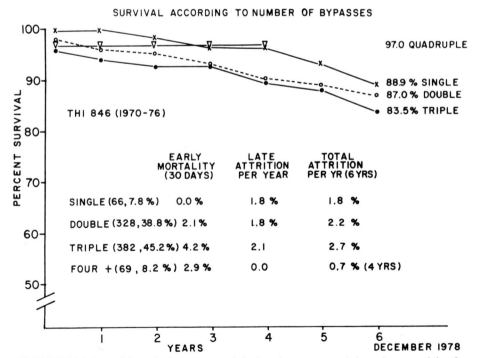

FIGURE 16-4 Actuarial survival curves reveal the best long-term result in patients receiving four or more bypasses. The life expectancies in other subgroups are very similar to each other.

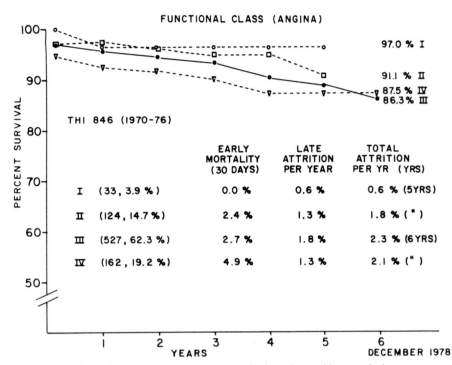

FIGURE 16-5 Survival curves show the best results in patients with no anginal symptoms at the time of surgery. The differences between long-term survival of patients with NYHA functional classes II, III, and IV are very minor.

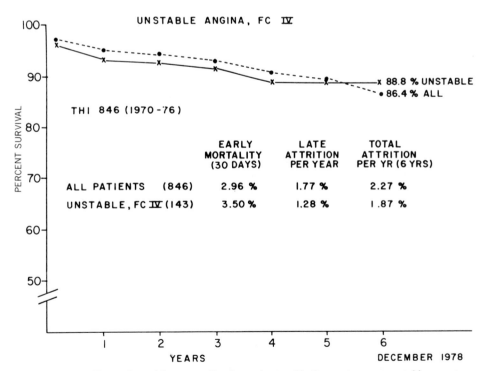

FIGURE 16-6 The early and late mortality for patients with the most severe unstable symptoms, i.e., recurrent angina at rest, is very similar to that of the entire group.

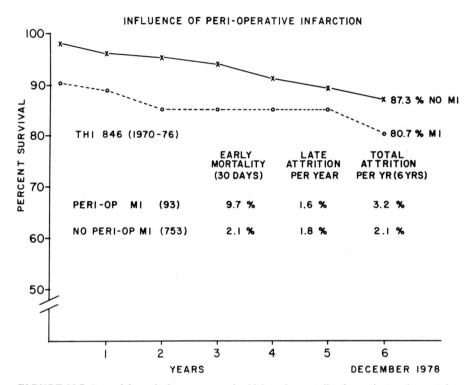

FIGURE 16-7 Actuarial survival curves reveal a high early mortality for patients who sustain a perioperative myocardial infarction, but the late attrition rate is similar to that of the rest of the population. Perioperative infarction was diagnosed if any of the following criteria were met: (1) diagnostic evolutionary changes in the electrocardiogram; (2) increase in enzymes beyond our accepted level for these surgical patients, i.e., SGOT >200, LDH >500, and CPK >500 units; and (3) postmortem evidence of new infarction in the fatal cases.

DISCUSSION

Survival

OVERALL SURVIVAL

In the entire group of our patients (Fig. 16-6), the early mortality was 2.96 percent, and the 6-year survival was 86.4 percent. After the 30-day period, the calculated late annual attrition rate was 1.8 percent per year. Studies of the natural history of patients with coronary artery disease have uniformly shown a much higher attrition rate. Data from several centers[65-75] summarized by Reeves in 1974,[76] Humphries in 1977,[77] and Green et al. in 1978[78] suggest that in patients with documented coronary disease, annual attrition is expected to be between 2 and 14 percent per year, depending on the extent of disease. In a recent report from the Cleveland Clinic, Proudfit et al.[61] found the 6-year survival to be 60 percent and the 10-year survival to be 43 percent in patients with documented coronary disease who were not operated on. In the multicenter VA cooperative study,[44] the overall survival of the patients randomized to "modern" medical treatment, although better than the Cleveland data,

was still far worse than that of our surgical series. The 4-year survival in the medically treated VA series was 83 percent as compared to 90.8 percent in our by-passed patients.

PATIENTS WITH LEFT MAIN CORONARY ARTERY DISEASE

The serious prognosis of patients with left main coronary disease was recognized early in the era of coronary angiography. The hazards during cardiac catheterization, the high mortality of medical treatment alone, and the improved survival with surgery were reported several years ago.[79-87] The results of the VA cooperative study confirmed the poor prognosis of the group who received "modern" medical treatment and revealed the superiority of surgical management.[46,88] In another randomized multicenter study initiated in 1972 and sponsored by the National Heart, Lung and Blood Institute,[30,89,90] all patients with critical stenosis of the left main coronary artery were excluded from randomization, and coronary bypass surgery was recommended because of the widespread belief even then that coronary artery bypass improved survival as well as quality of life in such patients. Our data (Fig. 16-3) support these observations. There were 68 patients who had critical stenosis of the left main coronary artery based on ≥75 percent luminal diameter reduction. Of these patients, associated critical disease in other major vessels was present in 65 (95 percent): one other vessel was involved in 12 patients, two other vessels in 18, and three in 35 patients. The early mortality was 1.5 percent, and the late attrition rate in the subsequent follow-up period was 3.2 percent per year. The 6-year survival was 79 percent. This compares favorably with less than 50 percent survival at 6 years reported from the Cleveland Clinic[61] for unoperated patients and about 65 percent survival at 4 years reported from the medically treated VA group.[44] The criterion for stenosis was ≥50 percent in the Cleveland Clinic and the VA series.

PATIENTS WITH TRIPLE-VESSEL DISEASE

Total group The survival rates of medically treated patients with triple-vessel disease have been uniformly poor in every reported study. In the patients randomized to medical therapy in the multicenter VA cooperative study,[44] 4-year survival was reported to be less than 75 percent, despite exclusion of several high-risk patient categories and the use of ≥50 percent stenosis as the criterion for critical disease. The survival rates in other medical series are worse, as has been pointed out in the VA report,[44] and Proudfit et al. report a survival of approximately 50 percent at 4 years and <40 percent at 6 years.[61] In comparison, using ≥75 percent diameter reduction as the criterion of stenosis, the survival in our surgical series of patients with triple-vessel disease is much better, being, among 393 such patients, 90.9 percent at 4 years and 81.9 percent at 6 years (Fig. 16-3). If ≥50 percent stenosis is used as the criterion of critical disease, there were 481 patients with triple-vessel disease whose survival was 91.3 percent at 4 years and 85.6 percent at 6 years (Table 16-8).

Group II The quality of both surgical technique and diagnostic studies has improved steadily during the last 10 years. This is reflected in the declining early mortality reported by many institutions,[91,92] including our own (Table 16-1), and an improved long-term sur-

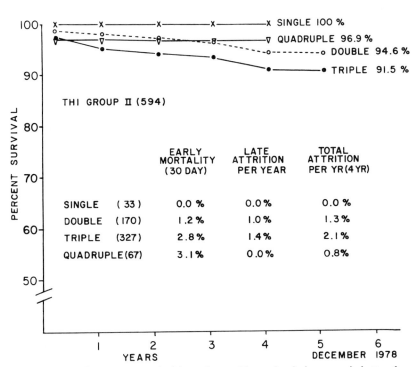

NUMBER OF BYPASSES

SINGLE 100 %
QUADRUPLE 96.9 %
DOUBLE 94.6 %
TRIPLE 91.5 %

THI GROUP II (594)

	EARLY MORTALITY (30 DAY)	LATE ATTRITION PER YEAR	TOTAL ATTRITION PER YR (4 YR)
SINGLE (33)	0.0 %	0.0%	0.0%
DOUBLE (170)	1.2%	1.0%	1.3%
TRIPLE (327)	2.8%	1.4%	2.1%
QUADRUPLE (67)	3.1%	0.0%	0.8%

YEARS
DECEMBER 1978

FIGURE 16-8 Long-term survival in patients with quadruple bypasses is better than survival in patients with double and triple bypasses, even though the disease in these patients is worse. This may be a reflection of more complete revascularization in patients receiving quadruple bypass surgery.

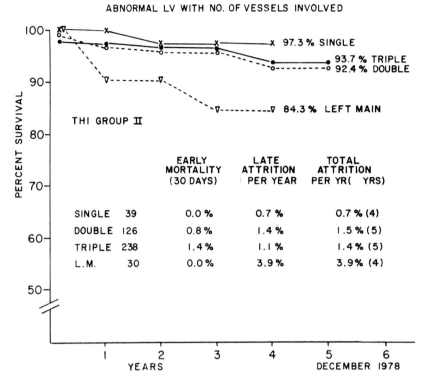

ABNORMAL LV WITH NO. OF VESSELS INVOLVED

		EARLY MORTALITY (30 DAYS)	LATE ATTRITION PER YEAR	TOTAL ATTRITION PER YR(YRS)
SINGLE	39	0.0 %	0.7 %	0.7 % (4)
DOUBLE	126	0.8%	1.4 %	1.5 % (5)
TRIPLE	238	1.4 %	1.1 %	1.4 % (5)
L.M.	30	0.0 %	3.9 %	3.9% (4)

FIGURE 16-9 Actuarial survival curves reveal very similar attrition rates in patients with single-, double-, or triple-vessel disease. All these patients are in Group II and have left ventricular contraction abnormalities.

vival (Table 16-5). Also, more complete surgical revascularization has been done in the last 5 years.[93] In Group II (March 1973 through June 1976), among the 594 patients, three or more bypasses were done in 394 patients (66.3 percent). This is in contrast to only 24.2 percent (61 of 252) of Group I patients who received three or more bypasses. Of 69 patients receiving four or more bypasses, 67 were in Group II (Fig. 16-8).

In 304 patients with triple-vessel disease in Group II (Table 16-7), the early mortality was 2.6 percent, and late attrition was only 0.9 percent per year; thus the 4-year survival was 93.8 percent. This long-term survival rate is strikingly better than the anticipated survival rate of nonoperated patients. The 4-year survival of 93.8 percent is so similar to the expected survival of "healthy" individuals in the same age group[55-59] that one finds it hard not to conclude that bypass surgery does prolong survival in this subset of patients with advanced disease. The data from several other surgical reports are remarkably similar to ours.[94-101]

Associated abnormal ventricle The unfavorable influence of abnormalities of left ventricular function on long-term survival has been well recognized.[66-77] Therefore, we studied this particular subset of patients

who are expected to have a poor prognosis. There were 238 patients in Group II with previous infarction and localized or generalized abnormality of left ventricular contraction and triple-vessel disease. The early mortality in this group was 1.4 percent, the late attrition was 1.1 percent per year, and the 5-year survival was 93.7 percent (Fig. 16-9). The survival in the nonsurgical series from Cleveland Clinic in patients with triple-vessel disease and abnormal ventricles ranges from approximately 18 percent to 52 percent at 5 years, depending on the degree of abnormality.[61] The data also were analyzed with respect to overall ventricular function (Fig. 16-10). There were 70 patients with three-vessel disease and moderate or severe left ventricular dysfunction whose ejection fraction was <0.45. There were no early deaths in this group, and late attrition was 1.4 percent per year, with a 5-year survival of 92.8 percent.

Associated severe symptoms Data are insufficient regarding the influence of severity of symptoms on the anticipated natural history of coronary artery disease. Webster et al. reported a relationship between the severity of angina and survival,[68] although Humphries et al. did not find such a correlation.[74] The recent report from Cleveland Clinic confirms that the worst prognosis is in the most symptomatic patients but reveals only minor differences between patients in functional classes II and III.[61] Our data (Fig. 16-11) reveal that following surgery, the 5-year survival is above 91 percent in all patients irrespective of preoperative functional class.

In the Cleveland Clinic group, there were 64 patients with triple-vessel disease and severe angina (functional classes III and IV), and 5-year survival was only 37.5 percent. In our total series, 254 patients had triple-vessel disease and functional class III angina; the ventricle was normal or mildly abnormal, with an ejection fraction ≥0.45 in 189 patients, while the ejection fraction was <0.45 in 65 patients. The 5-year survival in these two subsets was 89.3 percent and 72.0 percent, respectively (Table 16-7). In Group II, there were 190 patients with three-vessel disease and class III angina. The 5-year survival was 91.7 percent in those with an ejection fraction ≥0.45 (Fig. 16-12) and 87.6 percent in those with an ejection fraction <0.45 (Table 16-7). These data reflect remarkable survival rates following bypass among patients with severe anatomic and symptomatic disease, especially in those patients who were operated on during the second half of our study.

PATIENTS WITH ASSOCIATED SEVERE UNSTABLE ANGINA

The results of an additional subset of patients whose symptoms were unstable and who were in functional class IV were analyzed. Such patients generally have a poor prognosis.[102] There were 103 such patients in Group II who were operated on after March 1973. The early mortality in this latter group was 1.9 percent, late attrition was 1.3 percent per year, and five-year survival was 91.6 percent. This survival rate is so close to the overall rate (Fig. 16-13) that the poorer prognosis of these patients appears to have been neutralized by the surgical intervention, and life expectancy has been restored to a level expected before development of such symptoms.

PATIENTS WITH DOUBLE- AND SINGLE-VESSEL DISEASE

Because of our stringent criteria for coronary artery bypass, there were fewer patients with single- or double-vessel involvement (Table 16-4) than with triple-vessel disease. The actuarial survival rate of these patients was either similar to or better than that of

THREE VESSEL DISEASE (≥75% STENOSIS)

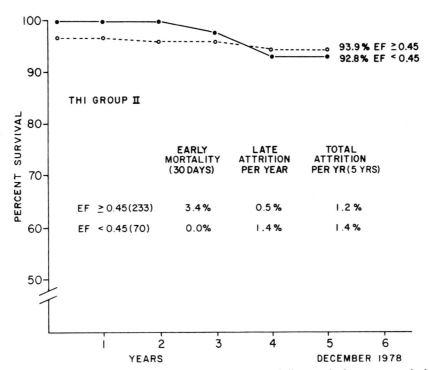

FIGURE 16-10 In Group II patients with three-vessel disease, the long-term survival rates are very similar whether ejection fraction is less than or greater than 0.45.

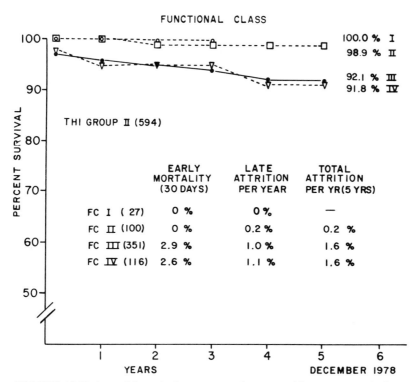

FUNCTIONAL CLASS

100.0 % I
98.9 % II
92.1 % III
91.8 % IV

THI GROUP II (594)

	EARLY MORTALITY (30 DAYS)	LATE ATTRITION PER YEAR	TOTAL ATTRITION PER YR(5 YRS)
FC I (27)	0 %	0 %	—
FC II (100)	0 %	0.2 %	0.2 %
FC III (351)	2.9 %	1.0 %	1.6 %
FC IV (116)	2.6 %	1.1 %	1.6 %

PERCENT SURVIVAL

YEARS   DECEMBER 1978

FIGURE 16-11 Actuarial survival curves reveal very good long-term survival rates even in patients with severe symptons. There is no difference in patients with NYHA functional class III or IV.

patients with triple-vessel disease (Table 16-7). The long-term survival was equally good in patients with low or adequate ejection fractions (Fig. 16-14). The survival rates were better than those of the nonsurgical patients from the Cleveland Clinic in all the categories analyzed.[61] The survival rate of our surgical patients was also better than that of the patients randomized to medical treatment in the VA cooperative study,[44] which as was pointed out in the VA report, was the best survival reported for medically treated patients. Our experience is very similar to that reported by other surgical centers. Since the prognosis in patients with single- and double-vessel disease treated medically is better than that of patients with triple-vessel or left main coronary artery disease, the difference in their life expectancy as compared to "normal" persons is less striking. Therefore, it will be necessary to follow these patients for a longer time to document improved life survival with surgery.

Is Improved Survival the Result of Coronary Artery Bypass?

While the data from our surgical series, as well as that from many other leading centers, leave little doubt that patients who undergo coronary artery bypass enjoy a

near normal life expectancy, a valid question is, What would have happened to these same patients if medical treatment alone had been continued? Because we did not have a control population in our series, we cannot answer that question precisely. We do know that in every reported series of patients with similar disease treated medically, survival has been much worse. Further evidence supporting prolongation of life after bypass surgery can be found by analyzing our data from two additional aspects: first, from analysis of the degree of completeness of revascularization, and second, from analysis of subsets of patients in whom progressive graduations of disease are known, from all previous studies, to adversely affect life survival. If such adverse effects upon survival are no longer evident following bypass surgery, a favorable influence of surgery must be strongly assumed.

LONGEVITY IN RELATION TO THE EXTENT OF REVASCULARIZATION

In every report dealing with the natural history of patients with coronary disease, the fact that survival is related to the extent of anatomic disease has clearly emerged. Our data reveal that not only is the life survival similar in patients receiving one, two, or three bypasses, but the best survival is in those who receive four or more bypasses and have the most complete revascularization in the presence of more extensive disease (Figs. 16-2, 16-4, and 16-8). Among Group II patients (Fig. 16-8), the subset of 67 patients with quadruple bypasses had a 4-year survival of 96.9 percent, an early mortality of 3.1 percent, and no late deaths.

LONGEVITY IN RELATION TO COMPLETE VERSUS INCOMPLETE REVASCULARIZATION

Of the 594 patients in Group II, 484 received the same number of bypasses as were planned. The 4-year survival in this group was 94.0 percent, with an early mortality of 2.1 percent and a late attrition rate of 0.8 percent per year (Fig. 16-15). In comparison, there were 62 patients in whom one less bypass was performed than planned because of poor accessibility of that vessel, even though it was considered suitable angiographically. In this group, the early mortality was 4.8 percent, late attrition was 1.4 percent per year, and 4-year survival was 88.4 percent.

If the same data are examined in another manner, there were 370 patients who received a bypass to every diseased major vessel and 130 patients in whom one major diseased vessel was not bypassed. The 5-year survival in the former was 95.1 percent and that in the latter was 86.7 percent (Fig. 16-16). We have not performed angiography routinely after surgery to ascertain the frequency of patent bypasses and true complete revascularization. It is interesting that despite this, a difference between results of patients undergoing attempted complete versus incomplete revascularization is noticeable. Boake et al. have reported similar observations.[93]

PROGNOSIS OF PATIENTS WITH SINGLE-, DOUBLE-, OR TRIPLE-VESSEL DISEASE

As previously mentioned, and according to every major report,[65-78] the survival of medically treated patients correlates with the number of vessels involved. If bypass surgery did not influence survival, this relationship should still hold true following bypass. In the patients operated upon in the second half of our

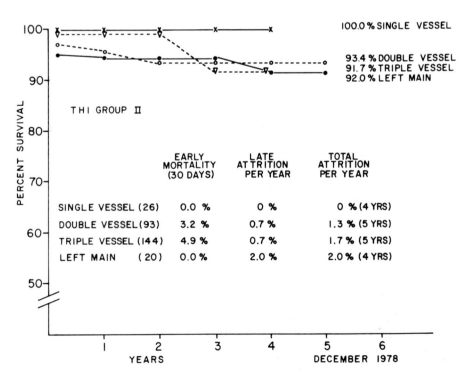

FUNCTIONAL CLASS III WITH >EF 0.45

	EARLY MORTALITY (30 DAYS)	LATE ATTRITION PER YEAR	TOTAL ATTRITION PER YEAR
SINGLE VESSEL (26)	0.0 %	0 %	0 % (4 YRS)
DOUBLE VESSEL (93)	3.2 %	0.7 %	1.3 % (5 YRS)
TRIPLE VESSEL (144)	4.9 %	0.7 %	1.7 % (5 YRS)
LEFT MAIN (20)	0.0 %	2.0 %	2.0 % (4 YRS)

100.0 % SINGLE VESSEL
93.4 % DOUBLE VESSEL
91.7 % TRIPLE VESSEL
92.0 % LEFT MAIN

THI GROUP II

DECEMBER 1978

FIGURE 16-12 Long-term survival rates in patients with NYHA functional class III angina are plotted here, according to the number of vessels involved (only those with ejection fraction ≥ 0.45). The attrition rates are similar for patients with left main, triple- or double-vessel disease.

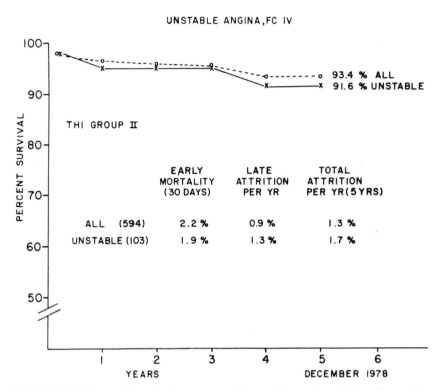

UNSTABLE ANGINA, FC IV

THI GROUP II

	EARLY MORTALITY (30 DAYS)	LATE ATTRITION PER YR	TOTAL ATTRITION PER YR (5 YRS)
ALL (594)	2.2 %	0.9 %	1.3 %
UNSTABLE (103)	1.9 %	1.3 %	1.7 %

93.4 % ALL
91.6 % UNSTABLE

YEARS — DECEMBER 1978

FIGURE 16-13 Actuarial survival curves reveal the attrition rate in patients with unstable and severe NYHA FC IV symptoms to be very similar to that in the total population of Group II patients.

study period, the 4-year survival for those with single-, double-, and triple-vessel disease was, respectively, 96.9 percent, 93.0 percent, and 93.8 percent (Table 16-7). In patients with abnormal ventricles and single-, double-, and triple-vessel disease, the 4-year survival figures were 97.3 percent, 92.4 percent, and 93.7 percent (Fig. 16-9). Thus, even with abnormal ventricles, patients with triple-vessel disease survive as long as patients with double-vessel disease and almost as long as patients with single-vessel disease. The elimination of the anticipated difference is strongly suggestive of the favorable influence of bypass surgery.

PROGNOSIS OF PATIENTS WITH NORMAL AND ABNORMAL VENTRICLES

Another fact that has emerged from the natural history studies is that patients with coronary artery disease and normal ventricles have a better prognosis than those with varying degrees of dysfunction.[67-77] If bypass surgery has no role in improving survival, these differences should persist following surgery. While this appears to hold true in the first few years of bypass experience,[62] particularly among patients operated on

in the first half of our study, this difference appears to have been eliminated in the second half of our study with improved diagnostic and surgical techniques and efforts at more complete revascularization. We analyzed this aspect of the data in several ways. As shown in Fig. 16-17, the 5-year survival for patients with normal left ventricles is 94.3 percent, and for those with abnormal ventricles, it is 93.1 percent. If patients with triple-vessel disease are considered, the 4-year survival is 93.7 percent in those with normal as well as in those with abnormal ventricles (Table 16-7)—a remarkable finding. Based on ejection fraction, Group II patients with normal (≥ 0.60), mildly abnormal (≥ 0.45 to <0.60), or moderately abnormal (≥ 0.30 to <0.45) ventricular function have similar long-term survival rates. The 4-year survival rates are 94.5 percent, 93.5 percent, and 93.9 percent, respectively (Table 16-7). In patients with severe abnormality (<30), the 3-year survival rate is 91.9 percent but falls to 76.6 percent in the fourth year (Table 16-7). In patients with triple-vessel disease, the 4-year survival rates were 93.9 percent and 92.8 percent for patients with ejection fractions of ≥ 0.45 and <0.45, respectively (Fig. 16-10).

PROGNOSIS IN PATIENTS WITH OR WITHOUT PREVIOUS INFARCTION

Patients with symptomatic coronary disease who have sustained a previous myocardial infarction are expected to carry a poorer prognosis than patients without prior infarction.[103-105] When the data from the present series are examined, this difference was eliminated. In the total series, the 6-year survival rates were 85.9 percent for patients with and 87.9 percent for patients without prior infarction (Fig. 16-18). In Group II, the 5-year survival rates were 93.8 percent and 92.5 percent for similar patients (Fig. 16-19). We have further analyzed the patients with prior infarction in Group II according to ejection fraction. As seen in Fig. 16-20, the long-term survival is similar in all the patients in this population regardless of the overall ventricular function.

All these observations suggest that the survival rates for all patients who undergo coronary bypass surgery tend to be close—approximately 92 to 95 percent at 5 years—irrespective of the extent and type of disease present before surgery. We believe this serves as strong circumstantial evidence that coronary bypass favorably influences survival in patients whose natural history would predict it to be worse.

Why Have the Randomized Studies Not Confirmed Improved Survival?

A compelling argument against the claim of improved survival following bypass surgery is the failure of randomized studies to confirm it. The results of two multicenter[43-46,89,90] and three single-institution prospective randomized studies[17,18,106-108] in this country have been reported, and short-term results from others abroad also have been reported.[109-112]

VETERANS ADMINISTRATION COOPERATIVE STUDY

In the often quoted VA cooperative study, the data pertaining to the group with the most severe disease, namely left main coronary artery disease, have confirmed the improved survival experienced by the surgical cohort.[43-46,88] The data from one hospital that contributed 20.3 percent (121 of 596) of patients for the study also suggest improved survival in the surgical group as a whole, after excluding patients with left main disease.[113] Why do the data from the other contributing VA hospitals fail to confirm this difference? Following publication of the results, many of the

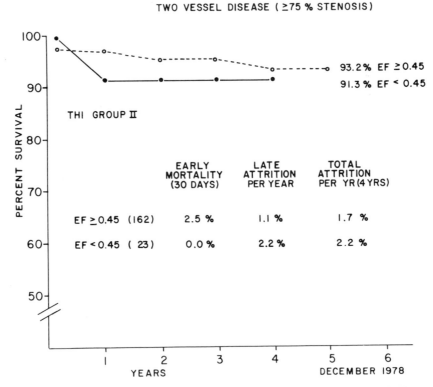

TWO VESSEL DISEASE (≥75 % STENOSIS)

FIGURE 16-14 Long-term survival for patients with two-vessel disease is plotted. There is no difference between the two subsets based on ejection fraction.

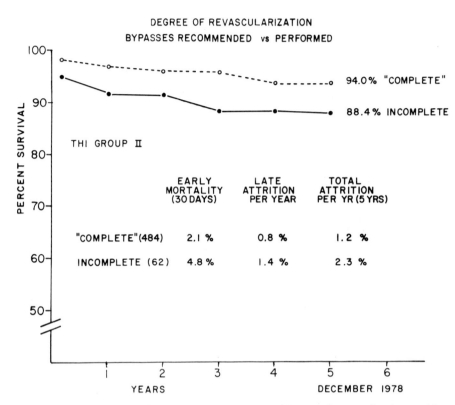

DEGREE OF REVASCULARIZATION

BYPASSES RECOMMENDED vs PERFORMED

	EARLY MORTALITY (30 DAYS)	LATE ATTRITION PER YEAR	TOTAL ATTRITION PER YR (5 YRS)
"COMPLETE" (484)	2.1 %	0.8 %	1.2 %
INCOMPLETE (62)	4.8 %	1.4 %	2.3 %

FIGURE 16-15 Actuarial survival curves show that the early mortality as well as late attrition rate is lower in patients who undergo more complete revascularization.

shortcomings of the study have been discussed in the correspondence section of various medical journals.[38] The criteria for inclusion in the VA cooperative study were very stringent in order to select a homogenous, well-definable population. The insistence on complete stability for the previous 6 months and exclusion of several associated ailments had the net effect, although unwanted, unforeseen, and inadvertent, of excluding many of the higher risk candidates for such surgery. Thus the randomized population, although extremely well defined, is not representative of the average candidate for coronary bypass. The devastating effects of such exclusion criteria are obvious from two pertinent points. First, although 5,538 patients were screened for inclusion in the study, only 1,015 were randomized;[15] the reported data are from 686 patients (from 3,659 screened patients) who were randomized between 1972 and 1974.[43-46,88] Second, considering the participation of 13 hospitals, each hospital could find only an average of 1.5 patients per month to fit the criteria for randomization. In these same hospitals during this same period, many more patients were undergoing coronary bypass but could not or did not undergo randomization, thus rendering the randomized population nonrepresentative of the overall

coronary bypass candidates. Unless the indications for surgery and the results of these other operated on patients are known, one cannot know how the randomized population differed from the nonrandomized, but operated, population.

Another factor that weakens the impact of the VA cooperative study data is that 80 patients died between screening and randomization.[45] Had randomization into two treatment modes been performed earlier after screening and before the death of some of these 80 patients (11.7 percent of 686), the survival rates of the medically managed patients would definitely have been influenced unfavorably. Another criticism of the VA study was the choice of 50 percent luminal diameter reduction as the criterion of critical stenosis rather than 75 percent, allowing patients with lesser disease to enter the randomized group. Exclusion from randomization because of patient unwillingness or other unexplained reasons had an additional negative impact upon the representative nature of the VA study. These factors explain why the medically randomized patients experienced better survival than anticipated. In addition, many of the patients randomized to medical therapy (17 percent) subsequently crossed over to surgery, and it is likely that the medical survival curve would have been adversely influenced if these progressively symptomatic patients had remained in the medical follow-up group.

If the randomized population consisted of better risk patients, why did the surgical cohort not do better? One explanation may lie in the quality of surgery. Several critics have pointed out that the surgical mortality for this type of patient was too high, that the degree of revascularization may have been less than complete, and that graft patency was less than ideal.[38,40] In one of the participating hospitals that contributed a large number of patients, 20.3 percent (121 of 596), the surgical results were far better than in the total series.[113] The interhospital variability in the quality of surgery, the interobserver variability in selection of patients, and the angiographic interpretation[114-117] may also be partly responsible for the overall results being poorer than expected. It may take longer than the 4-year follow-up period to demonstrate differences between the medical and surgical groups, as has been pointed out by Green[118] and by Wukasch et al.[119] In the largest subset of the VA study, i.e., three-vessel disease with abnormal ventricle, the 30-month survival was approximately 86 and 87 percent for medical and surgical groups, respectively; however, at 54 months,

surgical survival was 85 percent as compared to 76 percent for the medical group.

Therefore, failure of the VA multicenter study to demonstrate improved survival with coronary bypass may be due to the selective inclusion of only better risk patients. This would result in better life expectancy of the medical cohort. The poorer life expectancy of the surgical cohort may be due to high surgical mortality and possibly poorer quality of surgery. In any case, the randomized study population is not representative of the average surgical candidate.

NATIONAL HEART, LUNG AND BLOOD INSTITUTE COOPERATIVE STUDY

The study sponsored by the National Heart, Lung and Blood Institute was designed to evaluate the role of coronary bypass in patients with unstable angina. As the preliminary results were reported, the authors unwittingly included late mortality figures as part of important results.[30] Many were given the impression that the results of this study revealed no prolonged survival with coronary bypass in such patients. As a result of

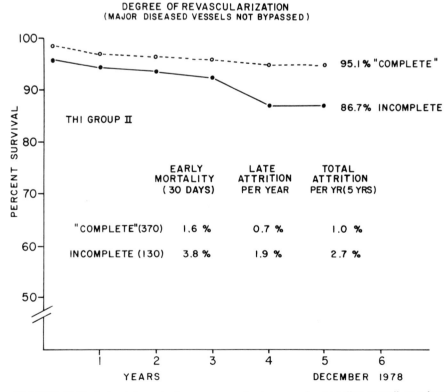

FIGURE 16-16 Actuarial survival curves reveal a lower early mortality as well as a late attrition rate for patients in whom all major diseased vessels are bypassed, as compared to the rates in those patients in whom one diseased vessel is left unbypassed.

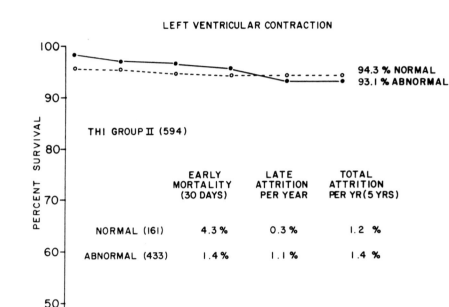

LEFT VENTRICULAR CONTRACTION

THI GROUP II (594)

	EARLY MORTALITY (30 DAYS)	LATE ATTRITION PER YEAR	TOTAL ATTRITION PER YR (5 YRS)
NORMAL (161)	4.3 %	0.3 %	1.2 %
ABNORMAL (433)	1.4 %	1.1 %	1.4 %

94.3 % NORMAL
93.1 % ABNORMAL

YEARS   DECEMBER 1978

FIGURE 16-17 Actuarial survival curves show no difference in long-term survival between patients with and without left ventricular contraction abnormalities.

widespread publicity in the lay press, some of the misunderstandings continued. In the first major published report, it was clarified that the purpose of the study was to determine whether patients with unstable angina pectoris are better treated with urgent coronary arterial surgery or with vigorous medical management.[90] The authors do not state whether the study of the influence of such surgery on long-term survival was one of the objectives. If the study was not designed to evaluate long-term survival, the results should not be used for that purpose. It is clearly stated in the conclusions that the large number of medically treated patients who later underwent surgery (36 percent of the medically treated patients later underwent surgery to relieve unacceptable angina during a follow-up period of 30 months) prevents the formulation of definitive conclusions about the relative effect of medical and surgical therapy on long-term mortality.

Another important aspect of the study is the total number of patients randomized. It is not clear from the published report how many eligible patients were screened to select the final study population and how many were excluded owing to patient or physician preference. In one institution, 228 patients satisfied clinical criteria, but only 141 patients received permission to enter the study; the therapy was dictated by the referring physician in the other 87 patients.[120]

Another 77 patients were excluded on the basis of cardiac catheterization findings, and only 64 were finally randomized. In the 4- to 5-year period from 1972 through December 1976, a total of 288 patients were entered into the study from nine university medical centers (originally eight); thus the average would be between 6.2 and 9.0 patients per year per hospital, depending upon the exact time period and the number of hospitals. Thus, each hospital could find less than 1 patient per month who was suitable for randomization as a result of either stringent and restrictive criteria or patient or physician preference. Therefore, the type of patient for whom the results of this study are valid is rarely seen in a university hospital.

OTHER RANDOMIZED STUDIES

In the Houston VA study of stable angina patients, Mathur and Guinn have reported sustained benefit and improved quality of life in the surgical group for up to 6 years.[121,122] The cardiac mortality during the follow-up period was 11 percent in the surgical and 20 percent in the medical group. At 5 years the crude survival rate was 88 percent in the surgical and 70 percent in the medical group. Although the trend has favored improved survival in the surgical group, the differences have not achieved statistical significance because of the size of the population (116 patients).

The randomized study from Portland revealed a similar trend.[108] There were 4 deaths among 51 surgical patients and 8 deaths among 49 medical patients, but the difference did not achieve statistical significance because of the small number. The death rate in the medical group was double that of the surgical group despite the fact that 8 medical patients were withdrawn from the study and underwent surgery as a result of refractory unstable symptoms.

The long-term results of the European trials are not yet available. In the shorter follow-ups, no definite conclusions can be drawn.[110-112]

DO THE TWO MULTICENTER STUDIES ON STABLE AND UNSTABLE ANGINA COVER MOST SURGICAL CANDIDATES?

When a patient is being evaluated for coronary artery bypass because of anginal symptoms, he or she is classified as either stable or unstable. Therefore, it is logical to assume that information about the life history of the stable angina patient should be available from the VA cooperative study of stable angina patients and that data about the natural life history of the unstable angina patients should be available from

the National Heart, Lung and Blood Institute (NHLBI) study. Careful scrutiny reveals that this is not the case. Each of these studies pertains to smaller subsets of patients, precisely defined in both studies, who constitute a relatively small fraction of the total population of angina patients who are candidates for possible coronary bypass surgery. On an average, only 18 patients meeting the VA criteria for stable angina present themselves per year to the major VA hospitals, and only 7 to 9 patients per year who meet the NHLBI study criteria for unstable angina present themselves to the major university hospitals. Thus, most patients with angina presenting to these institutions are neither stable nor unstable as defined by these studies. Therefore, it is imperative that in evaluating the results of coronary bypass, the overall data be examined, including every patient operated upon, in a consecutive manner. We believe our series satisfies this important point and is more representative of the patient who seeks a physician's opinion about symptoms of angina.

Can Improved Survival Be Expected Uniformly?

Should all patients expect prolonged survival following surgery, and should the results be identical in all institutions? The rationale for improvement following

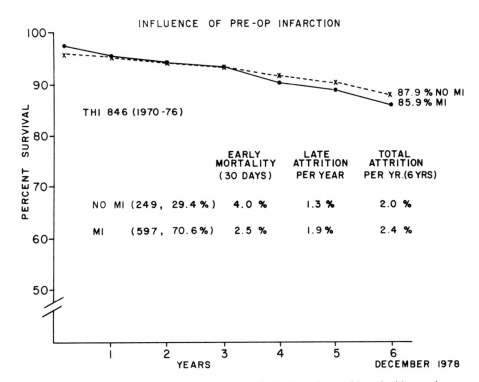

FIGURE 16-18 The long-term survival rates are similar in patients with and without prior myocardial infarction in the total group.

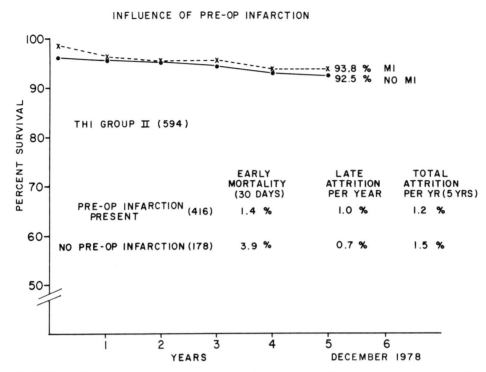

INFLUENCE OF PRE-OP INFARCTION

THI GROUP II (594)

	EARLY MORTALITY (30 DAYS)	LATE ATTRITION PER YEAR	TOTAL ATTRITION PER YR (5 YRS)
PRE-OP INFARCTION PRESENT (416)	1.4 %	1.0 %	1.2 %
NO PRE-OP INFARCTION (178)	3.9 %	0.7 %	1.5 %

YEARS   DECEMBER 1978

FIGURE 16-19 The long-term survival rates are similar in patients with and without prior myocardial infarction in Group II.

surgery is correction of the imbalance between myocardial blood supply and demand. Although there are exceptions,[17,123] the improvement in most patients is caused by increased myocardial blood flow through the patent bypass.[124] Therefore, long-term survival can be expected to improve with bypass only if surgery is adequate. This requires a low surgical mortality, good arterial anastomosis, adequate myocardial preservation with low perioperative myocardial infarction, and complete revascularization with bypasses to all the major stenosed vessels supplying viable, ischemic myocardium. In some patients, adequate surgery may not be feasible because of the nature of the coronary disease, and in others, it may not be achieved as a result of technical, diagnostic, or surgical problems. The results depend on the quality of surgery, the skills and experience of the surgical teams and support personnel, and the differences between institutions, which may be very real. In an earlier report from Duke University, the initial surgical mortality of 12 percent precluded the possibility of demonstrating improved survival during the next 2 years, although the survival in the medical group was poor.[125] In the current era, if diagnostic information and surgery of good quality can be offered to a patient with *severe* coronary artery disease, such a patient can expect an improved long-term survival.

For How Long Can the Improved Survival Be Expected?

Patients who develop coronary atherosclerosis are candidates for continued progression of disease, and some patients develop occlusive disease in the bypass grafts as well.[126-132] Many factors influencing these changes have yet to be recognized. The initial alarm about the rapid rate of occlusion of saphenous vein grafts is unfounded.[133] It is estimated that in patients with good surgery, the initial occlusion rate is approximately 10 to 15 percent, and an additional 2 percent per year can be expected to become occluded later. Bourassa et al. found enhanced progression of proximal disease in the bypassed arteries at the time of first postoperative study,[134] but in the repeat studies 5 to 7 years after surgery, progression was common in the nonbypassed arteries and very rare in the bypassed arteries.[135] Several early reports emphasized the phenomenon of enhanced progression of disease in the native circulation or occlusive disease in the bypass graft following surgery.[136-143] Mathur and Guinn found this not to be an important factor when every patient in their randomized study who received surgical or medical treatment was restudied.[144] In a recent report, Campeau et al. have emphasized the low rate of graft occlusion during a 5-year interval (0.7 percent per year) if the graft was patent 6 to 18 months following surgery in patients in their series II who were operated on prior to August 1972.[145] A very encouraging observation was that no late occlusion was found in grafts appearing to be normal at 1 year and that diffuse graft narrowing, noted during the first year, showed no further change during the subsequent 5 years. A recent report by Lawrie et al. supports this impression that enhanced progression of native disease, or an unacceptable rate of late graft closure, is not a major problem.[146]

With the data currently available, it is not possible to make a definite statement as to the duration of improved survival. Our data revealed that the survival curves in most subsets of patients do not show a sharp and steep downward slope within 6 years of operation; it is therefore likely that the benefit lasts for at least 6 years.

Palliative Rather than Curative Nature of Surgery

When assessing the results of coronary bypass surgery, it is important to keep the role of surgery in proper perspective. Coronary atherosclerosis is a progressive disease, the course of which continues unabated in most patients even after successful surgery. Evidence of progression can be detected in both surgically and medically treated groups.[144,147,148] The factors that control the rate of progression in individuals remain unclear. Such trends are detectable when longitudinal follow-up is extended for several years. In a randomized study, Mathur and Guinn found 70 percent of the patients who underwent operation to be asymptomatic after 2 years,[144] but only 52 percent remained asymptomatic after 6 years.[122] A study from our institution has revealed that results of treadmill tests are negative for ischemia in 80 percent of patients and that the exercise performance and maximal heart rates are significantly improved 1 year after surgery;[149] however, this declines gradually with time. At 4½ years the exercise duration remains unchanged, but the maximal heart rate declines slightly, and only 38 percent of the tests remain negative for ischemia. In addition to the effects of the continuing disease process, complications associated with surgery, although infrequent, can cause late deterioration and partially compromise the beneficial effects of surgery.[150-152]

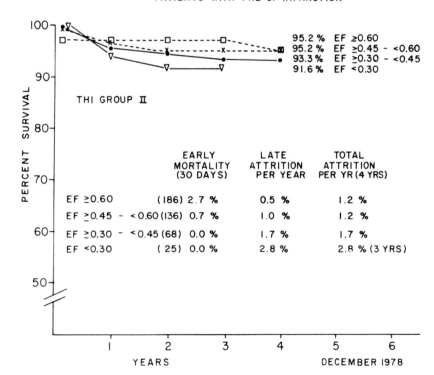

PATIENTS WITH PRE-OP INFARCTION

	EARLY MORTALITY (30 DAYS)	LATE ATTRITION PER YEAR	TOTAL ATTRITION PER YR (4 YRS)
EF ≥0.60	(186) 2.7 %	0.5 %	1.2 %
EF ≥0.45 - <0.60 (136)	0.7 %	1.0 %	1.2 %
EF ≥0.30 - <0.45 (68)	0.0 %	1.7 %	1.7 %
EF <0.30 (25)	0.0 %	2.8 %	2.8 % (3 YRS)

95.2 % EF ≥0.60
95.2 % EF ≥0.45 - <0.60
93.3 % EF ≥0.30 - <0.45
91.6 % EF <0.30

THI GROUP II

YEARS   DECEMBER 1978

FIGURE 16-20 Actuarial survival curves in Group II patients with prior infarction reveal similar long-term survival irrespective of ventricular function abnormality as judged by ejection fraction.

Should Bypass Surgery Be Recommended to Asymptomatic Individuals?

It is well known that the first clinical manifestation or event in many patients with coronary artery disease is sudden death or myocardial infarction. The 10-year experience from the Pooling Project involving 7,545 men revealed that 44 percent of the first coronary events were fatal.[37] Postmortem examination of such subjects generally reveals extensive coronary disease. It is logical to assume that such extensive disease was present for some time prior to the disastrous event. What is not known is the duration of severe latent disease. The observations of Vismara et al. that bypass surgery can reduce the incidence of sudden death are very encouraging.[153]

With the current emphasis on physical fitness and elaborate, routine clinical testing of many asymptomatic "healthy" individuals, serious coronary artery disease is being detected in an increasing number of people who have no recognizable symptoms. In some of these, angina is not present because of very sedentary life-style and absence of any provocations.

When an asymptomatic person with advanced coronary disease is identified, the physician faces the dilemma of whether or not to recommend bypass surgery. The risks of a potentially fatal disease have to be weighed against the risks of surgery. Also, we do not know when the disease will become manifest clinically, nor do we know the duration of improvement that the surgery will provide. We have some idea of natural life history of patients with severe disease *who have symptoms*,[65-77] but we do not know the life history of patients with severe disease *with no symptoms*. Our results indicate that surgery can be performed with a low risk of mortality and morbidity in such patients and that the long-term survival is at least as good or better (Figs. 16-5 and 16-11) than the long-term survival of more symptomatic patients who have been operated on. Based on these data, it is our opinion that life expectancy is likely to be improved with surgery in an asymptomatic patient with left main, triple-, double-, and possibly even single-vessel disease who also exhibits evidence of severe ischemia in the form of early or strongly positive treadmill test results, myocardial perfusion deficit with exercise (detected by thallium imaging), and regional or global ventricular wall motion abnormalities with exercise (detected by gated blood pool imaging). We hope that enough evidence will become apparent in the next 2 or 3 years to allow us to make this same prediction with more confidence. This might be a particular subset of patients for whom a randomized study may still be feasible and may provide important information.

SUMMARY AND CONCLUSIONS

We have reviewed the long-term survival data of a series of 846 consecutive, personally observed patients who underwent coronary artery bypass at our institution. The clinical and angiographic profile of these patients with predominantly severe disease and symptoms has been outlined. The overall survival rates were similar to the survival rates of the entire series of 13,004 patients who underwent such surgery at our institution. In addition, there is little variance in survival figures in accumulating data from many other centers.

Our results reveal that coronary artery bypass prolongs life in patients with left main coronary artery disease, triple-vessel disease, and probably, double-vessel disease. Patients with single-vessel disease also experience excellent results, but our experience with such patients is minimal, since they constitute only a small fraction of our patient population. The long-term survival in our series is superior to previously defined natural life history or historic controls. More reassuring is the fact that the survival rates are superior to those of patients randomized to modern medical treatment in two multicenter studies, namely the VA study for stable angina patients and the NHLBI study for unstable angina patients.

The conscientious physician is faced with the dilemma arising from an inherent objection to the use of historic controls and serious objections to the validity of the conclusions from the randomized studies. We have attempted to resolve this dilemma by demonstrating that the survival curve of selected subsets of patients in our series for whom the prognosis has been uniformly reported to be poor without surgery has been restored to near normal levels following coronary bypass surgery. We have also demonstrated that bypass surgery has eliminated the expected differences in long-term survival between patients with varying degrees of severity of disease and ventricular dysfunction, at least for the first 4 or 5 years after operation. We have noted this trend among patients with single-, double-, and triple-vessel disease; among those in functional classes I to IV; among patients with stable versus unstable symptoms; among patients with normal versus abnormal left ventricles; among those with and without prior infarction; and among those with better or worse ejection fractions. This is strong circumstantial evidence that life expectancy has been improved in patients with the worst prognosis. The long-term survival in patients operated on between March 1973 and June 1976 is so close to normal that it is hard to escape the conclusion that bypass surgery has prolonged life in these patients. Some of the reasons for the failure of randomized studies (although well conducted) to show prolonged survival have been discussed.

These observations have been derived from a population of patients who were nearly all symptomatic, and extrapolation of our conclusions to the asymptomatic patient is not necessarily valid. However, if high-quality surgery can be performed at a low risk, it may be justifiable to recommend surgery to those asymptomatic persons who have severe disease as well as evidence of significant ischemia.

The data from our institution, as well as that from others, support the conclusion that coronary artery bypass surgery prolongs life in patients with severe coronary artery disease. Further reduction of surgical mortality and progressive improvement of techniques of myocardial preservation during surgery should even further enhance long-term survival.

REFERENCES

1 Favaloro, R. G.: Saphenous Vein Graft in the Surgical Treatment of Coronary Artery Disease: Operative Technique, *J. Thorac. Cardiovasc. Surg.,* 58:178, 1969.

2 Johnson, W. D., Flemma, R. J., Lepley, D., Jr., et al.: Extended Treatment of Severe Coronary Artery Disease: A Total Surgical Approach, *Ann. Surg.,* 170:460, 1969.

3 Kerth, W. J.: Aortocoronary Bypass Grafts, *J. Thorac. Cardiovasc. Surg.,* 57:487, 1969.

4 Urschel, H. C., Jr., Miller, E. R., Razzuk, M. A., et al.: Aorta-to-Coronary Artery Vein Bypass Graft for Coronary Artery Occlusive Disease, *Ann. Thorac. Surg.,* 8:114, 1969.

5 Mundth, E. D., Harthorne, J. W., Buckley, M. J., et al.: Direct Coronary Arterial Revascularization for Segmental Occlusive Disease, *Surgery,* 67:168, 1970.

6 Morris, G. C., Jr., Reul, G. J., Howell, J. F., Crawford, E. S., Chapman, D. W., Beazley, H. L., Winters, W. L., Peterson, P. K., and Lewis, J. M.: Follow-up Results of Distal Coronary Artery Bypass for Ischemic Heart Disease, *Am. J. Cardiol.,* 29:180, 1972.

7 Hall, R. J., Dawson, J. T., Cooley, D. A., Hallman, G. L., Wukasch, D. C., and Garcia, E.: Coronary Artery Bypass, in J. H. Kennedy (ed.), "Cardiovascular Surgery 1972" (American Heart Association Monograph 41), *Circulation,* 47, 48 (suppl. 3):146, 1973.

8 Sheldon, W. C., Rincon, G., Effler, D. B., Proudfit, W. L., and Sones, F. M., Jr.: Vein Graft Surgery for Coronary Artery Disease: Survival and Angiographic Results in 1,000 Patients, in J. H. Kennedy (ed.), "Cardiovascular Surgery 1972" (American Heart Association Monograph 41), *Circulation,* 47, 48 (suppl. 3):184, 1973.

9 Alderman, E. L., Matlof, H. J., Wexler, L., Shumway, N. E., and Harrison, D. C.: Results of Direct Coronary Artery Surgery for the Treatment of Angina Pectoris, *N. Engl. J. Med.,* 288:535, 1973.

10 Hutchinson, J. E., III, Green, G. E., Mekhijian, H. A., Gallozzi, E., Cameron, A., and Kemp, H. G.: Coronary Bypass Grafting in 476 Patients Consecutively Operated On, *Chest,* 64:706, 1973.

11 Flemma, R. J., Johnson, W. D., Lepley, D., Jr., Tector, A. J., Walker, J., Gale, H., Beddingfield, G., and Manley, J. C.: Late Results of Saphenous Vein Bypass Grafting for Myocardial Revascularization, *Ann. Thorac. Surg.,* 14:232, 1972.

12 Mathur, V. S., and Guinn, G. A.: Prospective Randomized Study of Coronary Bypass Surgery (BS): Preliminary Report, *Circulation,* 47, 48 (suppl. 4):58, 1973. (Abstract.)

13 Mathur, V. S., Guinn, G. A., Anastassiades, L. C., Chahine, R. A., Korompai, F. L., Montero, A. C., and Luchi, R. J.: Surgical Treatment of Stable Angina Pectoris, *N. Engl. J. Med.,* 292:709, 1975.

14 Cannom, D. S., Miller, D. G., and Shumway, N. E.: The Long-term Follow-up of Patients Undergoing Saphenous Vein Bypass Surgery, *Circulation,* 49:77, 1974.

15 Kouchoukos, N. T., Kirklin, J. W., and Oberman, A.: An Appraisal of Coronary Bypass Grafting, *Circulation,* 50:11, 1974.

16 Sheldon, W. C., Rincon, G., and Pichard, A. D.: Surgical Treatment of Coronary Artery Disease: Pure Graft Operations, with a Study of 741 Patients Followed 3–7 Years, *Prog. Cardiovasc. Dis.,* 18:237, 1975.

17 Mathur, V. S., and Guinn, G. A.: Prospective Randomized Study of the Surgical Therapy of Stable Angina, *Cardiovasc. Clin.,* 8 (suppl. 2):131, 1977.

18 Kloster, F. E., Kremkau, E. L., Rahimtoola, S. H., Ritzmann, L. W., Griswold, H. E., Neill, W. A., Rosh, J., and Starr, A.: Prospective Randomized Study of Coronary Bypass Surgery for Chronic Stable Angina, *Cardiovasc. Clin.,* 8:145, 1977.

19 Anderson, R. P., Rahimtoola, S. H., Bonchek, L. A., and Staff, A.: The Prognosis of Patients with Coronary Artery Disease After Coronary Bypass Operations. Time Related Progress of 532 Patients with Disabling Angina Pectoris, *Circulation,* 50:274, 1974.

20 Dunkman, W. B., Perloff, J. K., Kastor, J. A., and Shelburne, J. C.: Medical Perspectives in Coronary Artery Surgery—a Caveat, *Ann. Intern. Med.*, 81:817, 1974.

21 Ross, R. S.: Ischemic Heart Disease. An Overview, *Am. J. Cardiol.*, 36:496, 1975.

22 Mundth, E. D., and Austen, W. G.: Surgical Measures for Coronary Heart Disease, *N. Engl. J. Med.*, 293:13,75,124, 1975.

23 McIntosh, H. D., and Garcia, J. A.: The First Decade of Aortocoronary Bypass Grafting, 1967–1977: A Review, *Circulation*, 57:405, 1978.

24 Loop, F. D., Proudfit, W. L., Sheldon, W. C.: Coronary Bypass Surgery Weighed in the Balance, *Am. J. Cardiol.*, 42:154, 1978.

25 DeBakey, M. E., and Lawrie, G. M.: Aortocoronary-Artery Bypass: Assessment after 13 Years, *J.A.M.A.*, 239:847, 1978.

26 Hultgren, H. N., Takaro, T., Detre, K. M., and Murphy, M. L.: Aortocoronary-Artery-Bypass Assessment after 13 Years, *J.A.M.A.*, 240:1353, 1978.

27 McIntosh, H. D.: Benefits from Aortocoronary Bypass Graft, *J.A.M.A.*, 239:1197, 1978.

28 Favaloro, R. G.: Direct Myocardial Revascularization: A Ten Year Journey. Myths and Realities, *Am. J. Cardiol.*, 43:109, 1979.

29 Cooley, D. A., Wukasch, D. C., Bruno, F., Reul, G. J., Sandiford, F. M., Zillgitt, S. L., and Hall, R. J.: Direct Myocardial Revascularization: Experience with 9364 Operations, *Thorax*, 33:411, 1978.

30 Conti, C. R., II, Gilbert, J. B., and Hodges, M.: Unstable Angina Pectoris—Randomized Study of Surgical vs. Medical Therapy, *Am. J. Cardiol.*, 35:129, 1974.

31 Pfeifer, J., Peduzzi, P., and Hultgren, H.: Medical Versus Surgical Therapy for Coronary Artery Disease—Effect on Symptoms, *Clin. Res.*, 26:259A, 1978.

32 Chalmers, T. C.: Randomization and Coronary Artery Surgery, *Ann. Thorac. Surg.*, 14:323, 1972.

33 Chalmers, T. C., Smith, H., and Kunzler, A. M.: A Comparison of Therapeutic Trials Employing Historical, Alternate and Randomized Controls, *Clin. Res.*, 24:475A, 1976.

34 Feinstein, A. R.: The Scientific and Clinical Tribulations of Randomized Clinical Trials, *Clin. Res.*, 26:241, 1978.

35 Lacher, M. J.: Physicians and Patients as Obstacles to a Randomized Trial, *Clin. Res.*, 26:375, 1978.

36 Ambroz, A., Chalmers, T. C., and Smith, H.: Deficiencies of Randomized Control Trials, *Clin. Res.*, 26:280A, 1978.

37 Vaisrub, S.: Random Thoughts on Randomization, *J.A.M.A.*, 239:858, 1978.

38 Special Correspondence: A Debate on Coronary Bypass, *N. Engl. J. Med.*, 297:1464, 1977.

39 Chalmers, T. C.: In Defense of the VA Randomized Control Trial of Coronary Artery Surgery, *Clin. Res.*, 26:230, 1978.

40 Proudfit, W. L.: Criticisms of the VA Randomized Study of Coronary Bypass Surgery, *Clin. Res.*, 26:236, 1978.

41 Loop, F. D., Proudfit, W. L., and Sheldon, W. C.: Coronary Bypass Surgery Weighted in the Balance, *Am. J. Cardiol.*, 42:154, 1978.

42 Hall, R. J., Garcia, E., Mathur, V. S., and de Castro, C. M.: Coronary Artery Bypass—Are Multicenter Cooperative Random Studies Misleading? *Cardiovasc. Dis., Bull. Texas Heart Inst.*, 5:12, 1978.

43 Murphy, M. L., Hultgren, H. N., Detre, K., Thomasen, J., and Takaro, T.: Treatment of Chronic Stable Angina: A Preliminary Report of Surgical Data of the Randomized Veterans Administration Cooperative Study, *N. Engl. J. Med.* 297:621, 1977.

44 Read, R. C., Murphy, M. L., Hultgren, H. N., and Takaro, T.: Survival of Men Treated for Chronic Angina Pectoris: A Cooperative Randomized Study, *J. Thorac. Cardiovasc. Surg.*, 75:1, 1978.

45 Detre, K., Hultgren, H., and Takaro, T.: Veterans Administration Cooperative Study of Surgery for Coronary Arterial Occlusive Disease: III. Methods and Baseline Characteristics, Including Experience in Medical Treatment, *Am. J. Cardiol.*, 40:212, 1977.

46 Hultgren, H. N., Takaro, T., and Detre, K. The Veterans Administration Cooperative Study of Surgical Treatment of Stable Angina: Preliminary Results, *Cardiovasc. Clin.*, 8 (suppl. 2):119, 1977.

47 The University Group Diabetes Program: A Study of the Effects of Hypoglycemic Agents on Vascular Complications in Patients with Adult-Onset Diabetes, *Diabetes*, 19 (suppl. 2):747, 1970.

48 Amsterdam, E. A., Wolfson, S., and Gorlin, R.: Effect of Therapy on Survival in Angina Pectoris, *Ann. Intern. Med.*, 68:1151, 1968.

49 Lambert, D. M. D.: Beta Blockers and Life Expectancy in Ischemic Heart Disease, *Lancet*, 1:793, 1972.

50 Wilhelmsson, C., Vedin, A., and Wilhelmssen, L.: Death and Non-fatal Reinfarctions During Two Years Follow-up, *Acta. Med. Scand.*, (suppl.), 575:19, 1975.

51 Fox, K. N., Chopra, M. P., Portal, R. S., and Abert, C. P.: Long-term Beta Blockade: Possible Protection from Myocardial Infarction, *Br. Med. J.*, 1:117, 1975.

52 Multicenter International Study: Improvement in Prognosis of Myocardial Infarction by Long-term Beta Adreno-receptor Blockade Using Practolol, *Br. Med. J.*, 3:735, 1975.

53 Lambert, D. M. D.: Effect of Propranolol on Mortality in Patients with Angina, *Postgrad. Med. J.*, 52 (suppl.):57, 1976.

54 Walker, W. J., Coronary Mortality: What Is Going On, *J.A.M.A.*, 227:1045, 1974.

55 Recent Trends in Mortality from Heart Disease, *Statistical Bull. Metropolitan Life*, 56:3, 1975.

56 U.S. Department of Health, Education and Welfare, Public Health Services, Health Resources Administration: "Health, United States, 1975" (DHEW Publication No. (HRA), 76-1232), National Center for Health Statistics, Rockville, Md. 1976, pp. 297, 299, 301.

57 Stamler, J.: "Introduction to Risk Factors in Coronary Artery Disease," Vol. 1, No. 3, E. R. Squibb & Sons, Inc., 1977.

58 Rogers, D. E., and Blendom, R. J.: The Changing American Health Scene—Sometimes Things Get Better, *J.A.M.A.*, 237:1710, 1977.

59 Stamler, J.: Life Styles, Major Risk Factors, Proof and Public Policy, *Circulation*, 38:3, 1978.

60 Braunwald, E.: Coronary-Artery Surgery at the Crossroad, *N. Engl. J. Med.*, 297:661, 1977.

61 Proudfit, W. L., Bruschke, A. V. G., and Sones, F. M.: Natural History of Obstructive Coronary Artery Disease: Ten-Year Study of 601 Nonsurgical Cases, *Prog. Cardiovas. Dis.*, 21:53, 1978.

62 Hall, R. J., Garcia, E., Mathur, V. S., Cooley, D. A., Gold, K. D., and Gray, A. G.: Factors Influencing Early and Late Survival After Aortocoronary Artery Bypass: A Preliminary Report, *Cardiovasc. Dis., Bull. Texas Heart Inst.*, 4:120, 1977.

63 Hall, R. J., Garcia, E., Mathur, V. S., Gold, K. K., Gray, A. G., and Cooley, D. A.: Long-term Survival After Coronary Artery Bypass (CAB) Surgery. Proceeding of the VIII World Congress of Cardiology, 1978, p. 210; 0489.

64 Cutler, S. J., and Ederer, F.: Maximum Utilization of the Life Table Method in Analyzing Survival, *J. Chronic Dis.*, 8:699, 1958.

65 Friesinger, G. C., Page, E. E., and Ross, R. S.: Prognostic Significance of Coronary Arteriography, *Trans. Assoc. Am. Physicians*, 83:75, 1970.

66 Bruschke, A. V. G., Proudfit, W. L., and Sones, F. M., Jr.: Progress Study of 590 Consecutive Non-surgical Cases of Coronary Disease Followed 5–9 Years: I. Arteriographic Correlations, *Circulation*, 47:1147, 1973.

67 Bruschke, A. V. G., Proudfit, W. L., and Sones, F. M., Jr.: Progress Study of 590 Consecutive Non-surgical Cases of Coronary Disease Followed 5–9 Years: II. Ventriculographic and Other Correlations, *Circulation*, 47:1154, 1973.

68 Webster, J. S., Moberg, C., and Rincon, G.: Natural History of Severe Proximal Coronary Artery Disease as Documented by Coronary Cineangiography, *Am. J. Cardiol.*, 33:195, 1974.

69 Burgraff, G. W., and Parker, J. O.: Prognosis in Coronary Artery Disease: Angiographic, Hemodynamic and Clinical Factors, *Circulation*, 51:146, 1975.

70 Gensini, G. G., Esente, P., and Kelly, A.: Natural History of Coronary Disease in Patients With and Without Coronary Bypass Graft Surgery, *Circulation*, 50 (suppl. 2):98, 1974.

71 Rosch, J., and Rahimtoola, S. H.: Progression of Angiographically Determined Coronary Stenosis, in S. H. Rahimtoola (ed.), "Coronary Bypass Surgery," F. A. Davis Co., Philadelphia, 1977, p. 55.

72 Rosch, J., Antonovic, R., and Trenouth, R. S.: The Natural History of Coronary Artery Stenosis, *Radiology*, 119:513, 1976.

73 Oberman, A., Jones, W. B., Riley, C. P., Reeves, T. J., Sheffield, L. T., and Turner, M. E.: Natural History of Coronary Artery Disease, *Bull. N.Y. Acad. Med.*, 48:1109, 1972.

74 Humphries, J. O., Kuller, L., Ross, R. S., Friesinger, G. C., and Page, E. E.: Natural History of Ischemic Heart Disease in Relation to Arteriographic Findings: A Twelve Year Study of 224 Patients, *Circulation*, 49:489, 1974.

75 Kimbiris, D., Lavine, P., and VanDenBroek, H.: Devolutionary Pattern of Coronary Atherosclerosis in Patients with Angina Pectoris, *Am. J. Cardiol.*, 33:7, 1974.

76 Reeves, T. J., Oberman, A., Jones, W. B., and Sheffield, L. T.: Natural History of Angina Pectoris, *Am. J. Cardiol.*, 33:423, 1974.

77 Humphries, J. O'N.: Expected Course of Patients with Coronary Artery Disease, in S. H. Rahimtoola (ed.), "Coronary Bypass Surgery," F. A. Davis Co., Philadelphia, 1977, p. 41.

78 Greene, D. G., Bunnell, L. L., Arain, D. T., Schimert, G., Lajos, T. Z., Lee, A. B., Tandon, R. N., Zimdahl, W. T., Bozer, J. M., Kolin, R. M., and Smith, G. L.: Long-term Survival After Coronary Bypass Surgery. (Scientific exhibit at the American College of Cardiology meetings, Anaheim, 1978.)

79 Lavine, P., Kimbiris, D., Segal, B. L., and Linhart, J. W.: Left Main Coronary Artery Disease: Clinical Arteriographic and Hemodynamic Appraisal, *Am. J. Cardiol.*, 30:791, 1972.

80 Cohen, M. W., Cohn, P. F., Herman, M. V., and Gorlin, R.: Diagnosis and Prognosis of Main Left Coronary Artery Obstruction, *Circulation*, 45, 46 (suppl. 1):57, 1972.

81 Talano, J. W., Scanlon, P. J., Meadows, W. R., Kahn, M., Pifarre, R., and Gunnar, R.: Influence of Surgery on Survival in 145 Patients with Left Main Coronary Artery Disease, *Circulation*, 51, 52 (suppl. 1):105, 1975.

82 DeMots, H., Bonchek, L. I., Rosch, J., Anderson, R. P., Staff, A., and Rahimtoola, S. H.: Left Main Coronary Artery Disease: Risks of Angiography, Importance of Coexisting Diseases of Other Coronary Arteries and Effects of Revascularization, *Am. J. Cardiol.*, 36:136, 1975.

83 Kisslo, J., Peter, R., Behar, V., Bartel, A., and Kong, Y.: Left Main Coronary Stenosis, *Circulation*, 47, 48 (suppl. 4):57, 1973. (Abstract.)

84 Oberman, A., Harrell, R. R., Russell, R. O., Jr., Kouchoukos, N. T., Holt, J. H., Jr., and Rackley, C. E.: Surgical Versus Medical Treatment in Disease of the Left Main Coronary Artery, *Lancet*, 7986:591, 1976.

85 Sung, R. J., Mallon, S. M., Richter, S. E., Ghahramani, A. E., Sommer, L. S., Kaiser, G. A., and Myerburg, R. J.: Left Main Coronary Artery Obstruction: Follow-up of Thirty Patients With and Without Surgery, *Circulation*, 51, 52 (suppl. 1):112, 1975.

86 Lim, J. S., Proudfit, W. L., and Sones, F. M.: Left Main Coronary Arterial Obstruction: Long-term Follow-up of 141 Nonsurgical Cases, *Am. J. Cardiol.*, 36:131, 1975.

87 Sharma, S., Khaja, F., Heinle, R., Goldstein, S., and Easley, R.: Left Main Coronary (LMC) Artery Lesions: Risk of Catheterization, Exercise Test and Surgery, *Circulation*, 47, 48 (suppl. 4):53, 1973. (Abstract.)

88 Takaro, T., Hultgren, H., and Lipton, M.: The VA Cooperative Randomized Study of Surgery for Coronary Arterial Occlusive Disease. II Subgroup with Significant Left Main Lesions, *Circulation*, 54 (suppl. 3):107, 1976.

89 Unstable Angina Pectoris Study Group: Unstable Angina Pectoris National Cooperative Study Group to Compare Medical and Surgical Therapy. I. A Report of Protocol and Patient Population, *Am. J. Cardiol.*, 37:896, 1976.

90 Unstable Angina Pectoris Study Group: Unstable Angina Pectoris: National Cooperative Study Group to Compare Surgical and Medical Therapy. II. In-hospital Experience and Initial Follow-up Results in Patients with One, Two and Three Vessel Disease, *Am. J. Cardiol.*, 42:839, 1978.

91 Kouchoukos, N. T., Oberman, A., Karp, R. B., and Russell, R. O., Jr.: Coronary Bypass Surgery: Assessment of Current Operative Risk., *Am. J. Cardiol.*, 39:285, 1977. (Abstract.)

92 Lajos, R. Z., Levinsky, L., Lee, A. B., Schimert, G., Greene, D. G., Bunnell, I. L., Arani, D. J., Visco, J., Tandon, R., Zimdahl, W. T., Kohn, R., and Bozer, J.: Refinements in Coronary Artery Surgery Contributing to Improved Survival. Proceedings of the VIII World Congress of Cardiology, 1978, p. 202; 0458.

93 Boake, W. C., Chopra, P., and Kahn, D. R.: Survival After Aorto-coronary Artery Bypass Graft Surgery in Relation to Completeness of Revascularization. Proceedings of the VIII World Congress of Cardiology 1978, p. 203; 0462.

94 Greene, D. G., Bunnell, I. L., Arani, D. T., Schimert, G., Lajos, T. Z., Lee, A. B., Tandon, R. N., Zimdahl, W. T., Bozer, J. M., Kohn, R. M., Visco, J. P., and Smith, G. L.: Actuarial Analysis of Survival of 875 Cases of Coronary Bypass Surgery. Proceedings of the VIII World Congress of Cardiology, 1978, p. 210; 0487.

95 Stiles, Q. R., Lindesmith, G. G., Tucker, B. L., Hughes, R. K., and Meyer, B. W.: Long-term Follow-up of Patients with Coronary Artery Bypass Grafts, *Circulation*, 54 (suppl. 3):32, 1976.

96 Lawrie, G. M., Lie, J. T., Morris, G. C., and Beazley, H. L.: Vein Graft Patency and Intimal Proliferation After Aortocoronary Bypass: Early and Long-term Angiopathologic Correlations, *Am. J. Cardiol.*, 38:856, 1976.

97 Lawrie, G. M., Morris, G. L., Jr., Howell, J. F., Tredici, T. D., and Chapman, D. W.: Improved Survival After 5 Years in 1,144 Patients After Coronary Bypass Surgery, *Am. J. Cardiol.*, 42:709, 1978.

98 Sheldon, W. C., Rincon, G., Pichard, A. D., Razavi, M., Cheanvechai, C., and Loop, F. D.: Surgical Treatment of Coronary Artery Disease: Pure Graft Operations with a Study of 751 Patients Followed 3–7 Years, *Prog. Cardiovasc. Dis.*, 18:237, 1975.

99 Loop, F. D., Irarrazaval, M. J., Bredee, J. J., Siegel, W., Taylor, P. C., and Sheldon, W.: Internal Mammary Artery Graft for Ischemic Heart Disease. Effect of Revascularization on Clinical Status and Survival, *Am. J. Cardiol.*, 39:156, 1977.

100 Cameron, A., Kemp, G. H., Shimomura, S., Santilli, E., Green, G. E., Hutchinson, J. E., and Mekhjian, E.: Coronary Bypass Surgery, a Seven Year Follow-up, *Circulation*, 58 (suppl. 2):19, 1978.

101 McCollum, W. T., and Greer, A. E.: Coronary Artery Bypass Surgery. Long-term Follow-up. Proceedings of the VIII World Congress of Cardiology, 1978, p. 209; 0485.

102 Gazes, P. C., Mobley, E. M., Jr., and Faris, H. M., Jr.: Preinfarctional (Unstable) Angina—A Prospective Study—Ten Year Follow-up, *Circulation*, 48:331, 1973.

103 Medilie, J. H., Kahn, H. A., Neufeld, H. N., Riss, E., Goldbourt, U., Perlstein, T., and Oron, D.: Myocardial Infarction over a Five-Year Period. I. Prevalence. Incidence and Mortality Experience, *J. Chronic Dis.*, 26:63, 1973.

104 Norris, R. M., Caughey, D. E., and Mercer, C. J.: Prognosis After Myocardial Infarction: Six Year Follow-up, *Br. Heart J.* 36:786, 1974.

105 The Coronary Drug Project Research Group: The Coronary Drug Project. Design, Methods and Baseline Results, *Circulation*, 47 (suppl. 1):1, 1973.

106 Selden, R., Neill, W. A., Ritzmann, L. W., Okies, J. E., and Anderson, R. P.: Medical Versus Surgical Therapy for Acute Coronary Insufficiency, *N. Engl. J. Med.*, 293:1329, 1975.

107 Neill, W. A., Ritzmann, L. W., and Okies, J. E.: Medical vs. Urgent Surgical Therapy for Acute Coronary Insufficiency—a Randomized Study, *Cardiovasc. Clin.*, 8 (suppl. 2):179, 1977.

108 Kloster, F. E., Kremkau, E. L., Ritzmann, L. W., Rahimtoola, S. H., Rosch, J., and Kanarek, P. H.: Coronary Bypass for Stable Angina. A Prospective Randomized Study, *N. Engl. J. Med.*, 300:149, 1979.

109 Bertolasi, C. A., Tronge, J. E., and Carerro, C. A.: Unstable Angina—Prospective and Randomized Study of Its Evolution, With and Without Surgery, *Am. J. Cardiol.*, 33:201, 1974.

110 Towers, M., Ahmed, M., Thompson, R., Fawzy, E.,

and Yacoub, M.: Survival After Coronary Bypass Grafting. Proceedings of the VIII World Congress of Cardiology, 1978, p. 212; 0495.

111 Yacoub, M., Thompson, R., Ahmed, M., and Towers, M.: Effect of Coronary Grafting on the Incidence and Prognosis of Myocardial Infarction in Patients with Stable Angina. A Prospective Randomized Study. Proceedings of the VIII World Congress of Cardiology, 1978, p. 207; 0476.

112 Varnauskas, E.: Report on the Controlled Studies in Progress: European Study. Long-term Results of Coronary Surgery. Presented at the VIII World Congress of Cardiology, 1978.

113 Pifarre, R., Loeb, H., Sullivan, H., Palac, R., Croke, R., and Gunnar, R.: Improved Survival After Surgical Therapy for Chronic Angina Pectoris. One Hospital's Experience in a Randomized Trial, *Circulation*, 58 (suppl. 2):96, 1978.

114 Gensini, G., quoted by Favaloro, R. G.: Direct Myocardial Revascularization: A Ten Year Journey, Myths and Realities, *Am. J. Cardiol.*, 43:109, 1979.

115 Towne, W. D.: Letter to the Editor, *N. Engl. J. Med.*, 297:1465, 1977.

116 Detre, K. M., Wright, E., Murphy, M. L., and Takaro, T.: Observer Agreement in Evaluating Coronary Angiograms, *Circulation*, 52:979, 1975.

117 Carey, J. S., Cukingnan, R. A., and Gabriel, G.: VA Coronary Cooperative Study: View from a Non-cooperating Hospital, *Circulation*, 58 (suppl. 2):85, 1978.

118 Greene, D. G.: Letter to the Editor, *N. Engl. J. Med.*, 297:1467, 1977.

119 Wukasch, D. C., Cooley, D. A., Hall, R. J., Reul, G. J., Sandiford, F. M., and Zillgitt, S. L.: Surgical Versus Medical Treatment of Coronary Artery Disease: Nine Year Follow-up in 9061 Patients, *Am. J. Surg.*, 137:201, 1979.

120 Priest, M. F., Curry, G. C., Smith, L. R., Rogers, W. J., Mantle, J. A., Rackley, C. E., Kouchoukas, N. T., and Russell, R. O., Jr.: Changes in Left Ventricular Segmental Wall Motion Following Randomization to Medicine or Surgery in Patients with Unstable Angina, *Circulation*, 58 (suppl. 1):62, 1978.

121 Mathur, V. S., and Guinn, G. A.: Sustained Benefit from Aortocoronary Bypass Surgery Demonstrated for 5 Years: A Prospective Randomized Study, *Circulation* 55,56 (suppl. 3):190, 1977.

122 Mathur, V. S., and Guinn, G.: Prospective Randomized Study of Coronary Bypass Surgery: Sustained Benefit in 3–6 Years Follow-up. Proceedings of the VIII World Congress of Cardiology, 1978, p. 211; 0490.

123 Griffith, L. S. C., Achuff, S. C., Conti, C. R., Humphries, J. O., Brawley, R. K., Gott, V. L., and Ross, R. S.: Changes in Intrinsic Coronary Circulation and Segmental Ventricular Motion After Saphenous-Vein Coronary Bypass Graft Surgery, *N. Engl. J. Med.*, 288:589, 1973.

124 Bittar, N., Kroncke, G. M., Rowe, G. G., et al.: Vein Graft Flow and Reactive Hyperemia in the Human Heart, *J. Thorac. Cardiovasc. Surg.*, 64:855, 1972.

125 McNeer, J. F., Starmer, C. F., Bartel, A. G., Behar, V. S., Kong, Y., Peter, R. H., and Rosati, R. A.: The Nature of Treatment Selection in Coronary Artery Disease: Experience with Medical and Surgical Treatment of a Chronic Disease, *Circulation*, 49:606, 1974.

126 Robert, E. W., Guthaner, D. F., Wexler, L., and Alderman, E. L.: Six-Year Clinical and Angiographic Follow-up of Patients with Previously Documented Complete Revascularization, *Circulation*, 58 (suppl. 1):194, 1978.

127 Kouchoukos, N. T., Karp, R. B., Oberman, A., Russell, R. O., Jr., Alison, H. W., and Holt, J. H., Jr.: Long-term Patency of Saphenous Veins for Coronary Bypass Grafting, *Circulation*, 58 (suppl. 1):96, 1978.

128 Winer, H. E., Glassman, E., and Spencer, F. C.: Mechanism of Relief of Angina by Bypass Grafting, *Circulation*, 58 (suppl. 2):16, 1978.

129 Jones, M., Conkle, D. M., Ferrans, V. J., Roberts, W. C., Levine, F. H., Melvin, D. B., and Stinson, E. B.: Lesions Observed in Arterial Autogenous Vein Grafts: Light and Electron Microscopic Evaluation, in J. H. Kennedy (ed.), "Cardiovascular Surgery 1972" (American Heart Association Monograph 41), *Circulation*, 47, 48 (suppl. 3):198, 1973.

130 Vlodaver, Z., and Edwards, J. E.: Pathologic Changes in Aorto-coronary Arterial Saphenous Vein Grafts, *Circulation*, 44:719, 1971.

131 Unni, K. K., Kottke, B. A., Titus, J. S., et al.: Pathological Changes in Aortocoronary Saphenous Vein Grafts, *Am. J. Cardiol.*, 34:526, 1974.

132 Spray, T. L., and Roberts, W. C.: Morphologic Observations in Biologic Conduits Between Aorta and Coronary Artery, in S. H. Rahimtoola (ed.), "Coronary Bypass Surgery," F. A. Davis Co., Philadelphia, 1977, p. 11.

133 Lesperance, J., Bourassa, M. G., Saltiel, J., Campeau, L., and Grondin, C. M.: Angiographic Changes in Aortocoronary Vein Grafts: Lack of Progression Beyond the First Year, *Circulation*, 48:633, 1973.

134 Bourassa, M. G., Goulet, C., and Lesperance, J.: Progression of Coronary Arterial Disease After Aortocoronary Bypass Grafts, in J. H. Kennedy (ed.), "Cardiovascular Surgery 1972" (American Heart Association Monograph 41), *Circulation*, 47, 48 (suppl. 3):127, 1973.

135 Bourassa, M. G., Lesperance, J., Corbara, F., Saltiel, J., and Campeau, L.: Progression of Obstructive Coronary Disease 5 to 7 Years After Aortocoronary Bypass Surgery, *Circulation*, 58 (suppl. 1):100, 1978.

136 Aldridge, H. E., and Trimble, A. S.: Progression of Proximal Coronary Artery Lesions to Total Occlusion After Aortocoronary Saphenous Vein Bypass Grafting, *J. Thorac. Cardiovasc. Surg.*, 62:7, 1971.

137 Maurer, B. J., Oberman, A., Hol, J. H., Jr., Kouchou-

kos, N. T., Jones, W. E., Russell, R. D., Jr., and Reeves, T. J.: Changes in Grafted and Nongrafted Coronary Arteries Following Saphenous Vein Bypass Grafting, *Circulation,* 50:293, 1974.

138 Frick, M. H., Valle, M., Harjola, P. T., and Korhola, D.: Changes in Native Coronary Arteries after Coronary Bypass Surgery: Role of Graft Patency, Serum Lipids, and Hypertension, *Am. J. Cardiol.,* 36:745, 1975.

139 Pasternak, R., Cohn, K., Selzer, A., and Langston, M. F., Jr.: Enhanced Rate of Progression of Coronary Artery Disease Following Aortocoronary Saphenous Vein Bypass Surgery, *Am. J. Med.,* 58:166, 1975.

140 Glassman, E., Spencer, F. C., Krauss, K. R., Weisinger, B., and Isom, O. W.: Changes in the Underlying Coronary Circulation Secondary to Bypass Grafting, *Circulation,* 49, 50 (suppl. 2):80, 1974.

141 Grondin, C. M., Lesperance, J., Bourassa, M. G., Pasternac, A., Campeau, L., and Grondin, P.: Serial Angiographic Evaluation in 60 Consecutive Patients with Aortocoronary Artery Vein Grafts 2 Weeks, 1 Year and 3 Years After Operations. *J. Thorac. Cardiovasc. Surg.,* 67:1, 1974.

142 Griffith, L. S. C., Bulkley, B. H., Hutchins, G. M., and Brawley, R. K.: Occlusive Changes at the Coronary Artery-Bypass Anastomosis: Morphologic Study of 95 Grafts, *J. Thorac. Cardiovasc. Surg.,* 73:668, 1977.

143 Lie, J. T., Lawrie, G. M., and Morris, G. C., Jr.: Atherosclerosis of Aortocoronary Bypass Grafts in Normal and Hyperlipoproteinemic Patients, *Am. J. Cardiol.,* 39:285, 1977. (Abstract.)

144 Mathur, V. S., and Guinn, G. A.: Prospective Randomized Study of Coronary Bypass Surgery in Stable Angina: The First 100 Patients, *Circulation,* 51, 52 (suppl. 1):133, 1975.

145 Campeau, L., Lesperance, J., Corbara, F., Hermann, J., Groudin, C. M., and Bourassa, M. G.: Aortocoronary Saphenous Vein Bypass Graft Changes 5 to 7 Years After Surgery, *Circulation,* 58 (suppl. 1):170, 1978.

146 Lawrie, G. M., Morris, G. C., Jr., Chapman, D. W., Winters, W. L., and Lie, J. T.: Patterns of Patency of 596 Vein Grafts Up to Seven Years After Aortocoronary Bypass, *J. Thorac. Cardiovasc. Surg.,* 73:443, 1977.

147 Ben-Zvi, J., Hildner, F. J., and Javier, R. P., Progression of Coronary Artery Disease, *Am. J. Cardiol.,* 34:295, 1974.

148 Bemis, C. E., Gorlin, R., and Kemp, H. G., Progression of Coronary Artery Disease, *Circulation,* 47:455, 1973.

149 Busch, U., Garcia, E., Hall, R. J., Mathur, V. S., DeCastro, C. M., Guttin, J., Dear, W. E., and Cooley, D. A.: Serial Graded Exercise Testing in Follow-up of Coronary Artery Bypass. A Preliminary Report, *Cardiovasc. Dis. Bull. Texas Heart Inst.,* 4:149, 1977.

150 Brewer, D. L., Bilbro, R. H., and Bartel, A. G.: Myocardial Infarction as a Complication of Coronary Bypass Surgery, *Circulation,* 47:58, 1973.

151 Shepherd, R. L., Itscoitz, S. B., Glancy, D. L., Stinson, E. B., Reis, R. L., Olinger, G. N., Clark, C. E., and Epstein, S. E.: Deterioration of Myocardial Function Following Aorto-coronary Bypass Operation, *Circulation,* 49:467, 1974.

152 Sternberg, L., Wisnecki, J. S., Ullyot, D. J., and Gertz, E. W.: Significance of New Q Waves After Aortocoronary Bypass Surgery. Correlation with Changes in Ventricular Wall Motion, *Circulation,* 52:1037, 1975.

153 Vismara, L. A., Miller, R. R., Price, J. E., Karem, R., DeMaria, A. N., and Mason, D. T.: Improved Longevity Due to Reduction of Sudden Death by Aortocoronary Bypass in Coronary Atherosclerosis, *Am. J. Cardiol.,* 39:919, 1977.

Acknowledgment and appreciation for technical assistance in the preparation of this manuscript are expressed to Ms. Christine Abrams, Ms. Joyce Staton, and Dr. Kenneth Gold and for statistical analysis to Dr. Albert Gray.

Chapter 17

Improved Survival in Patients with Chronic Angina Pectoris Treated Surgically: Report of a Randomized Prospective Study of Aortocoronary Bypass from Hines, Illinois*

ROLF M. GUNNAR, M.D., HENRY S. LOEB, M.D., ROBERT PALAC, M.D., and ROQUE PIFARRE, M.D.

INTRODUCTION

Although there have now been several studies to evaluate the effect of coronary surgery on longevity in patients with angina pectoris, there is apparently increasing confusion rather than increasing consensus. It is not surprising that the medical community looked upon aortocoronary bypass with skepticism despite excellent relief of angina. Previous surgical approaches to the disease had all given evidence of relief of pain. These procedures included poudrage of the pericardium, internal thoracic artery ligation, stenosis of the coronary sinus, sympathectomy, and finally, internal thoracic implantation. Despite the fact that each procedure gave relief of pain, there was no evidence that life was prolonged. The medical community was attuned to be skeptical of the efficacy of any treatment of angina because of the difficulty in evaluating results of drug therapy without carefully designed and vigorously controlled double-blind studies.

Aortocoronary bypass, however, had the advantage of logic and is analogous to revasculariztion of other organs. It also gives 90 percent incidence of improvement of symptoms,[1] which is certainly better than any previous surgical or medical approach. It is not surprising that it became popular when relief of pain became predictable and surgical mortality became very reasonable.

It was in the enthusiasm for studies of patients allocated to medical and surgical treatment by randomization to settle the question of the effect of this operation on longevity that we joined the Veterans Administration Cooperative Study of Surgical Treatment for Coronary Occlusive Disease.[2] To classify a study as prospective and randomized cloaks it with a great deal of validity which it may or may not deserve. One must understand what population is being randomized and what patients are being excluded either by design or by their own (or their physician's) decision. The clinical question to be answered by the prospective randomized study of chronic angina pectoris is whether the patient presenting for surgical treatment by aortocoronary bypass will live longer than if he or she were treated by standard medical regimens. In order to answer this question, one must randomize nearly all patients that fall into this broad category. If we only select for randomization a very few patients in whom clinical experience gives little enthusiasm for either form of therapy, the study will answer a question that is not being asked. The Veterans Administration study was labeled as a chronic stable angina study. If the angina were totally stable, there would probably be little consideration of the patient for surgery, since clinical experience would indicate that most patients who present for surgery have had some increase in the severity of their symptoms at the time they seek medical help. Therefore, in our group of patients, we did not deny entry into the study because of some increase in severity of symptoms, but only if the patient truly fit the definition of accelerating or unstable angina with continuation of pain after hospitalization.

The Veterans Administration study has the advantage of a very hard end point, which is death. This is easily definable. However, it can be divided into cardiac and noncardiac causes or disease-related and non-disease-related causes, and this softening of the end point can lead to misinterpretation. Because of this rather awesome end point, it was believed by our group that periodic review of the comparative status

*From the Department of Medicine, Section of Cardiology, Veterans Administration Edward J. Hines Medical Center and Loyola University Stritch School of Medicine, and the Department of Surgery, Section of Cardio-Thoracic Surgery, Veterans Administration Edward J. Hines Medical Center and Loyola University Stritch School of Medicine.

of the randomized patients was necessary. In 1973, we reviewed our experience with the patients who had left main coronary disease and found a significant increase in mortality in patients treated medically as compared to those treated surgically. It was our feeling that had this been a drug trial, wherein one form of therapy was found to be lethal even in one institution, some notification of the medical community should be made. We therefore reported our results to the VA study group. We did respect the agreement not to publish independently, and it was not until 18 months later that the report of the larger study was made, showing a significant increase in mortality in patients with disease of the left main coronary artery treated medically versus patients treated surgically.

From the time we entered the study, we understood that we would be allowed to publish our data by institution when a major end point had been published for the entire group. We believe that the release of the rather definitive "preliminary" report by Murphy et al.[4] allowed us to analyze and publish the findings of our subgroup. Since we think that we do represent a unique experience within a randomized cooperative study, we feel it is important that our data be made available for scrutiny by the medical community.

PATIENT POPULATION

The patients considered for this study were all males with chronic angina pectoris for at least 6 months and were under medical therapy for at least 3 months. Reasons for exclusion from the study were uncontrolled hypertension or diabetes, severe heart failure, significant cardiac or noncardiac disease that might influence longevity, and acute myocardial infarction within 6 months prior to randomization. The patients in the study were required to have an abnormal resting or exercise electrocardiogram. The patients were randomized after coronary arteriography and left ventriculography. The decision that the patient should be included in the randomized study was made by a medical and surgical team that worked together not only at the Veterans Administration Hospital but also at the University Hospital, where a large program of aortocoronary bypass was under way. Thus, one major consideration was whether or not the patient would be advised to have aortocoronary bypass had he presented to the University Hospital. Patients were not excluded from the study for poor ventricular function unless such function would have excluded them from consideration for aortocoronary bypass. Patients with a large, definable aneurysm that would qualify for resection were excluded from the study. Having determined the patients qualified for randomization, the ac-

tual randomization was done by the VA statistical center.

Between 1968 and 1974, we randomized 152 patients between medicine and surgery. Four patients were immediately dropped from the series. Three were excluded because they had Vineberg procedures, and 1 patient, on re-review after randomization, was not considered an operative candidate. This left 148 patients to represent the baseline group. Seventy-seven were in the medical series and 71 in the surgical series.

When we analyze the baseline characteristics of the 148 patients, there were no significant differences between the two groups. All patients were male by design of the study. The mean age in the medical group was 52.6 years, and in the surgical group, 50.8 years. There were no significant differences between the two groups in the duration of angina, the New York Heart Association classification, or incidence of previous myocardial infarction, hypertension, congestive heart failure, cerebrovascular accidents, or family history of cardiovascular disease. The percentage of patients with one-, two-, and three-vessel disease was not significantly different, although there were slightly more patients with three-vessel disease in the surgical group. There were a greater number of patients with left main coronary stenosis in the medical group, but these patients were eliminated for comparison of the survival curves between the two groups (Table 17-1).

TABLE 17-1

Baseline characteristics of 148 patients with coronary artery disease randomized to medical or surgical treatment between 1968 and 1974

Characteristics	Randomized to medicine	Randomized to surgery
Number of patients	77	71
Age	52.6 years	50.8 years
History of angina prior to randomization (interval in years):		
0–4	51 (66.2%)	47 (66.2%)
4–10	20 (26.0%)	16 (22.5%)
> 10	6 (7.8%)	8 (11.3%)
New York Heart Assoc. class.:		
Class I	0 (0.0%)	1 (1.4%)
Class II	27 (35.1%)	24 (33.8%)
Class III	45 (58.4%)	43 (60.6%)
Class IV	5 (6.5%)	3 (4.2%)
History of:		
Previous myocardial infarct	43 (55.8%)	36 (50.7%)
Hypertension	28 (36.4%)	28 (39.4%)
Congestive heart failure	8 (10.4%)	5 (7.0%)
Cerebral vascular accident	2 (2.6%)	2 (2.8%)
Family history of CV disease	43 (55.8%)	43 (60.6%)
Physical examination:		
Obesity	25 (32.5%)	25 (35.2%)

TABLE 17-1 *Continued*
Baseline characteristics of 148 patients with coronary artery disease randomized to medical or surgical treatment between 1968 and 1974

Characteristics	Randomized to medicine	Randomized to surgery
Blood pressure:		
Normotensive	51 (66.2%)	50 (70.4%)
Diastolic ≥ 95 mm Hg	10 (13.0%)	7 (9.9%)
Systolic ≥ 150 mm Hg	6 (7.8%)	8 (11.3%)
Systolic ≥ 150 mm Hg; diastolic ≥ 95 mm Hg	10 (13.0%)	6 (8.5%)
Lab data:		
Serum cholesterol < 280 mg/dl	53 (68.8%)	58 (81.7%)
Serum cholesterol ≥ 280 mg/dl	20 (26.0%)	12 (16.9%)
Not determined	4 (5.2%)	1 (1.4%)
Cardiothoracic ratio:		
≤ 0.50	64 (83.1%)	60 (84.5%)
> 0.50	8 (10.4%)	6 (8.5%)
Not measured	5 (6.0%)	5 (7.0%)
Coronary angiography (luminal obstruction 50% as critical stenosis):		
One-vessel disease	11 (14.3%)	12 (16.9%)
Two-vessel disease	33 (42.8%)	26 (36.6%)
Three-vessel disease	26 (33.8%)	29 (40.8%)
Left main coronary stenosis	7 (9.1%)	4 (5.6%)
Coronary artery score (0–6):		
1–3	30 (39.0%)	25 (35.2%)
4–6	47 (61.0%)	46 (64.8%)
Hemodynamics:		
LVEDP ≤ 12 mm Hg	42 (54.5%)	37 (52.1%)
LVEDP 13–23 mm Hg	27 (35.1%)	31 (43.6%)
LVEDP 24 mm Hg	4 (5.2%)	2 (2.8%)
Not measured	4 (5.2%)	1 (1.4%)
Left ventricular wall motion:		
Normal or mild hypokinesis	46 (59.7%)	45 (63.4%)
One-segment dys- or akinesis	18 (23.4%)	18 (25.4%)
Two-segment dys- or akinesis	10 (13.0%)	8 (11.3%)
Three-segment dys- or akinesis	2 (2.6%)	0 (0.0%)
Not done	1 (1.3%)	0 (0.0%)

The coronary stenosis was further analyzed by a scoring system that took into consideration the dominance of the vessels and gave greater emphasis to proximal lesions. This scoring system has been described elsewhere[5] and is graded 0 to 6, with 6 being the maximum score than can be allocated. There were 47 patients in the medical group with a score of 4 to 6 and 46 such patients in the surgical group. There were no significant differences in the hemodynamic measurements between the two groups. In analysis of wall motion abnormalities, there were no significant differences. There were 12 patients in the medical group with two- and three-segment wall motion abnormalities and only 8 in the surgical group with such

abnormalities. However, when analyzed for moderate or severe wall motion abnormalities or ejection fraction, the groups did not show significant differences.

Seven patients in the medical group had greater than 50 percent narrowing of the left main coronary artery. Five of these patients have died, 1 has been operated on and is alive, and only 1, whose left main lesion was the least severe, remains alive and continues to be treated medically. Four patients who had been randomized to surgery had greater than 50 percent narrowing of the left main coronary artery. All of these have been operated on, and all are alive.

RESULTS

In analyzing the mode of death of the medical patients, there were 28 deaths in the 77 patients randomized to medicine (Table 17-2). Of the 7 patients with stenosis of the left main coronary artery, 4 patients had sudden cardiac death and 1 patient died by suicide. Of the 70 patients randomized to medicine who did not have left main coronary artery stenosis, 54 remained in the medical series, and of these patients, 20 have died. Twelve had sudden cardiac deaths and 1 had nonsudden cardiac death. Three patients died of noncardiac causes (ruptured abdominal viscus, cerebrovascular accident, and metastatic carcinoma), 1 patient died by suicide, and 3 patients had complex illnesses and the cause of death was not easily classified. One of these unclassified patients called the hospital complaining of severe chest pain and several hours later was found dead. He had aspirated prior to death, and the autopsy report noted elevated blood alcohol levels. Another patient who frequently walked by the lake was found in the lake, but no suicide note was found. A third

TABLE 17-2

Status of patients with coronary artery disease on December 1, 1978, who had been randomized to medical or surgical treatment between 1968 and 1974

	Alive	Dead	Total
Randomized to medicine			
Left main coronary stenosis	2	5	7
Without left main stenosis			
Adherers	34	20	54
Operated	13	3	16
Total	49	28	77
Randomized to surgery			
Left main coronary stenosis	4	0	4
Without left main stenosis			
Adherers	55	8	63
Refused surgery	3	1	4
Total	62	9	71

patient died of cardiac failure 2 days after surgery for a bleeding peptic ulcer. The VA study group carries these 3 patients as noncardiac deaths, but we would prefer that they not be classified, since it is at least as likely that they were cardiac deaths. Sixteen of the medical patients crossed over to surgery, and 3 of these patients have died (2 suddenly and 1 during surgery). Of the 71 patients randomized to surgery, there have been 9 deaths, all in the 67 patients without left main coronary artery stenosis. Three were surgical deaths, 1 patient had a sudden cardiac death, and 2 patients died of cardiac disease but not suddenly. One patient had a noncardiac death, and 1 patient had a complex illness and the cause of death was not easily classified. This latter patient was hospitalized for a catatonic state, developed a febrile illness, became hypotensive, and died several days later. An electro-cardiogram recorded shortly before death showed no acute changes. This patient is classified as a cardiac death by the VA study group. However, we think it is more likely that this was septic shock, and we there-fore label the cause of death as nonclassified. There were 4 patients randomized to surgery who refused surgery. One of these patients died suddenly of a car-diac death, and the rest remain alive.

Of the 54 patients randomized to medicine and treated medically, 2 patients committed suicide, and 1 patient in the nonclassified group may have com-mitted suicide. The classification of suicide as to whether it is disease related or not is somewhat ob-scure. It is of interest that at last report all but 1 of the patients in the entire VA cooperative study who are classified as suicides were in the medical group. Since propranolol can cause depression, and since continued pain and limitation of life-style also tend to cause depression, it may well be that the suicides are related to the disease and medical treatment rather than being unrelated causes of death. Because of the ambiguities regarding mode of death, we have chosen to analyze our own results according to survival only, as was done in the published reports emanating from the VA total cooperative study.

Since it is difficult to completely justify any single mode of analysis of survival of patients in the medical series as compared to the surgical series, we have used several perspectives in analyzing our data, calculating cumulative survival rates by actuarial life-table meth-ods.[6] We have compared the groups by considering patients according to their randomization despite their mode of treatment, by considering mode of treatment irrespective of randomization, by analyzing only those patients who adhered to the treatment to which they were randomized, and finally by treating crossover patients as alive and having been lost to follow-up at time of crossover. The argument is quite persuasive that one should consider outcome on the basis of ran-domization despite the mode of treatment. The argu-ment is based on the high probability that patients who cross over, particularly when they cross over later in the study, do so because of acceleration of symptoms or at least failure of medical management to control their symptoms adequately. There is a discrepancy in numbers between the patients who cross over from the surgical group and those who cross over from the medical group, since once surgery has been performed the patient is no longer able to cross over. Thus, there are only 4 patients in the entire group who were ran-domized to surgery and actually refused the proce-dure. The countering argument, of course, is that if a patient randomized to medicine has surgery and dies at surgery, should he not be considered a surgical death and not a medical death. The logic of this ar-gument would require that patients in the medical se-ries who cross over to surgery and have a good out-come should therefore be credited to surgery. These arguments for various modes of analysis are not re-solvable and are each with strong advocates. In ana-lyzing our data by each method and showing that the significance of the difference remains between the sur-vival in the surgical group versus the medical group,

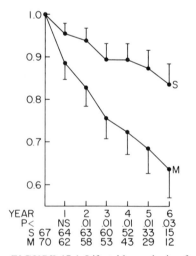

FIGURE 17-1 Life-table analysis of medical (M) and surgical (S) survival after randomization considering pa-tients as originally randomized despite ultimate therapy. The bar represents standard error of the mean. Numbers below the abscissa are: years after ran-domization, probability value, and numbers of patients at the beginning of each interval in the surgical or medical group. All patients were randomized between 1968 and 1974. Patients with left main coronary artery stenosis have been excluded from this analysis.

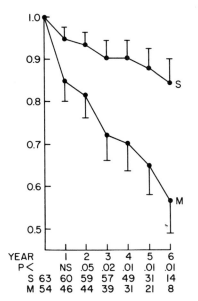

FIGURE 17-2 Life-table analysis considering only patients who adhered to the treatment group to which they were randomized. Notations as in Fig. 17-1.

we have a compelling substantiation that differences between the two groups are real.

The purest mode of analysis is to analyze by randomization treating crossover patients as originally randomized (Fig. 17-1). In this analysis of patients without left main coronary stenosis, there is a 5-year survival of 68.7 percent in the medical series and 87.4 percent in the surgical series. This difference is significant at the $p < .01$ level. In this analysis, there is a significantly improved survival in the surgical group in each of the years 2 through 6. If we analyze only those patients who remained in the series to which they were randomized, there are fewer patients for analysis, and some would argue that this is a fairer analysis. In this analysis (Fig. 17-2), the survival at 5 years in the medical series is 65.0 percent and 88.2 percent in the surgical series, with a difference significant at $p < .005$. Again, the difference in survival between the two groups is significant for years 2 through 6. If we analyze by treatment received (Fig. 17-3), i.e. those patients randomized to medicine who are eventually treated surgically are analyzed with the surgical group, we then have a survival of 65.7 percent at 5 years in the medical group and 86.8 percent in the surgical group. This shows significantly improved survival in the surgical group at 5 years with $p < .005$, and the difference is significant in the first and third through the sixth years. The final analysis (Fig. 17-4) is by randomization but eliminates the patients who crossed over from medicine to surgery, at which time

they are considered alive but lost to follow-up, and eliminates the surgical patients who refused surgery as lost to follow-up in the first year. By this analysis, the 5-year survival in the medical group is 70 percent and 88.3 percent in the surgical group. This difference is significant at $p < .02$, and the difference between medical and surgical survival shows significantly improved survival in the surgical group for years 3 through 6.

DISCUSSION

We have recently reported the 1972–1974 cohort of patients randomized in the Hines study,[5] and this can more easily be related to the other hospitals in the Veterans Administration study, as reported in their several reports.[4,7,8] The life-table analyses, as presented above, do not differ significantly from the 1972–1974 cohort.

How then do we differ from the combined data of the cooperative study? The Hines operative mortality of 4.5 percent is slightly better than the 5.6 percent reported for the cooperative study.[4] If, in the Hines group, we include the patients who crossed over from medical randomization, surgical mortality is 4.8 percent. The cumulative survival at 5 years of 88 percent, although third highest for the entire study, is only slightly better than the 84 percent survival at 5 years for the entire group. Therefore, there is no significant difference between the surgical survival at Hines and

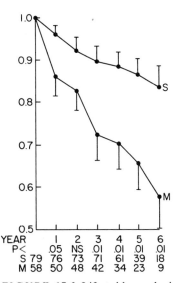

FIGURE 17-3 Life-table analysis considering patients as treated regardless of the group to which they were randomized. Notations as in Fig. 17-1.

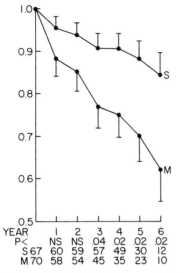

FIGURE 17-4 Life-table analysis considering patients as randomized, but in the medical group, crossover patients are considered alive and lost to follow-up at the time of surgery. In the surgical group, the patients who refused surgery are considered alive and lost to follow-up at 1 year. Notations as in Fig. 17-1.

the cumulative survival for the group. On the other hand, the medical survival is different in that the 60-month survival in our group is 67 percent, while the survival at this time is 80 percent in the entire group. There is only one other hospital in the VA cooperative study that has a similarly low survival rate in the medical group. Since there is no evidence of a significant difference in the method of medical therapy between hospitals, it would suggest that there are two populations within the study group. Six hospitals contributing a total of 89 patients randomized to medicine had no mortality in the first 3 years of this study. The mortality curves for all the hospitals except Hines and one other are above the mean for the entire cooperative study. The two hospitals with increased mortality had survival rates of approximately 75 percent in the medically randomized group at 3 years. The question must be asked, therefore, whether the method of randomization was different in these two hospitals. The data are not available at this point to determine the number of patients operated on outside of randomization in all the cooperating hospitals, but one would suspect that this information could give a clue to the inclusiveness of the patients to be studied within the randomized prospective project. We did analyze the data from Hines and have found that very few patients were excluded from randomization, except by very hard criteria. During the 1972–1974 period, there were 124 patients at Hines Hospital who had aortocoronary bypass outside of the randomized study. Forty of these patients were evaluated angiographically at other hospitals and were referred to Hines for surgery. It had been decided prior to initiating the study that these patients would not be considered for randomization. Nineteen patients were excluded because they had had a myocardial infarct within 6 months of study. Seventeen patients had associated valve disease which precluded them from the study. Fifteen patients had ventricular aneurysms considered large enough to qualify for aneurysmectomy. This left only 33 patients who had aortocoronary bypass with softer criteria for exclusion from randomization. Seventeen of these patients were considered to have such severe instability of their angina that they were excluded from randomization because of the preinfarction syndrome. Sixteen patients were excluded for miscellaneous causes, including inability to obtain informed consent.

To verify the validity of our proposal that we, in fact, randomized a clear cross section of the patients presenting with chronic angina who would be considered for aortocoronary bypass, we must now compare our group to other studies of the natural history of chronic angina pectoris.

The series of Block et al. encompassed 6,882 patients followed at Mayo Clinic for at least 5 years.[9] This was an extension of the series reported by Parker et al.[10] and encompassed patients entered between 1927 and 1944. The 5-year survival in this group was 58.4 percent as compared to our 5-year survival of 68.7 percent. Their series included 19.7 percent female patients who had significantly improved survival as compared to the males. The average age of 58.8 years in Block's series was slightly greater than the 52.6 years in our group. Block's group had a 33.8 percent incidence of hypertension as compared to a 33.7 percent incidence in our group. Cardiac hypertrophy was present in 27.3 percent of Block's patients and in 12.7 percent of our group. Fifty-five percent of our patients had had a prior myocardial infarction, while this had been reported in only 23.7 percent of Block's group. To compare the two groups, we must recognize that none of Block's patients had had angiographic documentation of their disease. From our experience[11] and that of others,[12] we would expect that 10 to 15 percent of Block's patients had normal coronary arteries and that 7 to 8 percent had left main stem coronary artery stenosis, conditions eliminated from our series that would bias the survival curves in opposite directions.

Richards et al. reviewed a series of 456 patients who had been diagnosed as having angina pectoris as a result of coronary atherosclerosis between 1927 and 1931.[13] All patients were followed to death or a minimum of 25 years. The 5-year survival of 64.5 percent in their series can be compared to the 68.7 percent survival in our series. Again, it must be realized that Richards' patients had not been documented by angiography and that the biases created by inclusion of patients with normal coronary arteries and patients with left main coronary stenosis would tend to cancel each other. Patients were slightly older in Richards' group, where the average age for males was 56.6 years. However, they showed only a slight but consistent bias favoring prolonged survival in the younger patients when they compared survival curves in patients 36 to 55 years of age to patients 56 to 80 years of age. The 3-year survival in male patients reported by Richards was 79.3 percent as compared to the 75.8 percent 3-year survival in our group and the 87 percent survival reported by Murphy et al. in the VA study.[4]

Friesinger, Page, and Ross were the first to report a group of patients with angina and relate the survival to angiographic analysis of the severity of the coronary disease.[12] Between 1960 and 1967, they selected 350 patients for coronary angiography from a group of more than 1,000 patients referred for evaluation of chest pain. After eliminating patients with associated diseases and unsatisfactory studies, and 40 patients who subsequently underwent coronary vascular surgical procedures, they had a population of 224, of whom 103 had significant coronary disease and who could be followed to evaluate the natural history of the disease as modified by current medical management. They devised a scoring system for location and extent of stenosis of 0 to 5 for each of the three major coronary vessels, with increasing numbers representing increasing severity of disease. Ten of 72 patients had typical angina pectoris but no significant coronary obstruction (13.9 percent). This percentage of patients with convincing histories is similar to our own experience at Loyola University Hospital[11] in patients with accelerating angina, is a fairly common percentage in such studies, and should be kept in mind as one analyzes data that are not substantiated by coronary angiography.

The 5-year survival in the 103 patients with significant coronary artery disease was 73 percent, but 40 patients had been removed for coronary surgical procedures. The 72 patients with typical angina pectoris in the group of Friesinger et al.[12] had a 5-year survival of 71 percent, which is very close to the 5-year survival of 68.7 percent in our group. Friesinger's patients with scores ≥ 10 had a 47 percent 5-year survival rate. The data according to the Friesinger score are difficult to apply to our group without re-review of all the arteriograms, but the score of ≥ 10 is probably similar to our own coronary score of 4 to 6, in which group the 5-year survival is 63 percent.

In 1974, Humphries et al. updated this series, which was now 12 years old and still had accurate status

information on 97 percent of the patients.[13] At entry, this group of patients had had a low incidence of Q waves, conduction defects, and arrhythmias because, at that time, patients of this type were not considered candidates for angiography. Eighty-three of the patients had abnormal ST-T waves, and these patients had a 26 percent mortality as compared to a 6.5 percent death rate for those with normal ST-T waves. They found the most important predictors of mortality were abnormal ST-T changes in patients with coronary obstruction and the severity of the coronary disease.

In their survival curve, it is interesting to note that at 5 years in this updated study, 53 percent of their patients with coronary scores ≥ 10 were alive, and from that time through 10 years the curve is fairly flat. In patients with scores of 5 to 9, 91 percent are alive at 5 years, but at 7 years, there is a sudden break in the curve, and at 9 years, only 53 percent are alive. This break, although later in time, is very similar to our own curves for patients with mild disease and perhaps indicates a critical phase of the progression of the disease. However, the number of patients is small as one gets to the end of the survival curve, and therefore, a single death has a greater effect on the curve.

Oberman et al. reported their experience at the University of Alabama in following 246 patients undergoing arteriography for chest pain between 1965 and 1970.[14] They excluded patients with associated disease and 55 patients who had a cardiovascular surgical procedure. All patients were entered before aortocoronary bypass was being performed at the University of Alabama, so it is most likely that the surgical procedures referred to, if for coronary disease, were internal thoracic implantations. The mean age of 46.8 years for the group was slightly younger than our series. Ninety-eight patients (39.8 percent) had no significant coronary obstruction, and these patients had an annual mortality of 1.4 percent per year. The patients with coronary disease were divided into 46 (31.3 percent) with single-vessel disease, 50 (33.8 percent) with double-vessel disease, and 52 (35.1 percent) with triple-vessel disease. These patients had an annual mortality of 2.0 percent, 13.0 percent, and 15.0 percent, respectively. If this mortality is applied to our own series and we use the 2-year statistics (since Oberman et al. reported a 22-month follow-up), we would anticipate a 2-year survival of 76 percent, as compared to an actual survival of 82.9 percent at 2 years in our medically randomized group. The survival rate of 91 percent in the entire VA group more closely resembles the single-vessel disease patients in the group of Oberman et al.

Kannel and Feinleib reported on 303 patients with angina pectoris from the Framingham study.[15] These patients were identified from a population that was free from cardiovascular disease at the time of entry, and a significant number of patients were identified as having angina by questions asked at routine follow-up. This undoubtedly differs from the presentation of the patient seeking surgical correction of his coronary disease. Thirty-four percent of our patients had had angina for more than 4 years at the time of randomization, and 50 percent of the medically randomized patients in the total VA study had had angina for more than 25 months. Previous myocardial infarction had been documented in 55.8 percent of our patients and in 59.3 percent of the total VA medical group. The patients followed by Kannel and Feinleib presented with angina de novo (53 percent) or following a myocardial infarction (47 percent), but in most instances, this would be the first infarct, since the patients entered the study healthy. The overall mortality for men was 4 percent per year whether angina was the initial cardiac event or followed another event. However, the initial year is without mortality and, if one takes the survival curve for years 1 through 9, then yearly mortality is 4.8 percent per year, which is in keeping with our medically randomized group, which had a 6.3 percent per year mortality for the first 5 years. We must take into consideration the late stage of the disease at which our patients entered the study and the fact that all our patients were documented angiographically, while the Framingham study probably has a significant number of patients with normal coronary arteries. Kannel and Feinleib's patients, despite the early stage of the disease, still show a higher mortality than the 3.5 percent per year (first 3 years) reported by the VA study after the Hines patients were removed, or the 3 percent per year mortality of the series after removing the Hines data and the one other hospital with a similar survival curve.

Bruschke et al. reported on 590 consecutive nonsurgical patients with documented coronary artery disease followed for 5 to 9 years at the Cleveland Clinic.[16,17] These patients had all been studied by selective coronary angiography between 1963 and 1965. They eliminated patients who had coronary surgery, but this was an era when only internal thoracic implantation was available, and this operation did not depend on the presence of bypassable vessels but rather on the intractability of the angina to medical management. It is most probable that this exclusion would be at least as likely to minimize the mortality of the remaining series as to accentuate it. Left main coronary stenosis occurred in 6.3 percent of their patients, and this group had a 5-year mortality of 56.8 percent.

In the study by Bruschke et al., 202 patients had single-vessel disease (36.5 percent), as compared to 14.3 percent in our series; 233 (42.1 percent) had double-vessel disease, as compared to 42.8 percent in our series; and 118 (21.3 percent) had triple-vessel disease, as compared to 33.8 percent in our series.[16] The 5-year mortality for one-, two-, and three-vessel disease in this series was 17.3 percent, 38.2 percent, and 55.1 percent, respectively. If we assign this death rate to our series based on the number of vessels involved, we could anticipate a 5-year survival (excluding left main lesions) of 58.9 percent, which compared to our actual 68.7 percent survival at 5 years. This improved survival in our group, when compared to expected survival, may well relate to the improvements in medical management that have occurred in the intervening years. The mortality of 3.5 percent per year in the first 3 years in the VA cooperative study after removing the Hines patients compared most favorably to the mortality in patients with single-vessel disease in the series of Bruschke et al.

Webster, Moberg, and Rincon, also from the Cleveland Clinic, studied the natural history of 469 patients with 80 to 100 percent proximal occlusions of one or more major coronary arteries.[18] A second vessel was considered involved if there was greater than 50 percent proximal narrowing. These patients were entered in the study between 1960 and 1965 and were followed for at least 6 years. The average age of their patients was 49.5 years, and one-, two-, and three-vessel disease was present in 40.5 percent, 38.4 percent, and 21.1 percent, respectively, after eliminating patients with left main coronary stenosis. Patients with one-, two-, and three-vessel disease had a yearly mortality of 3.4 percent, 6.8 percent, and 10.2 percent, respectively. If we apply these statistics to our own series, we would anticipate a 5-year survival of 62.4 percent, which compared to our actual survival of 68.7 percent at 5 years. The mortality in the VA medical group is almost identical to that in the single-vessel disease group in this series.

Russek reported on 133 patients with severe angina pectoris placed on an intensive therapeutic regimen of beta blocking agents and isosorbide dinitrate.[19] Only 32 of his patients were studied angiographically, and 26 of these (81 percent) had severe three-vessel disease. He separated 31 patients as poor risks for long-term survival on the basis of congestive heart failure, cardiac enlargement, multiple myocardial infarctions, gallop rhythm, refractory hypertension, atrial fibrillation, severe and uncontrolled diabetes, previous stroke or cerebrovascular insufficiency, or age over 70 years. Russek states that in his good-risk group the mortality is not unlike that of the general population of similar age. It is difficult to compare our series to his, since the modifiers of his criteria for "poor risk" are hard to interpret. Previous myocardial infarction was present in 55.8 percent of our group and in only 28 percent of his "good-risk" group. The 25 percent mortality per year in the "poor-risk" group, if applied just to our 10.4 percent of patients with congestive heart failure, would add a yearly mortality of 3.5 percent to our series, and we do not know how to apply the other criteria to our population to get an overall anticipated mortality figure. The overall yearly mortality for Russek's entire group was 4.5 percent, which suggests that with careful selection and intensive medical management, longevity can be increased in patients with severe angina pectoris, but this series suffers from lack of a control population. It also has the weakness of the early studies in that most patients did not have angiographic definition of their disease. Twenty-three percent of the patients were women, who have a better survival with angina pectoris.

Reeves et al. reviewed the natural history of angina[20] and, in addition to the series of medically treated patients reviewed above, also reviewed the series of Lichtlen and Moccetti[21] and Slagle et al.[22] reported in 1972. This review reinforced the need to look at subgroups of patients to understand and make meaningful comparisons of the natural history. They pointed out that electrocardiographic evidence of prior myocardial infarction increased 22-month mortality from 7 percent to 31 percent. In the Alabama study, 61 of the 148 patients had electrocardiographic evidence of prior myocardial infarction.[14] A history of congestive heart failure increased the 22-month mortality from 8 percent to 40 percent, and this was present in 36 of the 148 patients. He also noted increased mortality in patients with enlarged hearts, high resting heart rates, positive exercise tests, and ST-segment abnormalities. It appears that the patients in the Alabama series, although having no higher incidence of prior myocardial infarction, did have more evidence of congestive heart failure than the patients in our group or those in the combined Veterans Administration cooperative study. Reeves et al. concluded that it is difficult to justify surgery in patients with single-vessel disease.[20] However, patients with double-vessel disease (if there is evidence of ventricular dysfunction and ischemic pain) and those with triple-vessel disease deserve aortocoronary bypass. They also think that patients with very proximal left anterior descending disease may be candidates for surgery. It seems that these conclusions are not altered by our findings and will most likely survive the Veterans Administration cooperative study conclusions.

Vlietstra et al., in reviewing the recent experience at Mayo Clinic, emphasized the importance of ejection fraction in determining prognosis and felt that this was more important than severity or extent of coronary disease.[23] Unfortunately, their medical series was heavily weighted with patients with insufficient symptoms to be considered for operation or with ventricular function that was too poor for surgery. To compare our group, we would refer to the 1972–1973 cohort in whom more careful comparisons of left ventricular

function were made.[5] In this group, 29 percent of the medical and 20 percent of the surgical patients had ejection fractions of less than 0.45 ($p > .05$), and there were no significant differences in incidence of moderate or severe wall motion abnormalities which were present in 45 percent of the medical and 41 percent of the surgical patients.

From this review of the studies of the natural history and predictors of mortality of patients with angina pectoris resulting from coronary artery disease, we conclude that our medically randomized patients are representative of the population being considered for aortocoronary bypass and, therefore, are an excellent control group in our prospective randomized study of the effects of coronary artery surgery on longevity in patients with chronic angina pectoris. The somewhat improved survival in our group over most other historical control groups probably represents the effect of aggressive use of propranolol and longer acting vasodilators. We are at a loss to explain the benign nature of the disease and the excellent survival of the medical patients in the remainder of the Veterans Administration cooperative study. If the other hospitals have come upon a better method of medical treatment, it has not been made known to the rest of the group. If we consider the mortality of the patients in the entire study after subtracting the Hines experience and the experience of one other hospital with a similar survival curve, then survival is only slightly poorer than in males of similar age but without coronary disease.[14] It seems that these patients represent a group in whom there is little enthusiasm by patient or doctor for aortocoronary bypass, and therefore, they do not constitute a valid control group for evaluating the efficacy of this surgical procedure.

Green et al. constructed survival curves for medical management of patients with stable and unstable angina and separated out patients with lesions of the left main coronary artery.[24] They constructed these curves from a review of 3,009 patients reported in 24 various series, all patients having had angiography. The survival curve for the non-left main lesions shows a 72 percent survival at 5 years, which closely correlates with our own 5-year survival. Hurst et al. presented a review of the various methods of comparing medicine to surgery using matched series accumulated concurrently or sequentially, as well as reviewing the prospective randomized studies that are available.[25] Even when one separates out the survival curve into various severities of coronary artery disease, it appears that all except the Veterans Administration study of chronic stable angina[4] and the cooperative study of accelerating angina[26] have very similar curves. Therefore, the large majority of survival curves closely matched the survival curves of the Hines study.

In further validating our results, we must compare

them with results of other prospective randomized studies of angina pectoris—both stable and unstable—to see if treatment, base population, or method of randomization can explain discrepancies.

Mathur and Guinn randomized 116 patients to medicine or aortocoronary bypass surgery for stable angina pectoris between January 1972 and March 1975.[27-29] In their recent report, they have followed these patients for 13 to 52 months, with a mean of 38 months.[29] The two groups were very similar and were also very similar to our own group in that half of the patients had had myocardial infarctions. The distribution of one-, two-, and three-vessel disease was 15 percent, 39 percent, and 52 percent, respectively. There were 3 operative deaths in the surgical series and no other cardiac deaths following surgery. However, 1 patient died of bronchogenic carcinoma. In the medically treated group, there were 7 deaths, all cardiac, and in addition, 4 patients developed such severe angina that they had to undergo aortocoronary bypass. These patients are treated by Mathur and Guinn as lost to follow-up for analysis. Their 3-year survival rate is approximately 80 percent in the medical group and 88 percent in the surgical group. One of the patients in the surgical group had a noncardiac death and, if removed, the surgical survival rate at 3 years is 91 percent. Had the 4 patients with severe angina requiring surgery succumbed to the disease rather than being salvaged by transfer to surgery, the survival in the medical group at 3 years would have been 67 percent. Thus the true medical survival for this group at 3 years should be between 80 percent and 67 percent. Had the surgical mortality been held at the level of 4.5 percent, this series would appear very comparable to our own, except that there were fewer patients randomized in the Mathur and Guinn series. It is interesting to note the rather striking improvement in symptoms reported by this group, in which 52 percent of the surgical patients were asymptomatic at the point of last follow-up, while only 7 percent of the medically treated patients were asymptomatic. Only 38 percent of the nonsurgical group had experienced an uneventful 3-year course, while 75 percent of the surgical group were alive at 3 years without a major cardiac event. In the interim, these investigators also tested anginal threshold using atrial pacing and showed a significant improvement in the surgically treated group. They also demonstrated an improvement in exercise tolerance in 94 percent of the surgically treated group versus 43 percent of the medically treated group. It is therefore surprising that this series is quoted to negate the effect of aortocoronary bypass on longevity. The series certainly is a strong support for the symptomatic and functional improvement of this type of patient after aortocoronary bypass surgery. The investigators did exclude patients with left main coronary artery

disease from this study, and although they do not give the percentage of patients who refused to enter the study, the fact that they were able to randomize 116 patients in a 3-year period using a Veterans Administration population alone would suggest that the percentage of patients with angina meeting hard criteria who actually were randomized was quite high.

Kloster et al. reported on randomization of 100 patients to medical (49 patients) or surgical (51 patients) therapy for chronic stable angina at the University of Oregon Health Science Center and the Portland Veterans Administration Hospital.[30,31] This study had a 5-year entry period and an average follow-up of just over 3 years. Criteria for entry were similar to the criteria for the Veterans Administration study and the study of Mathur and Guinn. However, they did require chronic disabling angina pectoris for at least 1 year with no myocardial infarction or unstable angina within the 6 months prior to randomization. The two populations, medical and surgical, were very similar in their entry data base. There were only 5 females in the medical and 6 in the surgical group. The percentage of one-, two-, and three-vessel disease is quite similar to that of the study of Mathur and Guinn and of our own. The incidence of previous myocardial infarction was half the incidence of our own group.

The study had an end point of a "major event," either death, myocardial infarction, or unstable angina unresponsive to medical management. In order to compare these patients to other series, it is necessary to consider patients who were removed from the series at the period of new myocardial infarction and who later died within weeks or months as deaths in the series. Thus, there were 8 deaths in the medical group and 4 in the surgical group. Two deaths in the surgical group were associated with surgery and 2 occurred in the follow-up period.

There is little doubt that the surgically managed patients had less unstable angina, a better work capacity, and an improved functional capacity when compared to the medical group. The authors conclude that the death rate is not changed by aortocoronary bypass. However, if one includes all 8 medically treated patients who died in the 3-year follow-up, the mortality is 5.3 percent per year for the medical group. If one assigns a mortality to the patients in the medical series who were dropped from follow-up when they required surgery for refractory unstable angina, the mortality would be between 5.3 and 10.7 percent per year. Adding only 2 deaths would make the medical mortality significantly greater than the surgical. The operative mortality of 4 percent is not different from our own. (We have assigned surgical death to the patient who had postoperative cardiac arrest and who died 6 weeks later of the effects of brain damage.) The incidence of new myocardial infarcts in the surgical follow-up period is certainly an unusual feature of this particular series, but death from infarcts appears to be low in the surgical group.

This study, carefully done and fully reported, cannot be interpreted as a guide to care of the usual patient being considered for aortocoronary bypass for chronic angina. It must be a highly selected group, since the investigators only randomized 100 patients over a 5-year period. These patients were evenly distributed between the VA hospital and University of Oregon Hospital, where there is a large, ongoing surgical program. In the last 3 years of study, they randomized 18, 14, and 13 patients, respectively. This must represent only a small percentage of the patients undergoing aortocoronary bypass for chronic angina. The criteria for selection are not defined and must, from experience, be highly subjective. If this is true, then the patients randomized represent a rather select group who can be convincingly persuaded by the physician to enter the randomized study. The conviction and resultant persuasiveness of that physician may well relate to uncategorized characteristics of the clinical or angiographic presentation of the patient. The conclusions may also suffer from beta error, since doubling the numbers but leaving the proportion the same would bring the medical-surgical series just to the border of statistical significance.

Another prospective randomized study that is used to deny the efficacy of surgery in prolonging life in patients with angina is the frequently quoted cooperative study of unstable angina.[32,26] This study was begun in 1972 under the auspices of the National Institutes of Health. Between 1972 and 1976, 288 patients were entered into the study. The report of the inhospital and initial follow-up results has recently appeared in the *American Journal of Cardiology*.[26] Neither in the initial report of the protocol and patient population[32] nor in the current follow-up study do the investigators divulge the patient population from which the randomized patients were taken. In this study, they considered patients who were less than 70 years of age and, except for coronary disease, were in good health. They must not have had myocardial infarction within the previous 3 months, and they did, in fact, require evidence of ST-T wave changes during episodes of pain. Patients were randomized after angiography, with the elimination, at this point, of all patients who had significant obstruction of the left main coronary artery. Between coronary angiography and randomization, some proportion of the patients were directed to surgical or medical care. Thus, some patients were considered too sick to be included in the medical series and therefore were operated upon. However, the exact criteria for this decision remains obscure. It is implied that patients who continued to have pain on medical management made up at least part of this subset

of patients directed to surgery. Even after randomization to medicine, 36 percent of these patients later underwent surgery for relief of severe angina. Twenty percent of the patients with single-vessel disease, 33 percent of the patients with double-vessel disease, and 49 percent of the patients with triple-vessel disease randomized to medical treatment eventually underwent surgery. Over the years from 1972 to 1976 the surgical mortality declined from 21 percent to 3 percent. At the same time, the inhospital medical mortality declined from 11 percent to 2 percent. The decline in surgical mortality probably represents the improved surgical technique and perioperative management. The decline in medical mortality could mean better use of beta blocking agents but might well represent an improvement in the criteria used for electively removing the patients from randomization and directing them to surgery. The conclusions of this study are difficult to compare with previous reports. The investigators state that "medical therapy proved an acceptable alternative to urgent cardiac surgery because the rates of early mortality and myocardial infarction were lower than once thought."[32] However, we do not know the outcome of the patients who were treated outside randomization nor, in fact, the criteria that separated these patients. If, indeed, these patients were similar to the high-risk patients with unstable angina described by Gazes et al.,[33] then one would expect a 30-day myocardial infarction rate of 28 percent and a mortality of 20 percent. This could then change their entire statistical conclusions. The investigators do recognize the difficulty of analysis caused by the patients in the medical group who later crossed over to have surgery because of intractable angina, and they have treated these patients as lost to follow-up at the time of crossover. It is difficult, therefore, to assign a mortality to this group. It is of interest that at 3 years the survival rate of the patients who were randomized to medicine but later had surgery appears to be approximately 95 to 96 percent, while the survival of patients in the medical series who did not receive later surgery is approximately 85 percent.

Selden et al. reported a prospective randomized study of 40 patients with acute coronary insufficiency, and they required continued episodes of angina after 24 h of bed rest in the hospital for inclusion in the study.[34] There was no significant difference in mortality in the patients treated medically versus those treated surgically, but the analysis was at 4 months' follow-up. Of the 19 medical patients, 1 died at 4 months and 8 were operated on at 4 months. The series is too small and too short for adequate analysis but does indicate that early medical management in these patients is frequently possible.

Pugh et al. reported 50 patients with unstable angina in whom only 27 could be randomized to medical or surgical treatment groups.[35] They again showed a significant incidence of normal coronary vessels in this syndrome. Only 14 patients were eventually randomized to medical treatment, and 5 of these patients required surgical intervention 1 week to 6 months following randomization.

It is our conclusion from looking at these studies that unstable angina can well be treated medically if, in fact, the patient does not have obstruction of the left main coronary artery and if the patient's angina can easily be made quiescent while in the hospital. If angiography shows evidence of triple-vessel disease, it appears that there is no particular advantage in delaying surgery beyond that hospitalization. There is evidence from other studies that this method of using maximal medical management prior to surgery may well reduce the incidence of perioperative infarction, and it appears to be a consensus that there is no need to rush the patient to aortocoronary bypass until maximum medical management has been achieved. Our own feeling is that this would include intraaortic balloon counterpulsation to stabilize the patient prior to surgery. *However, once the patient is stable, there is disadvantage in delay of the procedure.*

Comparison of our surgical results to those of Lawrie et al.,[36,37] who recently reported 5-year results of 1,144 patients having aortocoronary bypass, reveals very similar follow-up statistics to our own. The clinical data between the two groups are remarkably similar. The number of patients with left main stem disease is almost identical. However, they did not exclude the 27 patients who had left ventricular aneurysms. Their patients had significant left ventricular abnormalities in 32.3 percent, which is very similar to our figure of 31 percent with an elevated left ventricular end-diastolic pressure, and 20 percent with an ejection fraction of less than 0.45. Lawrie et al. had a slightly higher incidence of single-vessel disease in their group. The operative mortality was 4.6 percent, which is essentially the same as our 4.5 percent. The survival at 5 years was 88.6 percent in Lawrie's group and 88 percent in our own group. It is of interest that in his analysis, Lawrie was able to make a 5-year survival prediction for the general population of identical age and sex and showed that this was almost identical to the survival after surgery of their patients with single-vessel disease and normal left ventricular function. The patients with two-vessel disease and normal left ventricular function had only slightly greater 5-year mortality than that expected for the general population. The data from this study would further confirm our thesis that the patient population randomized at Hines closely represents a cross section of the patient population presenting at large centers for aortocoronary bypass to relieve chronic angina pectoris. However, in his conclusions, Lawrie attacks the Veterans

Administration study for its surgical mortality, and again, as so frequently, the attack has been for the wrong reasons. The 5-year survival of the surgical group in the Veterans Administration study is 84 percent, which does represent a slightly higher mortality than the patients operated on in Lawrie's group. However, the major reason for the inability of the Veterans Administration study to show a significant difference is because of the benign nature of the disease in the patients subjected to randomization.

Kouchoukos et al. have reviewed the experience at the University of Alabama with patients referred for evaluation and treatment of ischemic heart disease between February 1967 and June 1975.[38] They had 53 patients with single-vessel disease of the left anterior descending coronary artery. Twenty-nine patients underwent aortocoronary bypass. The remaining 24 patients were treated medically. There were two cardiac deaths in the surgically treated group, and a single noncardiac death in the medical group. They evaluated 320 patients with two-vessel disease, 220 of whom had aortocoronary bypass. Ninety-three percent of the operated patients were alive at 2 years. The patients who were considered suitable for surgery but who did not undergo surgery had a lower survival of approximately 87 percent at 2 years. Patients with three-vessel disease could be followed for 36 months, and of the operated patients, 85 percent were alive. The operable but nonoperated patients had only 58 percent survival at 3 years. Of their 107 patients with greater than 50 percent stenosis of the left main coronary artery, 2-year survival in the operated group was 83 percent and was 62 percent in the nonoperated group. Thus, patients with two- and three-vessel disease and left main stem disease showed a significant improvement in survival with surgery when compared to medical therapy. The two- and three-vessel disease experience is very similar to our own. However, the single-vessel disease is somewhat different. We have not had any surgical mortality in the patients with single-vessel disease.

Hall et al. described a series of 846 consecutive patients operated on at the Texas Heart Institute between 1969 and 1976.[1] These patients were mostly male (88 percent). They did have a somewhat higher incidence of previous myocardial infarction than our group (63 percent). Fourteen percent of their patients had single-vessel disease, 8 percent had left main stem disease, and 44 percent had triple-vessel disease, giving a distribution very similar to our group. Eighteen percent of their patients had ejection fractions of less than 0.45, again suggesting that our patients had at least as much ventricular dysfunction. Hall et al. demonstrated a changing pattern of the angina in the 60 days prior to the operation in 61 percent of their patients.[1] Since "changing pattern" is not defined well in their group or ours, it is difficult to evaluate whether there is a significant difference between the two groups. The early mortality or 30-day mortality was 3 percent in Hall's group, which is somewhat less than the overall 4.5 percent for our group. Their long-term survival at 5 years was 88.2 percent, taking into account all forms of death, and this again is almost identical to our series. At the end of 5 years 90 percent of the patients were asymptomatic or had few symptoms. It is interesting that Hall's group, very much like Seides' report,[39] shows a progressive increase in evidence of ischemia as time approaches 5 years, suggesting continued progression of the disease. Sheldon reviewed still another 741 patients followed between 6 and 10 years after aortocoronary bypass.[40] These patients had an average 5-year survival of 89.4 percent. His series had an inordinately high number of patients with single-vessel disease, accounting for 56 percent of the patient population. The patients with left main disease constitute 8.5 percent of the series and have a 5-year survival rate of 85.5 percent. Sheldon did compare his series to Proudfit's et al.[41] series of medically treated patients who were, by his estimate, surgical candidates. These admittedly were collected at a different time, and in no way were these patients matched with Sheldon's group. However, they had an average 5-year survival of 70 percent, which was very close to our own medical series. Proudfit's series showed a 29 percent incidence of single-vessel disease and a 9 percent incidence of left main disease. Again, there was a slight increase in single-vessel disease as compared to the Veterans Administration cooperative study but a similar incidence of left main stem lesions.

Vismara et al. attempted to assess whether or not coronary bypass surgery affected the incidence of sudden death in patients with coronary artery disease.[42] They analyzed 172 consecutive patients undergoing elective aortocoronary bypass and 112 consecutive patients treated medically for coronary artery disease during the same period of time. These patients were all entered in the study between 1970 and 1973. They dropped patients from each of the groups because of noncardiac death and then attempted to match the two groups as closely as possible. The final follow-up involved 121 patients who had undergone surgery and 96 patients who were treated medically. All patients had had cardiac catheterization and were proven to have two- or three-vessel coronary artery disease. Sudden death was defined as death occurring within 6 h of the onset of symptoms and clinically attributed to unexpected arrhythmias not related to shock or congestive heart failure. There was no significant difference in the symptoms, extent of coronary disease, or hemodynamic findings at time of entry into the study. The mean follow-up period was 39 months. *During this period of time, 7 of the 121 patients in the surgical group died suddenly, while 23 of the 96 in the medical group died suddenly.* This difference was significant ($p < .001$). Thus the annual mortality resulting from sudden death in this group of patients with two- and three-vessel disease was 7 percent. When they added back the 8 deaths resulting from congestive heart failure, the overall mortality was 10 percent per year. Since 62 percent of the patients had three-vessel disease and 6 percent had left main lesions, the mortality is consistent with other reported series. It is further evidence of the validity of the statistics developed by Bruschke[16,17] and Oberman[14] and supports the validity of our own medical series.

The incidence of ventricular arrhythmias in patients treated medically or surgically has been studied within the Veterans Administration cooperative study by two groups. De Soyza has reported on the group of patients at Little Rock and found that in follow-up there was no difference in the incidence or severity of arrhythmias in the patients who were treated surgically versus those treated medically.[43] There was a decreased usage of antiarrhythmic agents and beta blockers in the surgically treated patients. Lehrman et al. of the Palo Alto Veterans Administration Hospital have reported on exercise-induced arrhythmias and found a somewhat increased incidence of ventricular ectopic activity during exercise in the surgically treated patients.[44] However, the surgically treated patients achieved higher exercise levels.

Since Vismara et al. have found a decreased incidence of sudden death in patients treated surgically versus those treated medically with chronic angina pectoris,[42] it becomes a question of whether the exercise protocol used in the Veterans Administration reports truly predicts dangerous ectopic activity. It also must be noted that in the Veterans Administration study, patients were not operated on primarily for ventricular arrhythmias in ischemic heart disease. Patients with well-defined ventricular aneurysms were excluded from the study, and it is in these patients that surgery may be most beneficial for elimination of ectopic activity.

Hammermeister et al. studied the effects of aortocoronary bypass on sudden death in a nonrandomized series and showed that the incidence of sudden death in the medically treated patients was 1.8 to 10.9 times greater than that of matched subgroups of surgically treated patients.[45] However, the patients in their medically treated group tended to have more extensive ventricular contraction abnormalities, somewhat increased end-diastolic volume, and fewer graftable distal vessels. Since ventricular ectopy does relate best to the severity of ventricular dysfunction,[46] this increased incidence of sudden death in the medical group might well be expected. It is also difficult to relate deaths primarily to arrhythmias, since the sudden death group included all deaths within 24 h of the onset of the symptoms and not just sudden arrhythmic deaths.

CONCLUSION

Our experience, and our review of the experiences of others, convinces us that never again can a meaningful randomized study of the effect of aortocoronary bypass on longevity in symptomatic patients with coronary disease be done. Therefore, we must make the best possible use of the data available in the Veterans Administration study. It becomes evident that two populations of patients exist in this study, and we conclude from review of well-documented studies of the natural history of angina pectoris that the population we randomized is representative of the clinical problem presented by patients seeking surgery for this syndrome. The surgical results, although representative of the time, must be interpreted in view of the current, very low operative mortality (1 to 2 percent) in this disease. Therefore, the improved survival in the surgical group is even more meaningful and should not be obscured by those who would have this operative procedure denied to many patients whose lives could not only be improved but also prolonged.

REFERENCES

1 Hall, R. J., Garcia, E., Mathur, V. S., Busch, U., Cooley, D. A., Gold, K. A., and Gray, A. G.: Long-term Follow-up After Coronary Artery Bypass, *Cleve. Clin. Q.*, 45:162, 1978.

2 Detre, K., Hultgren, H., and Takaro, T.: Veterans Administration Cooperative Study of Surgery for Coronary Arterial Occlusive Disease. III. Methods and Baseline Characteristics, Including Experience with Medical Treatment, *Am. J. Cardiol.*, 40:212, 1977.

3 Takaro, T., Hultgren, H. N., Lipton, M. J., and Detre, K. M.: The VA Cooperative Randomized Study of Surgery for Coronary Arterial Occlusive Disease. II. Subgroup with Significant Left Main Lesions, *Circulation*, 54 (suppl. 3):107, 1975.

4 Murphy, M. L., Hultgren, H. N., Detre, K., Thomsen, J., and Takaro, T.: Treatment of Chronic Stable Angina. A Preliminary Report of Survival Data of the Randomized Veterans Administration Cooperative Study, *N. Engl. J. Med.*, 297:621, 1977.

5 Loeb, H. S., Pifarre, R., Sullivan, H., Palac, R., Croke, R. P., and Gunnar, R. M.: Improved Survival After Surgical Therapy for Chronic Angina Pectoris. One Hospital's Experience in a Randomized Trial, *Circulation*, in press.

6 Colton, T.: Longitudinal Studies and Use of the Life Table, in "Statistics in Medicine." Little, Brown, and Company, Boston, 1974, p. 237.

7 Read, R. C., Murphy, M. L., Hultgren, H. N., and Takaro T.: Survival of Men Treated for Chronic Stable Angina Pectoris. A Cooperative Randomized Study, *J. Thorac. Cardiovasc. Surg.* 75:1, 1978.

8 Detre, K., Murphy, M. L., and Hultgren, H.: Effect of Coronary Bypass Surgery on Longevity in High and Low Risk Patients. Report from the V.A. Cooperative Coronary Surgery Study, *Lancet*, 2:1243, 1977.

9 Block, W. J., Jr., Crumpacker, E. L., Dry, T. J., and Gage, R. P.: Prognosis of Angina Pectoris. Observations in 6,882 Cases, *J.A.M.A.*, 150:259, 1952.

10 Parker, R. L., Dry, T. J., Willius, F. A., and Gage, R. P.: Life Expectancy in Angina Pectoris, *J.A.M.A.*, 131:95, 1946.

11 Scanlon, P. J., Nemickas, R., Moran, J. F., Talano, J. V., Amirparviz, F., and Pifarre, R.: Accelerated Angina Pectoris. Clinical, Hemodynamic, Arteriographic, and Therapeutic Experience in 85 Patients, *Circulation*, 47:19, 1973.

12 Friesinger, G. C., Page, E. E., and Ross, R. S.: Prognostic Significance of Coronary Arteriography, *Trans. Assoc. Am. Physicians*, 83:78, 1970.

13 Humphries, J. O., Kuller, L., Ross, R. S., Friesinger, G. C., and Page, E. E.: Natural History of Ischemic Heart Disease in Relation to Arteriographic Findings. A Twelve Year Study of 224 Patients, *Circulation*, 49:489, 1974.

14 Oberman, A., Jones, W. B., Riley, C. P., Reeves, T. J., Sheffield, L. T., and Turner, M. E.: Natural History of Coronary Artery Disease, *Bull. N.Y. Acad. Med.*, 48:1109, 1972.

15 Kannel, W. B., and Feinleib, M.: Natural History of Angina Pectoris in the Framingham Study. Prognosis and Survival, *Am. J. Cardiol.*, 29:154, 1972.

16 Bruschke, A. V. G., Proudfit, W. L., and Sones, F. M. Jr.: Progress Study of 590 Consecutive Nonsurgical Cases of Coronary Disease Followed 5-9 Years. I. Arteriographic Correlations, *Circulation*, 47:1147, 1973.

17 Bruschke, A. V. G., Proudfit, W. L., and Sones, F. M., Jr.: Progress Study of 590 Consecutive Nonsurgical Cases of Coronary Disease Followed 5-9 Years. II. Ventriculographic and Other Correlations, *Circulation*, 47:1154, 1973.

18 Webster, J. S., Moberg, C., and Rincon, G.: Natural History of Severe Proximal Coronary Artery Disease as Documented by Coronary Cineangiography, *Am. J. Cardiol.*, 33:195, 1974.

19 Russek, H. I.: The "Natural" History of Severe Angina Pectoris with Intensive Medical Therapy Alone: A Five Year Prospective Study of 133 Patients, *Chest*, 65:46, 1974.

20 Reeves, T. J., Oberman, A., Jones, W. B., and Sheffield L. T.: Natural History of Angina Pectoris, *Am. J. Cardiol.*, 33:423, 1974.

21 Lichtlen, P. R., and Moccetti, T.: Prognostic Aspects of Coronary Angiography, *Circulation*, 45, 46 (suppl. 2):7, 1972.

22 Slagle, R. C., Bartel, A. G., Behar, V. S., Peter, R. H., Rosati, R. A., and Kong, Y.: Natural History of Angiographically Documented Coronary Artery Disease, *Circulation*, 47, 46 (suppl. 2):60, 1972.

23 Vlietstra, D. E., Assad-Morell, J. L., Frye, R. L., Elveback, L. R., Connolly, D. C., Ritman, E. L., Pluth, J. R., Barnhorst, D. A., Danielson, G. K., and Wallace, R. B.: Survival Predictors in Coronary Artery Disease. Medical and Surgical Comparisons, *Mayo Clin. Proc.*, 52:85, 1977.

24 Green, D. D., Bunnell, I. L., Arani, D. T., et al.: Longterm Survival After Coronary Bypass Surgery. Buffalo General Hospital, State University of New York (brochure for exhibit at American Heart Association Meeting, Miami, 1977).

25 Hurst, J. W., King, S. B., III, Logue, R. B., Hatcher, C. R., Jones, E. L., Craver, J. M., Douglas, J. S., Jr., Franch, R. H., Dorney, E. R., Cobbs, B. W., Jr., Robinson, P. H., Clements, S. D., Jr., Kaplan, J. A., and Bradford, J. M.: Value of Coronary Bypass Surgery. Controversies in Cardiology: Part 1, *Am. J. Cardiol.*, 42:308, 1978.

26 Russel, R. O., Jr., Moraski, R. E., Kouchoukos, N., Karp, R. et al.: Unstable Angina Pectoris: National Cooperative Study Group to Compare Surgical and Medical Therapy. II. In-hospital Experience with Initial Followup Results in Patients with One, Two and Three Vessel Disease, *Am. J. Cardiol.*, 42:839, 1978.

27 Mathur, V. S., and Guinn, G. A.: Prospective Randomized Study of Coronary Bypass Surgery in Stable Angina. The First 100 Patients, *Circulation*, 51, 52 (suppl. 1):133, 1975.

28 Guinn, G. A., and Mathur, V. S.: Surgical Versus Medical Treatment for Stable Angina Pectoris: Prospective Randomized Study with 1-to 4-Year Follow-up, *Ann. Thorac. Surg.*, 22:524, 1976.

29 Mathur, V. S., and Guinn, G. A.: Prospective Randomized Study of the Surgical Therapy of Stable Angina, *Cardiovasc. Clin.*, 8:131, 1977.

30 Kloster, F. E., Kremkau, E. L., Rahimtoola, S. H., Ritzmann, L. W., Griswold, H. E., Neill, W. A., Rösch, J., and Starr, A.: Prospective Randomized Study of Coronary Bypass Surgery for Chronic Stable Angina, *Cardiovasc. Clin.*, 8:145, 1977.

31 Kloster, F. E., Kremkau, E. L., Ritzmann, L. W., Rahimtoola, S. H., Rösch, J., Starr, A., and Kanarek, P. H.: Coronary Bypass Surgery for Stable Angina: A Prospective Randomized Study, *N. Engl. J. Med.*, in press.

32 Russell, R. O., Moraski, R. E., Kouchoukos, N. T., Karp, R., et al.: Unstable Angina Pectoris: National Cooperative Study Group to Compare Medical and Surgical Therapy. I. Report of Protocol and Patient Population, *Am. J. Cardiol.*, 37:896, 1976.

33 Gazes, P. C., Mobley, E. M., Jr., Faris, H. M., Jr., Duncan, R. C., and Humphries, G. B.: Preinfarctional (Unstable) Angina—a Prospective Study—Ten Year Follow-up. Prognostic Significance of Electrocardiographic Changes, *Circulation*, 48:331, 1973.

34 Selden, R., Neill, W. A., Ritzmann, L. W., Okies, J. E., and Anderson, R. P.: Medical Versus Surgical Therapy for Acute Coronary Insufficiency. A Randomized Study. *N. Engl. J. Med.*, 293:1129, 1975.

35 Pugh, B., Platt, M. R., Mills, L. J., Crumbo, D., Poliner, L. R., Curry, G. C., Blomqvist, G. C., Parkey, R. W., Buja, L. M., and Willerson, J. T.: Unstable Angina Pectoris: A Randomized Study of Patients Treated Medically and Surgically, *Am. J. Cardiol.*, 41:1291, 1978.

36 Lawrie, G. M., Morris, G. C., Jr., Howell, J. F., Ogura, J. W., Spencer, W. H., III, Cashion, W. R., Winters, W. L., Beazley, H. L., Chapman, D. W., Peterson, P. K., and Lie, J. T.: Results of Coronary Bypass More than 5 Years After Operation in 434 Patients. Clinical, Treadmill Exercise and Angiographic Correlations. *Am. J. Cardiol.*, 40:665, 1977.

37 Lawrie, G. M., Morris, G. C., Jr., Howell, J. F., Tredici, T. D., and Chapman, D. W.: Improved Survival After 5 Years in 1,144 Patients After Coronary Bypass Surgery, *Am. J. Cardiol.*, 42:709, 1978.

38 Kouchoukos, N. T., Oberman, A., and Karp, R. B.: Results of Surgery for Disabling Angina Pectoris, *Cardiovasc. Clin.*, 8:157, 1977.

39 Seides, S. F., Borer, J. S., Kent, K. M., Rosing, D. R., McIntosh, C. L., and Epstein, S. E.: Long-term Anatomic Fate of Coronary-Artery Bypass Grafts and Functional Status of Patients Five Years After Operation, *N. Engl. J. Med.*, 298:1213, 1978.

40 Sheldon, W. C.: Effect of Bypass Graft Surgery on Survival. A 6- to 10-Year Follow-up Study of 741 Patients, *Cleve. Clin. Q.*, 45:166, 1978.

41 Proudfit, W. L., Bruschke, A. V. G., and Sones, F. M., Jr.: Natural History of Obstructive Coronary Artery Disease: Ten-Year Study of 601 Nonsurgical Cases, *Prog. Cardiovasc. Dis.*, 21:53, 1978.

42 Vismara, L. A., Miller, R. R., Price, J. E., Karem, R., DeMaria, A. N., and Mason, D. T.: Improved Longevity Due to Reduction of Sudden Death by Aortocoronary Bypass in Coronary Atherosclerosis. Prospective Evaluation of Medical Versus Surgical Therapy in Matched Patients with Multivessel Disease, *Am. J. Cardiol.*, 39:919, 1977.

43 de Soyza, N., Murphy, M. L., Bissett, J. K., Kane, J. J., and Doherty, J. E., III: Ventricular Arrhythmia in Chronic Stable Angina Pectoris with Surgical or Medical Treatment, *Ann. Intern. Med.*, 89:10, 1978.

44 Lehrman, K., Tilkian, A., and Hultgren, H. N.: The Effect of Coronary Artery Bypass Surgery on Exercise-induced Arrhythmias: A Randomized Study, *Circulation*, 57, 58 (suppl. 2):238, 1978.

45 Hammermeister, K. E., DeRouen, T. A., Murray, J. A., and Dodge, H. T.: Effect of Aortocoronary Saphenous Vein Bypass Grafting on Death and Sudden Death. Comparison of Nonrandomized Medically and Surgically Treated Cohorts with Comparable Coronary Disease and Left Ventricular Function, *Am. J. Cardiol.*, 39:925, 1977.

46 Califf, R. M., Burks, J. M., Behar, V. S., Margolis, J. R., and Wagner, G. S.: Relationships Among Ventricular Arrhythmias, Coronary Artery Disease, and Angiographic and Electrocardiographic Indicators of Myocardial Fibrosis, *Circulation*, 57:725, 1978.

Chapter 18

Improved Survival After Coronary Bypass: A Long-term Perspective from Baylor College of Medicine*

GERALD M. LAWRIE, M.D.,
and GEORGE C. MORRIS, JR., M.D.

Although the coronary bypass procedure has gained wide acceptance as a highly effective form of therapy for the relief of angina pectoris secondary to coronary atherosclerosis, there has been continuing doubt (with the notable exception of patients with left main stenosis) as to the effect of operation on the late survival of these patients.

There are two basic approaches to answering the question of whether coronary bypass influences late survival. One is to determine whether operation favorably modifies the pathophysiologic mechanisms responsible for death in these patients. The other approach is to compare surgical survival rates with similar patients treated medically or with the general U.S. population of identical age, race, and sex distribution.

It is important to recognize that successful surgical procedures are conceived from an accurate knowledge of clearly identifiable anatomy, physiology, and pathology of a particular condition. All enduring surgical procedures have had such a foundation. Those that have fallen by the wayside either never had such a foundation (e.g., internal thoracic artery ligation) or with the passage of time the basic scientific foundation was found to be partly or completely incorrect (e.g., the Beck I and II procedures).

Thus, unlike drug therapy, which acts at the molecular level with sometimes unpredictable side effects, the outcome of the majority of surgical procedures can be accurately predicted if the fundamental characteristics of a disease are well understood and if a well-designed and skillfully executed surgical procedure is employed to correct the condition.

As for regarding the use of the randomized prospective study as an indispensable research tool, it is of interest that the conclusions drawn relatively early from retrospective reviews of nonrandomized coronary bypass series in regard to relief of angina, prevention of coronary events, improved exercise tolerance, and in the case of left main disease, prolongation

of life by operation have all been confirmed subsequently by prospective studies, emphasizing the accuracy of traditional methods of assessing results of surgical therapy. Similarly, we believe that the evidence for prolongation of life by operation is available already and that eventually, randomized prospective studies will again confirm what already is known from retrospective analyses.

The fundamental mechanism responsible for death as a result of coronary artery disease is myocardial ischemia producing either fatal arrhythmias, acute myocardial infarction and its complications, or progressive ischemic cardiomyopathy and congestive heart failure. Therefore, the actual mechanism whereby coronary bypass improves survival must relate to the successful long-term alleviation of myocardial ischemia and resultant preservation of left ventricular function.

Direct evidence of improved myocardial perfusion after operation has been obtained from studies of preoperative and postoperative myocardial lactate production,[1] from studies of regional myocardial blood flow,[2] and from thallium radionuclide scanning and radionuclide wall motion studies. Possibly of even greater significance has been the demonstration by radionuclide techniques that coronary bypass eliminates ischemic depression of left ventricular function during exercise.[3] It would be expected that protection of the ventricle from acute ischemia during stress would have a beneficial influence on late survival.

Indirect evidence of prevention of myocardial ischemia has been obtained from several sources. In the Baylor College of Medicine randomized prospective trial of coronary bypass for stable angina conducted at the Houston Veterans Administration Hospital, treadmill exercise performance showed superior improvement in surgical patients. Furthermore, fewer cardiac events such as myocardial infarction and unstable angina occurred in operated patients—27 percent versus 51 percent.[4] In the National Heart, Lung and Blood Institute's randomized study on unstable angina, recurrence of severe unstable angina was so

*From Baylor College of Medicine, Houston, Texas.

221

common that 36 percent of patients in the medical group ultimately required operation. Class III-IV angina was present in 40 percent of the medical group with multivessel disease and in only 14 percent of the surgical group at the time of follow-up, providing striking clinical evidence of a significant reduction in the incidence of ischemic insults in surgical patients.[5]

The concept of ischemic cardiomyopathy is now well established, and its association with recurrent myocardial infarction, arrhythmia, and congestive heart failure has been documented.[6] It is clear that successful revascularization does preserve myocardium by preventing such ischemic insults.

The importance of ventricular arrhythmias as a factor in sudden death is well recognized. The influence of coronary bypass on ventricular arrhythmias is at present unclear. Some ventricular arrhythmias observed after operation represent persistence of preoperative arrhythmias of heterogeneous etiology, only some of which will respond to the improved myocardial perfusion. New postoperative ventricular arrhythmias may occur secondary to very small amounts of ischemic damage arising either spontaneously or from iatrogenic causes.

There is some evidence that the incidence of sudden death in patients with multivessel coronary disease can be reduced by coronary bypass. In a prospective study of 286 patients, 114 of whom were treated medically and 172 surgically, sudden death occurred in 24 percent of the medical group and in 6 percent of the surgical group ($p < .05$).[7]

Another approach we have employed in order to determine whether coronary bypass affects survival has been to examine the influence of completeness of revascularization on late survival in our patients, that is, whether the presence or absence of functioning grafts act as an independent variable affecting survival. To determine this, we have reviewed the fate of 792 consecutive patients operated upon between 1968 and 1972 and determined the relationship between completeness of revascularization and late survival.[8]

We compared the initial 250 patients with the sub-

sequent 542 patients. The two groups were of similar age and sex and had a similar distribution of coronary disease and impaired left ventricular function. Perioperative mortality fell from an initial 6.8 percent (17 of 250) to 4.8 percent (26 of 542). The number of grafts per patient was initially 1.5 but later increased to 1.8. Graft patency beyond 5 years in 105 patients was 88.6 percent (148 of 167) overall and was comparable in the two groups, and 96.2 percent of all patients had at least one patent graft. Initially, the crude 5-year survival rate was 78.0 percent (195 of 250) in the earlier, less well revascularized group, but the survival rate was 87.8 percent (476 of 542) in the later group in which revascularization was more complete. Patients who had no residual unbypassed lesions after operation had a 91.4 percent (287 of 314) survival, while those with two residual lesions had a 66.7 percent (14 of 21) survival. (Table 18-1) Those patients with a preoperative end-diastolic pressure of less than 15 mm Hg and no localized abnormality of contraction had a 5-year crude survival rate of 92.1 percent (316 of 343) overall, whereas the patients with poor ventricular function had a survival of 81.8 percent (108 of 132) overall.

Thus, although preoperative left ventricular function remained an important determinant of late survival after operation, at a given level of ventricular function, patients with one-, two-, or three-vessel disease who had no residual lesion all achieved similar and normal survival rates that were superior to those of patients with two to three residual lesions. (Table 18-1) These findings suggest that coronary bypass does favorably influence late survival and that improved late survival occurs because the coronary bypass grafts effectively eliminate the functional significance of proximal coronary lesions. Thus the majority of patients with double- or triple-vessel disease or left main stenosis are converted by operation to a state functionally equivalent to no significant coronary lesions or to single-vessel disease, both of which have a good prognosis (Table 18-2).

It is well recognized that patients with known cor-

TABLE 18-1

Absolute five-year survival rates of 474 patients* according to extent of residual disease and left ventricular function

	No. of residual lesion (474 pts.)†		
Left ventricular function	0–66.2% (314/474)	1–29.1% (138/474)	2–4.4% (21/474)
Good	93.5% (202/216)	88.6% (62/70)	72.2% (13/18)
Poor	86.7% (85/98)	64.8% (57/88)	33.3% (1/3)
Overall	91.4% (287/314)	75.3% (119/158)	66.7% (14/21)

*Left main disease and left ventricular aneurysm resection excluded.

†One patient had three residual lesions.

SOURCE: Lawrie et al.[8]

TABLE 18-2
Comparison of the completeness of revascularization achieved by operation in the initial and subsequent experiences

Vessels involved	1968–1971		1971–1972	
	Preop	**Postop***	**Preop**	**Postop***
0	—	55.2% (129/235)	—	66.2% (329/497)
1	24.7% (58/235)	30.0% (71/235)	20.7% (103/497)	29.0% (144/497)
2	47.2% (111/235)	15.0% (35/235)	45.7% (227/497)	4.4% (22/497)
3	28.1% (66/235)	—	33.6% (167/497)	0.4% (2/497)

*Postoperative figures include results of graft patency in 251 patients.
SOURCE: Lawrie et al.[8]

onary atherosclerosis are at greater risk of myocardial infarction and death from major surgery. In one study of 587 patients with previous myocardial infarctions who underwent various operations, 6.1 percent (36 of 587) of patients had recurrent myocardial infarctions, and the operative mortality was 4.3 percent (25 of 587).[9]

In contrast to these results has been the very favorable outcome in relation to mortality and myocardial infarction in patients with functioning coronary bypass grafts who have undergone subsequent major surgical procedures. In a review of a series of 358 such patients operated upon at Baylor College of Medicine, perioperative (30-day) mortality was 1.1 percent, and the incidence of perioperative myocardial infarction was 1.6 percent.[10] We have also reviewed our experience with the treatment of coexistent carotid and coronary artery disease.[11] Of those patients with a history of angina and documented coronary disease who did not undergo coronary bypass prior to carotid endarterectomy, operative mortality was 18.2 percent (14 of 77), almost all due to myocardial infarction. However, in patients who underwent prior or simultaneous coronary bypass and then carotid endarterectomy, operative mortality was reduced to 3 percent (4 of 135) and was largely the result of noncardiac causes. Others have had similar experiences.[12]

When considering the long-term future of these patients, it is clear that their ultimate fate will depend on good long-term surgical results in relation to graft patency, progression of disease in the native circulation, and preservation of ventricular function. In order to examine these important questions more closely, we reviewed our experience at Baylor College of Medicine between 1968 and 1972 of 434 patients and performed follow-up angiography in 131 patients more than 5 years after operation.[13] The patency rate was 90.7 percent (176 of 193) beyond 5 years, with 96.2 percent (126 of 131) of patients having at least one graft patent and 82.9 percent (109 of 131) having all grafts patent. In our other studies, histological examination of graft specimens obtained up to 10 years after

operation indicate that the changes of intimal proliferation occurred in all grafts but rarely caused occlusion.[14] Atherosclerosis in our experience is rare, and its overall incidence up to 7 years after operation has been only 0.5 to 1 percent per year.[15] Furthermore, it has occurred mainly in patients with severe hyperlipmias. Thus, in our experience, graft function has remained excellent beyond 5 years.[13-16]

We examined in detail the late changes in the native coronary circulation and found that significant progression of disease was rare in grafted vessels (less than 1 percent per year) and, while still infrequent, was more common in ungrafted vessels (4 percent per year).[13]

In our own experience, left ventricular function as assessed by end-diastolic pressure and left ventriculogram has been stable over a 5-year interval. Furthermore, because our patients have continued to have good treadmill performance beyond 5 years, we feel that the operation is effective in long-term relief of myocardial ischemia.[13]

The second major approach to the question of survival is to determine and then make comparisons with the actual long-term survival rates achieved. Analyses of the observed survival rates of surgically treated groups of patients are directed at answering two questions. The first is whether coronary bypass influences survival at all, that is, whether it has any effect on the adverse natural history of the disease, and second, whether the influence of coronary bypass is superior to modern medical therapy.

The late survival of symptomatic patients with coronary artery disease has been shown to be determined predominantly by the extent and severity of coronary artery involvement and the degree of impairment of left ventricular function.[17-20] Thus, for reports of survival rates of patients with angiographically proven coronary disease to be useful for comparisons of survival between different forms of treatment, it is clear that the minimum information required is the number of major vessel stenoses and their severity (preferably percentage of luminal diameter reduction) and ventriculographic data, ideally including the ejection fraction, the left ventricular end-diastolic pressure, and some description of the extent and severity of wall motion abnormalities. Thus, because the most useful medical survival data have been reported in this fashion,[17-20] data of patients undergoing operation should be presented similarly by subgroups according to the presence of one-, two-, or three-vessel disease or left main stenosis and according to left ventricular function in each subgroup. Data reported only according to the number of vessels diseased, without reference to ventricular function or, even worse, only according to the number of grafts attached at operation and not the preexisting disease cannot be compared directly to other series.

Furthermore, at a given level of severity of coronary stenoses, quality of left ventricular function is the dominant determinant of late survival. Thus, an accurate description of this variable is essential, since in some nonconsecutive retrospective and prospective studies, populations with superior ventricular function (and therefore a better prognosis regardless of treatment) have been selected.

Patients with coronary disease highly selected in relation to good left ventricular function have annual attrition rates in milder forms of coronary stenosis as low as 1 to 2 percent. Therefore, studies to determine the relative effects of medical and surgical treatment on late survival may be seeking differences in annual attrition rates on the order of only 1 to 5 percent, which, though small on an annual basis, may represent striking differences in mortality in the long term.

Thus, it is necessary to follow large groups of patients so that each subgroup defined according to number of stenoses and level of ventricular function will be of adequate size for meaningful statistical analysis. Furthermore, even in a large group of patients, the absolute number of deaths will be relatively small in the short term, and not all will be related to coronary disease. Thus, in addition to large number of patients, it is necessary to follow the group over a long period of time to generate sufficient attrition for an unequivocal difference to be obtained between different forms of treatment. The two major current randomized prospective studies of survival[4,21] suffer from these problems of small numbers and short follow-up periods and are further aggravated by substantial numbers of crossovers from medical to surgical treatment.

In order to overcome some of these difficulties and obtain meaningful objective data on late survival after coronary bypass, we determined the fate of 1,144 consecutive patients, all of whom were followed for a minimum of at least 5 years after operation.[22] In order to eliminate the risk of retrospective selection of a good-risk patient population from our overall experience, we included all patients treated primarily for

coronary disease in our consecutive series of 1,144 patients regardless of the severity of the preoperative clinical status or the degree of impairment of left ventricular function. Both elective and emergency operations were included in the series. We included deaths from all causes, even those clearly not related to a cardiac event, such as cancer or accidents. Furthermore, although initially our group of patients was free of other serious disease such as cancer, the 5-year interval of follow-up was sufficiently long to expose our group to the risk of developing these diseases comparable to the risk of the general population.

We elected to follow up a large group of patients in all cases for more than 5 years in order to be able to determine absolute 5-year survival rates. We considered that the advantages of this approach outweighed the fact that this confined us to reviewing the fate of patients operated upon between 1971 and 1972 when our surgical results, although good by the then prevailing standards, were not representative of our later results, which have been consistently improving over the last 6 years despite poorer clinical material. By adopting this approach, we were able to obtain subgroups of adequate size and duration of follow-up for meaningful analysis.

Of the 1,144 patients, 1,000 were men (87.4 percent). The mean age was 50.1 years (range 24 to 75). Operation was performed for angina pectoris in 1,101 patients (96.2 percent). We chose coronary lesions of > 70 percent luminal diameter reduction to ensure that truly severe coronary disease was present in each category. Forty-three patients (3.8 percent) had congestive heart failure without angina. Unstable angina was present in 149 patients (13 percent). Previous myocardial infarction had occurred in 675 patients (59 percent). Single-vessel disease was present in 226 patients (19.8 percent), double-vessel disease in 442 (38.6 percent), triple-vessel disease in 376 patients (32.9 percent), and greater than 50 percent stenosis of the left main coronary artery was present in 100 patients (8.7 percent).

Preoperative left ventricular function was classified as either good or poor by means of the preoperative left ventricular end-diastolic pressure and ventriculogram. Good left ventricular function was defined as the presence of an end-diastolic pressure of less than 15 mm Hg and the absence of a contraction abnormality as defined above.

Patients with even significant elevations of end-diastolic pressure (up to 55 mm Hg) were not excluded. Further subjective evaluation of the left ventriculogram by visual estimation of end-diastolic volume, ejection fraction, or myocardial contractility was not employed in classifying left ventricular function. Unfortunately, in this early experience, objective measurements of the ejection fraction were not available.

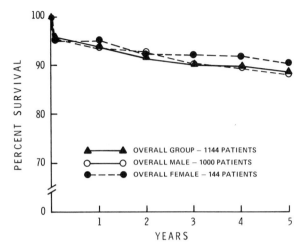

FIGURE 18-1 Survival of overall group in the study. The late survival rates of men and women are almost identical. *(From G. M. Lawrie et al., Improved Survival After 5 Years in 1144 Patients After Coronary Bypass Surgery, Am. J. Cardiol., 42:709, 1978.)*

By the objective criteria defined, reasonably good left ventricular function was present in 67.7 percent (775 of 1,144) of patients, while poor left ventricular function was present in 32.3 percent (369 of 1,144). Of these patients, 31.7 percent (117 of 369) had end-diastolic pressures in the range of 25 to 55 mm-Hg. Left ventricular aneurysms consisting of areas of paradoxical motion as shown by left ventriculography were present in 7.3 percent (27 of 369), and left ventricular aneurysm resection was performed in 3.0 percent (11 of 369). Thus, no patient was excluded retrospectively from this series, regardless of the severity of impairment of left ventricular function. Had we employed the additional criteria of ventricular function mentioned, only 28.6 percent (237 of 1,144) of patients would have had normal left ventricular function.

The overall operative mortality was 4.6 percent (52 patients). With exclusion of patients with left main coronary artery disease, this rate was 3.8 percent (40 of 1,144) and the overall crude 5-year survival rate was 89.1 percent (930 of 1,144). The survival rates of men and women were comparable (Fig. 18-1). Among men, the respective survival rates for each subgroup and for those with good left ventricular function within that subgroup were as follows: one-vessel disease, 92.9 percent (169 of 182) and 94.9 percent (130 of 137) (Fig. 18-2); two-vessel disease, 90.3 percent (352 of 390) and 94.3 percent (248 of 263) (Fig. 18-3); three-vessel disease, 85.7 percent (293 of 342) and 90.9 percent (189 of 208) (Fig. 18-4); left main coronary artery disease, 81.4 percent (70 of 86) and 90.6 percent (48 of 53). The graft patency rate in 157 patients was 86.4 percent (247 of 286 grafts), and 149 patients (94.9 percent) had at least one patent graft.

The first comparison we made with our surgical data was with the survival rates reported for the medical control group of the VA cooperative study which represents the best results ever reported for a medically treated group of symptomatic patients.[20,23] These patients were a highly selected group. The presence of any of the following conditions led to exclusion from the VA study: myocardial infarction less than 6 months before operation; persistent diastolic hypertension despite treatment; marked cardiac enlargement; presence of left ventricular aneurysm or other significant cardiac disease such as valvular heart disease; presence of any other major disease making major surgery inadvisable or limiting life expectancy to less than 5 years; previous operation for angina pectoris; unstable angina or angina of increasing severity suggesting "impending infarction"; or the presence of congestive heart failure unless clinically compensated for at least 3 weeks.

Following qualification by these rigorous clinical criteria for entry into the VA cooperative study, coronary angiography and left ventriculography were performed on 2,084 patients. At this point, 11 percent (308 of 3,804) of patients were rejected because of abnormalities of ventricular function: poor myocardial contractility in 134 patients, left ventricular aneurysm in 160 patients, or marked elevation of end-diastolic pressure in 14 patients. That is, 42 percent (308 of 733) of all patients who were rejected after angiography were excluded because of impairment of left ventricular function.[20]

This selection process led to a very low incidence

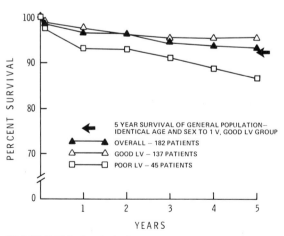

FIGURE 18-2 Survival of men with single-vessel (1V) disease according to preoperative left ventricular function (LV). The expected 5-year survival rate of a sample group from the general U.S. population of identical age and sex distribution is indicated. *(From G. M. Lawrie et al., Improved Survival After 5 Years in 1144 Patients After Coronary Bypass Surgery, Am. J. Cardiol. 42:709, 1978.)*

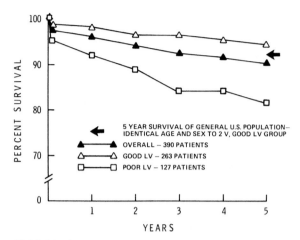

FIGURE 18-3 Survival of men with double-vessel (2V) disease according to preoperative left ventricular function (LV). Data from the general population as in Fig. 18-2. *(From G. M. Lawrie et al., Improved Survival After 5 Years in 1144 Patients After Coronary Bypass Surgery, Am. J. Cardiol., 42:709, 1978.)*

of poor (as opposed to abnormal) left ventricular function in the final group selected as further indicated by a low incidence of a history of congestive heart failure (6.9 percent), left ventricular aneurysm (2 percent), and an ejection fraction < 45 percent in only 15 percent of patients. The left ventricular end-diastolic pressure was > 14 mm Hg in 33.4 percent of patients, but the magnitude of elevation was not specified. Patients with ''excessive elevations'' of end-diastolic pressure were specifically excluded.[20]

It is important to note also that in the VA study the angiographic criterion chosen for significant coronary stenosis was only a > 50 percent luminal diameter reduction, compared with our use of a > 70 percent reduction as our criterion for classification of one-, two-, and three-vessel disease groups.

The foregoing considerations notwithstanding, it is apparent from Table 18-3 that our surgically treated patients with multivessel disease have 5-year survival rates that are superior to the 4-year survival rates of

the medically treated groups of the VA cooperative study. Furthermore, the overall annual attrition rates of our surgical patients are consistently lower than those of the corresponding VA medical groups (Table 18-4), suggesting an increasing advantage for our surgical group with the passage of time.

In contrast to our favorable late survival rates with operation, the preliminary medical and surgical survival results of the VA cooperative study have been interpreted as showing that medical and surgical therapy for chronic stable angina will achieve comparable late survival rates.

Leaving aside the highly selected patient population, the major problem with the VA cooperative study has been the poor surgical results obtained. The extensive exclusions from the VA study leave a group of patients whose operative risk should have been extremely low. Despite suggestions to the contrary, an operative mortality of 5.6 percent was excessive in such a group of patients even between 1972 and 1974. In our own experience between 1971 and 1972 (Table 18-4) with a group of patients in which none of these exclusionary criteria were employed and in which patients with severe impairment of left ventricular function, congestive heart failure, and unstable angina were all included, the operative mortality was 3.8 percent, and the major proportion of the mortality was in patients with severely abnormal ventricular function, most of whom would have been excluded from the VA study. This is even more apparent when one considers that in our initial experience between 1968 and 1971, which represented one of the earliest reported surgical series,[13] the operative mortality was only 5.5 percent (excluding left main stenosis) compared with 16 percent for the initial VA period between 1970 and 1972. Others have also reported operative mortalities of 3 to 6 percent for the same period in unselected series that included poorer risk patients.[24] The report by Conley and associates on the influence of patient selection on mortality also suggests that for such a good-risk group, an operative mortality of 5.6 percent was excessive.[25]

These poor results are also reflected in an inadequate overall graft patency rate of only 69 to 71 per-

TABLE 18-3

Comparison of survival rates of the Baylor surgical group[22] with survival rates reported for the VA cooperative study medical control group[20,23]

No. vessels diseased	2-year surgical Baylor	5-year surgical Baylor	2-year medical VA (Detre et al.[20])	4-year medical VA (Read et al.[23])
1—Good LV	97%	95%	97%	—
Overall	96%	93%	94%	97%
2—Good LV	97%	94%	94%	—
Overall	94%	90%	90%	87%
3—Good LV	94%	91%	90%	—
Overall	90%	86%	88%	74%

TABLE 18-4

Comparison of the surgical results of the VA cooperative study (VA) with those of the Baylor College of Medicine surgical group's (BCM) initial (1968–1971) and subsequent (1971–1972) experiences

	VA 1972–1974	BCM 1968–1971	BCM 1971–1972
Operative mortality	5.6%	5.5%	3.8%
No. grafts/patient	1.9	1.5	1.8
Graft patency rate	69%	90.5%	84.3%
No. of patients with no grafts patent	12%	2.6%	7.4%
No. of patients with all grafts patent	54%	85.9%	74.1%
Crude survival at 36 months	88%	85.0%	92.2%
Overall average crude annual attrition rate	4.0%	5.0%	2.6%
Crude average annual attrition rate (excluding operative mortality	2.3%	3.1%	1.3%

SOURCE: Lawrie et al.[8]

cent.[23,26] This is considerably below the patency rate of 80 to 90 percent reported from experienced centers for patients operated on before the VA study began. Despite a number of grafts per patient comparable to our later experience, this low graft patency rate has resulted in complete surgical failure in 12 percent of the VA patients as compared with 3.8 to 7.4 percent in our experience. Perhaps more significantly, only 54 percent of VA patients had all grafts patent, as compared with 74.1 to 85.9 percent of our patients.[8,13,22]

It is obvious that patients who have no patent grafts represent individuals who have been exposed to a significant operative risk without resultant benefit. However, the low incidence of patients with all grafts patent is also of concern because, as we have stated previously, we believe that the mechanism whereby the coronary bypass operation enhances late survival is that patients are converted from high- to low-risk categories of coronary disease by elimination of the functional significance of a high-grade stenosis by a patent graft which, in effect, reduces the number of stenosed vessels, and this has not occurred with sufficient frequency in the VA study for survival differences to emerge so far. However, with the passage of sufficient time, we believe the VA study will begin to show major differences in survival.

The most interesting comparison we have made with our surgical results is with the survival of a sample of the general U.S. population of identical age and sex distribution. The design of this study is compared with a randomized prospective study in Fig. 18-5.

As cardiovascular mortality in the general U.S. population has been falling since 1963, it is important to compare surgical survival rates with the appropriate sample of the general U.S. population. Because the highest incidence of mortality was in the first 12 months of this study, 1973 was the mean time of death for the entire period of the study from 1971 to 1977. Selection of the mortality experience of the general U.S. population of 1973 enabled us to compare our mortality with the same population from which our patients were derived and of which they continued to constitute a portion (Fig. 18-5).

It should be emphasized that the figure for the expected deaths for each group of patients was calculated from the age and sex of each individual patient in the study and was not a rough approximation based on the mean age of each group but an exact application of the actual mortality experience of the 1973 general U.S. population to the exposure determined for our individual patients. It is also important to note that this comparison was made not with the death rates for a population sample with known cardiovascular disease but for the entire general U.S. population.[22]

In view of these observations, we were interested to find that patients with reasonably good (but not necessarily normal) preoperative left ventricular function (which constituted 68 percent of our patients) achieved a normal survival in relation to the general U.S. population as shown in Figs. 18-2 to 18-4.

That the coronary bypass grafting itself is responsible for this restoration of survival to normal is suggested by the convergence to a normal survival of all subgroups with good left ventricular function including

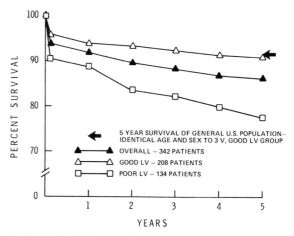

FIGURE 18-4 Survival of men with triple-vessel (3V) disease according to preoperative left ventricular function (LV). Data from the general population as in Fig. 18-2. (*From G. M. Lawrie et al., Improved Survival After 5 Years in 1144 Patients After Coronary Bypass Surgery, Am. J. Cardiol., 42:709, 1978.*)

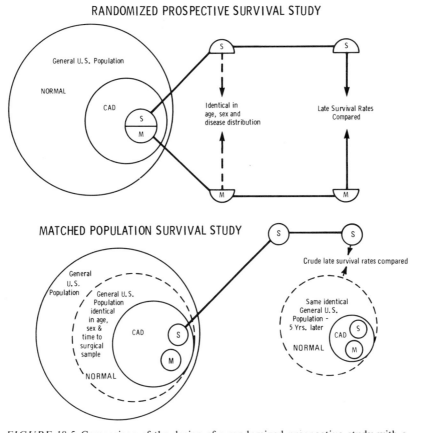

RANDOMIZED PROSPECTIVE SURVIVAL STUDY

MATCHED POPULATION SURVIVAL STUDY

FIGURE 18-5 Comparison of the design of a randomized prospective study with a matched population survival study. Note that in both cases, surgically (S) and medically (M) treated groups of patients are compared. However, in the matched population survival study, these patients are not specifically identified but form a part of the sample of identical age- and sex-matched population consisting of normal subjects, patients with untreated coronary disease (CAD), and patients with coronary disease on medical treatment (M).

those with double- and triple-vessel disease and left main stenosis. Following coronary bypass, the principal determinant of survival in this study was the status of preoperative left ventricular function, with the number of vessels diseased preoperatively influencing only the perioperative mortality but not late survival (Fig. 18-6).

Because it is now generally accepted that surgery prolongs life and is the treatment of choice for patients with left main coronary stenosis, we were interested to review our own long-term experience with this lesion.[27] Between 1968 and 1973, 134 patients with > 50 percent stenosis of the main left coronary artery underwent coronary bypass operation. The group consisted of 87 percent (117 of 134) men with a mean age of 56.0 years (range 37 to 70 years). In addition to left main stenosis, coexistent significant coronary disease was present in other vessels in 98 percent (131 of 134)

of patients, with multivessel disease in 81.4 percent (109 of 134).

Good left ventricular function as defined previously was present in 65.7 percent (88 of 134) of patients. Perioperative mortality in this early experience was 12.7 percent (17 of 134), but over the ensuing 5 years of follow-up, only 10 further patients died, for a late annual attrition rate (excluding perioperative mortality) of only 1.9 percent. Including perioperative mortality, overall annual attrition was 4.0 percent (Fig. 18-7).

A review of our results in a similar group of 73 patients operated on between 1976 and 1978 showed a perioperative mortality of 5.5 percent (4 of 73), and of these 4 deaths, 2 involved patients who had sustained cardiac arrests prior to arriving in the operating room and who had no spontaneous cardiac output prior to operation. In the 69 survivors of operation, there has been no late attrition up to 24 months after operation. As shown in Fig. 18-8, these results are superior to those obtained in three reports[28-30] of surgical candidates who were treated medically. We attribute these improved results to better medical stabilization of these patients preoperatively and to improved anesthetic and myocardial preservation techniques intraoperatively. The intraaortic balloon pump has not been used.

The low long-term attrition rates observed in this, the most severe form of operable coronary disease, are very encouraging evidence for a favorable influence of coronary bypass on late survival. In summary, we feel there can be little doubt that coronary bypass not only prolongs life in symptomatic patients with two- and three-vessel disease and left main coronary stenosis but also does so more effectively than modern medical therapy alone.

The influence of coronary bypass in prolonging life in patients with single-vessel disease is more difficult to determine because of the generally favorable prognosis with medical therapy. It is generally recognized, however, that patients with isolated involvement of the left anterior descending coronary artery have a worse prognosis than those with right or circumflex coronary lesions.[31] Furthermore, even isolated left anterior descending coronary lesions cannot be considered a homogeneous entity. In our own experience, lesions proximal to the first septal perforator are associated with more severe ventricular abnormalities

than those in the distal vessel.[32] Because operation in patients with single-vessel disease and reasonable ventricular function is extremely safe in experienced centers, we favor surgical treatment even in mildly symptomatic patients who have proximal left anterior descending coronary lesions for preservation of myocardial function and for probable, though as yet unproven, enhancement of survival.

Patients presenting with symptoms and signs of congestive heart failure secondary to coronary atherosclerosis have a poor prognosis. In clinical studies of the prognosis of patients with angina pectoris and congestive heart failure, death rates of around 12 to 16 percent per year have been reported,[19,33] and this represents about five times the mortality of patients with coronary atherosclerosis but without congestive heart failure. Thus it has long been recognized that a clinical diagnosis of congestive heart failure in patients with angina pectoris carries a bad prognosis.

More accurate stratification of risk has become possible using coronary angiography, left ventricular angiography, and more recently, radionuclide ventriculography. These studies have shown that for a given level of coronary arterial disease, abnormalities of left ventricular function influence prognosis adversely. Thus, one study showed 93 percent versus 58 percent survival for normal versus abnormal ventriculogram,[19] while another showed that patients with normal ventricles had a 75 percent 5-year survival, and 61 percent (153 of 253) of patients had two- or three-vessel dis-

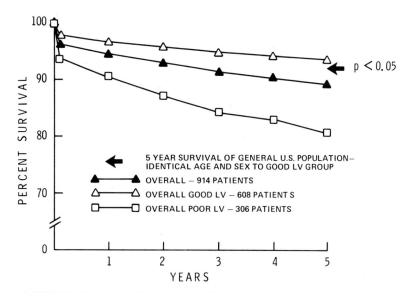

FIGURE 18-6 Survival of all men according to preoperative left ventricular function (LV). (Patients with left main coronary stenosis excluded.) Data from the general population as in Fig. 18-2. (*From G. M. Lawrie et al., Improved Survival After 5 Years in 1144 Patients After Coronary Bypass Surgery, Am. J. Cardiol., 42:709, 1978.*)

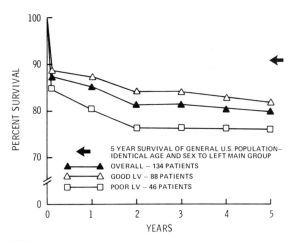

FIGURE 18-7 Survival of 134 patients with left main coronary stenosis operated upon between 1968 and 1973, according to preoperative left ventricular function. Data from the general population as in Fig. 18-2.

ease or left main disease, while 145 patients with localized scar had 69 percent survival, and 66 percent of patients had two- or three-vessel disease or left main disease. In the 79 patients with diffuse abnormality of ventricular function, survival was 31 percent, and 87 percent (69 of 79) of these patients had two- or three-vessel disease or left main disease.

When examining data relating to patients with poor

ventricular function, it is important to recognize that this is usually associated with a higher incidence of severe multivessel coronary disease, as the preceding data indicate. In our own study of 914 male patients, poor left ventricular function was present in 25 percent (45 of 182) of patients with single-vessel disease, in 33 percent (127 of 390) with double-vessel disease, in 39 percent (134 of 342) with triple-vessel disease, and in 37 percent (32 of 86) with left main coronary disease.[22] That is, 87 percent (293 of 338) of patients with poor ventricular function had multivessel coronary disease. The greater severity of coronary disease also makes surgical revascularization more difficult in patients with poor left ventricular function. In our study of 474 consecutive patients with one-, two-, or three-vessel disease, complete revascularization of all major vessels diseased was achieved in 66 percent (202 of 304) of patients with good left ventricular function, whereas in only 46 percent (85 of 189) of patients with poor left ventricular function was complete revascularization achieved by the same surgeon, reflecting a higher incidence of severe and diffusely diseased coronary arteries in these patients[8] (Table 18-1).

The possible beneficial effects of operation were first reported in patients with angina pectoris and congestive heart failure by Spencer et al.[34] and Mundth et al.[35] in 1971. These early encouraging results were further confirmed in the study of Morris et al. from Baylor College of Medicine reported in 1972.[36] There

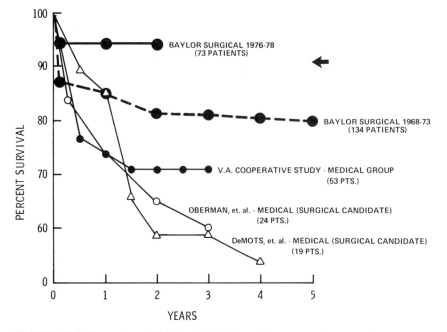

FIGURE 18-8 Comparison of initial (1968–1973) and later (1976–1978) survival of Baylor surgical group of patients with left main stenosis. Also shown are survival curves of three series[28-30] of medically treated surgical candidates with left main stenosis.

were 192 patients with symptoms of congestive heart failure who were on diuretics and had left ventricular end-diastolic pressure over 20 mm Hg and abnormal ventriculograms. Operation was performed with an initial perioperative mortality of 10.4 percent. In a later report,[37] perioperative mortality was 8.4 percent and at a follow-up of up to 6 years, annual attrition was 2.5 percent. In selected patients, quite significant improvement in left ventricular function was apparent on left ventriculography, while in others, no change could be discerned.[37] Relief of symptoms of congestive failure and angina and rehabilitation of these patients appeared to be very favorably influenced by operation.

However, because severe myocardial ischemia can induce reversible changes in ventricular compliance, the left ventricular end-diastolic pressure is not ideal for the accurate classification of severely impaired left ventricular function required for comparison of medical and surgical series. The best guide to prognosis in these patients for a given level of coronary disease has been the left ventricular ejection fraction.[38] Poor ventricular function is generally defined as the presence of an ejection fraction of < 30 to 35 percent.[39] However, at a given level of ejection fraction, patients with localized wall motion abnormalities (e.g., a left ventricular aneurysm) in general have a better prognosis than patients with diffuse impairment of left ventricular function.[18,39] Also influencing survival, as in patients with good left ventricular function, has been the number of vessels with significant stenosis.[18,39]

Thus, once again, for comparative analysis of medical and surgical results in patients with poor ventricular function, we feel that these are the minimal criteria that should be defined. There have been reports of three surgical series of patients with poor left ventricular function well defined by the ejection fraction. In one study, 72 patients with ejection fractions of < 35 percent were operated on with an operative mortality of 1.4 percent and an overall actuarial survival at 42 months of 92 percent.[40] However, mean follow-up was only 13.4 months.

In another study, 140 patients with ejection fractions of < 20 percent underwent operation with an overall mortality of 22 percent, which fell to 9 percent in the later experience between 1973 and 1976.[41] Overall actuarial 6-year survival was 59 percent.

In the study of Manley et al., operative mortality was initially 13 to 25 percent but later was 6 to 9 percent.[42] In patients with an ejection fraction of 31 percent (classes II-IV in this study), survival was 58 percent at 72 months. This study was of particular interest because of the comparison of the surgical group with a retrospectively matched medically treated control group. At all levels of ventricular function, survival of surgical patients was statistically superior ($p < .01$) to that of medically treated patients.

Almost all patients in these studies were operated upon primarily for angina pectoris. The question of appropriate therapy for patients with severe impairment of left ventricular function and no angina is a difficult one, and few data exist on this subject.

Preoperative and postoperative radionuclide ventriculography has been of interest in patients with poor ventricular function. In many patients, significant improvement has been observed even in the absence of preoperative angina (unpublished data). The value of the preoperative response of ejection fraction to nitroglycerin as a prediction of response to operation remains uncertain.

Our own approach with these patients has been to offer surgery to patients with significant symptoms either of angina and/or of congestive heart failure. Our primary requirement is the presence of good distal coronary arteries with high-grade proximal lesions. Patients with severe diffuse coronary disease or only mild to moderate stenosis, in our opinion, are not surgical candidates. Other lesions responsible for poor ventricular function, such as cardiomyopathy or valvular heart disease, require exclusion of these patients. Using current anesthetic and myocardial preservation techniques and, rarely, the intraaortic balloon pump, an operative mortality of much less than 10 percent can be achieved in these patients. Although conclusive evidence is not yet available, we feel that younger, well-selected patients will have improved survival following coronary bypass.

In the absence of symptoms of angina pectoris, the primary goals of operation are prolongation of life and preservation of myocardial function. Implicit in the decision to operate on a patient without symptoms of angina pectoris but with proven coronary atherosclerosis are the suppositions that there are asymptomatic subjects who are at risk from sudden cardiac death, that angina may not develop prior to a serious event, and that preservation of myocardial structure and function can be achieved by coronary artery bypass. Although we now consider the latter to have been well established, unfortunately, at present there is a paucity of good survival data on either medically or surgically treated asymptomatic patients with which to resolve the question of the value of operation under these circumstances.

However, there are a variety of data suggesting that absence of symptoms does not assure a normal prognosis in patients with angiographically proven significant coronary disease. The absence, presence, or severity of angina pectoris in patients in whom angiographic studies of coronary anatomy have been performed have shown a poor correlation between survival and angina as an isolated factor. Although increasing severity of angina pectoris has been shown to be associated with worsening survival,[43] this is due primarily to the higher prevalence of multivessel disease in groups of more symptomatic patients. In one study, 80 percent of New York Heart Association class I patients had single-vessel disease, whereas the large majority of patients who were class IV had double- or triple-vessel disease.[43] In a more detailed study of coronary anatomy, survival was shown to be related to the severity of coronary disease.[44] For a given arteriographic score of severity of coronary involvement, survival was uninfluenced by the severity of angina, although once again, patients with more severe angina generally had more severe coronary disease. This has been shown also in other studies.[19]

The unreliability of angina pectoris as a marker of severity of coronary disease has also been shown by the fact that myocardial ischemia without accompanying angina pectoris has been documented by exercise ECG studies in patients with angiographically proven coronary artery disease. In a study of 122 consecutive patients with an abnormal ECG response to exercise, Lindsey and Cohn reported that 36 percent of patients had no angina during the exercise test.[45] These patients were similar clinically and angiographically to patients who did experience pain. Of the "asymptomatic" group, 75 percent of patients had multivessel coronary disease but only 30 percent had an ejection fraction of < 50 percent. In another study, Bartel et al. found a 17 percent incidence of pain-free patients.[46]

The potential seriousness of asymptomatic coronary disease is emphasized by the fact that 30 to 60 percent of patients sustaining acute myocardial infarction have had no preceding angina, although other symptoms such as fatigue and dyspnea may have developed, causing the patient to consult a physician. Indeed, it is estimated that up to 25 percent of patients experiencing acute myocardial infarction complain of no anginal chest pain during the course of their acute event.[47] Of patients sustaining sudden cardiac death (within 1 h of the onset of the fatal event) about one-half had no prior angina.[18] Survivors of acute myocardial infarction who subsequently have no angina pectoris by current usage are included in the category of "asymptomatic" patients. Angiographic studies of such asymptomatic patients have shown a high prevalence of significant coronary disease.

In one angiographic study of 70 asymptomatic survivors of myocardial infarctions, 56 percent (39) of patients had three vessels with > 60 percent diameter reduction, 20 percent (14) had two-vessel disease, and 24 percent (17) had left main stenosis.[49] Of 210 vessels, 38 percent (80) were completely occluded and 93 percent (65 of 70) of patients had complete occlusion of at least one vessel.

In another study that included 88 asymptomatic patients with previous myocardial infarction, the incidence of single-vessel disease was 47 percent; double-vessel disease, 28 percent; and triple-vessel disease, 25 percent.

It is clear, then, that the occurrence of a myocardial infarction is a reasonably sensitive and specific indication of underlying significant coronary atherosclerosis. In view of the substantial late attrition in these patients of 5 to 10 percent per year,[51,52] we consider that the younger survivors of myocardial infarction should be considered for coronary angiography even in the absence of anginal symptoms. Indeed, we feel an event as serious as an acute myocardial infarction (overall mortality 30 to 50 percent) should be regarded as a pressing symptom of coronary atherosclerosis that is deserving of complete investigation.

An increasingly common clinical problem is the truly asymptomatic patient who is found to have a positive treadmill exercise test during a routine checkup. In one study, 900 presumably healthy policemen were followed after routine exercise stress testing.[53] Of these, 47 (mean age 42 years) had an abnormal ST response that was considered a false positive result by the authors' criteria. During a 7-year follow-up, no coronary events occurred. In 9 subjects, ST-segment abnormalities appeared after exercise, and 1 of these subjects had an acute myocardial infarction 5.5 years after his initial test. The remaining 8 remained stable. In a further 24 asymptomatic subjects with what was considered by the authors to be a true positive response during exercise, 10 had new coronary events: 7 developed angina, 2 others developed nonfatal myocardial infarction, and 1 died suddenly during exercise.

Thus, of this apparently healthy population, 3.6 percent (33 of 900) of subjects had positive treadmill exercise test results, and 1.2 percent (11 of 900) developed coronary events over a 7-year period. However, of the patients suspected of having coronary disease because of positive treadmill test results, 33 percent (11 of 33) developed significant coronary events, and there was one death.[53] The authors emphasized the particular significance of marked ST depression of prolonged duration following exercise.

In another study of 510 asymptomatic men 40 to 65 years of age, 11.9 percent (61 of 510) had positive exercise stress test results at initial examination.[54] During a 3-year follow-up interval, 25 percent (15 of 61) of men with positive stress test results developed clinical evidence of coronary atherosclerosis, 11 developed angina, 2 sustained myocardial infarction (1 of whom died) and 2 further patients experienced sudden death. Thus the mortality in this group was 4.9 percent (3 of 61) over 3 years. A further 11 patients with negative stress test results developed clinical problems, 2 with angina and 9 with infarctions, 2 of which were fatal, resulting in a mortality of 18 percent (2 of 11).

Thus, over a 3-year period, 5 percent (26 of 510) of an initially asymptomatic group of men developed evidence of coronary atherosclerosis, and 5 men died of coronary events. A higher incidence of risk factors was noted in the patients with abnormal stress tests who subsequently developed clinical coronary disease.

In another study, 2,014 apparently healthy males aged 40 to 59 were followed.[55] After excluding patients subsequently found to have clinical evidence of heart disease, diabetes, treated hypertension, or other disease, 86 percent of the eligible men were screened. In 115 patients, ischemic heart disease was suspected, primarily from exercise testing, and of 103 patients who underwent subsequent angiographic studies, significant coronary disease was found in 69 patients or 4.0 percent (69 of 1,732) of the overall group. Of these patients, 80 percent were 50 years old or older. The late fate of their patients was not described.

In another study, Froelicher reported on 76 asymptomatic aircrewmen who had undergone coronary arteriography following positive exercise stress test results.[56] Of the 76 apparently healthy men, 43.4 percent (33 of 76) subsequently were shown to have significant coronary atherosclerosis i.e., 50 percent stenosis in one or more coronary arteries. No survival data was reported.

Thus, in these studies of apparently healthy asymptomatic males in the 40 to 60 year age range, the prevalence of significant coronary disease was about 3 to 5 percent. Of those subjects who developed a positive response on their treadmill exercise test, about 25 to 33 percent developed clinical evidence of coronary atherosclerosis, and the mortality in this group with positive treadmills was around 4 percent over a period of several years.[53-56]

The treadmill exercise test has been shown to provide some quantitative guide to prognosis in groups of symptomatic patients. In symptomatic patients with no ST changes on treadmill exercise testing, the incidence of multivessel coronary disease is low and the prognosis is generally good, with an annual attrition rate of about 1 to 2 percent as compared with patients with definite ST-segment depression in whom annual attrition is up to 10 percent.[57] The time of onset of ischemic changes is also important; patients who experience changes in early stages of the test generally have a worse prognosis than those reaching stable class IV.[57] Angiographic correlation studies have indicated a higher incidence of multivessel and left main disease in patients with significant changes early in treadmill testing.[57]

It would seem likely, therefore, that the asymptomatic patient developing definite ischemia in the late stages of an exercise test will have a better prognosis, but primarily on the basis of the low incidence of mul-

tivessel coronary disease, not because of absence of symptoms alone. Unfortunately, no good data exist to show whether with a given level of coronary involvement, survival is worse in patients with strongly positive stress test results as compared to those with negative test results.

A problem is the significant incidence of false negative exercise stress ECG test responses. The introduction of exercise radionuclide angiography has provided a useful technique that has been shown to be more specific and sensitive than the stress ECG alone.[58,59]

The best available data on medically treated asymptomatic or minimally symptomatic patients are that of the NHLBI Prospective Coronary Artery Disease Natural History Study,[60] in which 105 patients referred to the National Institutes of Health for evaluation of coronary disease were followed for 6 to 40 months (average 22.5 months). The average age was 48 years. Symptoms were absent in 20 percent and mild in 80 percent. Ten patients with left main stenosis were excluded. Single-vessel disease was present in 24 percent of patients, double-vessel in 40 percent, and triple-vessel in 36 percent. Overall, left ventricular function was good, with ejection fractions of 55 percent in 65 percent of patients. Mortality was 2 percent per year overall and 2.4 percent per year for patients with double- and triple-vessel disease. Of the 4 deaths, 2 were sudden and 2 occurred following prior symptomatic deterioration. Symptoms subsequently progressed in 8 other patients. Thus, in this study, even in the absence of severe symptoms, patients with multivessel disease had an attrition rate about three times greater than that of the general U.S. population of age 48 years (7.9 of 1,000 per year).[61] However, this study again emphasizes the more favorable prognosis in asymptomatic or mildly symptomatic patients because of their younger age and generally good left ventricular function.

From all of the foregoing data, it would seem reasonable to assume that some determination of prognosis for asymptomatic patients with angiographically documented significant coronary disease can be made using the same clinical and angiographic criteria employed for those with symptomatic coronary disease, such as the presence or absence of abnormalities of resting ECG, hypertension, congestive heart failure, and the state of left ventricular function as assessed by radionuclide or angiographic evaluation. Thus, it is likely that for a given level of severity of angiographic coronary involvement and left ventricular impairment, these patients will have a prognosis similar to that of asymptomatic patients with comparably excellent clinical criteria and that the good prognosis expected for such asymptomatic patients arises not from lack of symptoms but from a correspondingly less severe and uncomplicated form of coronary atherosclerosis. It is important to emphasize again, however, the continued occurrence of myocardial infarction and sudden death in asymptomatic patients.

In asymptomatic patients in whom myocardial ischemia has been demonstrated by treadmill ECG and/or radionuclide stress ventriculography, we advocate early coronary angiography. Similarly, in younger survivors of myocardial infarction, we advocate coronary angiography and left ventriculography 6 weeks after hospital discharge.

In these two groups of patients, operation is considered if two- or three-vessel disease, left main stenosis, or proximal left anterior descending disease has been identified. We are less inclined to operate on patients with single-vessel disease because, although about 40 to 50 percent of acute myocardial infarctions are associated with single-vessel disease only, the majority of patients experiencing sudden death have severe multivessel coronary disease, are older, and usually have multiple associated risk factors for coronary atherosclerosis. Therefore, we feel that patients with single-vessel disease or, at times, double-vessel disease in whom no evidence of ischemia can be demonstrated by radionuclide stress ventriculography are at low risk of sudden death and can be followed and treated medically with reasonable safety. However, in three-vessel disease or left main stenosis, we are influenced to operate on the basis of anatomy alone.

It is important to recognize that just as the prognosis of asymptomatic patients is generally better than the overall group of symptomatic patients, so is surgery considerably safer in asymptomatic patients. We feel that surgery performed to prolong life alone is indicated primarily in younger patients in whom, in our experience, operation has been very safe.[62] Furthermore, these patients usually have superior left ventricular function. At operation, in our experience, the single most important problem with coronary disease has been the occurrence of acute myocardial ischemia and circulatory instability prior to and during induction of anesthesia. Patients in whom ischemia is mild or absent at rest also are much more stable during induction of anesthesia and operation. On the other hand, in older or poorer risk patients, the improvement in survival from operation must be weighed against the somewhat higher surgical risk.[62]

Although data are sparse as to the fate of asymptomatic patients undergoing coronary bypass, there are three reports of the late results of operation in a total of 125 asymptomatic patients, of whom 113 had severe (> 70 percent diameter reduction) two- or three-vessel disease or left main stenosis[63-65] (Table 18-5). These reports confirm the superior safety of operation in asymptomatic patients. Operative mortality was 0.8 percent (1 of 125), and late mortality (up to 7 years) was 1.6 percent (2 of 125). Of the 113 patients with multivessel disease, 99 percent (112 of 113) are alive at variable follow-up intervals beyond 19 months, which is a remarkably low late attrition rate.

These surgical data, although small in volume, are very encouraging. Because it is likely that the natural history of these asymptomatic patients, in regard to survival is reasonably good with medical therapy (although still substantially subnormal), it is crucial that if surgery is being undertaken for survival alone, it be performed by experienced surgeons capable of producing a negligible mortality, low perioperative infarction rate, and high graft patency.

CONCLUSION

Coronary artery disease remains a major source of morbidity and mortality in the United States despite many years of effort at preventing it or, if clinically manifest, controlling it with medical therapy. Although patients undergoing coronary angiography currently represent only a fraction of the overall population with coronary atherosclerosis, we feel nonetheless that based on the data presented here, we have available a safe, successful, and durable operation that will prolong life to a greater extent than medical therapy alone and that indeed may restore many of these patients to a relatively normal life expectancy as well as a normal life-style.

As a result of the need for long-term data in the study of survival, the surgical results presented here are from early experience with the operation and do not reflect the great advances in the safety of anes-

TABLE 18-5
Surgical results from three series[63-65] with a total of 125 patients in whom symptoms were minimal or absent

| Series | No. pts. | No. vessels diseased | | | | Perioperative mortality (no. pts.) | Late mortality (no. pts.) |
		1	2	3	LM		
Thurer et al.[63]	17	6	7	4	—	0	0
Johnson et al.[64]	88	5	25	58	—	1	1
Wynne et al.[65]	20	1	6	9	4	0	1
Total	125	12	38	71	4	1	2

thesia and surgery and resulting improvement in survival achieved over the last few years. There have been no correspondingly major improvements in the results of medical therapy, although progress is being made in some areas.

Until some simpler, cheaper, and more effective therapy than surgery becomes available, we feel that every effort should be made to identify patients at excessive risk of death from coronary disease and, when indicated, to offer them coronary bypass surgery not only for relief of symptoms but also for prolongation of life.

REFERENCES

1 Selden, R., Neill, W. A., Ritzmann, L. W., et al.: Medical Versus Surgical Therapy for Acute Coronary Insufficiency, *N. Engl. J. Med.*, 239:1329, 1975.

2 Korbuly, D. E., Formanek, A., Gypser, G., et al.: Regional Myocardial Blood Flow Measurements Before and After Coronary Bypass Surgery, *Circulation*, 52:38, 1975.

3 Kent, K. M., Borer, J. S., Green, M. V., Bacharach, S. L., McIntosh, C. L., Conkle, D. M., and Epstein, S. E.: Effects of Coronary-Artery Bypass on Global and Regional Left Ventricular Function During Exercise, *N. Engl. J. Med.*, 298:1434, 1978.

4 Mathur, V. S., and Guinn, G. A.: Prospective Randomized Study of Coronary Bypass Surgery in Stable Angina: The First 100 Patients, *Circulation*, 51, 52 (suppl. 1): 133, 1975.

5 Unstable Angina Pectoris: National Cooperative Study Group to Compare Surgical and Medical Therapy: II. In-hospital Experience and Initial Follow-up Results in Patients with One, Two and Three Vessel Disease, *Am. J. Cardiol.*, 42:839, 1978.

6 Danilevicius, Z.: Editorial: The Myocardium After Repeated Infarction, *J.A.M.A.*, 238:2637, 1978.

7 Vismara, L. A., Miller, R. R., Price, J. E., Karem, R., DeMaria, A. N., and Mason, D. T.: Improved Longevity Due to Reduction of Sudden Death by Aortocoronary Bypass in Coronary Atherosclerosis: Prospective Evaluation of Medical Versus Surgical Therapy in Matched Patients with Multivessel Disease, *Am. J. Cardiol.*, 39:919, 1977.

8 Lawrie, G. M., and Morris, G. C., Jr.: Factors Influencing Late Survival After Coronary Bypass Surgery, *Ann. Surg.*, 187:665, 1978.

9 Steen, P. A., Tinker, J. H., and Tarhan, S.: Myocardial Reinfarction After Anesthesia and Surgery, *J.A.M.A.*, 239:2566, 1978.

10 Crawford, E. S., Morris, G. C., Jr., Howell, J. F., Flynn, W. F., and Moorhead, D. T.: Operative Risk in Patients with Previous Coronary Artery Bypass, *Ann. Thorac. Surg.*, 26:215, 1978.

11 Ennix, C. L., Lawrie, G. M., Morris, G. C., Jr., Crawford, E. S., Howell, J. F., Reardon, M. J., and Weatherford, S. C.: Improved Results of Carotid Endarterec-

tomy in Patients with Symptomatic Coronary Disease: An Analysis of 1546 Consecutive Carotid Operations, *Stroke*, 10:122, 1979.

12 Mahar, L. J., Steen, P. A., Tinker, J. H., Vlietstra, R. E., Smith, H. C., and Pluth, J. R.: Perioperative Myocardial Infarction in Patients with Coronary Artery Disease With and Without Aorto-Coronary Artery Bypass Grafts, *Thorac. Cardiovasc. Surg.*, 76:533, 1978.

13 Lawrie, G. M., Morris, G. C., Jr., Howell, J. F., Ogura, J. W., Spencer, W. H., Cashion, W. R., Winters, W. L., Beazley, H. L., Chapman, D. W., Peterson, P. K., and Lie, J. T.: Results of Coronary Bypass More than 5 Years After Operation in 434 Patients: Clinical Treadmill Exercise and Angiographic Correlations, *Am. J. Cardiol.*, 40:665, 1977.

14 Lawrie, G. M., Lie, J. T., Morris, G. C., Jr., and Beazley, H. L.: Vein Graft Patency and Intimal Proliferation After Aortocoronary Bypass: Early and Long-term Angiopathologic Correlations, *Am. J. Cardiol.*, 38:856, 1976.

15 Lie, J. T., Lawrie, G. M., and Morris, G. C., Jr.: Aortocoronary Bypass Saphenous Vein Graft Atherosclerosis: Anatomic Study of 99 Vein Grafts from Normal and Hyperlipoproteinemic Patients up to 75 Months Post-operative, *Am. J. Cardiol.*, 40:906, 1977.

16 Lawrie, G. M., Morris, G. C., Jr., Chapman, D. W., et al.: Patterns of Patency of 596 Vein Grafts Up to Seven Years After Aorto-Coronary Bypass, *J. Thorac. Cardiovasc. Surg.*, 73:443, 1977.

17 Oberman, A., Jones, W. B., Riley, C. P., Reeves, T. J., and Sheffield, L. T.: Natural History of Coronary Artery Disease, *Bull. N.Y. Acad. Med.*, 48:1109, 1972.

18 Bruschke, A. V. G., Proudfit, W. L., and Sones, F. M., Jr.: Progress Study of 590 Consecutive Non-surgical Cases of Coronary Disease Followed 5-9 Years. I. Arteriographic Correlations; II. Ventriculographic and Other Correlations, *Circulation*, 47:1147, 1154, 1973.

19 Burggraf, G. W., and Parker, J. O.: Prognosis in Coronary Artery Disease: Angiographic, Hemodynamic, and Clinical Features, *Circulation*, 51:146, 1975.

20 Detre, K., Hultgren, H., and Takaro, T.: Veterans Administration Cooperative Study of Surgery for Coronary Arterial Occlusive Disease. III—Methods and Baseline Characteristics, Including Experience with Medical Treatment, *Am. J. Cardiol.*, 40:212, 1977.

21 Hultgren, H. N., Detre, K. M., Takaro, T., Murphy, M. L., and Thomsen, J. H.: The V.A. Cooperative Study of Coronary Arterial Surgery: Baseline Characteristics of Study Population and Survival in Subgroups with Medical Versus Surgical Treatment, in P. N. Yu and J. F. Goodwin (eds.), "Progress in Cardiology," Vol. 6, Lea and Febiger, Philadelphia, 1977, p. 67.

22 Lawrie, G. M., Morris, G. C., Jr., Howell, J. F., Tredici, T. C., and Chapman, D. W.: Improved Survival After 5 Years in 1144 Patients After Coronary Bypass Surgery, *Am. J. Cardiol.*, 42:709, 1978.

23 Read, R. C., Murphy, M. L., Hultgren, H. N., and Takaro, T.: Survival of Men Treated for Chronic Stable Angina Pectoris, *J. Thorac. Cardiovasc. Surg.*, 75:1, 1978.

24 Mundth, E. D., and Austen, W. G.: Surgical Measures for Coronary Heart Disease (3 Parts), *N. Engl. J. Med.*, 293:13, 75, 124, 1975.

25 Conley, M. J., Wechster, A. S., and Anderson, R. W.: The Relationship of Patient Selection to Prognosis Following Aortocoronary Bypass, *Circulation*, 55:158, 1977.

26 Murphy, M. L., Hultgren, H. N., Detre, K., et al.: Treatment of Chronic Stable Angina: A Preliminary Report of Survival Data of the Randomized Veterans Administration Cooperative Study, *N. Engl. J. Med.*, 297:621, 1977.

27 Lawrie, G. M., Morris, G. C., Jr., Howell, J. F., Hines, M., and Chapman, D. W.: Improved Survival Beyond 5 Years Following Coronary Bypass in 134 Patients with Left Main Coronary Stenosis, *Chest*, 74:342, 1978. (Abstract.)

28 Oberman, A., Kouchoukos, N. T., Harrell, R. R., Holt, J. H., Jr., Russell, R. O., Jr., and Rackley, C. E.: Surgical Versus Medical Treatment in Disease of the Left Main Coronary Artery, *Lancet*, 591, 1976.

29 Takaro, T., Hultgren, H. N., Lipton, M. J., Detre, K. M., and Participants in the Study Group: The V.A. Cooperative Randomized Study of Surgery for Coronary Arterial Occlusive Disease. II Subgroup with Significant Left Main Lesions, *Circulation*, 54 (suppl. 3):107, 1976.

30 DeMots, H., Rosch, J., McAnulty, J. H., and Rahimtoola, S. H.: Left Main Coronary Artery Disease in Coronary Bypass Surgery, in S. H. Rahimtoola (ed.), "Cardiovascular Clinics," F. A. Davis Company, Philadelphia, 1977, p. 201.

31 Abedin, Z., and Dack, S.: Editorial: Isolated Left Anterior Descending Coronary Artery Disease: Choice of Therapy, *Am. J. Cardiol.*, 40:654, 1977.

32 Kumpuris, A. G., Miller, R. R., Kanon, D., Lawrie, G. M., and Quinones, M. A.: Isolated Stenosis of the Left Anterior Descending Coronary Artery: A Heterogeneous Disease with Variable Surgical Implications, *Am. J. Cardiol.*, in press. (Abstract.)

33 Russek, H. I.: Prognosis in Severe Angina Pectoris: Medical Versus Surgical Therapy, *Am. Heart J.*, 83:762, 1972.

34 Spencer, F. C., Green, G. E., Tice, D. A., Wallsh, E., Mills, N. L., and Glassman, E.: Coronary Artery Bypass Grafts for Congestive Heart Failure: A Report of Experiences with 40 Patients, *J. Thorac. Cardiovasc. Surg.*, 62:529, 1971.

35 Mundth, E. D., Harthorne, J. W., Buckley, M. J., Dinsmore, R., and Austen, W. G.: Direct Coronary Artery Revascularization: Treatment of Cardiac Failure with Coronary Artery Disease, *Arch. Surg.*, 103:529, 1971.

36 Morris, G. C., Jr., Howell, J. F., Crawford, E. S., Reul, G. J., and Stelter, W.: Operability of End Stage Coronary Artery Disease, *Ann. Surg.*, 175:1024, 1972.

37 Morris, G. C., Jr.: Coronary Artery Surgery and Congestive Heart Failure, in J. C. Norman (ed.), "Coronary Artery Medicine and Surgery: Concepts and Controversies," Appleton-Century-Crofts, New York, 1975, p. 676.

38 Nelson, G. R., Cohn, P. F., and Gorlin, R.: Prognosis in Medically Treated Coronary Artery Disease, *Circulation*, 52:408, 1975.

39 Durairaj, S. K., and Haywood, L. J.: Long-term Follow-up of Patients with Poor Left Ventricular Function After Myocardial Infarction, *Cardiovasc. Med.*, 3:1227, 1978.

40 Jones, E. L., Craver, J. M., Kaplan, J. A., King, S. B., III, Douglas, J. S., Morgan, E. A., and Hatcher, C. R.: Criteria for Operability and Reduction of Surgical Mortality in Patients with Severe Left Ventricular Ischemia and Dysfunction, *Ann. Thorac. Surg.*, 25:413, 1978.

41 Zubiate, P., Kay, J. H., and Mendez, A. M.: Myocardial Revascularization for the Patient with Drastic Impairment of Function of the Left Ventricle, *J. Thorac. Cardiovasc. Surg.*, 73:84, 1977.

42 Manley, J. C., Kind, J. F., Zeft, H. J., and Johnson, W. D.: The "Bad" Left Ventricle: Results of Coronary Surgery and Effect on Late Survival, *J. Thorac. Cardiovasc. Surg.*, 72:841, 1976.

43 Webster, J., Moberg, C., and Rincon, G.: Natural History of Severe Proximal Coronary Artery Disease as Documented by Coronary Cineangiography, *Am. J. Cardiol.*, 33:195, 1974.

44 Humphries, J. O., Kuller, L., Ross, R. S., Friesinger, G. C., and Page, E. E.: Natural History of Ischemic Heart Disease in Relation to Arteriographic Findings, *Circulation*, 59:489, 1974.

45 Lindsey, H. E., Jr., and Cohn, P. F.: "Silent" Myocardial Ischemia During and After Exercise Testing in Patients with Coronary Artery Disease, *Am. Heart J.*, 95:441, 1978.

46 Bartel, A. G., Behar, V. S., and Peter, R. H.: Effects of Aortocoronary Bypass Surgery on Treadmill Exercise, *Circulation*, 46 (suppl. 2):24, 1972.

47 Uretsky, B. F., Farquhar, D. S., Berezin, A. F., and Hood, W. B.: Symptomatic Myocardial Infarction Without Chest Pain: Prevalence and Clinical Course, *Am. J. Cardiol.*, 40:498, 1977.

48 Gordon, T., and Kannel, W. B.: Premature Mortality from Coronary Heart Disease. The Framingham Study, *J.A.M.A.*, 215:1617, 1971.

49 Sanmarco, M. E., Hanashiro, P. K., Selvester, R. H., and Blankenhorn, D. H.: Clinical Arteriographic Correlations in Asymptomatic Men Post-Infarction, in J. C. Norman (ed.), ''Coronary Artery Medicine and Surgery: Concepts and Controversies,'' Appleton-Century-Crofts, New York, 1975, p. 255.

50 Proudfit, W., Shirey, E., and Sones, F. M.: Distribution of Arterial Lesions Demonstrated by Selective Cine-Coronary Arteriography, *Circulation*, 36:54, 1967.

51 The Anturane Reinfarction Trial Research Group: Sulfinpyrazone in the Prevention of Cardiac Death After Myocardial Infarction: The Anturane Reinfarction Trial, *N. Engl. J. Med.*, 298:289, 1978.

52 Szklo, M., Goldberg, R., Kennedy, H. L., and Tonaschia, J. A.: Survival of Patients with Nontransmural Myocardial Infarction: A Population-based Study, *Am. J.Cardiol.*, 42:648, 1978.

53 Morris, S. N., and McHenry, P. L.: Role of Exercise Testing in Healthy Subjects and Patients with Coronary Heart Disease, *Am. J. Cardiol.*, 42:659, 1978.

54 Cumming, G. R., Samm, J., Borysyk, L., and Kich, L.: Electrocardiographic Changes During Exercise in Asymptomatic Men: Three Year Follow-up, *Can. Med. Assoc. J.*, 112:578, 1975.

55 Erikssen, J., Enge, I., Forfang, K., and Storstein, O.: False Positive Diagnostic Tests and Coronary Angiographic Findings in 105 Presumably Healthy Males, *Circulation*, 54:371, 1976.

56 Froelicher, V. F., Yanowitz, F. G., and Thompson, A. J.: The Correlation of Coronary Angiography and the Electrocardiographic Response to Maximal Treadmill Testing in 76 Asymptomatic Men, *Circulation*, 48:597, 1973.

57 McNeer, J. F., Margolios, J. R., Lee, K. L., Kisslo, J. A., Peter, R. H., Kong, Y., Behar, V. S., Wallace, A. G., McCants, C. B., and Rosati, R. A.: The Role of the Exercise Test in the Evaluation of Patients for Ischemic Heart Disease, *Circulation*, 57:64, 1978.

58 Bodenheimer, M. M., Banka, V. S., Fooshee, C. M., Gillespee, J. A., and Helfant, R. H.: Detection of Coronary Heart Disease Using Radionuclide Determined Regional Ejection Fraction at Rest and During Handgrip Exercise: Correlation with Coronary Arteriography, *Circulation*, 58:640, 1978.

59 Botvinick, E. H., Taradash, M. R., Shames, D. M., and Parmley, W. W.: Thallium-201 Myocardial Perfusion Scintigraphy for the Clinical Clarification of Normal, Abnormal and Equivocal Electrocardiographic Stress Tests, *Am. J. Cardiol.*, 41:43, 1978.

60 Kent, K. M., and Epstein, S. E.: Prospective CAD Natural History Study of the National Heart, Lung, and Blood Institute, submitted for publication. (Abstract.)

61 Vital Statistics of the United States for 1973, U.S. Bureau of the Census, Statistical Abstract of the United States, 1975, 96th ed., U.S. Government Printing Office, Washington, D.C., 1975.

62 Lawrie, G. M., Morris, G. C., Jr., Murray, M. J., and Chapman, D. W.: Coronary Artery Bypass Surgery at the Extremes of Age, *Chest*, 70:432, 1976. (Abstract.)

63 Thurer, R. L., Lytle, B. W., Cosgrove, D. M., and Loop, F. D.: Asymptomatic Coronary Artery Disease Managed by Myocardial Revascularization: Five Year Results, *Circulation*, 58 (suppl. 2):60, 1978. (Abstract.)

64 Johnson, W. D., Hoffman, J. F., and Shore, R. T.: Myocardial Revascularization in the Absence of Cardiac Symptoms, *Am. J. Cardiol.*, 39:268, 1977. (Abstract.)

65 Wynne, J., Cohn, L. H., Collins, J. J., Jr., and Cohn, P. F.: Myocardial Revascularization in Patients with Multivessel Coronary Artery Disease and Minimal Angina Pectoris, *Circulation*, 58 (suppl. 1):92, 1978.

Chapter 19

Survival Analyses in Medically and Surgically Treated Patients with Coronary Disease: A Critical Review and Experience in Seattle Heart Watch, a Nonrandomized Series*

K. E. HAMMERMEISTER, M.D.,
TIMOTHY A. De ROUEN, Ph.D.,
and HAROLD T. DODGE, M.D.

INTRODUCTION

Whether or not late survival is improved by coronary artery bypass grafting in patients with coronary disease has been a topic of considerable interest and controversy in recent years. The controversy exists because, although many physicians expected (and logically so) that coronary artery bypass grafting would improve survival in patients with coronary disease, the one large, properly controlled study has failed to demonstrate improved survival, at least in a preliminary report.[1] Whether or not survival is improved by revascularization is a topic of considerable importance, since improved survival with surgical treatment could greatly broaden the indications for this already expensive and widespread operation.

It is the purpose of this chapter to review some of the data surrounding the controversy and critically to analyze the methodology used in studying the issue. We will emphasize that the randomized clinical trial, albeit the ideal way to study the question, is difficult to conduct. Accordingly, there have been few such studies on survival. Numerous studies have attempted to analyze survival data in nonrandomized cohorts of medically and surgically treated patients. We will examine some of the weaknesses of survival analyses of nonrandomized cohorts and propose methodology to correct these weaknesses. Finally, we will conclude by presenting our data from survival analyses in nonrandomized cohorts of patients from the Seattle Heart Watch, attempting to correct some of those shortcomings.

*From the Cardiovascular Disease Section, Seattle Veterans Administration Medical Center, and the Department of Biostatistics and Division of Cardiology, University of Washington.

   This work was supported by VA Institutional Research Funds and NHLBI Grant No. HL 18805-01

RANDOMIZED CLINICAL TRIALS

Gifford and Feinstein, in a paper assessing a series of studies on the use of anticoagulants in myocardial infarction, proposed eight criteria as important for drawing valid conclusions from studies comparing two forms of therapy.[2] These are (1) a statement of diagnostic criteria for the disease or population being studied, (2) an experimental trial, (3) the use of concurrent controls, (4) the random allocation of treatment, (5) the use of stratified prognostic correlation, (6) a statement of diagnostic criteria for end points, (7) blinding of patients and observers to form of treatment, and (8) interhospital coordination if the study involves more than one institution. Of these eight criteria, the randomized clinical trial has been recently emphasized as being essential to exclude selection bias. If randomization is not used, the selection of patients for one form of therapy may segregate patients with poorer or better risk characteristics to that form of therapy, thereby influencing the results. Later in this chapter, we will show data from Seattle Heart Watch clearly documenting that the patients who were selected for surgical therapy of coronary disease had baseline characteristics that differed from patients selected for medical therapy such that the surgically treated patients might be expected to have better survival even if they had been treated medically.

Other considerations aside, under ideal circumstances the randomized clinical trial is the best technique for studying whether or not coronary surgery prolongs survival. However, there are a number of practical and theoretical limitations to the use of this technique. First, one must recognize that surgery as a form of therapy has certain characteristics that make it less amenable to study by the randomized clinical trial than drugs or other less invasive forms of therapy. When drugs are studied using the randomized clinical trial (e.g., the VA hypertension studies), one is certain that the treatment to be given is homogeneous from patient to patient and from institution to institution. The degree of compliance in taking the drug can usually be monitored. On the other hand, the outcome from a surgical operation is highly dependent on the technique; there is a great opportunity for nonhomogeneity in the therapy given. Not only may there be variation from surgeon to surgeon or institution to institution, but the technique varies over time. The fall in operative mortality and the decrease in incidence of perioperative myocardial infarction for coronary artery bypass grafting since its institution in 1967 clearly indicate that the technique for performing this operation has changed over the years.

As a general rule, randomized clinical trials to evaluate a surgical procedure must involve a number of institutions in order to achieve a sample size that is adequate to provide sufficient statistical power to detect a difference in treatment effect if such exists.[3] The three randomized clinical trials of coronary bypass surgery from single institutions have been able to randomize fewer than 100 patients,[4-6] which is an inadequate sample size to get an acceptably small probability of making a type II error (not detecting a difference when it exists). The problems presented by the use of multiple institutions for studying a surgical procedure have not been fully resolved. It is difficult to get surgeons to agree on surgical technique. Documentation of standardization between institutions would be difficult to obtain. The fact that multiple institutions are used means that the quality and quantity will vary between institutions. There is no clear answer to the problem of what to do with low volume or low-quality participants once they have entered patients into a randomized clinical trial.

Physicians and patients may have biases either for or against a given procedure under study, making recruitment of study patients difficult. In the case of coronary artery bypass grafting, the symptomatic relief of disabling angina pectoris is widely known and accepted. This means that it is highly unlikely that another randomized clinical trial involving symptomatic patients with coronary disease will ever be carried out.

In the course of getting potential participants to agree on a common protocol, to prepare a careful, precise definition of the study population, and to exclude patients who might be adversely affected by participation in such a study, randomized clinical trials frequently end up studying relatively narrow spectra of patients. In most randomized clinical trials, only a minority of the patients initially screened with the diagnosis under study are finally randomized. Physicians reading the results of such trials often note the exclusion criteria and question whether the results of the randomized clinical trial are applicable to the broader spectrum of patients with the disease that they see in their practice.

Given these difficulties with randomized clinical trials and the fact that further randomized studies of broad groups of patients with symptomatic coronary disease are unlikely, we feel it is important that techniques for analyses of nonrandomized cohorts of medically and surgically treated patients be explored. In so doing, we must be fully aware of the pitfalls and weaknesses of survival analyses from nonrandomized cohorts. Again, we would emphasize that, where possible, the randomized therapeutic trial is the better technique.

PITFALLS IN SURVIVAL ANALYSES OF NONRANDOMIZED COHORTS OF MEDICALLY AND SURGICALLY TREATED PATIENTS

Selection Bias

The major difficulty in assessing the effect (survival) of a therapy (coronary artery bypass surgery) where the therapy is assigned nonrandomly is that the physicians may select patients for treatment with baseline characteristics such that the treated patients either respond exceptionally well or they would have done well regardless of the therapy given. This is known as selection bias. In the case of coronary artery surgery, this would mean selecting the better risk patient for surgery, while assigning the poorer risk patient to medical therapy. In fact, this selection bias is not only rather obvious, but is also good medical practice. One does not want to recommend an expensive, time-consuming surgical procedure for a patient who is likely to die regardless of the therapy. Most physicians and cardiologists select patients for surgical therapy of coronary disease on the basis of their being likely to survive the operation and also being likely to survive long enough so as to experience the symptomatic benefits of the operation.

While selection bias in the assignment of patients for medical or surgical therapy of coronary disease now seems rather obvious, it has not been clearly documented in the literature and has not been thoroughly considered in a number of the studies purporting to show that coronary surgery prolongs survival.[7-16] Since left ventricular performance has been demonstrated to be the variable most predictive of survival,[17,18] any study comparing survival of medically and surgically treated patients must compare the two cohorts by left ventricular function—preferably a quantitative assessment such as ejection fraction.

We have analyzed some of the baseline characteristics in patients in the angiography registry of Seattle

Heart Watch who had been selected by their physicians for medical or surgical therapy of their angiographically demonstrated coronary disease. These patients with suspected coronary disease were entered into Seattle Heart Watch on the basis of having had a coronary arteriogram and usually a left ventricular angiogram with quantitative analysis. The angiographic registry includes over 90 percent of the patients having coronary surgery in the city of Seattle during the 5-year period from 1969 to 1974 and approximately 40 percent of the patients undergoing coronary arteriography for suspected coronary disease and subsequently treated medically. The remainder of the medically treated patients having coronary angiography were not included owing to limitation in funding.

Tables 19-1 and 19-2 show the baseline variables that were statistically significantly different between the medically and surgically treated patients entered into the angiography registry of Seattle Heart Watch. We analyzed a total of 46 baseline variables from the history, physical examination, resting electrocardiogram, exercise stress test, and cardiac catheterization for all the patients entered into the angiography registry who had a stenosis or stenoses of ≥ 70 percent of one or more major coronary arteries. There were 450 medically treated patients and 1,864 surgically treated patients. More than half (28) of the 46 baseline variables were significantly different between the two treatment groups. This, of course, reflects the nonrandom selection of patients for one or the other form of therapy.

Although there are a large number of variables that are different between the two cohorts, the differences can be summarized relatively succinctly. The surgically treated patients were more symptomatic with regard to chest pain than the medically treated patients, as indicated by the limitations on treadmill exercise testing, the functional class, the frequency of use of beta blocking agents, and the frequency of chest pain and ST-segment depression on exercise testing. On the other hand, the medically treated patients exhibited evidence of more myocardial damage as indicated by the larger end-diastolic volume, lower ejection fraction, higher left ventricular end-diastolic pressure, and higher frequency of prior myocardial infarction, congestive heart failure, use of digitalis and diuretics, S_3 gallop and cardiomegaly, and subjective left ventricular contraction abnormalities. In addition, the medically treated patients had a higher frequency of ventricular arrhythmias on their resting electrocardiogram, more collateral vessels on the coronary arteriogram, and fewer vessels that were amenable to grafting. The variables relevant to myocardial performance all suggest that the surgically treated patients would have an intrinsically longer survival regardless of their form of therapy.

In conclusion, our experience from this communitywide study indicates that when physicians choose patients for coronary artery surgery, they generally select candidates with better baseline risk characteristics for survival than the patients they assign to medical therapy.

TABLE 19-1

Differences at entry between medically and surgically treated patients in the angiography registry of Seattle Heart Watch: continuous variables

Variable	Medically treated			Surgically treated			
	N	$\bar{X}$	S.D.	N	$\bar{X}$	S.D.	p
Clinical examination							
Risk factor index	450	1.20 ±	0.89	1,864	1.36 ±	0.89	<.001
Exercise test							
Duration of exercise (sec)	331	336 ±	152	673	281 ±	134	<.001
FAI (%)	333	36% ±	23%	683	44% ±	21%	<.001
Maximum heart rate	333	145 ±	23	669	136 ±	23	<.001
Change in heart rate	333	66 ±	23	662	59 ±	21	<.001
Maximum pressure rate product (× 1,000)	319	230 ±	63	642	217 ±	59	<.01
Cardiac catheterization							
Number of stenotic vessels	450	1.7 ±	0.8	1,864	2.1 ±	0.8	<.001
Vessels feasible for grafting	450	1.3 ±	1.0	1,863	2.0 ±	0.8	<.001
End-diastolic volume (ml/m²)	357	80.1 ±	29.2	989	71.5 ±	23.2	<.001
End-systolic volume (ml/m²)	357	40.2 ±	28.0	988	30.8 ±	19.1	<.001
Ejection fraction (%)	386	53.5 ±	16.2	1,232	58.6 ±	13.3	<.001
LVEDP (mm Hg)	408	13.9 ±	9.9	1,580	11.7 ±	7.3	<.001

Abbreviations: N, number of patients in which variable was measured; $\bar{X}$, mean; S.D., one standard deviation; p, significance of difference between means; FAI, functional aerobic impairment; LVEDP, left ventricular end-diastolic pressure.

TABLE 19-2
Differences at entry between medically and surgically treated patients in the angiography registry of Seattle Heart Watch: discrete variables

	Medically treated			Surgically treated			
	Variable present	Total N	%	Variable present	Total N	%	p
Clinical Examination							
Angina	374	449	83%	1,809	1,864	97%	<.001
MI	257	450	57%	793	1,864	43%	<.001
CHF	59	445	13%	134	1,848	7%	<.001
Functional class I	73	436	17%	74	1,840	4%	
II	191	436	44%	524	1,840	28%	
III	145	436	33%	1,000	1,840	54%	<.001
IV	27	436	6%	242	1,840	13%	
Use of digitalis	82	448	18%	205	1,817	11%	<.001
Use of diuretics	97	447	22%	317	1,814	17%	<.005
Use of beta blocker	71	447	16%	401	1,815	22%	<.001
Use of antiarrhythmic agent	50	450	11%	86	1,864	5%	<.001
S_3 gallop	42	447	9%	30	1,838	2%	<.001
Cardiomegaly	63	446	14%	77	1,836	4%	<.001
Ventricular arrhythmia (resting ECG)	52	446	12%	112	1,835	6%	<.001
Exercise test							
Chest pain	199	334	60%	555	689	81%	<.001
ST↓	149	335	44%	422	699	60%	<.001
Cardiac catheterization							
Collaterals present	304	420	72%	1,073	1,697	63%	<.001
No or poorly graftable distal vessels	95	450	21%	31	1,863	2%	<.001
No or minimal LV contraction abnormality	228	442	52%	1,163	1,719	68%	<.001

Abbreviations: N, total number of patients; MI, myocardial infarction; CHF, congestive heart failure, ST↓, ST-segment depression on exercise test ≥ 1 mm.

Early Medical Deaths

Another problem that comes up in the analysis of survival data from nonrandomized cohorts is that patients who die shortly after coronary arteriography without coronary surgery are usually all assigned to the medically treated cohort. Undoubtedly, some of these patients were intended to have surgical treatment of their coronary disease but did not survive until the time of surgery. Some physicians find it difficult to accept the logic that some of these patients should be assigned to the surgically treated cohort. Certainly, in a randomized therapeutic trial when the randomization is made shortly after the time of coronary arteriography, such patients would have been assigned to the surgical cohort. This practice of assigning these early deaths all to medical therapy gives an unduly poor survival to the medical cohort. In our survival analyses to be shown later in this chapter, we have excluded all patients from the medical cohort who, not having had coronary artery surgery, died within 30 days of their coronary arteriography. We did this because we did not know which of those patients were intended by their physicians to have undergone surgery but died while awaiting surgery and because the average length

of time from catheterization to surgery was 30 days. Our correction for these early medical deaths may be overly conservative, since not all the medically treated patients dying within 30 days of coronary arteriography were intended to have had coronary surgery. Nevertheless, we feel that it is important to correct for this bias.

Nonconcurrent Controls

Another problem raised by Gifford and Feinstein[2] is the use of nonconcurrent or historical controls. This has occurred in a number of the papers appearing in the recent literature on the survival analysis of medically and surgically treated coronary disease patients.[7-12] In some types of survival analyses where mean survival is short (e.g., cancer studies), the use of nonconcurrent controls is not only acceptable but necessary. However, in the assessment of coronary surgery, where mean survival is longer, this tactic produces potential for serious error. For example, in one of the early studies of the effect of coronary surgery on survival, the medically treated controls were drawn from a time period (1962 to 1967) prior to the general introduction of coronary care units and the widespread use of propranolol.[7] However, the surgically treated patients were drawn from a later time period (1967 to 1970) when these two advances in the care of coronary disease patients had come into relatively widespread use.

Data Analyses

We feel that the types of statistical analyses and the way in which the data are displayed are also important in making judgments about the quality of the data. Survival curves should be displayed with standard errors given at regular intervals so that the reader can immediately make a judgment regarding the significance of separated survival curves. Since the patients are almost always followed for variable periods of time, the numbers of patients followed for each interval should also be given on the survival curves. This enables the reader to make a judgment of the validity of the differences in survival, particularly in the later years of the study where the greatest separation in survival curves is frequently seen but the smallest number of patients have been followed. Finally, it is preferable to use a statistical test of significance that tests the differences in survival over the entire length of follow-up and weights the curves according to the number of patients followed for each interval. This would appear to be preferable to making tests of differences in survival at a fixed point in time (e.g., 2 and 4 years). In our studies, we have used the Mantel-Haenzel-Cox statistic,[19] which fulfills these criteria.

Use of Population Mortality Statistics

Several studies in the recent literature have made comparisons between the survival curves of surgically treated patients with coronary disease and the survival curve for the sex- and age-matched general population.[20,21] There is a major fallacy in this kind of comparison that has not been adequately emphasized in the literature. Coronary disease patients considered for coronary surgery (i.e., selected for coronary angiography) are in general free of other life-threatening disease such as chronic obstructive pulmonary disease, malignancy, renal failure, etc. The survival curves for the general population reflect deaths from all causes. In fact, coronary disease accounts for only about one-third of the deaths of males between ages 35 and 64,[22] the age group generally undergoing coronary surgery. The fact that patients being considered for coronary surgery (i.e., undergoing coronary angiography) are selected to be free of other life-threatening disease is documented by data from the Seattle

Heart Watch angiography registry.[23] For medically treated patients, only 10 percent (6 of 60) of the deaths were noncardiac from among the 748 patients followed an average of 29 months. Comparable figures for the 1,848 surgically treated patients were similar (10 percent, 11 of 108). Comparisons of survival of this select group of patients with the general population, two-thirds of whom will die of noncardiac causes, is inappropriate.

EXPERIENCE IN SEATTLE HEART WATCH—SURVIVAL ANALYSES IN NONRANDOMIZED COHORTS OF PATIENTS

Recognizing some of the pitfalls in the analysis of nonrandomized cohorts, but also recognizing the difficulties in carrying out randomized therapeutic trials, we have attempted to devise techniques to correct for some of the difficulties in survival analysis of nonrandomized cohorts. Our hypothesis was: if a population of coronary disease patients was adequately characterized by the variables predictive of survival, one could correct for the differences in baseline variables at entry and make meaningful conclusions regarding survival of medically and surgically treated cohorts. In our initial attempt, we selected the two variables then considered to be the most important predictors of survival (number of diseased coronary vessels and ejection fraction), and we subgrouped patients according to these two variables.[23]

Initial Survival Analyses of Seattle Heart Watch Registry

The characteristics of the Seattle Heart Watch angiography registry have been briefly defined earlier in this chapter. The survival analyses previously reported correcting for differences in ejection fraction and extent of disease[23] have been updated so that they represent a mean follow-up of approximately 41 months from the time of cardiac catheterization. Subjects are classified according to the extent of coronary artery disease and the level of ventricular performance. Extent of coronary disease is expressed as the number of vessels (right, left anterior descending, and left circumflex or marginal) with 70 percent or greater narrowing of the luminal diameter based on subjective interpretation. Narrowing of the left main coronary artery of 70 percent or greater is counted as two-vessel disease. Left ventricular performance is evaluated by the ejection fraction as determined from a cineven-

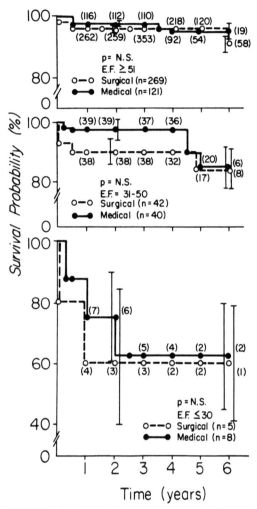

FIGURE 19-1 Survival curves for medically and surgically treated patients with single-vessel disease subgrouped according to ejection fraction.

triculogram. The subjects are classified into nine subgroups based on ejection fractions of $\geq$ 50 percent, 31 to 50 percent, and $\leq$ 30 percent and number of diseased vessels (one, two, or three). For the analyses and construction of life-table survival curves, only cardiovascular deaths are included. For the surgical group, deaths from the time of surgery, including operative deaths, were used for analysis. The average time from cardiac catheterization to surgery was 30 days. Accordingly, for the medical group, only those deaths that occurred after 30 days following cardiac catheterization were included in this analysis. There are 345 subjects in the medically treated and 1,196 in the surgically treated groups. The numbers of subjects in each of the subgroups and at various time intervals of follow-up are given in Figs. 19-1, 19-2, and 19-3.

Figure 19-1 shows the life-table survival curves for

subjects with single-vessel coronary artery disease grouped according to the three levels of ejection fraction. The survival curves up to 6 years for the medically and surgically treated groups are not statistically different for any subgroup. In the single-vessel disease group with an ejection fraction of 50 percent or greater, there is a very low mortality (less than 5 percent over 6 years in both the medically and surgically treated groups. The mortality in the medically treated group is so low that it would be difficult to demonstrate a reduced mortality from any therapeutic modality. In fact, this is lower than the age-predicted mortality for the general population. There was a substantial initial surgical mortality in the group with the moderately depressed ejection fraction (31 to 50 percent), but by 5 years the survival rate was similar for the medically and surgically treated groups. For the subjects with ejection fractions of $\leq$ 30 percent, there was a high mortality with both medical and surgical treatment, but the number of subjects is small.

The survival curves for the subjects with two-vessel disease are shown in Fig. 19-2. As with single-vessel disease, the subjects with the greatest ventricular damage as expressed by the ejection fraction had the highest mortality over 6 years. In comparison with Fig. 19-1, subjects with two-vessel disease had, in general, a lower 6-year survival than subjects with one-vessel disease and similar level of ejection fraction. For these subjects with two-vessel disease, the surgically treated patients had a significantly increased survival when compared to the medically treated patients for each of the ejection fraction subgroups ($p <$ .05).

For the subjects with three-vessel disease, as shown in Fig. 19-3, mortality during follow-up was much higher in the groups with depressed ejection fraction than in the group with ejection fractions of $\geq$ 51 percent. A comparison of the medically and surgically treated subjects showed no statistically significant difference for survival in the three-vessel disease groups with ejection fractions of $\geq$ 51 percent or $\leq$ 30 percent. The small medically treated subgroup with an ejection fraction of $\geq$ 51 percent had a 6-year mortality of only 5 percent. For the group with ejection fractions of $\leq$ 30 percent, there were so few subjects that the differences were not significant. However, for the subjects with ejection fractions of 31 to 50 percent, the surgical group had an increased survival over the medically treated group, and this difference was highly significant ($p <$ .01).

Accordingly, as is shown in Figs. 19-2 and 19-3, using a system of classification that considers only the number of significantly narrowed coronary arteries and the level of ejection fraction, it is possible to identify subgroups in whom survival within the surgically treated subjects is significantly improved over that in

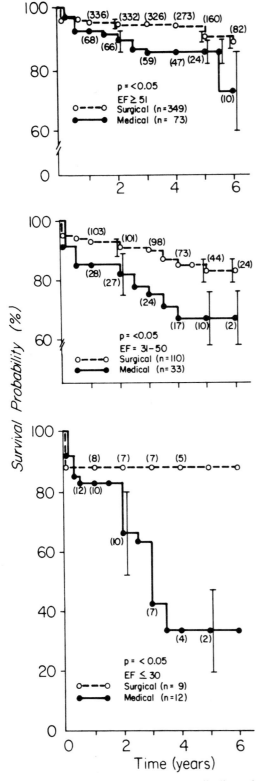

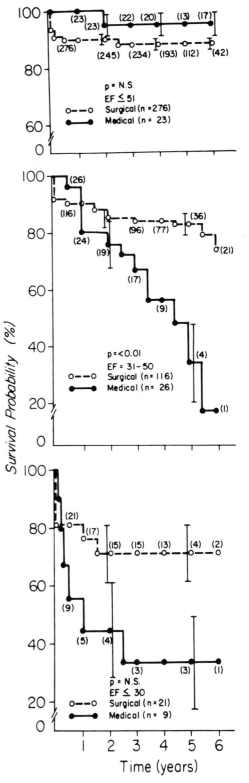

FIGURE 19-2 Survival curves for medically and surgically treated patients with two-vessel disease subgrouped according to ejection fraction.

FIGURE 19-3 Survival curves for medically and surgically treated patients with three-vessel disease subgrouped according to ejection fraction.

TABLE 19-3
Stepwise selection of covariates using Cox's regression model for survival analysis

Cohort	Step	Variable entered	X^2_1
Medical		$N = 550$	
	1	Ejection fraction	48.54
	2	Age	17.16
	3	Number of vessels with stenosis(es) $\geq$ 70%	7.36
	4	Ventricular arrhythmia	4.46
Surgical		$N = 913$	
	1	Ventricular arrhythmia	19.4
	2	Ejection fraction	13.22
	3	Heart murmur	10.96
	4	Left main stenosis	7.94
	5	Use of diuretics	5.38

N, number of patients used in each Cox's regression analysis.
SOURCE: Hammermeister et al.[18]

the medically treated subjects. However, this is not a randomized study, and to be confident that surgical therapy results in improved survival in these subgroups, one would need to demonstrate that subgroups are similar with respect to other variables or that the variables considered (number of coronary vessels significantly narrowed and the ejection fraction) are such powerful determinants of survival that other factors do not have an additional significant effect on survival. As was previously described in detail,[23] differences could be demonstrated between the medically and surgically treated subgroups when other variables were considered. In particular, the surgical subgroups were more symptomatic based on New York Heart Association functional class, had potentially more graftable vessels, had less ventricular damage based on an estimate of contraction grade, and had smaller end-diastolic volumes. These differences in baseline variables, particularly the differences in left ventricular performance, could have accounted for some of the differences in survival observed.

Multivariate Identification of Variables Predictive of Survival

Our next step was to use multivariate statistical techniques to identify a subset of the variables that contained most or all of the prognostic information with respect to survival. It is our thesis that the patients entered into the angiography registry of Seattle Heart Watch are as well characterized in regard to important baseline variables as any reported large population of coronary disease patients. Although the data are not 100 percent complete on all patients, most patients had relevant historical items, physical examination items,

resting ECG variables, and cardiac catheterization variables including scoring of the coronary arteriogram and quantitative angiographic analysis of the left ventricular angiogram included in their data base. We believe that this data base includes all the variables or the equivalents thereof known to be predictive of survival in patients with known coronary disease. The multivariate statistical techniques, which will not be described in detail here, were designed to sift out from this multitude of baseline variables those variables most predictive of survival when considered in conjunction with other variables. Many variables (e.g., end-diastolic volume and ejection fraction) carry similar prognostic information. In the multivariate statistical analyses, one of these will drop out. Our series of multivariate statistical analyses produced seven variables significantly predictive of survival,[18] as shown in Table 19-3. Note that the ejection fraction is by far the most important variable predictive of survival in the medically treated patients and is second in importance in the surgically treated patients. Ventricular arrhythmia on the resting electrocardiogram was an important prognostic variable, particularly in the surgical cohort. This may have important therapeutic implications, since it suggests that ventricular arrhythmia is relevant to survival independent of left ventricular function rather than being a manifestation of severe left ventricular dysfunction. Having identified the variables significantly predictive of survival, we used two techniques to make survival comparisons between medically and surgically treated patients: (1) the matched-pair technique and (2) Cox's regression analysis.

MATCHED PAIRS

For the matched-pair technique, we developed a computer program that randomly matched one surgically treated patient with one medically treated patient identical in the five discrete variables (number of vessels with stenosis or stenoses of $\geq$ 70 percent, ventricular arrhythmia, heart murmur, left main stenosis of $\geq$ 50 percent, use of diuretics) and within specified ranges for the two continuous variables (ejection fraction of $\leq$ 30 percent, ejection fraction of 31 to 50 percent, ejection fraction of $\geq$ 51 percent, and 5-year age ranges). In this way we identified medically and surgically treated patients who were identical or very similar in all of the seven variables found to carry most of the prognostic information that we had available to us. The results of the survival analyses in this matched-pair cohort are shown in Figs. 19-4 through 19-7. For the total group of 287 matched pairs, there is a highly significant ($p = .008$) difference between medically and surgically treated patients in favor of the surgically treated patients (Fig. 19-4). The estimated survival in the surgical cohort at 2 and 4 years is 0.96 ± 0.01

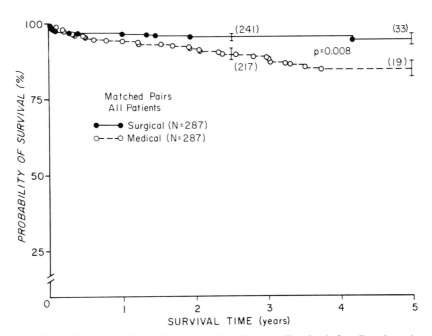

FIGURE 19-4 Actuarial survival curves based on cardiac death for all patients in matched-pair cohort showing improved survival (*p* = .008) in the surgically treated patients. *(From K. E. Hammermeister et al., Evidence from a Nonrandomized Study That Coronary Surgery Prolongs Survival in Patients with Two-Vessel Coronary Disease, Circulation, 59:431, 1979. Reproduced with permission of the American Heart Association).*

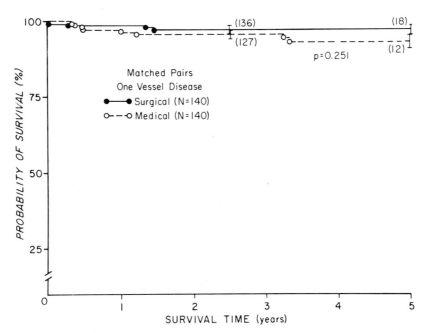

FIGURE 19-5 Actuarial survival curves based on cardiac death for the 140 matched pairs with single-vessel obstruction (≥70 percent) showing no statistical significant difference in survival between medically and surgically treated patients. *(From K. E. Hammermeister et al., Evidence from a Nonrandomized Study That Coronary Surgery Prolongs Survival in Patients with Two-Vessel Coronary Disease, Circulation, 59:431, 1979. Reproduced with permission of the American Heart Association).*

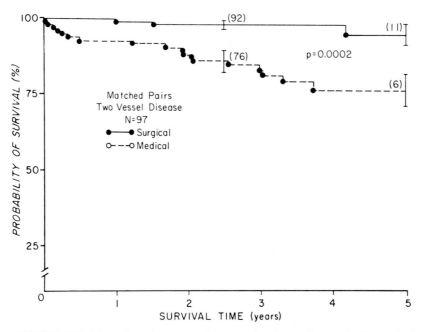

FIGURE 19-6 Actuarial survival curves based on cardiac deaths for the 97 matched pairs with two-vessel obstruction (≥ 70 percent) showing a highly significant (p = .0002) improvement in survival in the surgically treated patients. *(From K. E. Hammermeister et al., Evidence from a Nonrandomized Study That Coronary Surgery Prolongs Survival in Patients with Two-Vessel Coronary Disease, Circulation, 59:431, 1979. Reproduced with permission of the American Heart Association).*

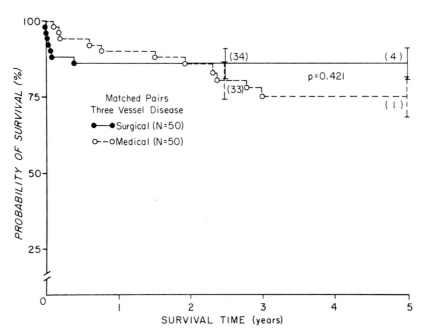

FIGURE 19-7 Actuarial survival curves based on cardiac death for the 50 matched pairs with three-vessel obstruction (≥ 70 percent) showing no significant (p = .421) difference in survival between the medically and surgically treated patients. *(From K. E. Hammermeister et al., Evidence from a Nonrandomized Study that Coronary Surgery Prolongs Survival in Patients with Two-Vessel Coronary Disease, Circulation, 59:431, 1979. Reproduced with permission of the American Heart Association).*

(standard error) and 0.96 ± 0.01, respectively. For the medical cohort the equivalent estimated survivals were 0.92 ± 0.02 and 0.86 ± 0.02, respectively. The overall operative mortality (30-day mortality) was 2.1 percent (6 of 287).

The patients with single-vessel disease showed no difference in survival between the medically and surgically treated patients (Fig. 19-5). The survival for both the medically and surgically treated patients was very good (0.97 ± 0.01 at 4 years in the surgical cohort and 0.93 ± 0.02 at 4 years in the medical cohort).

There was a significant difference in survival between medically and surgically treated patients with two-vessel disease in favor of the surgically treated patients (Fig. 19-6). This difference was highly significant statistically (p = .0002). The 2- and 4-year estimated survivals for the surgically treated patients were 0.98 ± 0.02 and 0.98 ± 0.02, respectively. Equivalent survivals for the medically treated patients were 0.88 ± 0.03 and 0.76 ± 0.05, respectively. The operative mortality in this group of 97 surgically treated patients was 0 percent (0 of 97).

There was no statistically significant difference in the survival of medically and surgically treated patients with three-vessel disease (Fig. 19-7). However, the number of matched pairs was small (50) as a result of the small number of medically treated patients with three-vessel disease available for matching. Also, the operative mortality in this small number of surgically treated patients was exceptionally high (10 percent, 5 of 50). Even given this high operative mortality, which is not representative of the current experience of 1 to 2 percent mortality, the survival curves have crossed over, with the surgically treated patients now appearing to be surviving longer than the medically treated patients (not yet statistically significant).

COX'S REGRESSION ANALYSIS

In the second type of analysis, we used Cox's regression analysis to test for the effect of therapy (medical vs. surgical) on survival in the presence of the seven variables previously identified to be predictive of survival. Cox's regression analysis is an analogue of multiple linear regression analysis applied to survival data. It has the advantage over the matched-pair technique of making use of all the survival data on all the patients in our registry who had known values for the seven covariates. The results of Cox's regression analysis (Table 19-4) show that the form of therapy (medical or surgical) was highly predictive of survival in the group of patients as a whole and in the subgroup of patients with two-vessel disease. The form of therapy (surgical vs. medical) was not predictive of survival in patients with single-vessel disease and triple-vessel disease. Thus, Cox's regression analysis in the total population

TABLE 19-4

Results of Cox's regression analysis testing for effect of mode of therapy on survival while correcting for other variables predictive of survival

Patient group	*N*	Variable	*p*
All patients	1,524	Ejection fraction	.0000002
		Ventricular arrhythmia	.002
		Use of diuretic	.005
		Number of stenotic vessels (≥ 70%)	.007
		Surgery	.008
		Left main stenosis	.026
		Age	.038
		Heart murmur	.116
Single-vessel disease	491	Ventricular arrhythmia	.025
		Use of diuretic	.035
		Ejection fraction	.045
		Heart murmur	.232
		Age	.446
		Left main stenosis	.487
		Surgery	.933
Two-vessel disease	585	Surgery	.0005
		Left main stenosis	.001
		Ejection fraction	.008
		Diuretic use	.021
		Age	.067
		Ventricular arrhythmia	.131
		Heart murmur	.920
Three-vessel disease	466	Ejection fraction	.0001
		Ventricular arrhythmia	.020
		Age	.293
		Heart murmur	.341
		Diuretic use	.341
		Surgery	.350
		Left main stenosis	.595

Abbreviations: *N*, number of patients in each group on whom all seven variables were known for Cox's regression analysis; *p*, significance of variable in predicting survival.
SOURCE: Hammermeister et al.[24]

of patients (n = 1,524) confirmed exactly the results observed in the matched pair cohort (574 patients).

Earlier in this chapter, we emphasized that the randomized clinical trial was the preferable technique for studying the effect of therapy, and we emphasized a number of pitfalls in survival analysis of nonrandomized cohorts. Our matched-pair analysis and use of Cox's regression analysis do not totally eliminate the possibility of the selection bias pitfall that we noted. There remains the possibility, and perhaps even the likelihood, of an additional unmeasured and/or as yet undescribed variable or variables that have prognostic significance. However, for such an unmeasured variable to alter our conclusions, it would have to carry additional prognostic information above and beyond (in a multivariate statistical sense) the 46 variables used in the study and also be distributed significantly differently between the medical and surgical cohorts. The difference in survival between medically and surgically treated patients with two-vessel disease are now of sufficient magnitude that such an unmeasured variable would have to be a powerful predictor of survival (probably more so than any of the seven used) and have a marked distribution difference between medically and surgically treated patients in order to invalidate surgical therapy as a cause of improved survival in this group. We believe this to be unlikely.

Comparisons with the VA Cooperative Study

Since the preliminary report of the randomized VA cooperative study showed no statistically significant difference in survival, we thought it would be useful to make comparisons between these two studies to identify where the differences lie. The VA cooperative study has classified left ventricular function differently than we have. Therefore, we reclassified the patients in our matched-pair cohort into normal or abnormal left ventricular function, following as closely as possible the criteria used by the VA cooperative study. The only differences between the two studies in variables used to define abnormal left ventricular function were that we defined an enlarged left ventricle quantitatively (end-diastolic volume of ≥ 105 ml/m^2) rather than qualitatively as was done in the VA cooperative study. Also, we used stenosis(es) of ≥ 70 percent to define significant obstruction, while stenosis(es) of ≥ 50 percent was used by the VA cooperative study.

Table 19-5 shows a comparison of 2-year survivals for the two studies. The largest difference between the two studies is seen in the subgroup of surgically treated patients with two-vessel disease and normal left ventricular function, where the Seattle Heart Watch patients appear to have significantly better survival. This subgroup in the VA cooperative study had a particularly poor 2-year survival rate, lower in fact than either their surgically treated patients with three-vessel disease and normal left ventricular function or their surgically treated patients with two-vessel disease and abnormal left ventricular function.

CONCLUSIONS AND THERAPEUTIC IMPLICATIONS

Single-Vessel Disease

None of the published studies to date has shown any difference in survival between medically and surgically treated patients with single-vessel coronary disease. All the studies have shown a good survival in these patients regardless of the form of therapy used. However, the follow-up intervals are still relatively short. *There remains the possibility that with follow-up of 5 to 10 years, differences in survival between medically and surgically treated patients may emerge. The failure to improve survival with surgery in patients with single-vessel disease does not negate the usefulness of this procedure in the relief of symptoms in this subgroup of patients.*

Severe Left Ventricular Dysfunction

Patients with severe left ventricular dysfunction (ejection fraction of less than 25 percent) have a poor survival regardless of the form of therapy applied.[23,25] *Since surgery does not generally improve left ventricular function in the chronic stable angina patient,[26] surgery should not be offered as a form of treatment for symptoms of congestive heart failure or fatigue*

TABLE 19-5

Comparisons of two-year survival probability of comparable patient groups between VA cooperative study and Seattle Heart Watch matched-pair analysis

Ventricular function	Number of diseased vessels*	Medically treated patients		Surgically treated patients	
		SHW	VA	SHW	VA
Normal	1	0.97±0.02	1.00±0.00	0.99±0.01	1.00±0.00
Normal	2	0.91±0.06	0.95±0.05	0.96±0.05	0.83±0.09
Normal	3	1.00±0.00	0.95±0.05	1.00±0.00	0.92±0.05
Abnormal	1	0.94±0.03	0.97±0.03	0.96±0.03	0.96±0.04
Abnormal	2	0.90±0.04	0.98±0.04	0.98±0.02	0.92±0.03
Abnormal	3	0.84±0.06	0.89±0.03	0.81±0.07	0.85±0.04

*Note that the definition of significant disease differs in the two studies: 70% diameter reduction in Seattle Heart Watch (SHW) and 50% in the VA Cooperative Study (VA).
SOURCE: Hammermeister et al.[24]

unless there is a correctable mechanical lesion such as a large ventricular aneurysm or mitral regurgitation. Similarly, surgery probably should not be offered with the sole hope of prolonging life, since this seems unlikely. However, in the rare patient with both severe left ventricular dysfunction and severe disabling angina, surgery may be considered, providing that both the surgeon and the patient are willing to accept the risk of significant operative mortality and recognize that even with successful surgery, subsequent survival may be short.

Left Main Stenosis

The VA cooperative study conclusively demonstrates that surgical therapy improves survival in symptomatic patients with left main coronary artery stenosis of ≥ 50 percent.[27] There are no data regarding the effect of surgery on survival in the asymptomatic patient with left main coronary artery obstruction. However, such patients must be rare. In general, we believe that the presence of significant obstruction of the left main coronary artery (equal to or greater than 50 percent) is an anatomic indication for surgery, providing that the distal vessels are adequate for bypass grafting and that other life-threatening disease is not present.

Two-Vessel Disease

Although our data strongly suggest that surgical therapy improves survival in patients with two-vessel disease, we are not yet ready to recommend that all patients with two-vessel disease should have surgery regardless of symptoms. Our population of patients was almost entirely symptomatic. Although we know of no data to indicate that asymptomatic patients with two-vessel disease might not also expect improved survival, the issue has not yet been studied. *We do believe that our data indicate that patients with two-vessel disease should not be required to have a prolonged period of medical therapy before being reluctantly offered surgery. This would seem to be particularly applicable to the younger patient with two-vessel coronary disease.*

Three-Vessel Disease

Our data are inconclusive in regard to three-vessel disease. *In the VA cooperative study, the surgically treated patients with three-vessel disease and abnormal left ventricular function are starting to show somewhat better survival than similar medically treated patients,*[28] *although the differences are not yet statistically significant.* Logically, if our data are correct for patients with two-vessel disease, one would also expect to find improved survival in patients with three-vessel disease treated surgically. Although our matched-pair analysis did not show improved survival in patients with three-vessel disease owing to small numbers and high operative mortality, our analysis of subgroups segregated by ejection fraction and extent of disease suggests that patients with three-vessel disease and moderately abnormal left ventricular function (ejection fraction of 31 to 50 percent) may have improved survival if treated surgically (Fig. 19-3). Our therapeutic conclusions with regard to the two-vessel disease patients would also seem to apply to patients with three-vessel disease. *That is, we would not require a period of prolonged medical therapy in patients with three-vessel disease and graftable distal vessels before moving toward surgery.* In particular, in the younger patient with three-vessel disease and good distal vessels, we feel that surgical therapy is probably indicated earlier rather than later.

The final answer on the effect of coronary surgery on survival in patients with coronary disease is not yet in. Important and relevant information can be anticipated from continued surveillance of the patients in the VA cooperative study and our Seattle Heart Watch patients. In addition, there are two additional randomized studies now under way that should shed further information on the topic. The European multicenter trial is just now beginning to analyze their survival data, and published results are expected soon. In the United States, the NHLBI-sponsored Coronary Artery Surgery Study (CASS) is randomizing mildly symptomatic or asymptomatic patients with coronary disease between medical and surgical therapy. Their period of patient entry is just now concluding. Results of survival analyses from this study may be anticipated in several years.

REFERENCES

1 Murphy, M. L., Hultgren, H. N., Detre, K., Thomsen, J., Takaro, T., and participants of Veterans Administration Cooperative Study: Treatment of Chronic Stable Angina. A Preliminary Report on Survival Data of the Randomized Veterans Administration Cooperative Study, *N. Engl. J. Med.,* 297:621, 1977.

2 Gifford, R. H., and Feinstein, A. R.: A Critique of Methodology in Studies of Anticoagulation Therapy for Acute Myocardial Infarction, *N. Engl. J. Med.,* 280:351, 1969.

3 Freiman, J. A., Chalmers, T. C., Smith, H., Jr., and Kuebler, R. R. L.: The Importance of Beta, the Type II Error and Sample Size in the Design and Interpretation of the Randomized Control Trial, *N. Engl. J. Med.,* 299:690, 1978.

4 Mathur, V. S., and Guinn, G. A.: Prospective Randomized Study of Coronary Bypass Surgery in Stable Angina: The First 100 Patients, *Circulation,* 52(suppl. 1):133, 1975.

5 Selden, R., Neill, W. A., Ritzmann, L.W., Okies, J. E., and Andersen, R. P.: Medical Versus Surgical Therapy for Acute Coronary Insufficiency. A Randomized Study, *N. Engl. J. Med.,* 293:1329, 1975.

6 Kloster, F. F., Kremkau, E. L., Rahimtoola, S. H., Ritzmann, L. W., Griswold, H. E., Neill, W. A., Rosh, J., and Starr, A.: Prospective Randomized Study of Coronary Bypass Surgery for Chronic Stable Angina, *Cardiovasc. Clin.,* 8:145, 1977.

7 Sheldon, W. C., Rincon, G., Effler, D. B., Proudfit, W. L., and Sones, F. M., Jr.: Vein Graft Surgery for Coronary Artery Disease. Survival and Angiographic Results in 1,000 Patients, *Circulation,* 48(suppl. 3):184, 1973.

8 Cannom, D. S., Miller, D. C., Shumway, N. E., Fogarty, T. J., Daily, A. O., Hu, M., Brown, F., Jr., and Harrison, D. C.: The Long-term Follow-up of Patients Undergoing Saphenous Vein Bypass Surgery, *Circulation,* 49:77, 1974.

9 Spencer, F. C., Isom, O. W., Glassman, E., Boyd, A. D., Engleman, R. M., Reed, G. E., Pasternack, B. S., and Dembrow, J. M.: The Long-term Influence of Coronary Bypass Grafts on Myocardial Infarction and Survival, *Ann. Surg.,* 180:439, 1974.

10 Cohn, L. H., Boyden, C. M., and Collins, J. J.: Improved Long-term Survival After Aortocoronary Bypass for Advanced Coronary Artery Disease, *Am. J. Surg.,* 129:380, 1975.

11 Tecklenberg, P. L., Alderman, E. L., Miller, D. C., Shumway, N. E., and Harrison, D. C.: Changes in Survival and Symptom Relief in a Longitudinal Study of Patients After Bypass Surgery, *Circulation,* 52(suppl. 1):98, 1975.

12 Ullyot, D. J., Wisneski, J., Sullivan, R. W., and Gertz, E. W.: Improved Survival After Coronary Artery Surgery in Patients with Extensive Coronary Disease, *J. Thorac. Cardiovasc. Surg.,* 70:405, 1975.

13 Vismara, L. A., Miller, R. R., Price, J. E., Karem, R., Demaria, A. N., and Mason, D. T.: Improved Longevity Due to Reduction of Sudden Death by Aortocoronary Bypass in Coronary Atherosclerosis, *Am. J. Cardiol.,* 39:919, 1977.

14 Kouchoukos, N. T., Oberman, A., Russel, R. O., Jr., and Jones, W. B.: Surgical Versus Medical Treatment of Occlusive Disease Confined to the Left Anterior Descending Coronary Artery, *Am. J. Cardiol.,* 35:836, 1975.

15 Oberman, A., Harrell, R. R., Russel, R. O., Jr., Kouchoukos, N. T., Holt, J. H., Jr., and Rackley, C. E.: Surgical Versus Medical Treatment in Disease of the Left Main Coronary Artery, *Lancet,* 2:391, 1976.

16 Campeau, L., Corbara, F., Crochet, D., and Petitclerc, R.: Left Main Coronary Artery Stenosis. The Influence of Aortocoronary Bypass Surgery on Survival, *Circulation,* 57:1111, 1978.

17 Vlietstra, R. E., Assad-Morell, J. L., Frye, R. L., Elveback, L. R., Connolly, D. C., Ritman, E. L., Pluth, J. R., Barnhart, D. A., Danielson, G. K., and Wallace, R. B.: Survival Predictors in Coronary Artery Disease. Medical and Surgical Comparisons, *Mayo Clin. Proc.,* 52:85, 1977.

18 Hammermeister, K. E., DeRouen, T. A., and Dodge, H. T.: Variables Predictive of Survival in Patients with Coronary Disease. Selection by Univariate and Multivariate Analyses from the Clinical, Electrocardiographic, Exercise, Arteriographic, and Quantitative Angiographic Evaluations, *Circulation,* 59:421, 1979.

19 Mantel, N.: Evaluation of Survival Data and Two New Rank Order Statistics Arising in Its Consideration, *Cancer Chemother. Rep.,* 50:163, 1966.

20 Lowrie, G. M., Morris, G. C., Jr., Howell, J. F., Ogura, J. W., Spencer, E. H. III, Cashian, W. R., Winters, W. L., Beazley, H. L., Chapman, D. W., Peterson, P. K., and Lie, J. T.: Results of Coronary Bypass More than 5 Years After Operation in 434 Patients, *Am. J. Cardiol.,* 40:665, 1977.

21 Lowrie, G. M., Morris, G. C., Jr., Howell, J. R., Tredici, T. D., and Chapman, D. W.: Improved Survival After 5 Years in 1144 Patients After Coronary Bypass Surgery, *Am. J. Cardiol.,* 42:709, 1978.

22 Fox, S. M. III, and Robins, M.: Incidence, Prevalence, and Death Rates of Cardiovascular Disease: Some Practical Implications, in J. W. Hurst (ed.), ''The Heart,'' McGraw-Hill Book Company, New York, 1978, p. 752.

23 Hammermeister, K. E., DeRouen, T. A., Murray, J. A., and Dodge, H. T.: Effect of Aortocoronary Saphenous Vein Bypass Grafting on Death and Sudden Death. Comparison of Nonrandomized Medically and Surgically Treated Cohorts with Comparable Coronary Disease and Left Ventricular Function, *Am. J. Cardiol.,* 39:925, 1977.

24 Hammermeister, K. E., DeRouen, T. A., and Dodge, H. T.: Evidence from a Nonrandomized Study That Coronary Surgery Prolongs Survival in Patients with Two Vessel Coronary Disease, *Circulation,* 59:430, 1979.

25 Yatteau, R. F., Peter, R. H., Behar, V. S., Bartel, H. G., Rosati, R. A., and Kong, Y.: Ischemic Cardiomyopathy: The Myopathies of Coronary Artery Disease, *Am. J. Cardiol.,* 34:520, 1974.

26 Hammermeister, K. E., Kennedy, J. W., Hamilton, G. W., Stewart, D. K., Gould, K. L., Lipscomb, K., and Murray, J. A.: Aortocoronary Saphenous Vein Bypass. Failure of Successful Grafting to Improve Resting Left Ventricular Function in Chronic Angina, *N. Engl. J. Med.,* 290:186, 1974.

27 Takaro, T., Hultgren, H. N., Lipton, M. J., Detre, K. M., and participants in the Study Group: The VA Cooperative Randomized Study of Surgery for Coronary Arterial Occlusive Disease. II. Subgroup with Significant Left Main Lesions, *Circulation*, 54(suppl. 3):107, 1976.

28 Read, R. C., Murphy, M. L., Hultgren, H. N., and Takaro, T.: Survival of Men Treated for Chronic Stable Angina Pectoris. A Cooperative Randomized Study, *J. Thorac. Cardiovasc. Surg.*, 75:1, 1978.

The authors gratefully acknowledge the efforts of John A. Murray, M.D., whose efforts were instrumental in the early organizational and data collection phases of the Angiography Registry of Seattle Heart Watch. The authors also acknowledge their debt to the cardiologists and cardiovascular surgeons in Seattle for freely contributing data on their patients to Seattle Heart Watch, to Ms. Verona Hofer and Ms. Gladys Pettet for ongoing data collection and analyses, and to Ms. Barbara Buck for manuscript preparation.

Chapter 20

The Prolongation of Life by Coronary Bypass Surgery: Experience at the Cleveland Clinic*

WILLIAM L. PROUDFIT, M.D.

Comparison of reported medical and surgical survival curves, as well as surgical survival at Emory University Hospital, has been reviewed in detail by Hurst and associates.[1] Kirklin has compared the experience at the University of Alabama with that of the VA.[2] Both of these reports involved analysis of subsets of patients. It was the conclusion of both that bypass operation is indicated for suitable candidates having left main artery obstruction and disease of three arteries. Hurst believed that surgical results are superior for two obstructed arteries, and Kirklin thought that this was probably true. There was agreement that surgery for single-artery obstructions had not been shown to improve survival but that further study was necessary. McIntosh and Garcia reviewed the literature and came to the conclusion that only patients who have left main artery lesions or "possibly other subsets" could be expected to show improved survival from bypass operation, and the "prudent physician, therefore, is advised to maintain an open mind even about these conclusions."[3] Various studies of the comparative survival after medical and surgical treatment are discussed in other chapters. Symptomatic improvement in the majority of surgical patients has been the universal experience.

Comparisons of long-term survival in large groups of surgical candidates treated nonsurgically are possible for the VA study and the subset of 388 surgical candidates in a group of 601 patients who had severe coronary artery disease documented by coronary arteriography at the Cleveland Clinic during a 2½-year period beginning in January 1963.[4,5] The patient selection was different in that the VA study consisted of men who had chronic stable angina pectoris, and the earlier study included all surgical candidates who were referred for coronary arteriography. The latter investigation included some patients at higher risk than those in the VA group. The VA study involved only men, whereas a small percentage of patients in the

Cleveland Clinic were women. No sex difference in survival has been found.[9] The number of arteries obstructed at least 50 percent in diameter was used for classification in both cases. The Cleveland Clinic's 1963–1965 medical patients would have been candidates for bypass operation if it had been available then; all were followed for at least 10 years or until death. Whatever benefit modern medical therapy confers was not available to these patients, especially during the first 6 or 7 years.

For surgical patients, the year 1973 was selected for comparison with the VA group because this was the middle year of the final VA study. The first 1,000 patients who had received bypass grafts at the Cleveland Clinic during that year were selected, and the total mortality was calculated, not just the cardiac mortality, which constituted about 56 percent of deaths in the surgical group. The operative mortality in the 1973 group was 0.4 percent (4 of 918), excluding 82 patients who had left main artery lesions, and 3.7 percent (3 of 82) for the latter group. Perioperative transmural myocardial infarction was diagnosed in 4 percent. Graft patency was 87 percent during this period. The VA study, excluding left main artery lesions, had 6 percent operative mortality, 18 percent perioperative infarction, and 69 percent graft patency.[6-8] Composite survival curves are shown in Fig. 20-1. It is evident that differences in operative mortality account for most of the disparity in the surgical groups during the first 2 years, but later divergence of the curves may be related to adequacy of revascularization. In view of the limited applicability of composite curves, further analysis is unnecessary.

If coronary bypass surgery improves longevity, proof would be easiest to obtain in the highest risk groups—those who have obstructions of the left main artery or involvement of three main arteries. Survival is significantly better in left main artery subset with bypass operation in both the VA study and in our experience, as shown in Fig. 20-2. There is general agreement that operation should be advised if a correctable lesion is demonstrated. Survival in obstruction of three main arteries, excluding the left main

*From Cleveland Clinic Foundation, Cleveland.

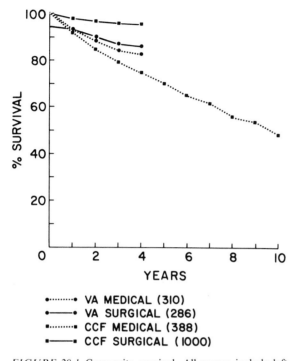

FIGURE 20-1 Composite survival. All curves include left main artery cases. Cleveland Clinic (CCF) medical data reported.[4,5] Cleveland Clinic surgical data for 1,000 consecutive patients in 1973. Numbers in parentheses refer to patients. Percentage at 0 years in surgical curves indicates operative survival in each figure. *(VA curves redrawn from Fig. 1 of R. C. Read et al., Survival of Men Treated for Chronic Stable Angina Pectoris: A Cooperative Randomized Study, J. Thorac. Cardiovasc. Surg., 75:1, 1978.)*

artery, is shown in Fig. 20-3. The VA figures shown are for patients who had left ventricular abnormalities, which seem to have constituted about 85 percent of the whole group. The early survival is higher than that for left main artery obstruction, but the long-term outlook is similar in our study. The VA report indicates a higher medical survival rate than ours and a lower surgical survival. The 4-year VA surgical survival of about 84 percent may be compared to the VA 93 percent surgical survival for left main artery cases, which is an unusual disparity. Much of the difference in the surgical groups having obstruction of three arteries is accounted for by difference in operative mortality (7.3 percent in the VA study and 0.9 percent for 429 patients in the Cleveland Clinic surgical group). The VA difference in survival of medical and surgical cases is approaching statistical significance, and the latter would be evident now if operative mortality had been lower. That the latter is attainable is evident by observation of our surgical curve for the 1973 patients. The reason for the disparity of the VA and our survival

curves for medical patients is not obvious, particularly in view of the fact that medical survival curves for left main artery lesions are similar. Differences in selection of patients for study, arteriographic interpretation, selection for operative candidacy, and perhaps changes in medical therapy may account for some of the variations. A preliminary report of the European cooperative study indicates that there was a significant difference at 2 years in survival of medical and surgical patients who had obstructions of three arteries.[9]

Lesions of two main arteries are associated with higher survival than those of three arteries, and this is evident in both the VA studies and our own (Fig. 20-4), although the difference is slight in the VA report at 3 years. Four-year survival for patients without left main artery lesions is not available in the VA reports, but only a few left main artery cases appear to be included in the two-artery subset. Differences in survival in the VA and our medical groups were not as great as in three-artery obstruction. The 4-year survival was higher in medical than in the surgical cases in the VA study, but our surgical patients had a 96

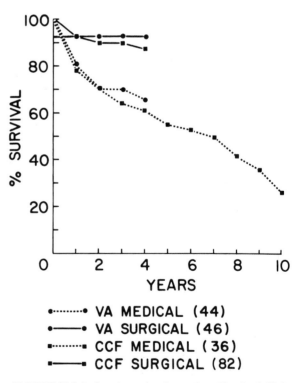

FIGURE 20-2 Left main artery obstruction. Cleveland Clinic (CCF) medical and surgical curves are shown for 1963–1965 and 1973 cases, respectively. *(VA curves redrawn from Fig. 8 of R. C. Read et al., Survival of Men Treated for Chronic Stable Angina Pectoris: A Cooperative Randomized Study, J. Thorac. Cardiovasc. Surg., 75:1, 1978.)*

percent survival at 4 years as compared to 81 percent in the VA study. Operative mortality excluding left main artery cases was stated to be 6.1 percent in the VA study, but there was no operative mortality in 324 patients in the Cleveland Clinic series. It is peculiar that the VA surgical survival at 4 years was higher for the three-artery cases than for the two-artery cases. The relatively high late death rate in the surgical subset is not characteristic of most surgical reports nor of the VA experience with left main or three-artery obstruction.

Analysis of the treatment of single-artery obstructions is complicated by the fact that early mortality is low, but mortality increases later, probably as a result of the subsequent development of the disease in other arteries (Fig. 20-5). In contrast to the opinion of many, however, obstructions of single arteries are not necessarily benign. Death can result from myocardial infarction, and about 15 percent of sudden deaths appear to be caused by obstruction of single arteries.[10-12] This

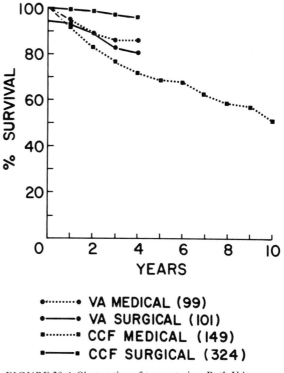

FIGURE 20-4 Obstruction of two arteries. Both VA curves include a few patients who had left main artery involvement apparently. Cleveland Clinic (CCF) data exclude left main artery involvement. *(VA medical curve redrawn from Fig. 6 and surgical curve from Fig. 3 of R. C. Read et al., Survival of Men Treated for Chronic Stable Angina Pectoris: A Cooperative Randomized Study, J. Thorac. Cardiovasc. Surg., 75:1, 1978.)*

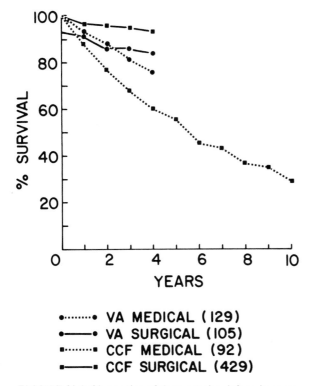

FIGURE 20-3 Obstruction of three arteries, left main cases excluded. Included are only those VA curves with abnormal left ventricular function (about 85 percent of total patients). Cleveland Clinic (CCF) medical and surgical curves show all patients. *(VA curves redrawn from Fig. 10 of R. C. Read et al., Survival of Men Treated for Chronic Stable Angina Pectoris: A Cooperative Randomized Study, J. Thorac. Cardiovasc. Surg., 75:1, 1978.)*

is a higher percentage of deaths than shown in the initial survival curve of patients who have had arteriographically demonstrated lesions. In the first 3 years of follow-up, only about 7 percent of deaths occurred in patients who had single-artery lesions in the Cleveland Clinic series and about 5 percent occurred in the surgical candidates. Some of these patients may have had progressive involvement of other arteries prior to death. Only surviving patients are studied arteriographically, so it is possible that death as an initial manifestation may bias the selection of patients. Survival was similar in the VA series for medical and surgical subsets (Fig. 20-5). Survival was better in the 1973 Cleveland surgical group than in the medical group at 5 years. It is possible to do single bypass operations with almost no operative mortality, but it would require study of a large group of patients followed for at least 5 years to show significant difference in survival. A recent report by Lytle and associates at the Cleveland Clinic indicated that the 5-year survival

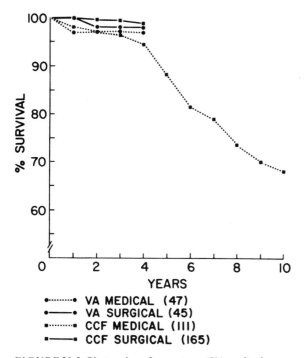

···· VA MEDICAL (47)

—— VA SURGICAL (45)

···· CCF MEDICAL (III)

—— CCF SURGICAL (165)

FIGURE 20-5 Obstruction of one artery. *(VA medical curve redrawn from Fig. 5 and surgical curve from Fig. 2 of R. C. Read et al., Survival of Men Treated for Chronic Stable Angina Pectoris: A Cooperative Randomized Study, J. Thorac. Cardiovasc. Surg., 75:1, 1978.)*

of 200 patients who had isolated disease of the anterior descending artery was 98 percent.[13]

Careful comparison of the survival curves for VA surgical cases in Figs. 20-2 to 20-4 reveals a peculiar anomaly. Most surgical series have shown a direct relation between the extent of arterial involvement and early and long-term mortality. In the VA series, except for single-artery disease, the operative mortality was about the same for all groups, and long-term mortality was inversely related to extent of arterial involvement, being highest for obstructions of two arteries, intermediate for three arteries, and lowest for the left main artery. This peculiarity in the case of a two-artery disease makes it evident that it would be difficult to prove nonsurgical treatment superior for this group.

SUMMARY

On the basis of personal experience and of reports of others, it is believed that bypass surgery for coronary disease improves longevity in suitable candidates who have obstruction of the left main artery or two or three major coronary arteries if operative mortality and perioperative infarction rate are low and graft patency is high. Single-artery lesions may be treated with almost no operative mortality and probable long-term benefit. In addition, angina pectoris is improved or eliminated in the majority of patients. Surgery does not cure coronary disease, and progression of obstruction in the native circulation distal to grafts or in ungrafted arteries appears to be the principal risk, rather than closure of grafts that are initially open. If progression of disease can be terminated or slowed by medical treatment, excellent long-term results should be expected to be even better than at present.

REFERENCES

1 Hurst, J. W., King, S. B., Logue, R. B., et al.: Value of Bypass Surgery: Controversies in Cardiology: Part I, *Am. J. Cardiol.*, 42:308, 1978.

2 Kirklin, J. W.: Research Related to Surgical Treatment in Coronary Artery Disease. Presented at the 30th Anniversary of the American Heart Association and National Heart, Lung and Blood Institute Scientific Symposium, "Current Horizons in Atherosclerosis and Hypertension," Washington, D.C., Feb. 9, 1978.

3 McIntosh, H. D., and Garcia, J.A.: The First Decade of Aortocoronary Bypass Grafting, 1967–1977, *Circulation*, 57:405, 1978.

4 Proudfit, W. L., Bruschke, A. V. G., and Sones, F. M., Jr.: Natural History of Obstructive Coronary Artery Disease. Ten-Year Study of 601 Nonsurgical Cases, *Prog. Cardiovasc. Dis.*, 21:53, 1978.

5 Proudfit, W. L., Bruschke, A. V. G., and Sones, F. M., Jr.: Natural History of Obstructive Coronary Artery Disease; Supplement to a 10-Year Study, *Clev. Clin. Q.*, 45:293, 1978.

6 Murphy, M. L., Hultgren, H. N., Detre, K., et al.: Treatment of Chronic Stable Angina. A Preliminary Report of Survival Data of the Randomized Veterans Administration Cooperative Study, *N. Engl. J. Med.*, 297:621, 1977.

7 Read, R. C., Murphy, M. L., Hultgren, H. N., et al.: Survival of Men Treated for Chronic Stable Angina Pectoris: A Cooperative Randomized Study, *J. Thorac. Cardiovasc. Surg.*, 75:1, 1978.

8 Proudfit, W. L.: Criticisms of the VA Randomized Study of Coronary Bypass Surgery, *Clin. Res.,* 26:236, 1978.

9 Varnauskas, E.: Personal Communication, 1978.

10 Romo, M.: Factors Related to Sudden Death in Acute Ischemic Heart Disease: A Community Study in Helsinki, *Acta Med. Scand.* [Suppl.], 547:1, 1972.

11 Myers, A., and Dewar, H. A.: Circumstances Attending 100 Sudden Deaths from Coronary Disease with Coroner's Necropsies, *Br. Heart J.,* 37:1133, 1975.

12 Bashe, W. F., Jr., Baba, N., Keller, M. D., et al.: Pathology of Arteriosclerotic Heart Disease in Sudden Death, III. The Significance of Myocardial Infarction, *Circulation,* 51, 52 (suppl. 3):63, 1975.

13 Lytle, B. W., Loop, F. D., Thurer, R. L., Groves, L. K., Taylor, P. C., and Cosgrove, D. M.: Isolated Left Anterior Descending Coronary Arteriosclerosis. Long-term Comparison of Internal Mammary Artery and Venous Autografts, *Circulation,* 58 (suppl. 2):17, 1978. (Abstract.)

Chapter 21

Medical Care Before, During, and After Coronary Bypass Surgery*

STEPHEN D. CLEMENTS, JR., M.D., and J. WILLIS HURST, M.D.

Although coronary bypass surgery has become commonplace, little has been written about the preparation and the proper care of the patient and the family before, during, and after the procedure. Many medical centers such as Emory University Hospital have achieved an operative mortality of about 1 percent. Although we can be proud of such an accomplishment, it is appropriate to consider each step of the procedure and to develop a plan that will ensure that the procedure is not only safe but also accompanied by as little fear and anxiety as possible.

The cardiologist who is involved in the care of the patient is often responsible for the continuity of medical care. Unfortunately, there is no single document that discusses the procedure and its complications for the cardiologist. Accordingly, the purpose of this chapter is to emphasize the emotional needs of the patient and his or her family, to highlight the complications of the procedure, and to discuss the flow of activity from the time the decision is made to operate until the patient has returned to work.

PREOPERATIVE CONSIDERATIONS

Let us assume that the decision has been made that coronary bypass surgery will be performed on a carefully selected patient. We must remember that the patient might have initially denied that he or she is seriously ill. This is often followed by acceptance of this fact, and this may be accompanied by fear and anxiety. At times, depending on the clinical situation, some patients may have less fear and anxiety because surgery is to be performed. Such patients may be less apprehensive because they believe that the alternative, i.e., no surgery, produces even more fear and anxiety. Such patients may believe as they do because a member of their family has died of the disease, the

*From Department of Medicine, Emory University School of Medicine, Atlanta, Georgia.

patients have had disabling symptoms for some time, or they feel better with a bold approach to the problem. On the other hand, another patient may develop more fear and anxiety because surgery is to be performed. This type of patient may have unreasonable fear of all types of surgery, may not understand the problem, may have been well until recently, may have few symptoms even though there is serious obstruction of the left main coronary artery, or may be emotionally disturbed or depressed at the time he or she learns of the new illness and the recommendation for surgery. In either case, the role of the physician is to lead the patient and his or her family through the procedure. In doing so, it is important to prevent and manage anxiety and to prevent or manage complications.

EDUCATION OF THE PATIENT AND FAMILY AND MEDICAL MANAGEMENT JUST PRIOR TO SURGERY

The medical problems should be explained to the patient and his or her family. Obviously, the patient should be asked to designate the family members that he or she wants to have involved in the discussion of the problem. The physician should have a reasonable view regarding which members are central to the emotional stability of the family. By educating the appropriate family members, they will assist in creating a calm home and hospital environment. Not to do so invites emotional turmoil.

The cardiologist, surgeon, and arteriographer should review the patient's medical problems and arteriograms and discuss the patient's condition and arrive at a common view regarding the solution to the problem. The surgeon then sees the patient and appropriate family members and collects any other medical data that is needed directly from the patient, states the risk of the procedure for the patient's particular problem based on the last 500 to 1,000 cases,* and answers any questions that the patient may have. Often the surgeon spends additional time with the spouse and answers additional questions that are asked.

When surgery is contemplated, the following steps are extremely helpful. The patient and the patient's spouse may wish to review the arteriograms with a knowledgeable member of the staff. Properly trained nurses should show and discuss the step-by-step sequence that occurs before, during, and after the surgery. The patient and family may visit the intensive care unit. All questions should be answered. Patients and their family members are reassured by seeing and talking with patients who have experienced and benefited from similar operations. It is better for the physician to take the lead in this effort and select an individual to whom the patient can talk. In this way, the physician can be assured that the patient will talk with a patient who had the same operation. If the patient seeks out someone to talk with, it is possible that he or she may select someone who has had open heart surgery for valve disease. In some locales the "Mended Hearts" organization helps patients who are to have heart surgery.

A maximum effort should be made preoperatively to detect potential neurologic problems. A thorough search for carotid bruits is imperative. If bruits are present, a complete four-vessel carotid and vertebral artery study should be done. The discovery of significant stenosis may force one to alter the surgical plans to include carotid artery surgery.

On the day prior to surgery, the patient is seen by a hematologist in order to review historical information related to a potential bleeding problem. A thorough coagulation survey is done and reviewed by the consulting hematologist.

The cardiac anesthesiologist also visits the patient on the day before surgery. Procedures are explained, including insertion of monitoring lines and endotracheal tube. Drug allergies are reviewed, and the anesthesia plan is explained.

Propranolol, isosorbide dinitrate, sulfinpyrazone (Anturane), and Nitrol Ointment may be given until 10 P.M. the night before surgery. Brittle cases with recurrent angina may require intravenous nitroglycerin drip prior to surgery. Aspirin should be stopped 10 days to 2 weeks prior to surgery.

OPERATIVE CONSIDERATIONS

During surgery the anxiety of family members is decreased by a flow of information from the operating room, particularly if favorable and steady progress is being made. A quiet, comfortable waiting area for the family is a necessity. A compassionate and knowledgeable person should remain in direct contact with the family and should receive information from the operating room and pass it on to the family members. We have learned that the family appreciates knowing exactly when the surgery begins, when the patient goes on cardiopulmonary bypass, when the distal ends of the grafts are anastomosed, when the proximal ends of the grafts are anastomosed, and when the patient goes off cardiopulmonary bypass.

Advances have been made in anesthesia for open heart surgery. Individuals with coronary disease need a smooth course from the time of induction to the initiation of cardiopulmonary bypass. Special attention is given to maintaining a low pressure–rate product and maintaining normal right and left atrial pressure.[1] If left ventricular dysfunction is present or likely to develop, a Swan-Ganz catheter allows monitoring of wedge pressures and administration of intravenous drugs such as nitroglycerin or nitroprusside to alter preloads and afterloads. Morphine anesthesia offers minimal myocardial depression and good relaxation.[2]

Special techniques during surgery are currently in use. The hypothermic state tends to preserve the myocardium.[3-5] At 28° to 30°C, oxygen consumption is about 50 percent of that at 37°, and when body temperature reaches 12° to 15°C, oxygen consumption is only 10 percent.[5,6] Potassium cardioplegia offers additional protection during surgery. A heart that is fibrillating uses more oxygen than a heart that is flaccid. Cardioplegia accomplishes this and allows the surgeon to have a motionless operative field.[6-8]

Areas of significant stenosis of carotid vessels are corrected prior to going on the heart-lung machine. If the patient is stable from the cardiac standpoint, then this is done as a separate procedure by the vascular surgeons. If the heart disease is severe, two teams of surgeons perform carotid endarterectomy and coronary bypass surgery simultaneously.[9] Sometimes the chest incision is made with bypass on standby, and the carotid procedure is done such that immediate pump assistance can be accomplished if problems arise during the carotid procedure.

Coming off the pump is always a critical time. A good myocardium and good surgical revascularization usually results in spontaneous cardiac rhythm and adequate cardiac output when adequate preload is present. When preload is low, transfusion from the pump will usually increase the arterial pressure. High preload, low cardiac output, and low arterial pressure suggest the need for sympathetic agents such as dopamine or epinephrine. Failure of dopamine or epinephrine to elevate systemic pressure leads to a trial of vasodilator therapy with intravenous nitroglycerin or nitroprusside.[11-13] Inadequate cardiac output and

---

*Note that the risk of the procedure could not be given unless a data bank for answering such questions has been developed.

hypotension with maximum pharmacologic effort require the use of the intraaortic balloon assist pump.[14]

If rhythm problems arise, they are treated as indicated. Bradycardia may require either atrial, ventricular, or sequential atrioventricular pacing. Leads are left on the epicardial surface and exit through small skin incisions and later can simply be pulled out with gentle traction.[15]

The referring physician should be called by the cardiologist when the surgery is completed. When this is not possible, it is often our practice to have the surgeon send a Mail-O-Gram letter which is received the next day and can become part of the referring physician's record.

POSTOPERATIVE CONSIDERATIONS

After leaving the operating room, the patient is transferred directly to the intensive care unit for 24 to 48 h of monitoring. An intraarterial line permits direct pressure determination by digital reading and also allows frequent blood gas measurements. Central venous pressure and pulmonary capillary wedge pressure are monitored, as is cardiac rhythm. Other important parameters such as the level of consciousness and fluid intake and output are recorded. The patient usually stays on the volume ventilator overnight.

Immediately after arrival at the intensive care unit, a portable chest x-ray is obtained to check lung expansion and tube positions. Baseline blood studies are drawn, an electrocardiogram is obtained, and the rewarming procedure is initiated. The problems that may occur in the immediate postoperative period are listed in Table 21-1.

Excessive bleeding from the mediastinal tubes is a particularly bothersome problem. As a rule, there should be about 100 to 150 ml of blood loss or less from the mediastinal tubes each hour for about 3 h. Persistent bleeding at a rate of 200 ml/h or more in the first 3 h despite correction of clotting factor deficits may require surgical intervention. Approximately 1 in 50 patients has to return to the operating room for surgical exploration for excessive bleeding. It is common immediately after surgery to have platelet counts in the 50,000 range. Platelet transfusions are commonly used in this setting if bleeding is a problem. Heavy bleeding usually means that a small artery, a graft anastomotic site, or aortotomy site is bleeding. More commonly, however, diffuse oozing from a large surface results in excessive bleeding. The cauterization of several small areas usually solves the problem.

After a few hours in the intensive care unit, a falling arterial pressure with a rising right atrial pressure suggests *cardiac tamponade*. The arterial pulse tracing

TABLE 21-1
Problems that may arise in the immediate postoperative period

Excessive bleeding from mediastinal tubes
Hemodynamic alterations
   Preload abnormality
   Hypotension
   Hypertension
Neurologic deficits
Electrocardiographic changes
   Rhythm disturbances
   Depolarization and repolarization
   abnormalities
Hypokalemia
Fever

may or may not show pulsus paradoxus. Mediastinal tubes should be checked for clots and perhaps even irrigated. If the situation becomes critical, the lower part of the incision must be opened under sterile conditions, and the pericardial area should be explored. This may occur despite leaving the pericardium open. The cardiac tamponade may be due to anterior mediastinal clots, and it may not be possible to aspirate blood to relieve the tamponade. Unfortunately, one problem that can present with similar hemodynamics is right ventricular failure resulting from infarction.[17] This is a serious problem and requires maximum volume loading, unloading of both left and right ventricles, and sometimes inotropic agents and vasopressor drugs. These two situations, cardiac tamponade and right ventricular failure, can be so similar that exploration through the lower portion of the incision is often required to absolutely exclude tamponade.

Hemodynamic alterations may begin in the immediate postpump period and continue in the intensive care units. Very high filling pressures in the left ventricle and borderline systemic pressures often respond to intravenous nitroglycerin.[12] Low filling pressures and low systemic pressures require volume expansion. Elevated filling pressures and systemic hypertension require more potent agents such as nitroprusside. Extreme tension on the aortic suture line sets the stage for aortic dissection, so systemic hypertension is promptly treated.[16] Unfortunately, an occasional patient exhibits poor left ventricular function in the face of optimal filling pressures. Systemic pressure and cardiac output may be low. When dopamine, and epinephrine, and vasodilating agents fail and volume expansion is maximum, the intraaortic balloon pump is necessary.[12]

Neurologic deficits are sometimes obvious in the operating room but most commonly become manifest during the first few hours after arrival in the intensive care unit. Failure to become alert after a few hours may indicate a problem. Hemiparesis is a dreadful finding. Seizure activity is an ominous sign requiring prompt treatment and usually indicates a serious underlying problem.

Seizure disorder or hemiparesis usually indicates particle embolization either from an intracardiac source or from the proximal graft sites. Air embolism usually results in a transient neurologic defect.

A neurologic deficit after coronary bypass surgery should be viewed with some optimism, since it is frequently completely clear. Occasionally, a period of unusual drowsiness and confusion is present for several days before clearing. This is commonly caused by sedatives and pain medication. An occasional patient will also complain of recent memory difficulties. Some patients complain of pain or a transient numbness in the arms along the ulna nerve distribution. This is probably due to compression of the ulna nerve against the proximal portion of the humerus in patients whose surgical position requires extreme abduction of the arms.[10] This difficulty usually clears after several days.

Many patients note a numbness along the medial aspect of the legs at the vein harvest sites. This is often painful but usually is a numb sensation and rapidly clears. An occasional patient will complain of this a year or more after surgery.

Electrocardiographic abnormalities may be either rhythm disturbances or depolarization and repolarization abnormalities (see Table 21-2).

Occasionally, function of the sinus node and the activity of the atrioventricular node junctional area are sluggish after coming off bypass. Myocardial preservation solutions containing potassium in addition to hypothermia aggravate this problem. In these situations, atrial and ventricular wires are used for pacing. Atrial pacing, ventricular pacing, or atrioventricular sequential pacing can be temporarily used to overcome this condition.[15] Persisting difficulties with sinus node dysfunction are unusual after 24 h. Atrioventricular block requires the avoidance of digitalis preparations and propranolol until improvement occurs. Again pacing is required. Occasionally, especially

when there were prior clues to atrioventricular block either at the junctional area or in the fascicles, a permanent pacemaker may be implanted at the time of surgery or a pacemaker wire may be left in place.

Heart rates of a 150 to 160 should immediately bring to mind atrial flutter with 2:1 conduction. Atrial fibrillation results in a chaotic ventricular response and loss of "atrial kick." Both of these rhythms disturb atrial transport, which may lead to serious hemodynamic consequences. If digitalis, propranolol, and quinidine do not control rates promptly and restore sinus rhythm, then electrical cardioversion can be used. A precipitating factor may be atrial irritation from pericarditis. Treatment of this problem with a 4-mg bolum of dexamethasone often helps control the situation. This requires follow-up with either aspirin, indomethacin, or a tapering course of corticosteroids.

Ventricular premature beats occur with variable frequency in the postoperative period. If they are present preoperatively, they usually return postoperatively. The basic therapeutic approach to these premature beats is similar to the approach in the coronary care unit. More than six ventricular premature beats per minute, closely coupled ventricular premature beats, bigeminal and trigeminal patterns, or couplets warrant a bolus of lidocaine or procainamide hydrochloride followed by a continuous infusion. Runs of ventricular tachycardia deserve the same treatment unless cardioversion is needed. An occasional patient will experience ventricular tachycardia or ventricular fibrillation in the first few postoperative hours. Freshly closed median sternotomy incisions are commonly disrupted by external cardiac massage. This cannot be withheld, but prompt electrical defibrillation should be accomplished if possible. Occasionally, a thump on the chest will revert these rhythms to normal.[18]

Intraventricular conduction defects are common upon arrival in the intensive care unit. The hypothermic state, shifting potassium levels, and myocardial ischemia are all contributing factors. Hemiblocks may cause shifts in the electrical axis, and bundle branch blocks may widen the QRS complexes. They are usually transient and by 24 h have reverted to the preoperative status. Left anterior hemiblock and left bundle branch block can sometimes result in bothersome ST-T wave changes in the precordial leads that suggest the "hyperacute" changes (tall peaked T waves) of infarction. These changes must be interpreted only in combination with a follow-up tracing 12 to 24 h later. These abnormalities also commonly disappear.

ST and T wave changes are influenced by a number of factors. Potassium levels are usually low. Pericardial irritation is always present. Two to three millimeters of ST-segment elevation in the precordial leads or in leads II, III, and aV$_F$ is a bothersome finding, especially if these changes are in a grafted area. Many times, however, these changes, too, are reversible.

TABLE 21-2
Electrocardiographic abnormalities

Rhythm disturbances
    Sinus node dysfunction and slow junctional rhythms
    Atrioventricular block
    Atrial flutter and fibrillation
    Ventricular premature beats and tachycardia
    Ventricular fibrillation
Intraventricular conduction defects
ST-segment and T wave abnormalities
Infarction patterns

Infarction patterns may become apparent in the immediate postoperative period. Significant new Q waves, in addition to associated ST and T changes, usually mean perioperative infarction. Typical evolution of these changes occur in the postoperative period. The incidence of such changes ranges from 10 to 15 percent at most.[19] The incidence of perioperative infarction in our own patients at Emory University Hospital is 4.6 percent.

Hypokalemia occurs during cardiopulmonary bypass.[20] The correction of hypokalemia is imperative, since arrhythmias may be precipitated by potassium depletion.

Fever occasionally occurs while the patient is in the intensive care unit. Antibiotics, usually antistaphylococcal agents, are routinely started preoperatively and continued for 5 days postoperatively. It is frequently difficult to determine the source of fever. Blood transfusions can provoke a febrile response, and atelectasis can result in pulmonary congestion and infection. We usually make an effort to keep body temperature in the normal range in the postoperative period in order to avoid the extra work requirements of the heart that are brought about by fever. We sometimes use acetaminophen (Tylenol) and even thermal blankets in order to lower elevated temperatures. It is unusual to identify active infection requiring additional antibiotics during the first 24 to 48 postoperative hours. Pericarditis is common and occasionally responds to previously mentioned therapy.

Special mention should be made of the 12 to 24 h spent on the volume ventilator after coronary bypass. Many patients have a great fear of the endotracheal tube and become agitated and hypertensive postoperatively. Sedation with small doses of intravenous morphine is helpful in this situation. Frequent blood gas determinations allows one to know if respiration is properly controlled. Considerable tracheobronchial secretions and a painful throat sometimes follow extubation. Vocal cord edema is sometimes a problem, especially after prolonged intubation. Hoarseness may persist for several days. Pneumothorax can occasionally occur and will become tense if the patient is on the respirator when it develops.

Bedside examination of patients in the immediate postoperative period may lead to confusion. Neck veins are often constricted from being cold, and heart sounds may be barely audible because of superimposed mediastinal crunches and tube rubs. If blood pressure, filling pressures, urine output, and chest tube drainage are satisfactory and if the patient is awake and communicates, then the situation is progressing satisfactory. Basic blood studies including hematocrit value, blood gases, and serum potassium level should be in correct range. This is one situation where neck vein assessments and auscultatory findings can be confusing and must be interpreted in light of the patient's general appearance and the monitored parameters.

Moving to the postoperative surgical ward from the intensive care unit represents progress. Occasionally, a patient will become fearful of this move because of a sense of dependency on nurses and monitoring devices. Encouragement by floor nurses and friendly visits from the intensive care unit nurses and family members will overcome this fear. Steady anticipated progress is always encouraging. It is comforting to know that the surgeon and cardiologist are only a few minutes away and will promptly come if problems arise.

Mediastinal tubes are usually removed 48 h postoperatively if drainage is minimal, and pacing wires are capped and removed on the fifth or sixth day. Antibiotics are started orally after 24 to 48 h and are continued for a total of 5 days postoperatively. Percodan* is ordered for pain if not relieved by Darvocet N.† Propranolol is restarted postoperatively as soon as the patient can swallow. Propranolol is given indefinitely, especially for those patients on large doses preoperatively and those who have incomplete revascularization. We usually give digoxin to the patients who receive propranolol. We continue antiarrhythmic drugs such as procainamide as long as ventricular arrhythmias are a problem.

While on the postoperative surgical ward the patient and family are given a booklet[21] that outlines progress in detail from the immediate postoperative period to full recovery. Also, complications are listed with associated symptoms and signs. Landmarks of progress are underlined, such as going back to work and driving a car. All this puts things into perspective and decreases anxiety. Family members are usually well ahead of the patient in the educational process—they have more time to read the material and usually sit at the bedside and comment on when this or that will occur.

While on the postoperative surgical ward, some patients receive chest physical therapy to keep secretions moving. A maximum effort is made preoperatively to identify patients who might have pulmonary problems postoperatively, and these patients have pulmonary medicine consultation and chest physical therapy. The patient who is young and has no pulmonary disease may not need this therapy.

Patients sit in a chair on the second and third postoperative day and by the fourth postoperative day are ambulating about the room and halls with help. Knee-length support stockings are used until about a month postoperatively to minimize the occurrence of pulmonary embolism, which rarely occurs in these pa-

*Endo Laboratories, Inc.
†Eli Lilly and Co.

tients, and to decrease lower extremity edema. Usually by the seventh postoperative day the patients are walking in the hallway and are ready to go home.

The cardiologist should be alert to several complications that may occur while the patient is recovering on the postoperative surgical ward. Some of these are listed in Table 21-3.

Pericarditis occurs in nearly all patients. Symptomatic pericarditis requiring treatment occurs in 15 to 30 percent of patients after coronary bypass surgery. This may manifest itself as chest pain, fever, unexplained tachycardia, atrial tachyarrhythmias, swallowing difficulties, hiccups, or sleeplessness. The chest pain may be quite variable. It is commonly retrosternal with a left shoulder component and is aggravated by inspiration. There may or may not be a pericardial friction rub. The absence of a friction rub should not cause the physician to withhold therapy if the subjective data suggest pericarditis. Experienced nurses regularly make this diagnosis and call the physician to ask for therapy for pericarditis. Atrial fibrillation or flutter with 2:1 conduction are commonly precipitated by pericarditis, and therapy for the underlying pericarditis should accompany the digitalis and propranolol. We usually give 4 mg of dexamethasone intravenously for pericarditis. This can be followed up with indomethacin orally, and after 1 to 6 h the patient and family will think a miracle has been performed! We usually continue indomethacin for several weeks postoperatively and then taper this off slowly. Those patients who are refractory to indomethacin are treated with tapering doses of oral corticosteroids (prednisone) and then tapering doses of indomethacin. There should be no hesitation in making this diagnosis, for this problem can make the patient miserable for hours. Pericarditis can recur days, weeks, months, or years after surgery. Pericarditis is one of the more aggravating complications of the postoperative period and unfortunately often goes unrecognized. It is rarely mentioned in the medical literature. Constriction rarely occurs.

Arrhythmias may be detected after discharge from the intensive care unit. Atrial tachyarrhythmias, including atrial flutter and fibrillation, are common and often mean that pericarditis is present. As a general rule, frequent ventricular premature beats should be treated with antiarrhythmic drugs. Sometimes propranolol keeps these suppressed and also serves other previously mentioned purposes. A rare patient will have a serious life-threatening arrhythmia after discharge from the intensive care unit. The frequency of this problem is extremely low, and thus we have not chosen to use telemetry routinely in those patients who have left the intensive care unit and are progressing well on the postoperative ward.

Infection is a dreaded complication of coronary bypass surgery but fortunately is quite rare. These individuals have already been treated with antistaphylococcal agents and thus are prone to develop gram-negative infections. Persistent fever in a spiking pattern in addition to a leaking sternal wound indicates *mediastinitis*. This usually takes several days to develop, since mediastinal tubes drain this area. Fever persisting to the seventh postoperative day should make one consider mediastinitis. Small pustules in the suture line that communicate through the sternal incision signal the diagnosis and the need for surgical exploration. Treatment with continuous mediastinal lavage is often required,[22] and a prolonged hospital course follows. The condition is life threatening and is emotionally disturbing to the patient, family, and physician. Continued infection that requires open drainage, removal of the sternum, and skin grafting is devastating to the patient. Aortic rupture and pulmonary infection account for high hospital mortality. Mediastinitis is rarely discussed in large series but obviously occurs in a few patients who have this procedure and is associated with high mortality and morbidity.

Cellulitis along any suture line occasionally occurs and requires local treatment in addition to antibiotics. This is particularly common at the vein harvest sites in the presence of diabetes.

Pneumonia may occur but must always be differentiated from pulmonary emboli. Individuals with underlying lung disease are prone to pulmonary infection and deserve special preoperative and postoperative chest physical therapy.

Pleural effusion and pulmonary embolization may be aggravating factors in the recovery period. Blood that is not adequately drained from the mediastinum may spill over to the pleural spaces and result in pleuritis and more fluid accumulation. This can be helped by thoracentesis if the effusion is large. Pulmonary embolus may be the cause of pleural effusion and should be vigorously investigated. If found, heparin can be instituted after a few days of healing. A careful watch for mediastinal bleeding and cardiac tamponade

TABLE 21-3
Complications occurring while recovering on the postoperative surgical ward

Pericarditis	Phlebitis
Arrhythmias	Digitalis intoxication
Infections	Ileus
Mediastinitis	Rash
Cellulitis	Hypertension and
Pneumonia	hypotension
Pleural effusions	Aortic dissection
Pulmonary embolization	Disruption of sternal wires
Drowsiness, confusion	
Stroke	

should be instituted if heparin is started. This can be devastating when unrecognized and occasionally requires bedside opening of the lower part of the incision and release of accumulated mediastinal blood.

Drowsiness and confusion sometimes follow in the first several days after surgery. This requires discontinuation of sedatives and medication used for pain. The condition usually clears. Occasionally, a patient will complain of persistent memory problems after surgery. Most of this is reversible. The patients who are drowsy commonly will be amnesic for a few days following surgery. Confusion is a bothersome problem to the patient, physician, and family but usually clears in a few days. The worry, of course, is that something permanent is present. Family members need reassurance that this will usually clear.

Stroke sometimes occurs after a delayed period. We commonly think of this as being due to particle embolization from the aorta at proximal graft sites or the cross-clamp site. Patients with "eggshell" aortas are at risk for this complication. A mural thrombus in the atrium or ventricle can give rise to an embolus and subsequent stoke.

Phlebitis sometimes occurs at the vein harvest sites and, of course, delays discharge from the hospital. It is remarkable that the condition is so rare. The treatment includes heparin, elevation, heat, and rest, hoping that pulmonary embolus will not occur. Coumadin therapy should follow for about 6 months.

Digitalis intoxication occasionally occurs. It is especially likely to occur in small, elderly individual patients. Anorexia, nausea, lethargy, and lack of taste or bad taste should signal the cessation of this medication. Arrhythmias, of course, may be present.

Ileus can occur. This may aggravate breathing and require a nasogastric tube. Hypokalemia is commonly an aggravating factor. Hiccups can appear and be very irritating, lasting sometimes 2 or 3 days. They are often resistant to therapeutic efforts.

Rashes of all kinds occur. Usually maculopapular rashes result from the penicillin drugs. They are irritating and sometimes require assistance from the dermatologist.

Hypertension or hypotension sometimes develop in the postoperative period. Hypertension should be treated in order to lessen tension on suture lines. Hypotension requires a search for bleeding, tamponade, infarction, pulmonary embolus, hypovolemia, and sepsis. This is a serious problem and requires prompt attention.

Aortic dissection develops in the rare patient. The dissection begins at the proximal graft sites in the aorta.[16] This rare but dreaded complication can be fatal.

Disruption of sternal wires may follow prolonged vigorous coughing or sneezing. Chronic lung disease and some degree of osteoporosis is the usual setting in which this problem occurs. It is best to rewire these as soon as possible, since pseudoarthrosis develops and repair is more difficult. One can expect some movement of the sternum early after operation, but no gross motions should be present. An occasional patient will experience loosening of costochondral joints, and the anterior chest plate will move paradoxically on inspiration. This usually poses no significant problem.

INSTRUCTIONS AT TIME OF DISCHARGE

Instructions about activity should be reviewed at the time of discharge from the hospital. Activity should be gradually increased over the next month. The patient can usually walk ½ mile in the morning and evening. This should be gradually increased until the patient is walking 1 mile twice a day by 1 month after discharge. Avoiding driving is a clear and definite goal. Lifting should be avoided. Returning to work should be discussed after a month of convalescence. If the individual does manual labor, a 2- to 3-month recovery period may be required. A treadmill test prior to returning to work is a good idea in this situation.

We usually continue propranolol and digitalis postoperatively. Aspirin, 650 mg twice daily, or Anturane, 200 mg four times a day is used for its antiplatelet effect. Indomethacin or prednisone are continued in tapering doses for several weeks if pericarditis was present.

The cardiologist and surgeon see the patient at 4 to 6 weeks and assess the progress the patient is making as compared to other patients. The patient is then seen by the cardiologist when the referring physician thinks it is appropriate.

PROBLEMS OCCURRING DURING CONVALESCENCE AT HOME

During the 1- or 2-month period of convalescence at home, several problems may occur that require attention (Table 21-4). Because of this potential, we always recommend an early visit to the patient's referring physician so that a baseline examination can be obtained.

Pericarditis having its onset after leaving the hospital is common. As mentioned earlier, presenting symptoms are chest pain with an inspiratory component associated with fever and/or arrhythmia. Treatment has already been mentioned. Constriction occurs rarely.

TABLE 21-4
Problems occurring during convalescence at home

Pericarditis
Wound infection
Pulmonary embolus
Recurrence of angina pectoris
Hepatitis
Chest wall pain
Impotence
Emotional problems

Drainage from the sternal wound and fever suggests mediastinitis and requires prompt antibiotic treatment and surgical exploration.

Pulmonary embolus may occur after ambulation is well underway. The combination of bed rest plus manipulation of leg veins sets the stage for this complication. We have been surprised at the relatively low incidence of this problem.

Angina pectoris may recur as activity increases, especially in patients who had less than satisfactory revascularization. Small vessels that were borderline for revascularization may not accept the graft, giving rise to potentially ischemic areas. Propranolol continued in these settings helps to prevent or control symptoms. We advise patients to keep nitroglycerin and use it if they think it is indicated.

A rare patient will develop *hepatitis* from previous transfusions but this is generally uncommon.

Commonly, as activity is increased, all types of *chest wall pain* may occur. Point tenderness at a sternal wire or at a costochondral junction is often irritating but usually clears with time. Skeletal muscles that have been inactive ache as they bear the load of resumed activity.

Multiple medication plus the emotional burden of such a procedure sometimes results in *impotence*. As medications are withdrawn and the overall situation improves, this problem disappears.

Occasionally, *profound depression* follows coronary bypass surgery and may extend into the convalescent period at home. Inactivity, recognition of the presence of an underlying disease, restriction of activity, and medication all play a role. Steady progress is a key factor in overcoming this problem.

RETURNING TO WORK

The objective of the rehabilitation of patients who undergo coronary bypass surgery is to have them return to work. This is usually accomplished in patients who are self-employed and where surgery has not been delayed inordinately. The patient and family should be led to understand that the patient must return to work. The physician should not entertain any other thought. Patients who have already retired or are already receiving disability insurance should be advised to be more active than they were prior to surgery. Whenever possible the retired person or the patient who is already on disability insurance at the time of surgery should be encouraged to seek employment. If the patient continues to be truly disabled from angina pectoris or if moderately severe chronic heart failure develops, then the patient may not be able to work. The latter state is actually rare compared to the number of patients who do not return to work because they have already retired, they are already on disability insurance, they have been squeezed out of their job, etc.

CONCLUSIONS

The cardiologist who is involved in the care of the patient is often responsible for the continuity of the patient's care during the hospitalization for coronary bypass surgery. The cardiologist is responsible for the total care of the patient and the patient's return to the referring physician. Regrettably, there is no single document that discusses the procedure and its complications for the medical cardiologist or internist. The purpose of this chapter has been to discuss the emotional needs of the patient and family, the complications of the procedure, and the medical conditions that may occur from the time the decision is made to operate until the patient has returned to work.

REFERENCES

1 Waller, J. L., Kaplan, J. A., and Jones, E. L.: Anesthesia for Coronary Revascularization, in J. A. Kaplan (ed.), "Cardiac Anesthesia," Grune & Stratton, Inc., New York, 1979, p. 260.

2 Lowenstein, E., Hallowell, P., and Levine, F.: Cardiovascular Responses to Large Doses of Morphine Sulfate in Man, *N. Engl. J. Med.*, 281:1389, 1969.

3 Bigelow, W. G., Lindsay, W. K., and Greenwood, W. F.: Hypothermia: Its Possible Role in Cardiac Surgery: An Investigation of Factors Governing Survival in Dogs at Low Body Temperatures, *Ann. Surg.*, 132:849, 1950.

4 Niaz, S. A., and Lewis, F. J.: Tolerance of Adult Rats to Profound Hypothermia and Simultaneous Cardiac Standstill, *Surgery*, 36:25, 1954.

5 Gordon, A. S., Jones, J. C., Luddington, L. G., and Meyer, B. W.: Deep Hypothermia for Intracardiac Surgery: Experimental and Clinical Use Without an Oxygenator, *Am. J. Surg.*, 100:332, 1960.

6 Gay, W. A., Jr.: Intraoperative Myocardial Protection. *Cardiovasc. Med.*, 3:1057, 1978.

7 Gay, W. A., Jr., and Ebert, P. A.: Functional, Metabolic and Morphologic Effects of Potassium-Induced Cardioplegia, *Surgery*, 74:284, 1973.

8 Ellis, R. J., Pryor, W., and Ebert, P.A.: Advantages of Hypothermia and Potassium Cardioplegia in Left Ventricular Hypertrophy, *Ann. Thorac. Surg.*, 24:299, 1977.

9 Mehigan, J. T., Buch, W.S., Pipkin, R. D., and Fogarty, T. J.: A Planned Approach to Coexistent Cerebrovascular Disease in Coronary Artery Bypass Candidates, *Arch. Surg.*, 112:1403, 1977.

10 Hopkins, L. H.: Personal communication.

11 Chatterjee, K., Parmley, W. W., and Swan, H. J.: Beneficial Effects of Vasodilating Agents in Severe Mitral Regurgitation, *Circulation*, 48:684, 1973.

12 Dunbar, R. W., Kaplan, J. A., and King, S. B.: Vasodilator Treatment of Heart Failure After Cardiopulmonary Bypass, *Anesth. Anal.*, 54:842, 1975.

13 Brown, D. R., and Sterek, P.: Sodium Nitroprusside Induces Improvement in Cardiac Function in Association with Left Ventricular Failure, *Anesthesiology*, 41:521, 1974.

14 Buckley, M. T., Craver, J. M., Gold, H. K., et al.: Intraaortic Balloon Pump Assist for Cardiogenic Shock After Cardiopulmonary Bypass, *Circulation*, 47 (suppl.3):90, 1973.

15 Waldo, A. L., MacLean, W. A. H., Cooper, T. B., Kouchoukos, N. T., and Karp, R. B.: Use of Temporarily Placed Epicardial Atrial Wire Electrodes for the Diagnosis and Treatment of Cardiac Arrhythmias Following Open-Heart Surgery, *J. Thorac. Cardiovasc. Surg.*, 76:500, 1978.

16 Nicholson, W. J., Crawley, I. S., Logue, R. B., Dorney, E. R., Cobbs, B. W., and Hatcher, C. R.: Aortic Root Dissection Complicating Coronary Bypass Surgery, *Am. J. Cardiol.*, 41:103, 1978.

17 Cohn, J. N., Guiha, N. H., Broder, M. I., and Constantios, J. L.: Right Ventricular Infarction, *Am. J. Cardiol.*, 33:209, 1974.

18 Pennington, J. E., Taylor, J., and Lown, B.: Chest Thump for Reverting Ventricular Tachycardia, *N. Engl. J. Med.*, 283:1192, 1970.

19 Munath, E. D., and Austen, W. G.: Surgical Measures for Coronary Heart Disease, *N. Engl. J. Med.*, 293:13, 75, 124, 1975.

20 Logue, R. B., Robinson, P. H., Hatcher, C. R., and Kaplan, J. A.: Medical Management in Cardiac Surgery, in J. W. Hurst (ed.) "The Heart," McGraw-Hill Book Company, New York, 1978, p. 1790.

21 Burrows, S. G., and Garrert, C. A.: "Moving Right Along," Pritchett and Hall Associates, Inc., Atlanta, 1976.

22 Craver, J. C., and Jones, E. L.: Personal communication.

Chapter 22

The Cost of Coronary Bypass Surgery*

JOHN J. COLLINS, JR., M.D.

Growing public concern over the cost of medical care has resulted in close scrutiny of the cost/benefit ratios of complex treatment programs. Because of the very large number of persons affected by coronary heart disease, there has been anxiety that proliferation of coronary bypass surgery, an apparently expensive therapy, may result in such massive expenditure that other medical programs will be impossible to support without an unacceptable rise in total health care costs. A frequently employed illustration of the magnitude of cost involved in coronary bypass surgery has been the calculation of total dollars represented by multiplying the estimated number of operations performed by the estimated "average" cost of each. A formidable product results, since there are probably about 80,000 such operations performed annually in the United States at a cost of about $12,000 to $15,000 each. Such a calculation has led one editorialist to refer to coronary bypass surgery as a billion dollar industry.[1]

To appreciate properly the cost of coronary bypass surgery, a far more complex analysis is needed. The means for assessing costs of technological advances and changes have been carefully studied, and a variety of techniques have been developed. Unfortunately, there are major differences between the results of medical therapy and the products of industrial production, and the examination of one by techniques of the other is not easily done. While it may be possible to calculate the value of an automobile or refrigerator, it is repugnant to many, if not most persons, to place some finite value on life or health. Concern with the possible consequences of public disclosure of the techniques of determining such values has been expressed by many, although some need for value judgments in medical care clearly exists.[2]

The general principles of cost/benefit analysis as applied to problems of surgical care have been outlined by Pliskin and Taylor.[3] Consideration must be given to the questions of what costs and what benefits

should be included in the analysis, how the costs and benefits should be valued, what are appropriate discount rates, and what are the relevant constraints. To provide answers to these questions is a complex and difficult task. For example, if one chooses to examine hospitalization costs for coronary bypass surgery, it will be found that a great variation exists in various areas of the United States and throughout the world.[4] In addition, quoted costs are dependent upon accounting procedures of the various hospitals, and these procedures may be remarkably complex and may substantially influence comparisons between one form of hospital service and another because revenue generated from one hospital department is often used to defray expenses in another. If services received are subsidized by contributions from other departments, costs will be artificially low. Conversely, costs for laboratory examinations, expendable supplies, x-ray services, and operating room utilization will become artificially inflated because surplus from these departments is often used to bolster inadequate room rate compensation. Patients undergoing coronary bypass surgery may therefore appear to have higher hospitalization costs because of greater utilization of "profit-making" services than patients whose primary expense is related to occupation of a hospital bed.

By whatever technique of calculation, the cost of cardiac surgical operations will be found high in comparison with other surgical procedures, and some attempt to discover whether such costs are justified is reasonable. A useful approach involves comparison of costs and benefits of medical and surgical therapy of coronary obstructive disease, considering both costs and benefits to be direct, indirect, or intangible. Direct costs include actual money expended for hospitalization, medication, and physician fees, and direct benefits include reduction of these costs as a result of therapy. Indirect costs include loss of productivity, while indirect benefits are realized when a person, unemployed by virtue of medical disability, returns to work or continues to work following treatment. Intangible costs include pain, fear, grief, and death. Intangible benefits result when some degree of freedom from these miseries is achieved.

---

*From Department of Surgery, Harvard Medical School, Boston.

Additional comments regarding the cost of coronary bypass surgery may be found in Chapter 12, "The Perils of Waiting".

COMPARISON OF DIRECT COSTS AND BENEFITS FOR MEDICAL AND SURGICAL TREATMENT OF CORONARY OBSTRUCTIVE DISEASE

General Considerations

Neither medical nor surgical therapy can be started until patients requiring intervention are identified. Therefore, there is a certain unavoidable case-finding cost for both modes of therapy. The general problem of costs versus benefits and costs versus effectiveness of diagnostic studies has been investigated and well described.[5]

The majority of persons with coronary artery disease are introduced into therapeutic programs because of development of symptoms. Some, however, have been identified by analysis of risk factors in screening tests or routine examinations with or without stress testing. Initial symptoms may be angina pectoris or pain of myocardial infarction in most persons. Since many of those with myocardial infarction may have premonitory symptoms for days, weeks, or even months that have been unrecognized as harbingers of heart attack, there is reason to believe that education and widespread availability of diagnostic facilities may reduce the incidence of myocardial infarction if interventions available actually can prevent infarction. Patients presenting in this phase of illness are said to have preinfarction angina, but certainty that infarction will ensue can only be established in retrospect. At present, there are no data available as to the cost of identification of patients with preinfarction angina.

There are also no reliable data available concerning the costs of caring for persons who sustain myocardial infarction. It is estimated that more than 400,000 myocardial infarctions occur each year in the United States, and the average hospital stay for each event probably averages more than 3 weeks. With daily charges for hospitalization averaging $300 per day, the simple product indicates at least the possibility that direct costs of well over one billion dollars each year may be involved. Actual charges probably are considerably higher, particularly when it is appreciated that most of these persons will spend at least 4 or 5 days in a coronary care unit. If it should be possible to prevent the occurrence of a substantial number of myocardial infarctions by some intervention, it is possible that even a high-cost intervention would result in lower overall health care expenses by reducing subsequent hospitalization for treatment of infarction.

Chronic angina pectoris is a very common affliction of adults in technologically advanced societies. Medical care costs for this large group of persons are un-known. The expected rate of hospitalization for patients with angina also cannot be readily ascertained. The development of more sophisticated means for evaluation of myocardial ischemic syndromes increases diagnostic costs but may make possible ultimate savings if patients at higher risk for serious complications can be identified and spared these costly illnesses.

Myocardial Infarction

About 60 to 70 percent of persons suffering myocardial infarction may be expected to survive the acute episode when treated medically (including risk of prehospitalization death). Although occasional reports of surgical management of uncomplicated myocardial infarction have been published, there are no adequate data by which costs for care of acute episodes or subsequent direct costs may be estimated. There are also no data to indicate whether early revascularization surgery for uncomplicated infarcts may reduce mortality.

Myocardial infarctions complicated by arrhythmias or congestive heart failure often prompt surgical consideration. There are numerous reports of successful operations with restoration of capability for an active life, but such reports have not been directed toward assessment of costs involved. Intensive care required for either medical or surgical management of patients with complicated myocardial infarction is very expensive, but a comparison of costs is presently impossible. In many cases the distinction between medical and surgical care may become unclear. When an intraaortic counterpulsation balloon is employed, should the expense be considered medical or surgical? If medical, costs for "conservative" management of complicated myocardial infarction may be quite high, and careful analysis would be needed to discover whether an early attempt to achieve definitive improvement by surgery may be more economical in many patients.

Unstable Anginal Syndromes

Most patients with unstable angina pectoris improve with hospitalization and medication. Earlier reports indicated that such patients were at high risk for recurrence of symptoms, often leading to myocardial infarction after the initial episode had apparently been controlled.[6,7] Since utilization of beta blocking drugs and more efficient long-acting vasodilators, the prognosis for medically managed patients seems to have improved.[8] Although there is widespread belief that the extent and location of coronary artery obstruction bears an important relation to prognosis in these patients, precise data are lacking. There is general agreement that patients with unstable angina and main left coronary obstruction have a grim outlook with medical management but fare better with surgical therapy which has a 5 to 10 percent risk of associated death.[9] Although exact data are not yet available, it appears likely that longevity is improved and the hazard of myocardial infarction is less after revascularization in many patients with unstable angina.[10,11]

In an economic analysis of 85 patients randomized for surgical or medical therapy of unstable angina pectoris as part of the National Cooperative Study Group at the University of Birmingham, Kronenfeld and associates investigated relationships of modes of therapy and costs with particular attention to discriminating between patients who could be "successfully" managed by medical therapy and those who became "medical failures" requiring surgery after a trial of medical management. Direct costs in the first 2 years after selection for medical or surgical therapy averaged $6,226 (SD $2,967) for medical patients and $10,416 (SD $2,146) for surgical patients, including both hospital charges and physicians' fees. Patients initially selected for medical management who later required surgery because of failure to control progression of symptoms had a mean cost of $20,059 (SD $10,748) for the 2-year period. Thus, although surgery was more expensive than medical management over the first 2 years after selection for patients whose medical management proved adequate, the total cost of care for medical therapy was raised by the substantially greater overall cost for those later requiring surgery. Discriminant function analysis showed the number of vessels diseased, severity of angina, presence of congestive heart failure, hypertension, and the duration of anginal symptoms to be significant predictors ($p < .01$) for patients who later required surgery. Using these data, the authors were able to predict a substantial savings in health care costs by more accurate selection of patients for initial surgical management.

Chronic Angina Pectoris

Chronic angina pectoris may be unremitting and predictable or may be episodic with periods of more severe disability. During severe episodes, hospitalization may be required for control or to rule out myocardial infarction. Some patients may have stable mild angina for many years, while progression of severity is characteristic of others. Many patients are treated with office or clinic visits alone, while others may be hospitalized for initial evaluation and to establish a treatment program. Because premonitory symptoms of myocardial infarction are often mild, many physicians tend to hospitalize patients with recent on-

set of angina for diagnostic studies. To discover the cost of medical management in these patients may be quite difficult, and no reliable data are available.

Direct costs of coronary bypass surgery for patients having chronic angina pectoris have recently been investigated. At the Peter Bent Brigham Hospital, analysis was conducted of costs of hospitalization before and after coronary bypass surgery in 100 consecutive patients with chronic angina pectoris.[12] In this group were 81 men, with an average age of 50.1 years, and 19 women, with a mean age of 56.0 years. There were 8 patients with single-vessel disease, 37 patients with two-vessel disease, and 55 patients with three or more coronary branches involved by 70 percent or greater obstruction. There were 12 patients who had a single bypass graft, 50 patients who had two grafts, and 38 patients who had three or more bypass grafts. As a result of surgery, 79 patients were completely revascularized, 19 patients were left with one vessel not grafted, and 2 patients were left with two vessels not grafted. The incidence of hospital admissions for cardiac problems, not including diagnostic angiography, is shown in Fig. 22-1. There were 46 patients who had no hospital admission during the 2 years prior to surgery. A single hospital admission was necessary for 27 patients, two hospital admissions for 17 patients, three hospital admissions for 6 patients, four hospital admissions for 2 patients, and five hospital admissions for 2 patients. In Fig. 22-2 is shown the incidence of hospitalization during 2 years following coronary bypass surgery. There were 13 patients requiring hospitalization in this interval, and only 1 patient required

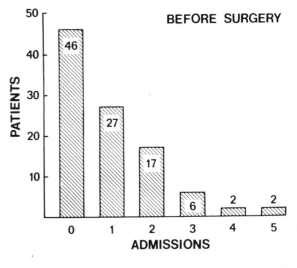

COST OF CORONARY SURGERY 1978

FIGURE 22-1 Incidence of hospitalization (not including diagnostic angiography) during 2 years before coronary bypass surgery in 100 patients with chronic angina pectoris.

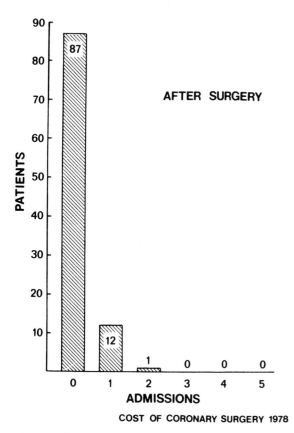

AFTER SURGERY

COST OF CORONARY SURGERY 1978

FIGURE 22-2 Incidence of hospitalization (not including diagnostic angiography) during 2 years after coronary bypass surgery in 100 patients with chronic angina pectoris.

two episodes of hospitalization. The reasons for hospital admission during the 2 years following coronary bypass surgery included angina in 9 patients, pericarditis in 1 patient, pleural effusion in 1 patient, a broken pacing wire in 1 patient, and an episode of pulmonary embolism (nonfatal) in 1 patient. The average requirement for hospitalization during the 2 years before coronary bypass surgery in these patients was 7.7 days per patient per year and was reduced to 1.8 days per patient per year during the 2 years subsequent to surgery. The difference of 5.9 days per patient per year, considering $300 per day as an average hospital expense, represents a saving of $1,770 per patient per year. Under these circumstances, the $8,000 hospital cost for performance of the surgery in these patients would be amortized in about 4.5 years. If only those patients requiring hospitalization during the 2 years prior to surgery are analyzed, it was noted that the average hospitalization during 2 years prior to surgery was 15.5 days per patient per year and 1.4 days per patient per year during the 2 years following operation. This difference of 14.1 days per patient per year represents a savings during 2 years after surgery of $4,230

per year for an amortization rate of 1.9 years. These data suggest, at least over a short term of years, that coronary bypass surgery may actually be a less expensive form of therapy than medical management for patients with angina pectoris, particularly if the angina is severe enough to require hospitalization. Similar data were found in the Veterans Administration study of the influence of surgery on the course of coronary obstructive disease as reported by Takaro and associates.[13] In this study of patients with left main coronary obstructive disease, it was found that a significant decrease in hospitalization requirement was observed in those patients who were operated on compared to those who were treated medically.

Hammermeister and associates, in an analysis of 287 matched pairs of medically and surgically managed patients from the angiography registry of Seattle Heart Watch, also found a reduction in hospitalization rate (hospitalizations per 1000 man-years) in the surgical patients.[14]

From these reports, it appears that direct costs on a short-term basis (up to 5 years) do not so clearly favor medical therapy, as has been thought by many. It may be contended that any savings realized for surgical survivors will be lost subsequently as the disease progresses and recurrence of angina or myocardial infarction negates the initial therapeutic benefits of revascularization. No one can deny that this may occur—and, in fact, will occur in certain patients, particularly those with significant metabolic risk factors resistant to therapeutic manipulation such as diabetes mellitus and familial hyperlipidemia. But in many patients the progression of atherosclerotic obstruction may be alterable by certain life-style changes such as stopping smoking and by therapeutic programs such as platelet function alteration and diet regulation. In patients with severe proximal obstruction in multiple arteries, bypass grafts may continue to function for many years if disease progression can be slowed.

COMPARISON OF INDIRECT COSTS AND BENEFITS

Myocardial Infarction

Although there has been perhaps as much study and writing devoted to myocardial infarction as to any single adverse medical occurrence, there has been little attention given to the change in productivity that results. Such changes may be related not only to cessation of employment but also to change of jobs or realignment of ambitions or opportunities. Many job changes or alterations in hours worked may be based upon physicians' prognosis. Workman's Compensation laws may also be operative in removing from employment persons whose infarction occurred while at work. In sum, however, it must be observed that few facts are available to judge the economic impact of myocardial infarction. Thus the value of prevention of infarction cannot be readily calculated.

Angina Pectoris

There are no significant data available on loss of productivity as a result of angina pectoris in patients managed medically. Several studies have suggested that demonstration of improved productivity after surgery may be difficult or impossible, not because the potential for productive living has not been improved, but because the sociopolitical system in which we live brings about behavior styles after surgery in which improved productive capacity may be effectively masked. Change in work status after coronary bypass surgery in 350 patients was analyzed by Barnes and associates.[15] These patients, operated on at the University of Alabama, Birmingham, between July 1970 and August 1974 were interviewed 1 year after surgery to evaluate job status and hours worked and to ascertain the influence of such variables as the number of hours worked each week before surgery, extent of symptom relief, severity of disease, number of bypass grafts placed, and level of education. In the group as a whole, there was no detectable increase in work activities after surgery. A decrease in hours worked each week was noted in 44 percent, an increase in 32 percent, and no change in 24 percent of patients. The factor showing highest correlation ($p < .001$) with hours worked each week after surgery was hours worked before. Of 218 patients working full-time before surgery, 144 (66 percent) returned to full-time employment after operation, and an additional 13 percent were working part time at 1 year after operation. The reasons for change of work status and the number of nonworking or reduced-work patients whose physical condition would have allowed them to work were not specified. Other factors with significant correlation included relief of angina ($p < .001$), absence of symptoms of congestive heart failure after operation ($p < .003$), and level of education ($p < .001$), as well as the extent of disease, and the number of grafts placed when preoperative angina status was taken into account. No significant correlation with postoperative employment status was found with such factors as sex, age, marital status, and occupation. In discussing these findings, the authors note that many circumstances modify a patient's ability or desire to return to employment after coronary bypass surgery. These include lack of financial incentive as well as the fear that occupational stress may predispose to recurrence of anginal symptoms or progression of atherosclerotic

obstruction. The latter consideration may or may not be realistic but is often initiated or reinforced by physician's advice.

The importance of analyzing specific reasons for changing work status, rather than simply correlating change with persistence of symptoms, age, and such factors, is demonstrated by the experience of David from the Montreal Heart Institute who found that patients' decisions to retire after coronary bypass surgery were influenced by physicians' advice in over 60 percent.[16] There is also a frequent influence from the employer's consultant physician. Many employers, and carriers of Workman's Compensation insurance as well, seem to have more concern about patients after coronary bypass surgery than after myocardial infarction, virtually without regard to published prognostic indexes.

The problem of negative financial incentive for return to work after myocardial revascularization surgery is understandable. A person who has worked in an occupation for many years in which he or she has no deep personal interest may be quite willing to retire for "medical disability" when the opportunity arises. There may be sufficient compensation to nearly equal average working pay, and income may be supplemented by part-time employment unreported to the insurance carrier or to the physician. Such a practice probably occurs quite frequently. As every physician knows, it is difficult or impossible to assure a patient or employer that return to work is "safe." In addition, patients may describe a variety of specific or nebulous symptoms that are impossible to ignore, although also impossible to correlate with defective myocardial blood supply. Physicians who assiduously pursue diagnostic studies to "prove" that a patient is sufficiently healthy to return to work may lose rapport with the patient and will almost certainly see these efforts fail. In addition, there is a realistic concern for liability of the physician should a patient be "forced" to return to work and later experience recurrence of complications of coronary artery obstruction. These psychosocial and economic considerations are well known to workers in the field of rehabilitation and have an important influence upon the indirect cost of surgery.

COMPARISON OF INTANGIBLE COSTS AND BENEFITS

Intangible costs of coronary artery obstructive disease include death, grief, pain, and fear. Intangible benefits, of course, are realized when these possibilities are eliminated, postponed, or ameliorated.

The influence of intangible benefits upon cost of coronary bypass surgery is, of course, difficult to estimate. How can a monetary value be placed upon relief of angina pectoris? The unique aspect of angina pectoris when compared with discomfort of most injuries and illnesses is its association with the fear of imminent death. This oppressive aspect of angina has been described by many observers and is an important consideration. What is it worth to be free of angina? And what is it worth to preserve an active life-style for the average person?

The question of improved longevity following coronary bypass surgery is still hotly debated, although evidence is accumulating that persons with left main coronary obstruction and multiple-vessel (including left anterior descending coronary artery) obstruction have a greater probability of prolonged survival with surgery.[12,17,18] Estimation of the possible superiority of longevity after revascularization surgery is difficult primarily because of lack of survival data for medically managed patients. The several randomized prospective studies thus far attempted have not clarified matters very much, and the Veterans Administration cooperative study on surgery for chronic stable angina pectoris has proved so controversial as to be detrimental to the cause of further studies in this area.[19] There seems no doubt, however, that persons with severe multiple-vessel coronary artery obstruction who survive revascularization surgery can have a life expectancy over the ensuing 5 to 6 years (and probably longer) that is not significantly different from that of the general population. In Figs. 22-3, 22-4 and 22-5 are shown actuarial curves illustrating probability of post-

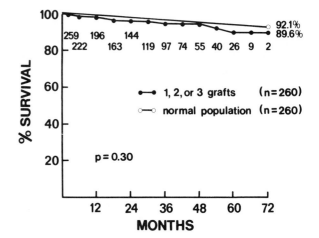

FIGURE 22-4 Probability of survival for patients with angina pectoris and two-vessel coronary obstructive disease. (*Reprinted with permission from J. J. Collins, Jr. et al., The Influence of Coronary Bypass Surgery on Longevity in Patients with Angina Pectoris, in D. T. Mason (ed.), "Advances in Heart Disease—1978," Grune & Stratton Publishers, Inc., New York, in press.*)

operative survival of patients with one-vessel, two-vessel, and three-vessel coronary artery obstruction. Operative mortality risk in these patients was 1.6 percent and is included in the curves. Note that although the overall survival probability is slightly lower for these surgical patients than for a theoretical age- and sex-matched "normal" population, the difference is small and abolished if only surgical survivors are included. Several formulas have been devised to relate additional years of life to some monetary value. The artifacts of such manipulations are so great as to make the results nearly, if not entirely, meaningless. For most human beings, a year or two of additional life is very worthwhile without regard to cost, particularly if a reasonably active life-style can be maintained.

With publication of studies of survival probability after coronary bypass surgery, the prognosis for persons with various combinations of coronary obstructive disease is gradually becoming clear. Unfortunately, the prognosis for medically managed patients with similar disease characteristics is far from clear. The early studies of Friesinger[20] and Bruschke[21] indicated that there was a direct relationship between the likelihood of death and the number of significantly obstructed coronary arteries. In addition, and to some extent independently, the integrity of left ventricular function has a bearing on survival.[22] Because of the very high mortality of patients with severely embarrassed left ventricular contractility, it is not surprising that this factor often outweighs the extent of coronary obstruction as a risk factor in the first several years after diagnosis. For these patients, alteration in life

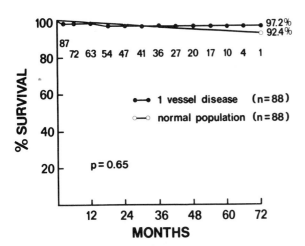

FIGURE 22-3 Probability of survival for patients with angina pectoris and single-vessel coronary obstructive disease. (*Reprinted with permission from J. J. Collins, Jr. et al., The Influence of Coronary Bypass Surgery on Longevity in Patients with Angina Pectoris, in D. T. Mason (ed.), "Advances in Heart Disease—1978," Grune & Stratton Publishers, Inc., New York, in press.*)

expectancy by coronary revascularization is likely to be less evident than for those with better left ventricular function for whom extent of coronary obstruction is the primary life-limiting factor. The report of Vlietstra and associates from the Mayo Clinic comparing survival in medically and surgically managed patients with various degrees of coronary obstructive disease indicated that both groups had excellent 4-year survival (91 percent medical and 96 percent surgical) when the left ventricular ejection fraction was 50 percent or greater and that both groups had poor 2-year survival (33 percent medical and 40 percent surgical) when the ejection fraction was under 25 percent.[23] In 86 patients with ejection fractions between 25 and 49 percent, there was a significant improvement in survival ($p < .05$) at 3 years in the 56 surgical patients as compared to 30 medically managed patients. The authors suggest on the basis of these data that coronary bypass surgery may have a greater role in prolonging life in patients with moderately impaired left ventricular function than in those with relatively intact or severely impaired left ventricular function. Under the circumstances of this study, such a conclusion seems valid, but it may be that with longer follow-up, a similar or greater benefit may be observed in patients with better left ventricular function. Only time will tell.

Assignment of economic value to relief of pain and fear in patients with angina pectoris is probably impossible. Still, the remarkable symptomatic relief, particularly in patients refractory to medical management, is a worthwhile benefit of surgery. It is common for patients to state "I can't go on living this way," and although they may not precisely mean what they say, it is evident that they perceive their disability as very severe.

DECISION ANALYSIS FOR CORONARY BYPASS SURGERY

Weinstein, Pliskin, and Stason have proposed the utilization of decision analysis to provide for a systematic approach to problems involving multiple variables, multiple possible outcomes, and "substantial uncertainty."[24] The general principles of decision analysis and application to surgical problems are discussed by Pliskin and Taylor.[3] The construction of a decision tree is needed, and choices and risks must be carefully specified. There must be consideration also of degrees of uncertainty in estimation of risks, and techniques are needed for estimating the significance of uncertainty factors as they modify the final decision. If a decision tree is constructed based solely on medical probabilities, a decision may be reached indicating that a particular therapy is optimal, and the extent to

which the chosen mode is superior to other possibilities may be estimated. Such a decision analysis may not take into account the financial or sociologic cost of such therapy, however, or the very important possibility that the patient may prefer to have some other therapeutic decision than would be indicated strictly on the basis of medical probability of success. As long as people are free to choose, there will be substantial uncertainty introduced into such decision analysis. In many instances, the physician may strongly advise the patient, and may present arguments, to persuade the patient that a particular type of treatment is in his or her best interest, but in the final analysis, the patient must make the decision.

Further modification of the decision may be introduced by other factors including preferences determined by circumstances unrelated to purely medical considerations. For example, if one recommends coronary bypass surgery for a patient with single-vessel right coronary obstruction based upon a decision tree that indicates superior longevity by 4 to 5 percent and enhanced comfort by 4 to 5 percent, one might be dissuaded by a cost difference between this and the next preference (if only slightly worse) which makes the more optimal medical decision socially unacceptable. It is this consideration that seems to trouble many observers about coronary bypass surgery. As Braunwald has intimated, even if myocardial revascularization surgery should be found preferable to medical therapy, some consideration must be given to the possibility that the cost of a nationwide program

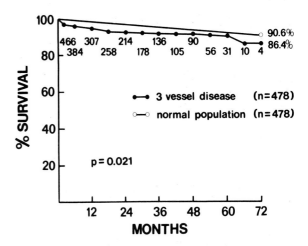

FIGURE 22-5 Probability of survival for patients with angina pectoris and three-vessel coronary obstructive disease. (*Reprinted with permission from J. J. Collins, Jr. et al., The Influence of Coronary Bypass Surgery on Longevity in Patients with Angina Pectoris, in D. T. Mason (ed.), "Advances in Heart Disease—1978," Grune & Stratton Publishers, Inc., New York, in press.*)

to provide such operations for all patients in categories likely to be helped would be prohibitively expensive. As indicated by the data presented in this chapter, the assumption that myocardial revascularization surgery is more costly than ''conservative'' management is open to question, and more information is needed to establish the relative costs of care for patients with various syndromes of coronary obstructive disease.

One of the most important questions relevant to the cost of coronary bypass surgery is whether, by some manipulation of the manner of distribution, such services might be made available to all persons in need at less cost than would be estimated by summation of present cost per unit. In other words, is the present cost of coronary bypass surgery artificially high? And, if so, is this related to hospital charges, surgeons' fees, or the cost of supplies and equipment or some combination of these? Is there some rearrangement that might result in a substantial reduction of costs to allow wider distribution of services?

Preston has pointed out that medical services, when provided on a fee-for-service basis, may be independent of the ''economic laws and influences of the marketplace.''[25] He maintains that the physician has a basic conflict of interest because the physician's income is derived from procedures she or he orders for patients. Therefore, a physician or surgeon may be influenced by need or desire for additional income in advising a particular therapeutic approach for a given disease process. It has been asked, for example, why coronary bypass procedures are more commonly performed in countries with a fee-for-service system than in those where there is no economic incentive for the performance of such operations. To respond to the implication that desire for personal gain is a major motivating force in the selection of medical therapy is difficult because it is impossible to deny that the opportunity for such misbehavior exists under such a system. Of equally obvious significance, however, is the possibility that indicated operations are delayed or not recommended under circumstances where the effort necessary for such operations is not compensated and, therefore, not expended. Even a casual perusal of waiting times for surgical operations in socialized systems is sufficient to indicate that the best interests of many may not be well served.

It may be that some system intermediate between unlimited fee-for-service and compensation without regard to productivity may be best for patients. The large clinics in the United States have used such an approach with apparent success for many years, although these institutions are not entirely free of economic pressures either. The prepaid health insurance systems have been considered an appropriate answer by some, and such systems are operating in apparently successful configurations in various areas of the country. Experience has shown that health care costs, particularly those directly related to physicians' fees and hospital costs, may be substantially reduced with a prepaid health insurance program. An intangible cost to patients in both the clinic system and the prepaid insurance system is the loss of some features of personal physician–patient rapport characteristic of a fee-for-service system. Perhaps, for complex care such as cardiac surgery, this sacrifice may be worthwhile and of less impact than would be loss of a personal relationship with a general practitioner or family physician.

Another approach to cost containment for complex health care procedures is regionalization of facilities with regulation of facility proliferation by use of federal and state guidelines and certificate-of-need procedures. These measures, designed to improve utilization of existing equipment, hospitals, and personnel have proved to have an effect in many instances antagonistic to their intent. Those institutions with busy and heavily utilized surgical programs, for example, may be effectively prohibited from expanding because of higher than allowed capital expenses, while underutilized (and often inefficient) programs are encouraged to increase their number of operations (without regard to medical indications) or lose accreditation. There is thus a strong influence toward increasing the number of operations exerted by regulations designed to limit costs.

It seems evident that no system for distribution of complex surgical care in current use, or likely to be devised, will prove free of imperfections. However, the cost of cardiac surgery, as well as the cost of other complex, inhospital therapies could almost certainly be greatly reduced by a combination of regionalization, reduction of nonessential costs, and improved hospital utilization. Whether a more ideal system for providing surgical services can be devised without major changes in the structure of private medical practice remains to be seen. Such a system would demand a great deal more cooperation among surgeons, among hospitals, and among insurance carriers than currently exists, but it is theoretically possible. That greater efficiency will be achieved by closer government regulation seems very doubtful unless a spirit of cooperation among the principal providers of services can be achieved.

SUMMARY

Consideration of the cost of medical care has been a serious concern for government policymakers in the United States for a relatively short time. In other countries where publicly financed comprehensive medical care has a long history, there is greater familiarity with the difficulty of assimilating technological advances in a rigid financial system. The easiest and most frequently utilized approach to cost containment in most countries is limitation of access of the population to complex therapeutic programs. For example, an age limit may be placed on acceptance of patients for dialysis programs, or for consideration of cardiac surgery, or for intensive therapy of major burns. Or some other restrictive criteria may develop simply as a result of lack of available resources. There has been no need, fortunately, for such restrictions in the United States up to the present time, but the expression of fears of ever-increasing costs now make such a possibility likely.

Under these circumstances, it is helpful to remember that the primary purpose of medical practice is to relieve suffering and prolong comfortable life for all the people. If the capability for achieving these goals is to be limited, it is better that the limitation is imposed only after all available means for achieving efficiency in equitable distribution have been exhausted. Furthermore, it is necessary that careful analysis be conducted to ascertain what benefits may be lost and what costs saved by such measures. The addition of bureaucratic regulatory agencies to the expense of health care does not seem likely to improve efficiency of health care distribution without the active cooperation of the health care professions, and if such cooperation is achieved, the bureaucracy is unnecessary.

Only a beginning has so far been made to understand the impact of myocardial revascularization surgery upon health care costs. Many, if not most, of the data needed for reaching rational decisions as to the costs and benefits of coronary surgery are unavailable. The initial impression that expense is increased by such surgery may not be substantiated by careful analysis, as shown by the few studies so far reported, at least for those persons whose clinical course and disease characteristics promise great difficulty with medical management.

REFERENCES

1 Braunwald, E.: Coronary Artery Surgery at the Crossroads, *N. Engl. J. Med.,* 297:661, 1977.

2 Hapgood, F.: Risk-Benefit Analysis. Putting a Price on Life, *Atlantic Monthly,* January 1979.

3 Pliskin, N., and Taylor, A. K.: General Principles: Cost-Benefit and Decision Analysis, in J. P. Bunker, B. A. Barnes, and F. Mostellar (eds.), "Costs, Risks, and Benefits of Surgery," Oxford University Press, New York, 1977.

4 Marty, A. T., Matar, A. F., Danielson, R., and O'Reilly, R.: The Variation in Hospital Charges: A Problem in Determining Cost-Benefit for Cardiac Surgery, *Ann. Thorac. Surg.,* 24:409, 1977.

5 McNeil, B. J., Collins, J. J., Jr., and Adelstein, S. J.: Rationale for Seeking Occult Metastases in Patients with Bronchial Carcinoma, *Surg. Gynecol. Obstet.,* 144:389, 1977.

6 Gazes, P. C., Mobley, E. M., Jr., Faris, H. M., Jr., Duncan, R. C., and Humphries, G. B.: Preinfarctional (Unstable) Angina—A Prospective Study—Ten-Year Follow-up, *Circulation,* 48:331, 1973.

7 Krauss, K. R., Hutter, A. M., Jr., and DeSanctis, R. W.: Acute Coronary Insufficiency: Course and Follow-up, *Circulation,* 45, 46:66, 1972.

8 Hutter, A. M., Jr., Russel, R. O., Jr., Resnekov, L., et al.: Unstable Angina Pectoris—National Randomized Study of Surgical Versus Medical Therapy: Results in 1, 2, and 3 Vessel Disease, *Circulation,* 55, 56:60, 1977.

9 Cohn, L. H., Koster, J. K., Jr., Mee, R. B. B., and Collins, J. J., Jr.: Surgical Management of Stenosis of the Left Main Coronary Artery. *World J. Surg.,* in press.

10 Hultgren, H. N., Pfeiffer, J. F., Angell, W. W., Lipton, M. J., and Bilisoly, J.: Unstable Angina: Comparison of Medical and Surgical Treatment, *Am. J. Cardiol.,* 39:734, 1977.

11 Cohn, L. H., Alpert, J., Koster, J. K., Jr., Mee, R. B. B., and Collins, J. J., Jr.: Changing Indications for the Surgical Treatment of Unstable Angina, *Arch. Surg.,* 113:1312, 1978.

12 Collins, J. J., Jr., Cohn, L. H., Koster, J. K., Jr., and Mee, R. B. B.: The Influence of Coronary Bypass Surgery on Longevity in Patients with Angina Pectoris, in D. T. Mason (ed.), "Advances in Heart Disease—1978," Grune & Stratton Publishers, Inc., New York, in press.

13 Takaro, T., Hultgren, H. N., Lipton, M. J., Detre, K. M., and participants in the Study Group: The VA Cooperative Randomized Study of Surgery for Coronary Arterial Occlusive Disease. II. Subgroup with Significant Left Main Lesions, *Circulation,* 54 (suppl. 3):107, 1976.

14 Hammermeister, K. E., DeRouen, T. A., Curci, H., Blake, B., and Dodge, H. T.: Evidence for Reduction in Rate of Hospitalization for Cardiac Causes as a Result of Coronary Bypass Surgery, *Circulation,* 57, 58 (suppl. 2):18, 1978.

15 Barnes, G. K., Ray, M. J., Oberman, A., and Kouchoukos, N. T.: Changes in Working Status of Patients Following Coronary Bypass Surgery, *J.A.M.A.,* 238:1259, 1977.

16 David, P.: Contributing Factors Preventing Return to Work of Cardiac Surgery Patients, *Cleve. Clin. Q.,* 45:177, 1978.

17 Lawrie, G. M., Morris, G. C., Jr., Howell, J. F., Tredici, T. D., and Chapman, D. W.: Improved Survival After 5 Years in 1,144 Patients After Coronary Bypass Surgery, *Am. J. Cardiol.,* 42:709, 1978.

18 Cooley, D. A., Wukasch, D. C., Bruno, F., Reul, G. J., Jun, G. J., Sandiford, F. M., Zillgitt, S. L., and Hall, R. J.: Direct Myocardial Revascularization: Experience with 9,364 Operations, *Thorax,* 33:411, 1978.

19 Murphy, M. L., Hultgren, H. N., Detre, K., Thomsen, J., Takaro, T., and participants in the VA Cooperative Study: Treatment of Chronic Stable Angina. A Preliminary Report of Survival Data of the Randomized Veterans Administration Cooperative Study, *N. Engl. J. Med.,* 297:621, 1977.

20 Friesinger, G. C., Page, E. E., and Ross, R. S.: Prognostic Significance of Coronary Arteriography, *Trans. Assoc. Am. Physicians,* 83:78, 1970.

21 Bruschke, A. V. G., Proudfit, W. L., and Sones, F. M., Jr.: Progress Study of 590 Consecutive Nonsurgical Cases of Coronary Disease Followed 5–9 Years. I. Arteriographic Correlations, *Circulation,* 47:1147, 1973.

22 Bruschke, A. V. G., Proudfit, W. L., and Sones, F. M., Jr.: Progress Study of 590 Consecutive Nonsurgical Cases of Coronary Disease Followed 5–9 Years. II. Ventriculographic and Other Correlations, *Circulation,* 47:1154, 1973.

23 Vlietstra, R. E., Assad-Morell, J. L., Frye, R. L., et al.: Survival Predictors in Coronary Artery Disease. Medical and Surgical Comparisons, *Mayo Clin. Proc.,* 52:85, 1977.

24 Weinstein, M. C., Pliskin, J. S., and Stason, W. B.: Coronary Bypass Surgery: Decision and Policy Analysis, in J. P. Bunker, B. A. Barnes, and F. Mostellar (eds.), "Costs, Risks, and Benefits of Surgery," Oxford University Press, New York, 1977.

25 Preston, T. A.: "Coronary Artery Surgery: A Critical Review," Raven Press, New York, 1977.

Index

Page references in *italic* indicate illustrations or tables.